Studies in Fuzziness and Soft Computing 302

Editor-in-Chief

Prof. Janusz Kacprzyk
Systems Research Institute
Polish Academy of Sciences
ul. Newelska 6
01-447 Warsaw
Poland
E-mail: kacprzyk@ibspan.waw.pl

For further volumes:
http://www.springer.com/series/2941

Rudolf Seising and Marco Elio Tabacchi (Eds.)

Fuzziness and Medicine: Philosophical Reflections and Application Systems in Health Care

A Companion Volume to Sadegh-Zadeh's Handbook of Analytical Philosophy of Medicine

Springer

Editors
Dr. Rudolf Seising
European Centre for Soft Computing,
Edificio de Investigación,
Asturias,
Spain

Dr. Marco Elio Tabacchi
Università di Palermo,
Department of Matematics and Informatics,
Palermo,
Italy

ISSN 1434-9922 e-ISSN 1860-0808
ISBN 978-3-642-36526-3 e-ISBN 978-3-642-36527-0
DOI 10.1007/978-3-642-36527-0
Springer Heidelberg New York Dordrecht London

Library of Congress Control Number: 2013931275

Printed on acid-free paper

Springer is part of Springer Science+Business Media (www.springer.com)

Preface

Towards the end of 2010, the Iranian-German physician and philosopher of medicine Kazem Sadegh-Zadeh was putting the final touches to his *Handbook of Analytical Philosophy of Medicine*, to which the volume you are reading is intended as a critical companion. One of the editors happened to have the chance to read a very advanced draft of the Sadegh-Zadeh's opus, and while convinced that the systematization presented in it was certainly helping to put some definitive words on topics argued about since the eighties, also appreciated how the book contained many different starting points for new discussions and a fresher debate. With Sadegh-Zadeh's consent, the editor assembled a group of philosophers and scientists from different disciplines, such as mathematics, logics, social sciences, computer sciences, linguistics, to comment and discuss various parts, subjects and propositions from the *Handbook*. A lively discussion of such topics, under the label of the *I. International Symposium on Fuzziness, Philosophy and Medicine*, was held at the European Centre for Soft Computing (ECSC) in Mieres, Asturias (Spain) on March 2011, immediately followed by the *I. International Open Workshop on Fuzziness and Medicine*, in which further theories, and methods, developments and challenges, application systems, tools and case studies were presented and debated. The beneficial exchange continued in the following months, more scientists were added to the roster, and all the written contributions to the debate were collected in the present volume. We hope that readers of Sadegh-Zadeh's *Handbook* from all the facets of science and humanities will also enjoy this snapshot of a debate.

As far as our duties are concerned, first of all we really are indebted with Kazem Sadegh-Zadeh for letting us and the authors have a sneak peek to his *Handbook*, and for all the encouragement we have received in organizing the Symposium and the International Open Workshop. Without his ideas and writing, and his enthusiasm, this book would not exist.

We would like to express our gratitude to the Foundation for the Advancement of Soft Computing, the Scientific Committee of the ECSC and, especially, to the General Director of the ECSC, Luis Magdalena, the two emeritus researchers Claudio Moraga and Enric Trillas of the unit of "Fundamentals of Soft Computing" and the affiliated researcher Settimo Termini for their help in the development of the International Symposium, the following International Open Workshop and this companion volume project.

We are also very grateful to Springer Verlag (Heidelberg) and in particular to Dr. Thomas Ditzinger, Leontina Di Cecco, and Holger Schäpe for helping this edition find its way onto the publisher's list, and likewise to Janusz Kacprzyk (Warsaw), who accepted the book into the series *Studies in Fuzziness and Soft Computing*. Finally, our thanks go to all of the participants to the International Symposium on Fuzziness, Philosophy and Medicine and the International Open Workshop on Fuzziness and Medicine for their enthusiastic contribution and for creating with us a rich and stimulating companion to Kazem Sadegh-Zadeh's Handbook of Analytical Philosophy of Medicine.

Rudolf Seising and Marco Elio Tabacchi
Mieres (Asturias), Spain and Palermo, Italy
September, the 30th, 2012

Abstracts

Fuzziness, Philosophy, and Medicine
Rudolf Seising and Marco Tabacchi

In his *Handbook of Analytic Philosophy of Medicine*, a book that in our view is qualified to be the starting point of a new discourse in the fields of Theoretical Medicine and Philosophy of Medicine, Kazem Sadegh-Zadeh uses two scientific theories that are studied and regarded in many specific sectors of hard and human sciences but not globally well-known in Philosophy of Medicine: Fuzzy Set Theory and Structuralism. This opening contribution briefly discusses those approaches, and introduces the musing, ideas, counterpoints and contributions from many other authors, among them philosophers, logicians, mathematicians and researchers from different and competing disciplines, that constitute the rest of this volume.

The Construction of Fuzziness
Kazem Sadegh-Zadeh

The nature of fuzzy logic is briefly discussed. It is argued that fuzzy logic is a scientific conceptualization of vagueness and a methodology of how to cope with it. The basic notion of vagueness is briefly explicated to show that fuzzy logic reconstructs vagueness as what has come to be called fuzziness, i.e., what is representable as, or by, a fuzzy set. While vagueness is an attribute of real-world entities, fuzziness is a construct provided by fuzzy logic. Otherwise put, "fuzzy" and "fuzziness" are theoretical terms of fuzzy logic.

A "Goodbye to the Aristotelian Weltanschauung" and a *Handbook of Analytical Philosophy of Medicine*
Rudolf Seising

Almost 50 years ago Lotfi A. Zadeh founded the theory of *Fuzzy Sets and Systems* based on his works in system and information technology and continuing Norbert

Wiener's research in cybernetics. In the 1970s, Mario Bunge published a system theoretical approach in philosophy of medicine that he named *Iatrophilosophy* and in the 1980s Kazem Sadegh-Zadeh opened the door to use fuzzy system's concepts in this area and to define a patient's state of health as a linguistic variable. Sadegh-Zadeh demonstrated that these concepts "are not amenable to classical logic and he rejected the conceptual opposition that an individual could be either healthy or ill. Then he created a fuzzy theoretic approach toward a novel theoretical framework of these concepts: "health is a matter of degree, illness is a matter of degree, and disease is a matter of degree". In this paper we will follow the historic path of fuzzy theoretic thinking in medicine until the appearance of his epoch-making *Handbook of Analytical Philosophy of Medicine*.

Specificities and Vagaries of Medicine from the Viewpoint of Hard Sciences
Settimo Termini and Marco Elio Tabacchi

Among many other beautiful reflections on the ontology of medicine, in his Handbook of Analytic Philosophy of Medicine, Sadegh Zadeh promotes Fuzzy Sets Theory among the basic instruments of logic for medical understanding, highlights the importance of vagueness in the medical language and as an intrinsic property of medical epistemology, and invokes the clear advantages of a medical fuzzy taxonomy to overcome the binary concept of being healthy/ill. We briefly discuss these aspects, relating them to the peculiarity of Fuzziness as the only purely scientific notion among the foundational tools needed to define an analytic philosophy of medicine more concerned with an explicatum of the notions of health, illness, and disease than with precision and accuracy.

Medical Ethics, Fuzzy Logic and Shared Decision Making
Julia Inthorn

Medical practice is often viewed as a series of complex decisions bringing together normative aspects as well as factual knowledge. Sadegh-Zadeh's reconstruction of medicine as a deontic discipline is taken as a starting point for an analysis of shared decision making processes in medicine. The focus lies on shared responsibility within patient-physician-interaction from an ethical point of view. It is argued that shared decision making processes need a good basis in facts and information provided to the patient on the one hand side, where fuzzy logic might help. On the other hand the normative dimension of decisions cannot be reduced but relies on personal interaction and processes of deliberation. The involvement of the patient in a decision making process can be seen as an aim in itself and should be structured along the individual needs of the patient.

Health, Illness, and Disease – Adjusting the Coordinates
Lukas Kaelin

"Medicine is not concerned with illness and disease, but with suffering human beings called patients." (Sadegh-Zadeh, p. 148) Rather than understanding the patient from illness, Kazem Sadegh-Zadeh takes the inverse trajectory. A comprehensive theory of the patients sheds light on the concepts of health, illness, and disease. In such a perspective disease is not the opposite of health, and needs to be construed as a nonclassical concept based on a number of prototype diseases. Dwelling upon Wittgenstein's family resemblance theory and Eleanor Rosch's theory of categorization, Sadegh-Zadeh's theory of prototype diseases allows for gradual membership in the category of diseases. The boundary of diseases and non-diseases thus becomes blurry and is construed as a matter of social definition depending on the cultural context. Such a social construction of disease reorients the basic coordinates of the philosophy of medicine. This paper will track the way the coordinates are reoriented and test them from perspectives at the edge respectively critical to orthodox medicine such as Arthur Kleinman's medical anthropology and Michel Foucault's archeology of medical institutions.

What Does It Mean to Be an Individual? The Patient as a Vague Object in Medicine and Research
Karin Hutflötz

This paper wants to point out the problem of taking the patient generally as an object, even if it is considered to be a vague object based on an individual and fuzzy concept of person. Taking the individual patient as an object in medicine and research is strictly speaking a category mistake. The only thing to be taken as an object is empirical data, a detailed description or a quantified model of a measurable symptom. Reducing the fact of being individual to some measurable variables, generates the problem of misdiagnosis, and denotes a loss of self-respect and privacy in medical care situations, what could have an unrecoverable impact on rehabilitation and healing. The thesis to put forward in this paper is that we do not really need a better theory of the patient, but some new tools and fuzzy set models to quantify his needs and interests in the situation of being a patient. That shed light on the need for a renewed practice in medicine traced back to the first person's perspective, instead of a more precise theory of the concept of 'person', Sadegh-Zadeh argued for. Application of fuzzy sets to medical diagnosis and therapy, as proposed in this paper especially in order to measure and formalize the patient's degree of pain and context-dependent needs, could pave the way for improving diagnostics and therapy actually for individuals. That requires a new understanding of the person as a dynamic and social embedded system, in order to confirm the integrity of the individual in conflict with the primacy of the third person's perspective in medicine and science.

Epistemology of Medical Knowledge
Clara Barroso

The attempts of the Positivist School to establish the logical and methodological requisites of scientific knowledge at the beginning of the 20th Century stimulated the creation of epistemological discourses on the statute of knowledge. The view of science that the positivists bequeathed to us is still very important in the scientific community today. We continue to establish differences between "objective data and "subjective data"; what we consider basic science and what we consider to be applications of that science. Beyond the valuable contribution of positivism, science today does not question the legitimacy of objective knowledge, but rather seeks to adapt it so that it can be used to analyze and resolve problems through the consideration of "valid knowledge". This knowledge is not assessed exclusively for its objectivity or neutrality, but rather from the perspective of what the knowledge contributes to the understanding of problems facing humans and its capacity to generate solutions to those problems. We are going to examine the implications of this assertion for the discipline of Medicine from an epistemological point of view.

A Fuzzy-Logic Approach to Bioethics
Txetxu Ausín

Virtually any term, whether properties or states of affairs, involved in the bioethical debate - as in everyday life and in most sciences - is likely to have fuzzy edges and as regards borderline cases, without precise lines of demarcation. That is the case to face euthanasia, abortion, embryonic research, hybrids, animal experimentation, etc. etc. Thus, there is a profound disagreement between a continuous and gradual reality, riddled with nuances and transitions, a reality in gray, and a logic (an analysis and description of it) bivalent, between sheer truth and complete falsehood, in "all-or-nothing" terms, black or white. As an alternative to the 'principle of bivalence' that permeates the standard approach to reality in general and bioethics in particular, we maintain the 'principle of gradualism', which says that everything is a matter of degree and therefore a fuzzy-logic approach is an appropriate theoretical method in bioethics. So, the fuzzy approach to bioethics entitles us to soften the sharp dichotomies usually stated on bioethical issues in three main fields: about facts and definitions; about reasons and arguments, concretely in analogies and slippery slope arguments; and about norms and values (deontics). The main consequence of the fuzzy approach to bioethics is that it allows us to cope with thousands of dilemmas that arise in our discipline in a way less wrenching, traumatic, and arbitrary than the "all-or-nothing" approach. Consequently, similar behaviours and situations can receive a similar normative (ethical and legal) treatment, in the sense of the elementary principles of fairness and proportionality.

A Philosophical Anthropology of Medicine: The Split Subject

José Lázaro and Juan C. Hernández-Clemente

Spain's most distinguished philosopher of medicine, Pedro Laín Entralgo (1908-2001), believed that philosophical anthropology should be the fundamental basis of any history and theory of medicine, since it could give us a general theory of the human being as a whole, including both the biological and cultural dimensions of human essence; this general anthropology should be both philosophical and medical, multidimensional and systematic, deeply trans-disciplinary. The aim of this contribution is to pose a hypothesis about the double sidedness of human thinking and language, a basic point for any medical-philosophical-anthropology. This hypothesis is based on three classic 19th and 20th Century authors from quite different disciplines: a novelist (Marcel Proust), an anthropologist (J.G. Frazer) and a linguist (Roman Jakobson). From very different points of view, they all present the same basic idea: human thinking and language is the combination of two different processes coming from two different levels of the human mind. The first level, which we shall call "classical rationality", allows us to communicate in a clear and distinct way. It is the component of human language that transmits voluntary information. Its ideal models are mathematical and logical language. The second level, which I shall call "associative rationality", allows us to introduce the poetical dimension of language, particularly metaphors and metonyms. It is the component of human language that transmits partly involuntary information. Its purer models are dreams, delusions and some expressions of children's language. The final product of the indivisible activity of both simultaneous processes would be what we call "human rationality". If this problematic hypothesis were true, medical philosophy, like any product of human logos, could only be understood as the synthetic result of these two essential components of reason and language.

Automatic Linguistic Report on the Quality of the Gait of a Person

Alberto Alvarez-Alvarez and Gracian Trivino

Gait analysis has been explored thoroughly during the last decade as a behavioral biometric measurement. Some areas of application include: access control, surveillance, activity monitoring and clinical analysis. Our work aims to contribute to the field of human gait modeling by providing a solution based on the computational theory of perceptions. Our model differs significantly from others, e.g., based on machine learning techniques, because we use a linguistic model to represent the subjective designer's perceptions of the human gait process. This model is easily understood and provides good results. Using accelerometers included in a smart phone, we propose a method for producing a linguistic report about the quality of the gait in terms of homogeneity and symmetry. This type of reports could be used to analyze the evolution of the human gait after a recovery treatment and also for preventing falls in elderly people.

Fuzziness in Medical Image Processing. Representation and Models
Miguel Pagola, Aranzazu Jurio, Daniel Paternain, and Humberto Bustince

This work discusses Fuzziness in Medical Image Processing. We start summarizing different techniques of medical image acquisition and their main features. Examining the specialized literature, we discuss the fuzziness present in these images, including Fuzziness in pixel information and Fuzziness in model representation. Further, we present a review of the most popular fuzzy techniques for medical image segmentation which is one of the main steps in the processing of medical images. The work finishes with an example of a MRI brain image segmentation problem.

Medical Concept Representation and Data Mining
Mila Kwiatkowska and Najib T. Ayas

Medical data stored in clinical files and databases, such as patient histories and medical records, as well as research data collected for various clinical studies, are invaluable sources of medical knowledge. The computer-based data-mining techniques provide a tremendous opportunity for discovering patterns, relationships, trends, typical cases, and irregularities in these large volumes of data. The patterns discovered from data can be used to stimulate further research, as well as to create practical guidelines for diagnosis, prognosis, and treatment. Thus, a successful data-mining process may result in a significant improvement in the quality and efficiency of both medical research and health care services. Many studies have already demonstrated the practical values of data-mining techniques in various fields. However, in contrast with more traditional areas of data mining, such as mining of financial data or mining of purchasing records, medical data-mining presents greater challenges. These challenges arise not only from the complexity of the medical data, but more fundamentally from the difficulty of linking the medical data to medical concepts or rather medical concepts to medical data. Thus, although computerized medical equipment allows us to store increasingly large volumes of data, the problem lies in defining the meaning of the data and even more so in defining the medical concepts themselves. This paper will address issues specific to medical data and medical data mining in the context of Dr. Kazem Sadegh-Zadeh's discussion of the typology of medical concepts. In his *Handbook of Analytic Philosophy of Medicine*, Dr. Sadegh-Zadeh outlines four main classes of medical concepts: individual, qualitative (classificatory), comparative, and quantitative. Moreover, he introduces a novel distinction between classical and non-classical concepts. We will explain how his typology can be utilized for conceptual modeling of medical data. Specifically we will illustrate how this typology can pertain to data used in the diagnosis and treatment of sleep disorders.

Application of Knowledge-Engineering Methods in Medical Knowledge Management
von Krzysztof Michalik, Mila Kwiatkowska, and Krzysztof Kielan

This paper deals with knowledge engineering (KE), clinical decision support systems (CDSS), and expert systems (ES) as essential methods and tools supporting the knowledge management (KM) process in medicine. Specifically, we focus on the main component of the CDSS, knowledge base (KB). We demonstrate a hybrid approach to the creation, modification, verification, and validation of KB, which combines a fuzzy rule system with data mining. We describe the design and implementation of KB for two CDSS systems. The first system, which supports the evaluation of clinical depression, uses a combination of three methods: (1) creation of fuzzy rules based on expert clinicians' knowledge and standard guidelines, (2) construction of artificial neural networks (ANN) based on patients' data, and (3) implementation of a CAKE (Computer Aided Knowledge Engineering) tool. The second system, which supports the diagnosis of obstructive sleep apnea, uses a combination of two methods: (1) creation of fuzzy rules derived from the medical literature and the expert clinicians' knowledge and (2) induction of decision trees from large clinical data sets. Based on these two clinical studies, we demonstrate that KE methods should be regarded as valuable methods and tools which can be successfully used in medical KM for the creation, validation, and maintenance of KB.

A Layperson Reflection on Sorites
Enric Trillas and Itziar García-Honrado

This paper just contains some reflections on the well known classical 'Sorites Paradox', under which it appears that some imprecise linguistic terms cannot have a crisp extension, that there is no any subset containing the elements in the universe verifying the term. Such reflections are conducted from a typically layperson's point of view that heaps are not definable by means of the number of grains of sand they have, but mainly by its three-dimensional shape. Representing imprecise terms *P* by means of fuzzy sets, or contextual membership functions, it is shown that the Black's separation point is sometimes uniquely determinable, and that it always exists a crisp subset whose elements are 'more' *P* than either not *P*, or an opposite of *P*. Additionally, some considerations on the case of heaps once compared with the shape of either a pyramid, or a circular cone, are done.

Fuzziness in Medical Measurement and Approximate Reasoning
Ernesto Araujo

Fuzziness in measurement and approximate reasoning is presented as an alternative for dealing with the vague, conflicting, and not definitive decisions in medicine and health care. Conditional restrictions work as a fuzziness mechanism of measure concerning the possibility an evidence can occur. Represented as fuzzy sets, they are elastic restrictions associated to information that is simultaneously imprecise and uncertain. The human reasoning able to capture the subjectivity, vagueness, and inexact information is accomplished by fuzzy logic. The difference and similarities among fuzzy measure and fuzziness in measure are presented, demonstrating how important these approaches assume in medicine and health care. Being a feasible structure for emulating the human reasoning, fuzzy systems are natural mechanisms for helping in deciding how to obtain a safer, more effective, more efficient, higher quality, and lower costs in medical and healthcare risk analysis, assessment, analysis, classification, decision, diagnosis, and therapeutic conduct.

Approaching What-, How- and Why-Questions Using a Medical Example
Alejandro Sobrino and Cristina Puente

The aim of this paper is to approach causal questions in a medical domain. Causal questions par excellence are what-, how- and why-questions. What-questions usually ask for information related to data. How-questions generally involve the specification of a mechanism. Lastly, why-questions are related to scientific explanations. Although cover law explanation is characteristic of physical sciences, it is less common in the medical domain. In medicine, it seems that doctors express their knowledge using mechanisms instead of natural laws. In this paper we will approach causal questions with the aim of: (1) answering what-questions as identifying the cause of an effect; (2) answering how-questions as selecting an appropriate part of a mechanism that relates pairs of cause-effect (3) answering why-questions as identifying the prior and ultimate causes as well as the central nodes in the graph representing a mechanism. To accomplish this task, graph centrality measures are taken into account.

On Examination of Medical Data with Approximate Reasoning
Vesa Niskanen

We consider how computational intelligence may be applied to quantitative medical research, and this study is inspired by Lotfi Zadeh's recent work and the ideas of Kazem Sadegh-Zadeh. In particular, we consider the role of computational intelligence in statistical research in the light of medical data. Our methods stem from fuzzy extended logic, fuzzy cluster analysis and fuzzy modeling in general, and then we apply them to regression analysis. We also provide some ideas for applying our models to analysis of covariance, clustering techniques and discriminant analysis.

Statistical Procedures for Fuzzy Data in Medical Research
Takehiko Nakama

In medical research, there has been an increasing interest in statistical analysis of inherently imprecise, uncertain, or linguistic observations such as perceived breathlessness, general fatigue, or self images. Fuzzy sets can effectively encode them, and a variety of statistical procedures have been developed to analyze fuzzy data. In this paper, we review some of the procedures and explain how they can be applied to medical research.

Probability, Fuzziness and Information: Defining Missions in Medicine
Luis Argüelles Méndez

Aristotelian logic has played, and is still nowadays playing, an essential role in health sciences, resulting in sharp classifications where symptoms, diseases and treatments seem to be clearly defined. However, this schema suffers from uncertainty since every human being is an extremely complex biological individual and, for example, some symptoms associated to a given disease can show only mildly or even be absent in a sick person, health conditions usually express themselves with variations into a given set of patients and treatments almost always need to have some sort of personalization. Even in some cases, drugs must be administrated by trial and error attempts. In a traditional way, both probability theories and statistics are a major toolbox of mathematical assistance in health sciences, since they help to describe observed cases into a context of population. In particular, probability is useful as a tool for forecasting and we can say: "prognosis of patient A is X with probability p", but it is not useful for describing intrinsic phenomena in states that are vague in nature, as, for example, in the following sentence: "Patient B, located in room 212, is rather ill", where "rather ill" is an imprecise linguistic slab of information. Fuzzy sets theory, introduced by Lofti Zadeh back in 1965, sheds new lights in the very paradigm of classifications, logic and thus medicine. In this work we shall introduce the concepts of Life Illness Curves (LIC) and Life Quality Curves (LQC) that will help us to redefine missions in medicine where human perceptions must be also taken into account for a better representation of the information handled by physicians.

Medical Decision Making as a Group Choice Process: Consensual Dynamics in Fuzzy Diagnosis
Silvia Bortot and Mario Fedrizzi

In this paper we present an approach to medical diagnosis based on the collective choice paradigm introduced in the middle of 20th century by Kenneth Arrow. Starting from a GDSS architecture introduced to support collaborative medical decision making we focus on the representation of the consensual dynamics based on the minimization of a cost function and aiming at selecting the most agreeable diagnosis profile. The model is based on a set of individual fuzzy preference relations and combines a soft measure of collective dissensus with an inertial mechanism of opinion changing aversion.

Towards an Interpretation of the Medical Expert System CADIAG2

David Picado Muiño, Agata Ciabattoni, and Thomas Vetterlein

The present paper responds to an attempt to interpret the inference process and ultimately the output of the medical expert system CADIAG2. We first provide a formalization of the inference process by means of a set of logical rules and later attempt to provide an interpretation (i.e., semantics) for them. Two semantics are taken as reference for our purpose: probabilistic semantics and fuzzy (*t-norm*-based) semantics.

Electronic Health Records Interoperability by Archetype Based Contexts

Belén Prados-Suárez, Carlos Molina, Miguel Prados de Reyes, and Carmen Peña-Yañez

This research is focused on the use of contexts of access as a means to provide the interoperability between different Electronic Health Records Systems (EHRS), as mandated by the european standard ISO 13606. In this standard the interoperability is posed in two levels: at structural level, by the so called "reference model", and at logical and conceptual level, by the "archetype model". The interoperability at the first level is quite difficult to achive, due to the huge variability of EHRS implementations. However the use and the needs of access are very similar in most of the hospitals, since the pathological processes, the protocols, the medical specialities, etc. and the information required for each of them is very similar in most of the cases. This is why we propose to define archetypes in the second model of the standard, based on the different contexts of access and the information pertinent to each of them, determined using fuzzy logic. This way when a doctor accesses from a given context to the EHRS of a different hospital, he/she receives the information that this hospital has determined pertinent for that context .

Fuzzy Pain Assessment in Musculoskeletal Disorder

Ernesto Araujo and Leandro Lazzareschi

A fuzzy decision support system for the evaluation of musculoskeletal pain based on fuzzy unidimensional pain scales and fuzzy multidimensional professional-social-sexual scale is presented. The subjective, inaccurate, unclear, and vague pain perception is described by using fuzzy set theory and fuzzy logic. The proposed approach advantages by its ability to explain the direct relationships of musculoskeletal pain that are not linguistically well understood and the freedom of movement leading to an effective pain assessment tool. The Fuzzy Musculoskeletal Pain Scale (FUMPS) is submitted to the evaluation of amplitude of movement concerning shoulder flexion and shoulder extension rating the intensity of the pain. The proposed fuzzy musculoskeletal pain assessment dealing with Flexion–Extension (FE) Shoulder Range of Motion Analysis (FE–FUMPS) is characterized by being comprehensive and consistent to clinical practice. The Fuzzy Pain Assessment for

Patients with Musculoskeletal Disorder becomes an affordable and comprehensive approach to deal with the complexity associated to the clinical aspects of pain.

Fuzzy Logic in Diagnostics of Rare Diseases
Tatiana Kiseliova, Maka Korinteli, and Karaman Pagava

Background. Rare disease (RD) is any disease that affects a small percentage of the population, with a prevalence of about 1 in every 2000 people. Diagnostic of RDs is hindered by the lack of knowledge predetermined by the multitude of these diseases, which can lead to medical mistake and even medical failure. It may also occasion the omission of the necessary investigations and vice-versa – the prescription of a multitude of unnecessary and potentially hazardous invasive diagnostic interventions and/or delay in performing them. Quite frequently the correct diagnosis is belated, sometimes it is not made at all. The generally accepted way for RD diagnosing is usage of search machines, but this way is reasonable only when some outstanding symptoms/signs, like dismorphological signs, mental retardation, etc. occur. Very often the RDs mask as common diseases. In such cases the problem is to suspect the RD. There are no special algorithms which give rise to a suspicion for the RD. Objective. Elaboration of the model/algorithm for revealing cases suspicious of RDs (if they present under the mask of a common disease). Methods. We need to have an approach which will help us to suspect the RD to use the search machines afterwards as usually. We assume to suspect a RD when the clinical picture and course of a disease are atypical. But the point is that the border between typical (normal) and atypical (abnormal) is not crisp: the fuzzy methodologies can be used here. Results. We present an algorithmic approach for the implementation within a framework of a computer program, that would allow to suspect RD, and therefore serve as a basis of a decision support system. Examples from medical practice illustrate our approach. Conclusions. For the group of common diseases (syndromes), e.g. pneumonia, bronchitis, rheumatic fever, etc., we propose to prepare medical electronic records (including complains, anamnesis aegroti/vitae, anamnesis morbi, status presence, etc.), which would reveal the signs/symptoms which deviate from the normal clinical course (by frequency, intensity, time of manifestation, duration, etc.). When deviation reaches some level, the program would signal that there is some suspicion of the non-common disease (e.g., RD) which masks as a common one.

Category Theoretic Ontology for Representation of Assessment Scales and Consensus Guidelines in Elderly Care
Patrik Eklund

In this paper we show how category theoretic ontology provided by generalized general logic can be used for decision-making with assessment scales and consensus guidelines in social and health care of older people. Computerized decision-making in social and health care is traditionally views ontologies not as part of underlying logics for decision-making, but rather as standards and terminologies including skeletons and frameworks of informal logic structures. Programming in logic is manipulation of terms, and substitution with terms. Classical terms won't suffice. An ontology building upon classical terms, trying to enhance missing parts in the underlying structures by being clever about inference, becomes logically sterile and basically useless in formal frameworks. We also need to make a distinction between imprecise or vague information, and being formal and accurate in reasoning with vague values. Furthermore, a value may be vague as produced by a crisp operation, or a value is vague since the underlying operation is vague. From formal point of view this is all about underlying categories and monads, and in this paper we will continue investigations showing how the signatures reside in term monads over chosen categories. Our approach is thus monadic, and we consider monads over suitable categories.

Fuzzy Cognitive Map Decision Support System for Successful Triage to Reduce Unnecessary Emergency Room Admissions for the Elderly
Voula C. Georgopoulos and Chrysostomos D. Stylios

This work presents a Fuzzy Cognitive Map Medical Decision Support System (FCM-MDSS) for the hospital admission procedure of elderly patients. The FCM-MDSS is applied to the Emergency Department (ED), where elderly patients arrive requesting medical assistance. Here a new hybrid methodology is introduced to develop FCM-MDSS exploiting human experience and accompanied by available bibliographic information. It is based on the widely applied Triage complex decision-making process and the generally accepted procedures while trying to minimize unnecessary admissions as well as over/under-triaging. The FCM-MDSS is evaluated for known cases of real patients arriving at the ED from the literature.

Contents

Part III: Models, Methods, and Representation

Part I

Introductory Chapters

1

Fuzziness, Philosophy, and Medicine

Rudolf Seising and Marco Tabacchi

From the 1980s, the Iranian-German physician and philosopher of medicine Kazem Sadegh-Zadeh discussed the nature of health, illness, and diseases and the meaning of these notions in medical sciences. He has just published the *Handbook of Analytic Philosophy of Medicine* [3] (to which the book you are reading is a companion) where, in more than 700 dense and detailed pages, he presents the work of his lifetime; in our view this book is qualified to be the starting point of a new discourse in the fields of Theoretical Medicine and Philosophy of Medicine!

In his *Handbook*, Sadegh-Zadeh uses two scientific theories that, while studied and regarded in many different sectors of hard and human sciences, are not globally well-known in Philosophy of Medicine: Fuzzy Set Theory and Structuralism. The following sections will briefly discuss those approaches.

1.1 Fuzzy Logic and Medicine

Fuzzy Set Theory is a discipline that was founded in 1964/65 by the electrical engineer Lotfi A. Zadeh (Berkeley). This theory was applied for decades in many parts of science and technology (such as Control, Data Mining, Economy, and many others) and there are many researchers in mathematics and other fields who continue the theoretical framework of this theory. In the 1970/80s some scientists created approaches an methods to use Fuzzy Sets in modelling Medical Knowledge and building Medical Knowledge-based Systems (or Medical Expert Systems) – e.g CADIAG – but, as far as we know, Kazem Sadegh-Zadeh was the only scientist in Theoretical Medicine who used this theory for a new approach to Analytical Philosophy of Medicine. That kind of perspective could be very beneficial to the Philosophy of Medicine as a whole.

Kazem Sadegh-Zadeh demonstrated that concepts such as health, illness, or disease "are not amenable to classical logic", and adopted a fuzzy-theory approach to postulate a novel theory of these concepts: "health is a matter of degree, illness is a matter of degree, and disease is a matter of degree". He rejected the conceptual opposition that an individual could be either healthy or ill. In fact, health and illness are, in this philosophy, particular fuzzy states of health. In Sadegh-Zadeh's

R. Seising and M.E. Tabacchi (Eds.): *Fuzziness and Medicine*, STUDFUZZ 302, pp. 3–8.
DOI: 10.1007/978-3-642-36527-0_1

philosophy of medicine, also disease entities "may be conceptualized as fuzzy sets" and "symptoms, and signs would then belong to an individual disease to particular extents. Thus, an individual disease would appear as a multidimensional cloud rather than a clear-cut phenomenon". Sadegh-Zadeh introduced the term "disease" not with a linguistic but a social definition: There are complex human conditions "that in a human society are termed diseases", and he specifies potential candidates "like heart attack, stroke, breast cancer, etc. Such complex human conditions are not, and should not be, merely confined to biological states of the organism. They may be viewed and represented as large fuzzy sets which also contain parts that refer to the subjective, religious, transcendental and social world of the ill, such as pain, distress, feelings of loneliness, beliefs, behavioural disorders, etc." Thus, Sadegh-Zadeh's fuzzy approach to philosophy of medicine is oriented to the actual lives, needs and interests of people in their communities. This philosophy of medicine is in conformity with Ludwik Fleck's philosophy of medicine, published in the 1920s and 1930s, whose fame and acceptance was hindered by National Socialism.

In the *Handbook*, Sadegh-Zadeh now devotes a sizable part of his analysis to the role of fuzziness, beginning with a simple but powerful assertion: speaking of the classic binary logic for the description of illnesses he affirms that "[Using bivalent logic] requires that medical statements be capable of possessing determinate truth values and be true or false. This presupposition of bivalence could be satisfied only if medical terms had precise meanings and denoted crisp sets, i.e., classical sets with sharp boundaries, so that one may determine whether a particular object does or does not fall within a particular class. We know, however, that this is not the case. Almost all medical terms are vague." [3, p. 603] This problem of a clear lack of precision in medicine is worsened by the pretension of a sturdy application of probability: "probability theory and logic can be meaningfully applied only under the assumption that the events to which probabilities are assigned are crisp events. However, due to the above-mentioned vagueness of most real-world classes, there are virtually no such events." [3, p. 603] A solution can be found, as already stated in the "Goodbye"-article, by resorting to a Fuzzy approach: "The only remedy to the above-mentioned difficulties is to use fuzzy logic in medicine." [3, p. 603f]

In the spirit of a true handbook, useful to medical students that do not necessarily have a strong background in mathematics and logic, Sadegh-Zadeh gives a full instructional treatment to Fuzziness when applied to medicine, starting with a full section devote to fundamentals of Fuzzy Logic, and extending both Etiology and Epistemology in the same direction. This approach has an important role in the dissemination of the ideas behind Fuzziness in fields that are usually less inclined — if not actually reluctant — to embrace a way of thinking that embrace uncertainty and imprecision, and has certainly to be commended for its outreaching nature: instead of limiting himself to some short remarks and a bulk of references, Sadegh-Zadeh decided to embed the necessary notions in full, exposing future physicians and medical operators to the powerful instruments of fuzziness.

1.2 The Structuralist View

The *Structuralist View* on scientific (empirical) theories is an approach to Philosophy of Science that was founded by the mathematician and philosopher Patrick Suppes (Stanford). It has been elaborated and continued by Joseph D. Sneed, Wolfgang Stegmüller, C. Ulises Moulines and Wolfgang Balzer and others. In a certain way this theory acts as a bridge between Philosophy of science and History of science and in this book it is used to model the "Architecture of Medical Knowledge". After the discussions concerning the different views in history of sciences in the first six decades of the 20th century, in later years we can find two trends in obtaining systematic rational reconstructions of empirical theories: Carnap's approach and Suppes's approach[1]. In both, the first step consists of an axiomatization that seeks to determine the mathematical structure of the theory in question. However, whereas in the Carnap approach the theory is axiomatized in a formal language, the Suppes approach uses informal set theory. Thus, in the Suppes approach, one is able to axiomatize real physical theories in a precise way without recourse to formal languages. This approach can be traced back to Suppes' proposal in the 1950s to include the axiomatization of empirical theories of science in the metamathematical programme of the French group Bourbaki [1]. In the 1970s, one of Suppes' Ph D.-students, the US-American physicist Joseph D. Sneed (born 1938), developed informal semantics meant to include not only mathematical aspects, but also application subjects of scientific theories in the framework, based on this method. In [7] he presented the view that all empirical claims of phys- ical theories have the form "x is an S", where "is an S" is a set-theoretical predicate (e.g., "x is a classical particle mechanics"). Every physical system that fulfills this predicate is called a model of the theory. For example, the class M of a theory's models is characterized by empirical laws that consist of conditions governing the connection of the components of physical systems. Therefore, we have models of a scientific theory, and by removing their empirical laws, we get the class M_p of so- called potential models of the theory. Potential models of an empirical theory consist of theoretical terms, i.e. observables with values that can be measured in accordance with the theory. This connection between theory and empiricism is the basis of the philosophical "problem of theoretical terms". If we remove the theoretical terms of a theory in its potential models, we get structures that are to be treated on a purely empirical layer; we call the class M_{pp} of these structures of a scientific theory its "partial potential models". Finally, every physical theory has a class I of intended systems (or applications) and, of course, different intended systems of a theory may partially overlap. This means that there is a class C of constraints that produces cross connections between the overlapping intended systems. In brief, this structuralist view of scientific theories regards the core K of a theory as a quadruple $K = < Mp, Mpp, M, C >$. This core can be supplemented by the class I of intended applications of the theory $T = < K, I >$. To make it clear that this concept reflects both sides of scientific

[1] These approaches are named after the German-US-American philosopher Rudolf Carnap (1891- 1970), and the American mathematician and philosopher Patrick Suppes (born 1922).

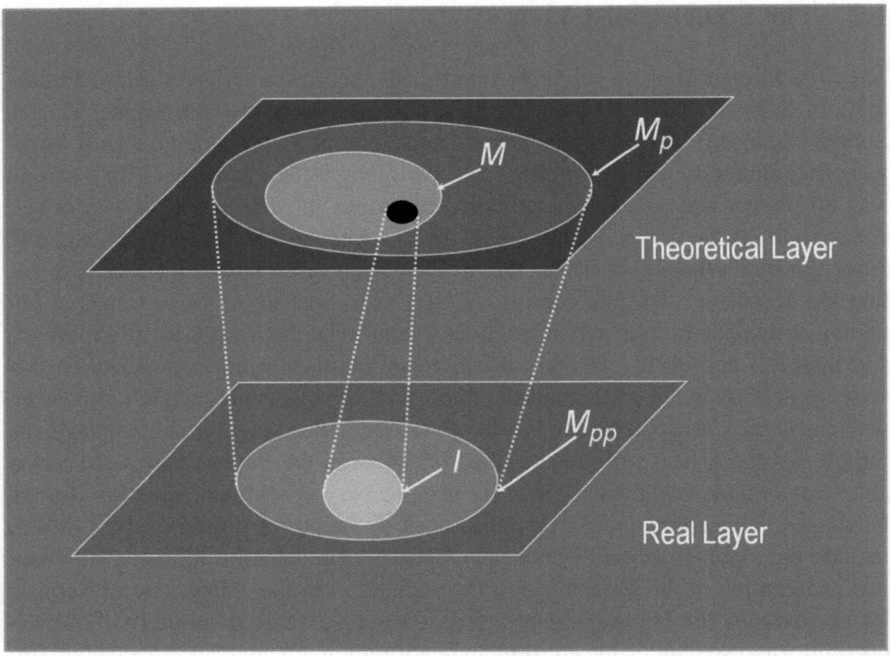

Fig. 1.1 Real and theoretical structural layers

theories, these classes of K and I are shown in Fig. 1.1. Thus we notice that M_{pp} and I are entities of an empirical layer, whereas M_p and M_{pp} are structures in a theoretical layer of the schema.

Referring to *The Structure and Dynamics of Theories* [8] by the Austrian philosopher of science Wolfgang Stegmüller (1923-1991), Sadegh-Zadeh stated in his article "The Fuzzy Revolution: Goodbye to the Aristotelian Weltanschauung"- that the concepts of Popper, Kuhn and their combatants "are still too vague and inadequate to be useful" [2, p. 3]

Now, in his *Handbook on Analytical philosophy of Medicine* (see Fig. 1.2 (a)) [3], he demands an "overhaul" to adapt the structuralist metatheory to fuzzy set theory [3, p. 439f]. He requires "to render the metatheory applicable to real world scientific theories, it needs to be fuzzified because like everything else in science, scientific theories are vague entities and implicitly or explicitly fuzzy. He then lists two ways of scientific theories' explicit fuzzifications:

1. Introduction of the theory's set-theoretical predicate as a fuzzy predicate ("x is a fuzzy S" instead of "x is an S").
2. In addition to 1. also any other component of the theory appearing in the structure that defines the predicate may be fuzzified.

Unfortunately, Sadegh-Zadeh does not go into details at this point but he concludes this section with an outlook: "Fuzzifications of both types will impact the application and applicability of theories as well as the nature of the knowledge produced by using them. This is true because fuzzification will change the conception of models; potential models; partial, potential models; and the core and intended applications of a theory, on the one hand; and the epistemological relationships between empirical claims of the theory and the 'real world', on the other, e.g., support, confirmation, falsification, etc." [3, p. 441] At the end of his chapter "The Architecture of Medical Knowledge" Sadegh-Zadeh (see Fig. 1.2 (b)) writes: "The above considerations suggest that the entities a theory is concerned with, be construed as vague entities. For similar analyses and assessments he referred to [4–6]." [3, p. 441].

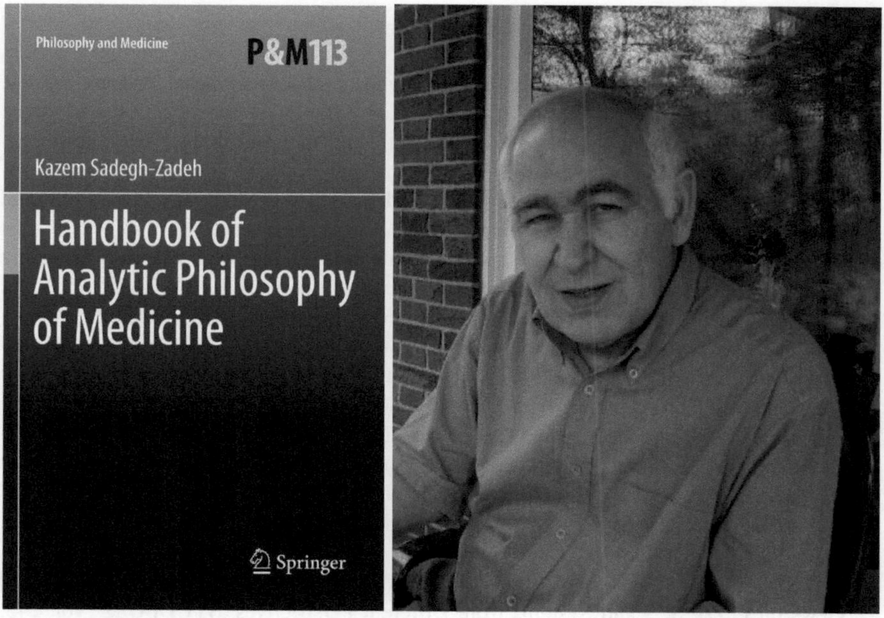

(a) (b)

Fig. 1.2 (a): Cover of the *Handbook* [3]; (b) Kazem Sadegh-Zadeh in 2011 in Tecklenburg, Germany

1.3 More Impressions from the Handbook

The two approaches highlighted in this brief introduction are neither exclusive nor even remotely exhaustive: many other authors, among them philosophers, logicians, mathematicians and researchers from different and competing disciplines have mused on the Handbook, each following on what they have found more interesting for their particular field of research. Their musing, ideas, counterpoints and contributions constitute the rest of this volume, divided in six thematic parts: the rest of this presents a contribution from the author of the *Handbook* on Fuzziness, followed by an historical perspective and some remarks on the future directions on Medicine and Philosophy. Part II will deal with the relationship between Ethics and Medicine. Part III will discuss the possible Models, Methods and Representation of medical facts; in Part IV the Reasoning and Questioning approach will be examined, while Part V and VI will deal respectively with Statistics and Data Analysis.

We hope the reader will find the debate around Philosophy of Medicine sparkled by the *Handbook* and summarized in this volume as entertaining, thought-provoking and as we have, and will join us and the other authors in what today, thanks to Sadegh-Zadeh's intuitions and systematizations, is a lively, interesting and fruitful discussion about the future of the role of Fuzziness in Medicine.

References

1. Bourbaki, N. (pseudo.): Elements of Mathematics: Theory of Sets. Addison-Wesley, Reading (1968)
2. The Fuzzy Revolution: Goodbye to the Aristotelian Weltanschauung. Artificial Intelligence in Medicine 21, 1–25 (2001)
3. Sadegh-Zadeh, K.: Handbook of Analytical Philosophy of Medicine. Philosophy and Medicine, vol. 113. Springer, Heidelberg (2012)
4. Seising, R.: Between Empiricism and Rationalism: A Layer of Perception Modeling Fuzzy Sets as Intermediary in Philosophy of Science. In: Castillo, O., Melin, P., Ross, O.M., Cruz, R.S., Pedrycz, W., Kacprzyk, J. (eds.) Theoretical Advances and Applications of Fuzzy Logic and Soft Computing. ASC, vol. 42, pp. 101–108. Springer, Heidelberg (2007); Proc. of the IFSA 2007 World Congress Theory and Applications of Fuzzy Logic and Soft Computing, Cancun Mexico. LNCS, June 18-21, vol. 4529 (2007)
5. Seising, R.: Scientific theories and the computational theory of perceptions: A structuralist view including fuzzy sets. In: Stepnika, M., Novák, V., Bodenhofer, U. (eds.) New Dimensions in Fuzzy Logic and Related Technologies. Proceedings of the 5th EUSFLAT Conference. European Society for Fuzzy Logic and Technology, Ostrava, Czech Republic, vol. 1, pp. 401–408 (2007)
6. Seising, R.: Fuzzy Sets and Systems and Philosophy of Science. In: Seising, R. (ed.) Views on Fuzzy Sets and Systems from Different Perspectives. STUDFUZZ, vol. 243, pp. 1–35. Springer, Heidelberg (2009)
7. Sneed, J.D.: The Logical Structure of Mathematical Physics. Reidel, Dordrecht (1971)
8. Stegmüller, W.: The Structure and Dynamics of Theories. Springer, New York (1976)

2

The Construction of Fuzziness

Kazem Sadegh-Zadeh

2.1 Introduction

I feel very honored to have the opportunity of speaking to you and to thank those of you in person who have been interested in my forthcoming *Handbook of Analytic Philosophy of Medicine* and have concerned themselves with one or another of its subjects.

Initially, when I was asked to present an introduction to this book, I wanted to write about an idea then that fuzzy logic might be an empirical science because it was concerned with something that existed in the experiential world and made statements about that empirical entity. But later, when I started writing this text, I didn't succeed to show that I was right. Therefore, I shall now slightly deviate from my initial intentions and shall discuss about the question whether fuzziness exists in the world out there or is something constructed by fuzzy logic. Concisely said, the topic of this introduction will be the ontological status of fuzziness. I shall deal with this topic by offering a few ideas on:

- The nature of fuzzy logic,
- The nature of vagueness, and
- The nature of fuzziness.

2.2 The Nature of Fuzzy Logic

Regarding the nature of fuzzy logic, we can first ask ourselves the question: What kind of science is fuzzy logic? Is it a theoretical science, a practical science, an empirical science, or what else? To answer such questions, I shall introduce some terminology. I shall first differentiate between theoretical or *pure science*, *applied science*, and *practical science*.

2.2.1 *Pure Science, Applied Science, and Practical Science*

A *pure science* is a scientific field which is not concerned with the question of whether, how, and for what purpose its results are actually applied or may be

R. Seising and M.E. Tabacchi (Eds.): *Fuzziness and Medicine*, STUDFUZZ 302, pp. 9–18.
DOI: 10.1007/978-3-642-36527-0_2

applied. Its subjects do not emerge from the human life world, for instance, from the desire to find an algorithm for solving a particular empirical problem. Examples are algebra, axiomatic set theory, and theoretical philosophy.

In contrast to a pure science, an *applied science* takes its subjects of research from the human life world, for example, from human illness and disease, or from traffic, from environmental pollution, and the like. Its aim is to find solutions for problems we are faced with in our experiential world. For instance, pharmacology and psychology are applied sciences. They try to solve empirical problems.

In addition to the term "applied science", we must also be aware that a particular science or theory such as algebra or the theory of probability may be applied in another field to solve some problems of this field. In this case, we have the *application of a science or theory*, but not an applied science. Such is the case, for example, when statistics is aplied in epidemiology to get a statistic of diseases or something like that.

Finally, a *practical science* is a science of *praxis,* i.e., a science of human action. Its concern is to find out what to do in particular circumstances. That is, to answer questions of the following form: If the circumstance is C and I want to achieve the goal G, what action should I perform to achieve this goal?

The term "practical science" does not mean that a science is a practical one when in this science one does something, one acts. This widespread view is inappropriate because every scientist does something in that she does scientific research. The term "practical science" means that a science is a *practical* one if it seeks rules of practice, i.e., rules of action of the following form in a particular domain:

> If the circumstance is $C_1 \& \cdots \& C_m$ and you want to achieve the goal G,
> then perform action $A_1 \& \cdots \& A_n$

with $m, n \geq 1$, and examines their efficiency. But I do not want to go into details here. For example, clinical medicine is a *practical science* not because physicians perform actions, but because it seeks action rules of the type above which physicians can follow in diagnostic-therapeutic decision-making [8]. Also all engineering sciences are practical sciences because they investigate what to do in order to produce some particular material, device, and the like. So, we have four concepts to differentiate:

- Pure science,
- Applied science,
- Application of a science or theory,
- Practical science.

The differentiation between the second and third categories, i.e., between *applied* and *application*, is easy. While an applied science *is doing* science, the application of a science *is using* a science to do something else.

Let us now turn to our initial question: What kind of science is fuzzy logic? Is it a pure science like algebra? Is it an applied science like pharmacology? Or is it a practical science like clinical medicine and engineering sciences? To talk about these questions, I should perhaps first clarify what I mean by the term "fuzzy logic".

2.2.2 What Does "Fuzzy Logic" Mean?

The term "fuzzy logic" has become ambiguous in the meantime. It is used to denote at least three different things. According to Lotfi Zadeh ([14] p. 2), it is appropriate to distinguish between:

- Fuzzy logic in the narrow sense, FLn for short, and
- Fuzzy logic in the wider sense, FLw for short.

Fuzzy logic in the narrow sense, FLn, is the logical, more or less formal system that deals with inexact, vague, or approximate *reasoning* concerned with rules of fuzzy inference such as the compositional rule of inference and others. In this sense, FLn is a particular extension of many-valued logic.

FLn is one of the branches of fuzzy logic in the wider sense, FLw, a subset of FLw, so to speak. FLw comprises, in addition to FLn, (i) fuzzy set theory; (ii) the theory of linguistic variables; (iii) the theory of fuzzy if-then rules; (iv) possibility theory; and (v) the theory of computing with words ([14] p. 2). FLw and fuzzy mathematics jointly yield what may be called Fuzzy Theory, or more appropriately, the theory of fuzziness. In what follows, by the term "fuzzy logic" I shall mean FLw.

A third variant that has emerged recently, in addition to FLn and FLw, is the *mathematical fuzzy logic* that is trying to develop a completely mathematical, axiomatized framework in the style of traditional, formal logic. It is in fact a mathematical, infinite-valued logic with truth values in the real, unit interval (see, e.g., [1]; [2]; [3], [4]; [5]; [9]). Lotfi Zadeh does not consider this approach a fuzzy logic at all (personal communication, 2005).

Now, turning to our original question:

2.2.3 What Kind of Science Is Fuzzy Logic?

We can observe that FLn is a pure science, whereas FLw is a mixed science. It is partly a pure science, namely FLn; partly an applied science; and partly a practical science. I would like to give a few examples:

- We have seen that FLn is a pure science;
- The theory of linguistic variables is an applied theory in that it is developed by analyzing a particular characteristic of natural languages such as English, Spanish, and German. Its goal is to investigate fuzzy set-theoretical correspondences and associations between qualitative and quantitative terms;
- Fuzzy control is a practical science in that it deals with fuzzy if-then rules of action to find out in what fuzzy circumstances $C_1, \ldots, C_m$ what actions $A_1, \ldots, A_n$ are to be performed to control real processes in the world out there, be they machines, biological processes, or others;
- The concern of your institute, i.e., *Soft Computing*, is partly a pure science, partly an applied science, and partly a practical science. It is thus a mixed science.

We have now come close to our question: What is the subject of fuzzy logic? There is no doubt that independently of whether we consider pure fuzzy logic, applied fuzzy logic, or practical fuzzy logic, the subject of all fuzzy logic is the so-called *vagueness,* be it vagueness of individual objects, classes, relations, structures, systems, processes, or actions. Fuzzy logic is a scientific conceptualization of vagueness and a methodology of how to cope with it. But what is vagueness?

2.3 The Nature of Vagueness

Is vagueness something *objective* that exists in the world out there, or is it something *subjective* that mirrors our uncertainty about objects and occurrences? There are those who maintain that it is something subjective, and those who say the opposite. To answer this question, it is expedient to differentiate between four types of vagueness:

1. Linguistic vagueness,
2. Epistemic vagueness,
3. Semantic vagueness,
4. Ontic vagueness.

As regards linguistic vagueness, phenomena such as unclarity of meaning, ambiguity, and polysemy are in principle remediable. They are not genuine vagueness. The remaining class of genuinely vague linguistic expressions such as "bald" and "young" which cannot be made precise, corresponds to ontic vagueness that will be discussed below.

Epistemic vagueness is in fact subjective uncertainty due to lack of information and knowledge. It is not genuine vagueness.

Semantic vagueness, or vague reference, is the representational vagueness, i.e., the unclear representation of an object y by a word or picture x when there is a relation of the form $Repr(x,y)$ such that x *represents* y. Examples are blurred pictures. Semantic vagueness as vagueness of reference is a vague relation, and as such, it also belongs to the following type of vagueness.

Ontic vagueness is the prototypical vagueness and the source of all other types of genuine vagueness.[1] It concerns the vagueness of individual objects, classes, relations, and states of affairs in 'the world out there'. Are there really such vague entities? And what does their vagueness look like?

Concisely, we cannot know how things are 'in themselves' irrespective of whether or how they are perceived, recognized, or represented, i.e., of the perspective from which they are viewed ([8], ch. 23). The world looks different depending on what glasses we put on. We may therefore be tempted to take the position that "we shall never know whether there is vagueness in the world out there and whether objects or states of affairs can be vague" . To assert or to deny vagueness in the world, will remain an ontological postulate in any case. From a practical perspective, however,

[1] The adjective "ontic" means "concerning the being". It originates from the Greek term *ον* (on) that derives from the present participle of the Greek verb *εiναι* (einai) for "to be".

it appears reasonable to prefer the affirmative. That means that it is more reasonable than not to suppose that there are vague objects, vague sets, including relations, and vague states of affairs. To give three corresponding examples, (i) a *frog* is a vague animal, i.e., an object with indeterminate spatio-temporal boundaries, because it is impossible to determine when it emerges from a tadpole. There is no abrupt end of being a tadpole and no abrupt start of being a frog. The transition is continuous. Similarly, (ii) the class of *bald* human beings has no sharp boundaries. It has a penumbral region of genuine borderline cases that imperceptibly vanishes into the set of non-bald people. Finally, (iii) there are also vague *states of affairs*, e.g., vague events. For, a state of affairs amounts to the belonging of an object to a class. For example, the state of affairs that *Picasso is bald* entails Picasso's membership in the class of bald people. If the class to which an object belongs, is a vague set, such as *bald*, and the object resides in its penumbra, the state of affairs turns out to be something indefinite. To elucidate, let us introduce an operator, symbolized by "Δ" and read "definitely". For instance, if α is a statement, $\Delta\alpha$ means "definitely α". Thus, "Δ(Picasso ist a Spanish artist)" says: Definitely, Picasso is a Spanish artist. With the aid of this operator, Δ, we can define the vagueness of classes in the following way:[2]

Definition 1. *A class C is vague if and only if* $\exists x \neg\Delta(x \in C) \wedge \neg\Delta(x \notin C)$.

For example, the individual Picasso shows that the class of bald people is vague because:

$$\neg\Delta(\text{Picasso is bald}) \wedge \neg\Delta(\text{Picasso is not bald}).$$

That means, it is indefinite whether Picasso is bald and it is indefinite as well whether he is not bald. Let α be any statement, the following sentence:

$$\neg\Delta(\alpha) \wedge \neg\Delta(\neg\alpha)$$

says that we neither know whether α is true nor know whether $\neg\alpha$ is true. This is equivalent to the following statement:

$$\neg\big(\Delta(\alpha) \vee \Delta\neg(\alpha)\big).$$

From this we can conclude that:

$$\neg\Delta(\alpha \vee \neg\alpha).$$

And that means that in the following disjunction contained in it:

$$\alpha \vee \neg\alpha$$

neither α nor its negation $\neg\alpha$ has a truth value. But this sentence is exactly the *Principle of Exluded Middle* of classical logic, and as such, a tautology. That is, it

[2] The definiteness operator Δ as well as the approach to vagueness using it I owe to Timothy Williamson ([10], 695 ff.).

should always be true according to classical logic. Thus, it seems that vagueness is in conflict with classical logic and vice versa. By the way, this fact has already been discovered in 1923 by one of the founders of classical logic himself [7].

The indeterminacy of being or not being a member of a vague class brings with it that objects can be members of a vague class to different extents. So, in characterizing their membership, linguistic hedges such as *more or less, very, very very,* and others come into play such that an object x may be stronger than another object y a member of a vague class C. While, for example, nobody has a brother of whom we could say *"he is a very brother"*, many of us have read some books of which one can say "this is a very interesting book". Thus, the class of *brothers* is not vague, whereas the class of *interesting books* is vague. The susceptibility to linguistic hedges is a typical characteristic of vague classes. It renders a vague class granular. We can thus say that a vague class is susceptible to linguistic hedges *and* granular.

As mentioned previously, fuzzy logic is a conceptualization and precise theory of vagueness, specifically, of ontically vague classes, including relations. The key notion of the entire system of fuzzy logic has been and still remains the concept of *fuzzy set*. Fuzziness is the property of a fuzzy set to be fuzzy. Therefore, it is appropriate to differentiate between *vagueness,* as sketched thus far, on the one hand; and *fuzziness*, on the other. Vagueness is not fuzziness, and fuzziness is not vagueness. But what is fuzziness exactly?

2.4 The Nature of Fuzziness

After we have approved the postulate that *vagueness* exists in the world out there, we can now ask the corresponding question whether *fuzziness* too exists in the world out there. To answer this question, I shall first make the notion of *fuzziness* a little bit more precise by constructing what I shall call a *fuzzy structure*. To this end we recall the concept of *fuzzy set.*

To obtain a fuzzy set, we need three things:

$$\begin{aligned} \Omega &= \text{a collection of objects} \\ \mu &= \text{a function that maps } \Omega \text{ to } [0, 1] \\ A &= \big\{\big(x, \mu(x)\big) \,|\, x \in \Omega\big\}. \end{aligned}$$

We need, first, a finite or infinite collection of objects, here symbolized by Ω and also called a base set or universe of discourse; second, a function, here symbolized by μ, which maps Ω to the unit interval; third, an emerging subset A in, or over, Ω which consists of pairs of objects such that the first object, x, is an element of Ω und the second object is the function value $\mu(x)$, referred to as the degree of membership of x in fuzzy set A.

We can use this basic terminology to introduce a new concept which will help us decide whether there exists fuzziness in the world:

Definition 2. *An object* ξ is a fuzzy structure *if and only if there are* Ω, A, *and* μ *such that:*

1. $\xi = \langle \Omega, A, \mu \rangle$,
2. *Ω is a non-empty set,*
3. *A is a fuzzy set over Ω,*
4. *μ is the membership function of A.*

That is, a fuzzy structure is a triple $\langle \Omega, A, \mu \rangle$ consisting of a universe of discourse Ω, a fuzzy set A over this universe, and its membership function μ. Now, our question whether fuzziness exists, reduces to the question whether there are fuzzy structures as just defined. Otherwise put, are there *models for* the set-theoretical predicate as defined in Definition 2? The answer to this question is twofold:

First: No, there are no fuzzy structures in the real world out there because a function from something to the unit interval such as a membership function μ is an abstract mathematical construct and does not exist in the empirical world.

Second: But of course, as *abstract mathematical structures*, fuzzy structures exist. What is needed for their existence, is only human beings to construct such membership functions as μ. Thus, fuzzy structures and their fuzziness are man-made formal entities, i.e., artifacts, like numbers in mathematics.

2.5 Concluding Remarks

Medicine as an application domain of fuzzy logic shows how fruitful even an abstract mathematical constcruct like the concept of fuzzy set can be. A few remarks here may suffice to realize the future impact of fuzzy logic on medicine:

Biomedical research, so-called, comprising cytology, physiology, biochemistry and other fields usually conducted on animals, is in fact zoology and *paramedical auxiliary.* Therefore, it should not be mistaken for medicine. It is true that this auxiliary paramedical research is based on natural-scientific principles of inquiry and is therefore a natural science discipline with its own methodology. Medicine as a healing profession, however, is not a natural science discipline. It is concerned with the health, illness, disease, therapy, life, and death of the patient as a human being, i.e., with something that is defined not by nature, but by human values, society, and culture. Accordingly, the statements that it produces and which control the behavior of the physician in diagnostic-therapeutic decision-making, are in the main conditional imperatives of the following form:

If A is $B_1 \& \cdots \& Z$ is B_m and you want to achieve the goal G,
then do $C_1 \& \cdots \& C_n$.

Insofar as medical thinking and practice has been concerned with this value-laden and action-theoretical subject rather than with zoology, it has taken place in a methodological vacuum until now. Medical students, doctors, and scientists have never been taught a methodology for their clinical decision-making and research simply because there is as yet no such methodology in medicine. A major obstacle to its emergence and development has been the fact that medical language and knowledge are inherently and irremediably vague and, therefore, not amenable to traditional methodological approaches that rely on precisionism. Consider, for example, the following description of pneumococcal lobar pneumonia:

> "In adolescents and adults the onset is sudden and may come 'out of the blue'; but often the patient has a cold or other upper respiratory infection and rapidly becomes much more ill, perhaps with an initial rigor but always with a sharp rise in temperature, usually to 101-103 F. Pleuritic pain usually develops over the affected lobe. The patient may become aware that he is breathing rapidly and certainly feels ill. Initially there may be a dry, painful cough but soon the cough becomes productive of sputum which is characteristically 'rusty' due to its content of altered blood from the foci of red hepatization; quite commonly, however, it is purulent or slightly blood-stained. It is often viscid and difficult to expectorate and this adds to the patient's pain" ([6], p. 18.28).

This passage from a standard medical textbook exemplifies the usual medical language and knowledge. Replete with vague, natural language terms such as *adolescent, adult, sudden, often, cold, rapidly, ill, much more ill, perhaps, rigor, usually* and so on, it conspicuously demonstrates that medicine is not mathematical physics or mathematical biology. It is an inexact action field because, first, the language and knowledge of the subjects constituting this field, i.e. the health care personnel and the patient, are vague and uncertain; and second, their goals and decisions based upon that language and knowledge are vague and uncertain as well. Fuzzy logic has enabled us to view this ubiquitous vagueness and uncertainty in medicine as an unavoidable consequence of the complexity and continuity of the 'real world out there', and to learn how to cope with it. Seen from this new perspective, the patient as the subject of medical language, knowledge, goals, and decisions appears as a highly complex bio-psycho-moral system that is primarily governed by continuous variables. Thanks to Zadeh's *incompatibility principle* ([11], p. 28), we have learned to realize that it is neither possible nor necessary to make precise every medical term and decision, and thereby awkwardly make discrete the given continuum. On the contrary, Zadeh's principle suggests that it is even desirable to fuzzify it, since significance is highly desired in medicine. This task is easily attainable in the following way.

The denotation of a medical term is a class X of any objects or processes. The Zadeh *fuzzifiability principle* which says that:

> Any crisp theory can be fuzzified by replacing the concept of a set in that theory by the concept of a fuzzy set ([12], p. 192; [13], p. 816; [13], p. 3)

will always enable us to reconstruct and treat the class X as a fuzzy set. It will thus be correct and advantageous to postulate that:

> Everything in medicine is fuzzy

rendering the entire medicine an application domain of fuzzy logic. Thus, about 2370 years after medicine's constitution as a discipline and profession by Hippocrates, it has eventually received a methodology. All logical, methodological, and epistemological problems associated with medical vagueness now appear tractable ([8]).

Due to its extended vagueness, medicine provides fertile ground for FLw and its subtheories from fuzzy set theory to possibilistic logic to fuzzy pattern recognition to fuzzy sensors and automata and additional yet-to-emerge methods and techniques. All of these conceptual frameworks and technologies will serve as a welcome medical intelligence enhancing tool and method. Research and practice of the following type have already advanced worldwide and may exponentially increase in the years ahead:

- Studies in the fuzzy foundations of medicine, e.g. concepts of fuzzy health, illness, disease, recovery, therapy, treatment efficacy, etc.;
- Applied fuzzy logic in all fields of medical research and practice, e.g. fuzzy anatomy, fuzzy physiology, fuzzy biochemistry, fuzzy pathology, etc.
- Fuzzy systems theory in medicine, e.g. theories of organism, consciousness, psyche, psychosomatic systems, infection systems, immune systems, etc.;
- Fuzzy signal processing, e.g. EEG, ECG, EMG, ERG;
- Fuzzy monitoring, e.g. in intensive care units;
- Fuzzy adaptive control, e.g. in anesthesia, intensive care units, therapeutic devices;
- Fuzzy image processing, e.g. in radiology, clinical anatomy, and clinical specialties;
- Fuzzy clustering, e.g. in nosology and epidemiology;
- Fuzzy pattern recognition, e.g. in genetics and genomics;
- Fuzzy organ support and prosthesis, e.g. in rehabilitation medicine;
- Fuzzy databases and data engineering, e.g. in hospitals and laboratories;
- Fuzzy analysis and interpretation of laboratory data, e.g. in pathology and clinical-chemistry laboratories;
- Fuzzy sensors in all medical domains;
- Fuzzy medical linguistics and terminology, yet to be developed;
- Fuzzy medical knowledge discovery, yet to be developed;
- Methodology of fuzzy concept and theory formation in medicine, yet to be developed;
- Fuzzy anamnestics, yet to be developed by utilizing branching questionnaires;
- Fuzzy medical knowledge engineering in every medical domain;
- Fuzzy clinical reasoning, e.g. in diagnostic-therapeutic decision-making.

An increasingly important role in this evolution will certainly play the latter two subdomains by utilizing the core fuzzy logic, i.e. fuzzy set theory plus linguistic variables plus FLn to contribute to the development of fuzzy artificial intelligence.

References

1. Roberto, C., D'Ottaviano Itala, M.L., Mundici, D.: Algebraic Foundations of Many-Valued Reasoning. Kluwer Academic Publishers, Dordrecht (2000)
2. Gottwald, S.: Mathematical fuzzy logic as a tool for the treatment of vague information. Information Sciences 172, 41–71 (2005)

3. Petr, H.: Fuzzy predicate calculus and fuzzy rules. In: Da, R., Kerre Etienne, E. (eds.) Fuzzy IF-THEN Rules in Computational Intelligence: Theory and Applications, pp. 27–36. Kluwer Academic Publishers, Dordrecht (2000)
4. Petr, H.: Metamathematics of Fuzzy Logic. Kluwer Academic Publishers, Dordrecht (2002)
5. Novák, V., Perfilieva, I., Močkoř, J.: Mathematical Principles of Fuzzy Logic. Kluwer Academic Publishers, Dordrecht (2000)
6. Reginald, P., Robson, J.S.: A Companion to Medical Studies, vol. 3, part I. Blackwell, Oxford (1975)
7. Russell, B.: Vagueness. Australasian Journal of Psychology and Philosophy 1, 84–92 (1923)
8. Sadegh-Zadeh, K.: Handbook of Analytic Philosophy of Medicine. Springer, Dordrecht (2011)
9. Esco, T.: Mathematics Behind Fuzzy Logic. Physica-Verlag, Heidelberg (1999)
10. Timothy, W.: Vagueness in Reality. In: Loux, M.J., Zimmermann, D.W. (eds.) The Oxford Handbook of Metaphysics, pp. 690–715. Oxford University Press, Oxford (2005)
11. Zadeh Lotfi, A.: Outline of a new approach to the analysis of complex systems and decision processes. IEEE Trans. Systems, Man and Cybernetics 3, 28–44 (1973)
12. Zadeh Lotfi, A.: The role of fuzzy logic in modeling, identification and control. Modeling, Identification and Control 15, 191–203 (1994)
13. Zadeh Lotfi, A.: The Birth and Evolution of Fuzzy Logic, Soft Computing and Computing with Words: A personal Perspective. In: Klir, G.J., Yuan, B. (eds.) Fuzzy Sets, Fuzzy Logic, and Fuzzy Systems. Selected Papers by Lotfi A. Zadeh, pp. 811–819. World Scientific, Singapore (1996)
14. Zadeh Lotfi, A.: Fuzzy Logic and the Calculi of Fuzzy Rules and Fuzzy Graphs. A Precis. International Journal of Multiple-Valued Logic 1, 1–38 (1996)

3

A "Goodbye to the Aristotelian Weltanschauung" and a *Handbook of Analytical Philosophy of Medicine*

Rudolf Seising

Abstract. In the 1960s Lotfi A. Zadeh founded the theory of *Fuzzy Sets and Systems* based on his works in system and information technology. In the 1970s, Mario Bunge published a system theoretical approach in philosophy of medicine that he named *Iatrophilosophy* and in the 1980s Kazem Sadegh-Zadeh opened the door to use fuzzy system's concepts in this area and to define a patient's state of health as a linguistic variable. He demonstrated that the concepts of health, illness, and disease "are not amenable to classical logic", he rejected the conceptual opposition that an individual could be either healthy or ill, and he created a new approach toward a novel theoretical framework of these concepts: "health is a matter of degree, illness is a matter of degree, and disease is a matter of degree". In the years before 2000 Sadegh-Zadeh fuzzified the "Fundamentals of clinical methodology" in a series of articles and he also started his research program from "Fuzzy Polynucleotide Spaces" to "Fuzzy Genomes". In 2001 he proclaimed a 'Goodbye to the Aristotelian Weltanschauung'. About one decade later he published "The Prototype Resemblance Theory of Disease" and his voluminous *Handbook of Analytical Philosophy of Medicine*. This introductory contribution delineates the historic path of fuzzy theoretic thinking in medicine.

3.1 Introduction

The German word 'Weltanschauung' has the meaning of 'world view'. Dictionaries show the literally translation "a comprehensive view of the world and human life". The *Oxford Dictionary of Philosophy* translates "Weltanschauung" to "a general world view; an overarching philosophy". [12] Therefore, the "Aristotelian Weltanschauung" is the all-world-embracing and completely independant philosophy of the ancient Greek philosopher Aristotle (384-322) that he had developed in opposite to the idealistic philosophy of his teacher Plato (428/427-348/347) and also to the atomic materialism of the epicurean, who followed Epicurus (341-270) and his

R. Seising and M.E. Tabacchi (Eds.): *Fuzziness and Medicine*, STUDFUZZ 302, pp. 19–76.
DOI: 10.1007/978-3-642-36527-0_3

teacher Democritos (ca. 460–ca. 370). Even if many of Aristotle's writings are lost, the historical traditional of his lifework seems to be the first comprehensive system of Western philosophy, encompassing morality, aesthetics, logic, science, politics, and metaphysics.

When the Iranian-German philosopher and physician Kazem Sadegh-Zadeh (born 1942 in Tabriz, Iran, Fig. 3.1 (a)) proclaimed his "Goodbye to the Aristotelian Weltanschauung" (Fig. 3.1 (b)) in the first year of our new millenium [69] he targeted the foundations of this world view that "had been laid by Aristotle himself in his *Metaphysics*, *Organon*, and *De Interpretatione*. They would constitute over more than two millenia the basic principles of classical reasoning in science, mathematics, philosophy, religion, politics, law, ethics, and all other areas" [69, p. 4], and Sadegh-Zadeh quoted the following text passages from the *Metaphysics* to represent its principles:

(A) This will be plain if we first define truth and falshood. To say that what is in not, or that what is not is, is false; but to say that what is is, and what is not is not, is true ([6], Book IV, 1011 b 26-27.)
(B) By demonstration I mean ..., e.g. "everything must be either affirmed or denied", and "it is impossible at once to be and not to be" ([6], Book III, 996 b 27-30.)
(C) ... that is the most certain of all principles. Let us next state what this principle is. "It is impossible for the same attribute at once to belong and not to belong to the same thing and in the same relation" ([6], Book IV, 1005 b 19-23.)
(D) Nor indeed can there be any intermediate between contrry statements, but of one thing we must either assert or deny one thing, whatever it may be ([6], Book IV, 1011 23-24.)
(E) Further, an intermediate between contraries will be intermediate either as grey is between black and white, or as "neither man nor horse" is between man and horse ([6], Book IV, 1011 b 29-32.) ... Again, there will also be an intermediate in all classes in which the negation of a term implies the contrary assertaion; e.g. among numbers there will be a number which is neither odd nor not-odd. But this is impossible ... ([6], Book IV, 1012 a 8-11.)
(F) Again, unless it is maintained merely for agument's sake, the intermediate must exist beside all contrary terms; so that one will say what is neither true nor false. And it will exist beside what is and what is not; so that there will be a form of change beside generation and destruction ([6], Book IV, 1012 a 5-8.)

Sadegh-Zadeh elucidated that (A) is the so-called correspondence concept of truth, that provided a basis for the correspondence theory of truth, and for Alfred Tarski's semantics of two-valued logic; the first part of (B) shows the principle of the two-valuedness; the second half of (B) and also (C) give Aristotle's version of the law of non-contradiction; in (B) and also in (D) we have formulations of the law of excluded middle; in (E) Aristotle advocated the two-valuedness because if theree would exist more than two values then we could suppose that there is no sharp border between its members and non-members. This, Aristotle said, is impossible! Finally, in (F) Aristotle refused the existence of something between being and nonbeing. This is called "Aristotelian ontology".

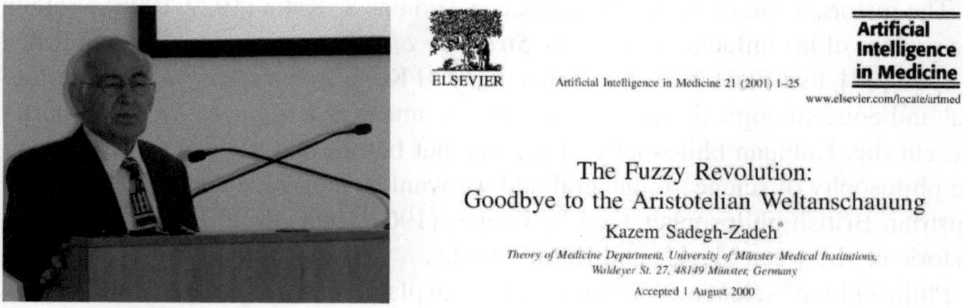
ELSEVIER Artificial Intelligence in Medicine 21 (2001) 1–25

Artificial Intelligence in Medicine

www.elsevier.com/locate/artmed

The Fuzzy Revolution:
Goodbye to the Aristotelian Weltanschauung

Kazem Sadegh-Zadeh*

Theory of Medicine Department, University of Münster Medical Institutions, Waldeyer St. 27, 48149 Münster, Germany

Accepted 1 August 2000

(a) (b)

Fig. 3.1 (a): Kazem Sadegh-Zadeh at the *1. International Symposium Fuzziness, Philosophy, and Medicine* at March 23-24, 2011 at the *European Centre for Soft Computing* in Mieres, Asturias (Spain); (b) his article [69].

To (A) - (F) Sadegh-Zadeh added the following "concept (G) of logical implication, consequence, or inference", that "represents the basic concept of the theory of deduction and proof underlying all classical mathematics, science, and technology and he called it "a modern derivative from the Aritotelian logic":

(G) A set of premises logically implies a conclusion if, and only if, whenever the premises are true the conclusion is true.

Sadegh-Zadeh characterized the concept of two-valuedness as "responsible not only for the emergence of individual theories, but for the very mode of scientific thinking and inquiry in all fields. In that generality we can say that the principles (A)-(F) together with (G) constitute the 'Aristotelian Weltanschauung' as a general 'world view' of scientific thinking!

3.1.1 Scientific World Views

Before we will return to this general concept we will consider the more restricted concepts of world views – "Weltanschauungen" – in science: "thought style" and "paradigm". The first was used by the Polish medical scientist and philosopher Ludwik Fleck (1896-1961) in his 1935 (in German) published book entitled *Genesis and Development of a Scientific Fact*. This book is currently regarded as a classic in history and philosophy of science, but was unknown in most parts of the world until it was translated into English language in the late 1970s [28]. In this book Fleck assumed that sciences grow as living organisms and that the development of a scientific fact is dependent on specific "styles of thought". He denied the existence of any absolute or objective criteria of knowledge; rather, he believed that different views could be true. He suggested that truth in science is a function of a particular way of thinking by the "thought collective", which was the name given to a group of scientists or persons "exchanging ideas or maintaining intellectual interaction".

The historian and philosopher of science Thomas S. Kuhn (1922-1996) wrote in the preface of his influential book *The Structure of Scientific Revolutions*, published in 1962 [38], that Fleck had anticipated many of Kuhn's own ideas on the sociological and epistemological aspects of the development of a science. We will shortly present this Kuhnian philosophy of science but before that we want to characterize philosophy of science in general and we want to introduce the work of the the Austrian-British philosopher Karl R. Popper (1902-1994) in a field that appeared historically between Fleck's and Kuhn's books.

Philosophy of science concerns scientific explanations of real systems and phenomena. Scientists observe these real systems and phenomena in natural environments and laboratories. They determine functions that represent the real system's properties and variables that characterize these systems. Scientists measure the values of the observed variables (observables) and therefore they collect a lot of data. Finally, scientists connect these real systems and phenomena with theoretical structures. They create these structures to have a "mapping" from the real world to the world of logics and mathematics. In this theoretical "paradise" they can define mathematical constants and variables and formulate axioms and laws that represent the real systems and phenomena. Scientists suppose that there is a connection between the real world and the logical-mathematical world – otherwise it doesn't make sense to speak about empirical science.

However, nobody can be sure that a scientific theory is true. In the 1930s, Karl R. Popper established the Critical Rationalism rejecting this classical empiricism. In principle, scientific theories are always tentative, and subject to corrections or inclusion in a yet wider theory [57].

Popper's *Logic of Scientific Discovery* was published already in 1934 in German but it became not influential before the English edition appeared in 1959. This work heralded a shift in differentiating between science and non-science, metaphysics or pseudo-science. In the "pre-Popper-times" philosophers tried to fix this demarcation in scientific language but in Popper's metatheory, named "Critical Rationalism", the decision of what is science and what is not science is related to theories and methods in these fields and not in the precision of the terms of language. Popper created such alternative concept in opposition to that of the Vienna Circle and the other Logical Empiricists who tried to analyze the constitution or the structure of scientific theories by using modern logic.

One of the main subjects of the Vienna Circle was the search for the greatest possible rapprochement between philosophy and science, by which they meant natural, social and psychological sciences. The "public" debut of the Vienna Circle was staged on November 23, 1928 in the ballroom of Vienna's Old Town Hall. The founding of the "Ernst Mach Society"[1] and the publication of the manifesto *Wissenschaftliche Weltauffassung — Der Wiener Kreis* provided the opportunity. Also these philosophers used the word "Weltauffassung" to describe their world view – and they emphasized it as scientific: *Scientific World View — The Vienna Circle*.

[1] The society's name even had an explanatory addition: Society to Spread Awareness of the Exact Sciences.

Particularly one member of the Vienna Circle, the German philosopher Rudolf Carnap (1891-1970), who later was a professor in the United States of America, wrote in 1928 *The Logical Structure of the World* [16] For Carnap and many others theories are sets of propositions and these propositions are built from data via induction. – Popper said: on the contrary! For Critical Rationalists scientific theories are not built from data by induction! There is no logical way from data to theory! Theories are hypotheses or conjectures and scientists test these hypotheses in experiments wich intend to refuse them. Even a great number of positive test results cannot confirm a scientific theory, but if there is only one outcome that is negative, this one counterexample shows that the theory is falsified. However, we can try to falsify our hypothesis and if we find one counterexample, then the hypothesis is refuted. Thus, in Critical Rationalism the falsifiability is the criterion of demarcation between what is scientific and what is not.

Another argument against the Logical Empirism is the following: it seems very clear that we can not reduce all our knowledge to sense experience. Therefore, we need so-called theoretical elements in addition to the empirical ones. These additional elements are being understood only in the context of a theory. They are more abstract, they are more distant from our perceptions than observational terms. To factor these elements in Logical Empiricism Carnap and the German philosopher Carl G. Hempel (1905-1997) introduced in the 1950s the so-called "double language model". [19, 32] Whereas observational and therefore non-theoretical terms are elements of the observation language, theoretical terms are elements of the theoretical language. Later, the US-American philosopher Willard van Orman Quine (1908-2000) joined in criticizing the empiricist differentiation between "analytical" and "synthetical". In short, the Logical Empiricism collapsed.

In *The Structure of Scientific Revolutions*. Kuhn criticized Popper's view on theory dynamics in science.[2] As he could show in many cases of his historical research work, no replacement of a theory by another happened because of falsification [38, 38]. He held the view that there is no linear accumulation of new knowledge in the development of scientific theories. Moreover, he claimed that science undergoes periodic revolutions. He proposed to distinguish three different stages of science: *Prescience* comes first with its lack of a central paradigm. Later, when scientists attempt to enlarge the central paradigm by "puzzle-solving" prescience is followed by *normal science*. Normal science reaches a crisis when anomalous results build up. At this point a new paradigm can emerge, which subsumes the old results along with the anomalous results into one framework. This new paradigm is termed *revolutionary science* [38]. Therefore, there are "paradigm shifts" in history of science, in which the nature of scientific inquiry within a particular field is transformed.

This new view on science development says that theory change in science is not a rational process and therefore we need assistance from sociology and psychology to explain the paths of science through history.

[2] Later he exemplified that the idea for this book went back to 1947 when he was asked as a graduate student at Harvard University to teach a science class for humanities undergraduates on historical case studies.

Most scientists in most periods have been "normal scientists". They are involved with puzzle-solving. Only if there were many anomalies in opposition to the current paradigm a crisis appeared and a scientific revolution could happen. Later, Kuhn introduced the notion "disciplinary matrix" to replace "paradigm" because of many criticisms for having used the notion "paradigm" extremely loosely.

When Sadegh-Zadeh said 'Goodbye to the Aristotelian Weltauffassung', he used this new Kuhnian terminology. After a brief sketch on Popper's, Fleck's, and Kuhn's views on theory dynamics in science he concluded to think that "all of these concepts are still too vague and inadquate to be very useful." Then he summarizes: "Science does not progress continuously and by accumulation knowledge. It does not add to an antecedent knowledge or theory T_i a subsequent knowledge or theory T_{i+1} of the same type such that one could reasonably consider science as the open, ordered series of related theories $T_1, T_2, \ldots, T_{i+1}$. Scientific ideas, theories, and worldviews evolve discontinuously in that a body of knowledge or theory, T_i, which is held over a particular period of time, is dislodged by another body of knowledge or theory T_j because the disciplinary matrix whithin which the foremer theory T_i had grown, changes to another disciplinary matrix which gives rise to the new theory, T_j, that is incompatible and incommensurable with its predecessor T_i. For example, the Hippocratic andf Galenic humoral pathology rooted in the pre-anatomical era of antiquity considered illness as an imbalance of four humours in the body, i.e. bile, phlegm, blood and urine, and lasted until the eighteenth century. After Andreas Vesalius' anatomy, *De Humanis Corporis Fabrica* (1543), and the then-emerging early empiricism conceptualized by Francis Bacon and John Locke had made a novel, empirical-anatomical disciplinary matrix abvailable within which illness appeared to have something to do with solid parts of the body, humoral pathology was replaced with the localized pathology of *De Sedibus et Causis Morborum* (1761) by Giovanni Battista Morgagni. By the end of the eighteenth century, it was complemented by Francois Xavier Bichat's tissue pathology. After the development of the microscope had enabled Theodor Schwann to discover the animal cell around 1838, localized pathaology was replaced by Rudolf Virchow's *cellular pathology* (1858), which considered diseases as cellular changes and disorders. With some alterations and additions, this view has been dominating medicine since. We are curretnly witnessing the emergence of a competing *molecular pathology*, e.g. genomics and pathobiochemistry, which explains and treats diseases as molecular processes in the body. Maybe our descendants will encounter *quantum pathology* or something like that in the near future ..." [69, p. 3f]

"Thought styles" or "paradigms" or "disciplinary matrices" represent scientific 'world views' (Weltanschauungen) but we have to consider their range of validity. Most of them root in just one scientific discipline (e.g. pathology, physics, or chemistry), they correspond to a self-contained excerpt of knowledge. Therefore, we have to cosinder what is the coverage of these thought styles or disciplinary matrices. As we mentioned already above, Sadegh-Zadeh identified the concept of two-valuedness as a disciplinary matrix of higher generality; he stated more precisely: "At the highest level of generality we presently encounter, to our surprise, a particular disciplinary matrix which has been nourishing all sciences and theories for the last 2300 years, i.e. the Aristotelian disciplinary matrix, because it contains the two-valued, classical logic whith which researchers reason and defend their work." [69, p. 4]

3.1.2 "Hello" to the "Fuzzy Revolution"

Saying "Goodbye to the Aristotelian Weltanschauung" Sadegh-Zadeh stated that the Aristotelian disciplinary matrix "is being eradicated by fuzzy theory" [69, p. 4]. In his article he said not only a "Goodbye" but also a "Hello" because its subtitle is headed by "The Fuzzy Revolution:". Consequently, Sadegh-Zadeh was also intended to show that there is a new scientific view that revolutionized our "Weltanschauung". He stated that the Fuzzy-view removes the fundamental principles (A) - (F) of the Aristotelian Weltanschauung: "The treatment of truth in fuzzy theory as a many-valued linguistic variable wiht a colorful and invigorating term set such as { true, not true, very true, completely true, more or less true, fairly true, false, very false, ..., etc. ... }, and the treatment of these terms as labels of fuzzy sets over the unit interval[3], is an ingenous andhighly esthetic dethronement of all existing theories of truth and oaf all simplistic semantics, including Aristotle's, Tarskis's Carnap's, and Kripke's perspectives, It goes without saying that whenever the simplistic concept of truth is lost, everything dependent will also vanish. That means that following the fall of A above, B - G will automatically collapse. Fortunately, there is a complete substitute for all of that, the fuzzy theory, which is capable of reigning immediately as the new disciplinary matrix. Its availablility as a more than perfect substitute is, thus, the reason of its success." [69, p. 6]

Sadegh-Zadeh replaced concept F, that he also named "Aristotelian ontology" and "Aristotelian doctrine of crisp existence", i.e. he replaced the refusal of the existence of something between being and nonbeing by the "Fuzzy ontology" that is on the contrary the permission of the existence of something between being and nonbeing. To this purpose he introduced the "fuzzy existence operator" as a new fuzzy quantifier:

$$\exists' \text{ that denotes "there is to some extent".} \tag{3.1}$$

Therefore, let (P, μ_P) be a fuzzy set and its membership function and let P be the corresponding predicate that signifies P, and $\exists' x(Px)$ means that *there is to some extent* an x such that x is P if and only if $\exists r(\mu_P(x) = r)$.

He named such an object x a "fuzzy object" and to measure the fuzzy existence of fuzzy objects he introduced the another operator:

$$_P\exists'_r x(Px) \text{ relative to } P \textit{ there is to the extent } r. \tag{3.2}$$

Therefore we have:

$$_P\exists'_r x(Px) \text{ if and only if } \exists r(\mu_P(x) = r). \tag{3.3}$$

[3] Here Sadegh-Zadeh refered to Zadeh's series of articles [112].

In Fuzzy ontology everything exists to an extent between 0 and 1. However, the Fuzzy ontolgy depends from the language in which the predicates are defined, or as Sadegh-Zadeh formulated, "first, that a language induces an ontology, and second, that being and nonbeing is relative to languages and logics.". [69, p. 7]

3.2 The Systems View on Science

In February of 1930, a "study group for scientific cooperation" led by Rudolf Carnap was founded under the auspices of the Ernst Mach Society and organized in the Vienna Chamber of Labor. The study group was intended "to bring about a harmonization of the special branches of science and a clarification of their place within the framework of science as a whole [...] by means of reports and discussions, particularly about the newer methods, problems, concept formations in the various specialist fields".[4] The Vienna Circle had shaped the concept of unified science, according to which there can only be pragmatic reasons for the separation of scientific disciplines, for they believed that unified scientific language and logic made it possible for everything to be described using this language.

Carnap elucidated this view in 1931 in a paper on The Physical Language as a Universal Language of Science. Here he contrasted the "generally widespread view" that the sciences "differ fundamentally in terms of their objects, their sources of perception, their methods" with the belief held by the "Wittgenstein faction" in the Vienna Circle: "By contrast, the view shall be expressed here that science forms one unit: All sentences can be expressed in one language, all facts are of one type, recognizable by one method."[5]

Carnap's book *The Unity of Science*, which was translated into English by Max Black [18] featured both his physical thesis, namely that all meaningful sentences can be translated into physical sentences, and the thesis that all events could be explained by physical laws. Even the laws of biology could be traced back to the laws of physics -- a thesis he admittedly could no longer substantiate later on, let alone prove.

The Austrian theoretical biologist Ludwig von Bertalanffy (1901-1972), who emigrated to Canada after the war, likely also no longer expected this when he called this view of a unity of the sciences in the mid-1950s "unrealistic". In his article "General Systems Theory" for the journal *Main Currents in Modern Thought*, he closed with some observations on the unity of science: "From our point of view, unity of science gains a more realistic aspect. A unitary conception of the world may be based, not upon the possibly futile and certainly far-fetched hope finally to reduce all levels of reality to the level of physics, but rather on the isomorphy of laws in different fields." [10, p. 8]

---

[4] [84, p. 382], quoted from *Erkenntnis*, 1, 1930–31, p. 79. See also [31, p. 74].

[5] "Demgegenüber soll hier die Ansicht vertreten werden, dass die Wissenschaft eine Einheit bildet: Alle Sätze sind in einer Sprache ausdrückbar, alle Sachverhalte sind von einer Art, nach einer Methode erkennbar." [17, p. 432].

He was not pleading for a reductionism but for a "perspectivism": "We can not reduce the biological, behavioral and social levels to the lowest level, that of the constructs and laws of physics. We can, however, find constructs and possibly laws within the individual levels." [10, p. 8]

"The whole is greater than the sum of its parts." This Aristotelian statement was interpreted by the Vitalists in the late 19th and early 20th century to mean that analytical-mechanistic examinations of life processes were not enough to explain them. Instead, everything organic was ruled by a "holistic causality" regulated by an "entelechy" that could be seen as a factor similar to the soul. This entelechy navigated life processes toward its goal. However, a nearly complete renunciation of the vitalist biologists was then made by British physiologist John Scott Haldane (1860–1936) in 1931. Mechanicism could not in turn explain the coordination in living systems. Only holism or organism — both terms were used in the 1920s — replaced vitalism as the "new paradigm".[6]

The natural philosopher and biologist Ludwig von Bertalanffy (Fig. 3.2 (a)) was familiar both with the mechanistic view, as well as with the newer philosophy of organism when he founded in the 1920s the so-called "General Systems Theory" as a "transdisciplinary" scientific view. Coming from the fact that the parts of the whole behave differently in isolation than in the dynamic of their context[7], Bertalanffy stated similar views with regard to psychology, medicine and the social sciences – Bertalanffy cited as examples *Gestalt psychology* und die *Psychosomatic medicine* – and "that these developments occurred independently of one another and usually without any knowledge of the parallel developments in other fields" [9, p. 8]. He saw this "parallelism" even in the "structurally similar models and sets of laws in completely different areas", e.g. the exponential law of growth and certain differential equations as examples. [9, p. 9]

However, constructions like this which encompassed all of the sciences were known in natural philosophy as 'world views', but the everincreasing differentiation and specialization made it difficult to devise an integrative system such as this in which every detail of even the most distant sub-discipline of a subject retains its classification. These philosophical observations on science and nature prompted Bertalanffy to proclaim a science that is superordinated wit respect to the sciences, with a system of sciences as its sub-systems. the sense of 'world views', but the everincreasing differentiation and specialization made it difficult to devise an integrative system such as this in which every detail of even the most distant sub-discipline of a subject retains its classification. These philosophical observations on science and nature prompted him to proclaim a science that is superordinated to the sciences, with a system of sciences as its sub-systems.

Despite the above mentioned sporadically occurring mathematically expressed rules, it was generally not possible to account for the circumstances of living systems using the traditional tools of physics-oriented mathematics. Therefore von

6 Organism was a term that had already been used in the social sciences by Auguste Compte (1798–1857), see [48, p. 40].

7 These formulations trace back to the philosophy of Georg W. F. Hegel (1770–1831). See e.g. [55].

Bertalanffy called "to expand our theoretical schemata in order to attain an exact set of laws in those fields where applying physical laws is not adequate or not even possible." [9, p. 8f] In order to identify "structural similarities", "isomorphies", "principles" that are true "absolutely" or "in general", in other words, to derive properties of "the systems of the most disparate kinds, be they mechanical, caloric, chemical or whatever," he required a "General Systems Theory".[9, p. 9] i.e. a "generalized science" as the cooperation of sciences where the different disciplines should be facilitated and fostered and multidisciplinary sets of laws should be sought, found and examined.

Bertalanffy's search for a more general theory could be seen in his 1928 opus *Modern Theory of Development* (*Kritische Theorie der Formbildung*) [8]: "Since the fundamental character of a life form lies in its organization, the usual examination of individual components and individual processes cannot provide a complete explanation of life phenomena. Instead, the laws of living systems must be examined at all levels of organization. We call this interpretation, when considered as research maxims, organismic biology and, as an attempt at explaining it, the systems theory of the organism [11, p. 20].

Also his concepts of "open systems", "dynamic equilibrium" and "feedback" can be found here. He employed these three interrelated fundamental concepts again in the 1950s to argue for *General Systems Theory*: First he separated the "open" from the "closed" systems and introduced his concept of "dynamic equilibrium": "Conventional physics is concerned with closed systems, that is, those that do not exchange any material with their environment. ... However, we find systems in nature that, by their essence and their definition, are not closed systems. Every living organism is an open system, for it maintains itself in a constant inflow and outflow, constant building up and breaking down of its components. As long as the organism lives, it is never in a state of rest, of chemical and thermodynamic equilibrium. Rather, it supports itself in a so-called dynamic equilibrium, i.e. a balance of import and export that is far removed from actual equilibrium. This is the essence of that basic phenomenon of life which we call metabolism."

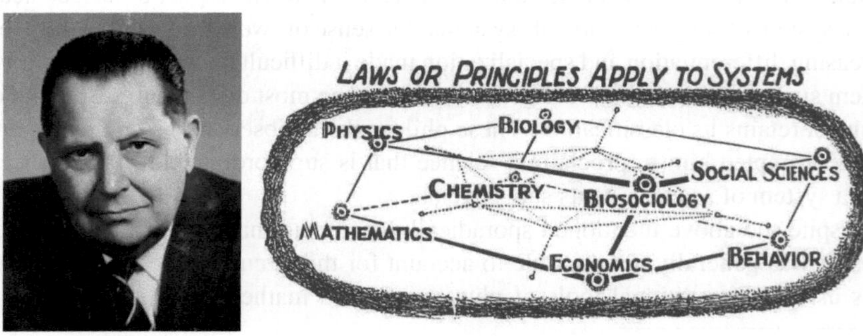

(a) (b)

Fig. 3.2 (a): Ludwig von Bertalanffy in the 1970s.; (b) his illustration to the *General Systems Theory*, [10, p. 8].

Bertalanffy was calling for a new view on science but he was not calling for a new "Weltanschauung," however. He wanted to turn attention to the interdisciplinary and transdisciplinary system structures of scientific principles.

One of the principles he found was the feedback principle, also central to Norbert Wiener's *Cybernetics or Control and Communications in the Animal and the Machine* [96] that appeared when the history of Ludwig von Bertalanffy's *General Systems Theory* was already 20 years old. The both melded in North America in the 1950s to a a new system theoretical approach in engineering sciences.

3.2.1 Iatrophilosophy – A System View on Medicine

Inspired by *Cybernetics* and *General Systems Theory* the Argentinian physicist and philosopher Mario Bunge (born 1919, Fig. 3.3 (a)) presented in the mid-seventies of the 20th century "Iatrophilosophy" as a new branch of epistemology. After he had emphasised that there are no generally accepted concepts of illness and health, he offered a general framework on the basis of Cybernetics and General Systems Theory that could contribute to build a theory of health and illness.

He picked the Greek word *iatros* for "physician", literally: the one who removes darts. "Iatrophilosophy" is the heading of a chapter of his book *Epistemología*, a collection of lectures and speeches that he has given in Mexico in 1975/76. [15] Hence, "Iatrophilosophy" is Bunge's new name for the field of philosophy of medicine.

Bunge started with the system-theoretical concept of a systems "state" that he transfered to the person as a patient in the field of medicine. He postulated that all the data gathered from a specific person at a specific time can be called his/her "medical status". This medical status is comprised of the various characteristics and symptoms of the person in question, such as his/her height, weight, body temperature, blood glucose levels, et cetera. The number of factors considered represents the number of parameters of the medical status. The relevance of individual symptoms to specific medical conditions can vary, but a person's medical status covers all of his/her attributes, providing a general overview of his/her condition.

Bunge's framework was the following system theoretic scheme: A concrete system a has a certain number of properties P_i, $i \in 1,\dots,n$ and we can find a function F_i to represent the property P_i, for example, if a is a human being, then F_i could be the glucose concentration in the blood, the blood pressure or the oral body temperature, the weight etc. In the easiest case, F_i is a function of the system a and of the time T. If H and $\mathbb{R}$ stand for the sets of human beings and the real numbers, respectively, than we have the following function:

$$F_i : H \times T \rightarrow \mathbb{R}^m. \tag{3.4}$$

We can imagine the n-tuple $\boldsymbol{F} = \langle F_1, F_2, \dots, F_n \rangle$ to be a vector in a n-dimensional Cartesian space and the value $s = \boldsymbol{F}(a,t)$ for a system a at time point t is called the state of this system at this time. During the times the state s moves in the state space S of the system a:

$$\sum(a) = \{F(a,t) \mid t \in T\}. \tag{3.5}$$

The arrowhead of the vector $\boldsymbol{F}(a,t)$ moves in the space S (a) on a trajectory that describes the history or the lifeline of the system a. If a is an organism, this lifeline starts at the birth and it ends at the death of the system.

The set of all possible states of a is restricted by some laws the components F_i have to observe, e.g. the heart frequency of a human is not between zero and infinity but between 30 and 200 beats per minute. Therefore, the allowed states of a build the subset $S_L(a)$ of $\sum(a)$ (Fig. 3.3 (b)).

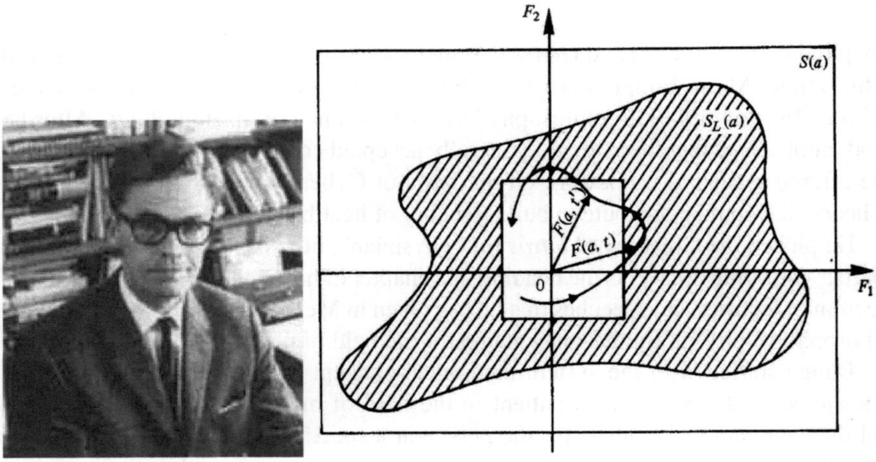

(a) (b)

Fig. 3.3 (a): Mario Bunge in the 1970s.; (b) his schema of an organism with two properties represented by functions F_1 and F_2 [15].

There are states of health and states of illness for every organism: if a biological system is in a state of health than the organism works optimally, if this is not the case, it is in a state of illness. Thus, in the case of a healthy organism the values of F_i i. e. the corresponding function of the system's property P_i is restricted to a subinterval of values of the interval of all possible F_i-values. Therefore, the states of health of a system a build a parallelepiped in the set $S_L(a)$ of all allowed states. Fig. 3.3 shows Bunge's fictive case of an animated system that is characterized by only two properties, represented by the functions F_1 and F_2. The hatched zone is the set of the ill (but living) states of the system a whereas the white rectangle in this zone is the set of all health states. The curve is the lifeline of the organism and we see that this organism is healthy for the most time of its life but some parts of the curve lay in the zone of ill states.

3.3 From the Systems View to the "New View" of Fuzzy Systems

As we mentioned already, in the 1950s, when *Cybernetics* and *System Theory* were rising scientific disciplines which concerned the general principles of characterizing input-output relationships. Engineers in that time were, in general, inadequately trained to think in abstract terms, but nevertheless, the electrical engineer Lotfi A. Zadeh (3.4 (a)) had been doing research in the fields of linear and nonlinear systems. In 1954, when he was an assistant professor at Columbia University in New York, he wrote an article entitled "System Theory" for the New York student publication *Columbia Engineering Quarterly* that he wanted to be an easily understandable introduction to this topic. Here, he described "System Theory" as a scientific discipline "to the study of systems per se, regardless of their physical structure". [99, p. 16] He believed that it was only a matter of time before system theory attains acceptance. He represented systems as block diagrams, i.e. graphical descriptions of the interrelationships between the variables associated with the system's objects. Thus block diagrams present in a graphical form the same information about a system as is conveyed by writing the input-output relationship:

$$v_1, \ldots, v_n = f(u_1, \ldots, u_m) \tag{3.6}$$

with inputs $u_1, \ldots, u_m$ and outputs $v_1, \ldots, v_n$, $(m, n \in N)$. In the case that these inputs and outputs are describable as time dependent functions the dynamic behavior of the system can be studied mathematically.

System theory became a well-known and important methodology in Electrical Engineering and after Zadeh became professor at the Unversity of California, Berkeley, he could describe problems and applications of System Theory and its relations to Network Theory, Control Theory, and Information Theory. Furthermore, he pointed out "that the same abstract 'systems' notions are operating in various guises in many unrelated fields of science is a relatively recent development. It has been brought about, largely within the past two decades, by the great progress in our understanding of the behaviour of both inanimate and animate systems—progress which resulted on the one hand from a vast expansion in the scientific and technological activities directed toward the development of highly complex systems for such purposes as automatic control, pattern recognition, data-processing, communication, and machine computation, and, on the other hand, by attempts at quantitative analyses of the extremely complex animate and man-machine systems which are encountered in biology, neurophysiology, econometrics, operations research and other fields" [101, p. 856 f.].

This quotation is from Zadeh's article "From Circuit Theory to System Theory" [101] to mark the 50th year of the Institute of Radio Engineers (IRE) where he described the successful developments in electrical engineering, and he specifically mentioned Bertalanffy's General Systems Theory.

Before we will refer to this interesting subject, let us consider an interesting event, i.e. the *Second Systems Symposium* that took place at the Case Institute of Technology in Cleveland (Ohio) in the spring of 1963. Entitled "Views on General

Systems Theory", this symposium was an interdisciplinary event where 17 speakers and over 200 participants included not only scientists represented General Systems Theory and Cybernetics but also engineering scientists and philosophers. The proceedings, published by Mihaljo D. Mesarović, were entitled *Views on General Systems Theory*. Indeed, this book contains very different views and approaches as the organizer emphasized in the preface:

"First of all, some of the participants took a definite stand, venturing to define a system and then discussing the consequences of such a definition. A second group of participants argued that the general systems theory should not be formalized since this very act will limit its generating power and make it more or less specific. A third group proposed to consider systems theory as a view point taken when one approaches the solution of a given (practical) problem. Finally, it was expressed that a broad-enough collection of powerful methods for the synthesis (design) of systems of diverse kinds should be considered as constituting the sought-for theory and any further integration was unnecessary. There were also participants that shared the viewpoints of more than one of the above groups." [49, p. xiv]

3.3.1 The "State" in System Theory

Zadeh based his contribution to this symposium on three concepts in System theory: the input, output and state of a system. While input and output were not expected to offer any difficulties, the concept of state appeared problematic. Zadeh noted that the idea of states had played an important role in the physical disciplines for a long time. It referred to a set of numbers that contain all of the information about a system's past and that determine its future behavior. The names of the French mathematician an physicist Jules Henri Poincaré (1854–1912), the US-American mathematician George David Birkhoff (1884–1944), the Russian mathematicians Andrei Andreyevich Markov (1856–1922) and Viktor Vladimirovich Nemytskii (1900-1967), and Lev Semenovich Pontryagin (1908–1988) stood for developments of more precise definitions of the concept of state in the fields where it was applied, such as dynamic systems and optimal control.

Zadeh's starting points to place a general notion of state in system theory were the fields of dynamical systems and of automata. As a simple example Zadeh presented the Turing machine: "Roughly speaking, a Turing machine is a discrete time ($t = 0, 1, 2, \ldots$) system with a finite number of states or internal configurations, which is subjected to an input having the form of a sequence of symbols (drawn from a finite alphabet) printed on a tape which can move in both directions along its length. The output of the machine at time t is an instruction to print a particular symbol in the square scanned by the machine at time t and to move in one or the other direction by one square. A key feature of the machine is that the output at time $t+1$ and the state at time $t+1$ are determined by the state and the input at time t." [101, p. 858].

If s_t, u_t, and y_t denote *state*, *input*, and *output* of the Turing machine at time t, respectively, and if f and g are functions on pairs of s_t and u_t, then the machine-operation is characterized by the following set of state equations:

$$s_{t+1} = f(s_t, u_t) \text{ and } y_t = g(s_t, u_t), \qquad t = 0, 1, 2, \ldots, \tag{3.7}$$

If the system is a differential system instead of a discrete-state system, *state*, *input*, and *output* of the system are represented by vectors $s(t)$, $y(t)$, and $u(t)$, respectively. With $\dot{s}(t) = d/dts(t)$ these *state equations* assume the forms

$$\dot{s}(t) = f((s(t), u(t)), \qquad y(t) = g(s(t), u(t)) \tag{3.8}$$

Some mathematicians and control theorists in the Soviet Union in the 1940s and 1950s – e.g. Pontryagin – used these state equations earlier than western scientists, and Zadeh took notice of the scientific progress in the Soviet Union after he migrated in the United States. He referred to the fact that "in the United States, the introduction of the notion of state and related techniques into the theory of optimization of linear as well as nonlinear systems is due primarily to Richard Ernest Bellman, whose invention of dynamic programming has contributed by far the most powerful tool since the inception of the variational calculus to the solution of a whole gamut of maximization and minimization problems." [101, p. 858]

"Among the scientists dealing with animate systems, it was a biologist — Ludwig von Bertalanffy -- who long ago perceived the essential unity of systems concepts and techniques in various fields of science and who in writings and lectures sought to attain recognition for "general systems theory" as a distinct scientific discipline. It is pertinent to note, however, that the work of Bertalanffy and his school, being motivated primarily by problems arising in the study of biological systems, is much more empirical and qualitative in spirit than the work of those system theorists who received their training in the exact sciences." [101, p. 857][8]

Then he demanded a new mathematics: "In fact, there is a fairly wide gap between what might be regarded as 'animate' system theorists and "inanimate" system theorists at the present time, and it is not at all certain that this gap will be narrowed, much less closed, in the near future. There are some who feel that this gap reflects the fundamental inadequacy of the conventional mathematics — the mathematics of precisely-defined points, functions, sets, probability measures, etc. -- for coping with the analysis of biological systems, and that to deal effectively with such systems, which are generally orders of magnitude more complex than man-made systems, we need a radically different kind of mathematics, the mathematics of fuzzy or cloudy quantities which are not describable in terms of probability distributions. Indeed, the need for such mathematics is becoming increasingly apparent even in the realm of inanimate systems, for in most practical cases the a priori data as well as the criteria by which the performance of a man-made system is judged are far from being precisely specified or having accurately-known probability distributions." [101, p. 857]

---

[8] For more details on *General Systems Theory* and *Cybernetics* in the history of the theory of Fuzzy Sets and Systesm see chapter III in [77].

When Zadeh established three years later the theory of Fuzzys Sets and Systems he proposed a solution for the problem: In his seminal article on Fuzzy Sets he introduced new mathematical entities that "are not classes or sets in the usual sense of these terms, since they do not dichotomize all objects into those that belong to the class and those that do not". He established a "way of dealing with classes in which there may be intermediate grades of membership." "... there may be a continuous infinity of grades of membership, with the grade of membership of an object x in a fuzzy set A represented by a number $f_A(x)$ in the interval $[0,1]$." [103].

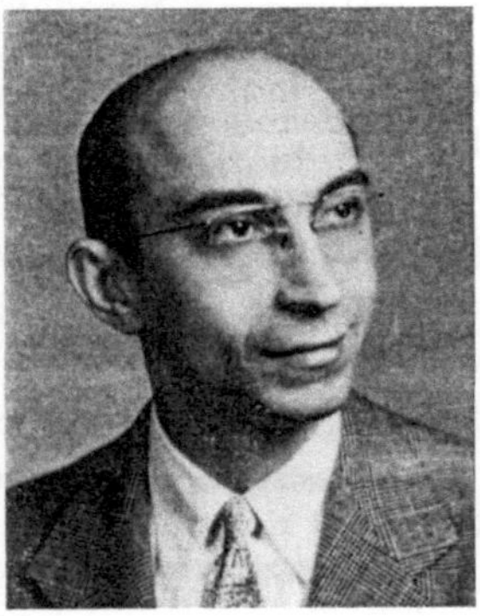

(a)

FUZZY SETS AND SYSTEMS*

L. A. Zadeh
Department of Electrical Engineering, University of California, Berkeley, California

The notion of fuzziness as defined in this paper relates to situations in which the source of imprecision is not a random variable or a stochastic process, but rather a class or classes which do not possess sharply defined boundaries, e.g., the "class of bald men," or the "class of numbers which are much greater than 10," or the "class of adaptive systems," etc.

A basic concept which makes it possible to treat fuzziness in a quantitative manner is that of a fuzzy set, that is, a class in which there may be grades of membership intermediate between full membership and non-membership. Thus, a fuzzy set is characterized by a membership function which assigns to each object its grade of membership (a number lying between 0 and 1) in the fuzzy set.

After a review of some of the relevant properties of fuzzy sets, the notions of a fuzzy system and a fuzzy class of systems are introduced and briefly analyzed. The paper closes with a section dealing with optimization under fuzzy constraints in which an approach to problems of this type is briefly sketched.

(b)

Fig. 3.4 (a): Lotfi A. Zadeh in the 1960s.; (b) Headline of his article in the year 1965 [104].

These new concepts provided a "convenient way of defining abstraction – a process which plays a basic role in human thinking and communication." To generalize various concepts of ordinary set theory, he defined equality, containment, complementation, intersection, and union relating to fuzzy sets A, B in any universe of discourse X as follows (for all $x \in X$):

- $A = B$ if and only if $A(x) = B(x)$,
- $A \subseteq B$ if and only if $A(x) \subseteq B(x)$,
- $\neg A$ is the complement of A if and only if $\mu_{\neg A}(x) = 1 - \mu_A(x)$,
- $A \cup B$ if and only if $\mu_{A \cup B}(x) = max(\mu_A(x), \mu_B(x))$,
- $A \cap B$ if and only if $\mu_{A \cap B}(x) = min(\mu_A(x), \mu_B(x))$.

3.3.2 *The Fuzzification of Systems*

In a talk at the Symposium on System Theory occurred in the Polytechnic Institute in Brooklyn in the same year Zadeh presented "A New View on System Theory", "which provide a way of treating fuzziness in a quantitative manner". In the symposium's proceedings there is a shortened manuscript version of the talk with the heading "Fuzzy Sets and Systems" ([104, p. 29], 3.4 (b)) where he introduced the concept of fuzzy systems for the first time:

Definition 3. *A system S is a fuzzy system if (input) $u(t)$, output $y(t)$, or state $s(t)$ of S or any combination of them ranges over fuzzy sets. [104, p. 33].*

Here, we have the same systems equations that hold for usual systems but with different meanings for u, y, and s as specified in their definition ($t = 0,1,2,\ldots$):

$$s_{t+1} = f(s_t, u_t) \text{ and } y_t = g(s_t, u_t) \tag{3.9}$$

Zadeh explained that "these concepts relate to situations in which the source of imprecision is not a random variable or a stochastic process but rather a class or classes which do not possess sharply defined boundaries." [104, p. 29]

In 1968, Zadeh presented "fuzzy algorithms", a concept that "may be viewed as a generalization, through the process of fuzzification, of the conventional (nonfuzzy) conception of an algorithm." [106, p. 94] Inspired by this idea, he wrote in the article "Fuzzy Algorithms" that all people function according to fuzzy algorithms in their daily life - they use recipes for cooking, consult the instruction manual to fix a TV, follow prescriptions to treat illnesses or heed the appropriate guidance to park a car. Even though activities like this are not normally called algorithms: "For our point of view, however, they may be regarded as very crude forms of fuzzy algorithms." [106, p. 95]

In 1973, in his "Outline of a New Approach to the Analysis of Complex Systems and Decision Processes" [110], he combined this concept of fuzzy algorithms with a new approach that was supposed to bring about a completely new form of system analysis based on his Fuzzy Set Theory: "The approach described in this paper represents a substantial departure from the conventional quantitative techniques of system analysis." [110, p. 28] This new way of going about system analysis differed from the conventional approach in the following new concepts:

- Linguistic variables: i.e. variables whose values are words or terms from natural or artificial languages. For instance, *not very large*, *very large* or *fat*, *not fat* or *fast*, *very slow* are terms of the linguistic variables size, fatness and speed. Zadeh represented linguistic variables as fuzzy sets whose membership functions map the linguistic terms onto a numerical scale of values (see Fig. 3.5.
- Fuzzy IF-THEN Rules: i.e. composite statements of the form IF *A* THEN *B*, where *A* and *B* are fuzzy expressions, "terms with a fuzzy meaning, e. g., 'IF John is nice to you THEN you should be kind to him,' are used routinely in everyday discourse. However, the meaning of such statements when used in communication between humans is poorly defined." [110, p. 29]

Zadeh often compared the strategies of problem solving by computers on the one hand and by humans on the other hand. In a conference paper in 1970 he called it a paradox that the human brain is always solving problems by manipulating "fuzzy concepts" and "multidimensional fuzzy sensory inputs" whereas "the computing power of the most powerful, the most sophisticated digital computer in existence" is not able to do this. Therefore, he stated that "in many instances, the solution to a problem need not be exact", so that a considerable "measure of fuzziness in its formulation and results may be tolerable. The human brain is designed to take advantage of this tolerance for imprecision whereas a digital computer, with its need for precise data and instructions, is not." [108, p. 132] He continued: "Although present-day computers are not designed to accept fuzzy data or execute fuzzy instructions, they can be programmed to do so indirectly by treating a fuzzy set as a data-type which can be encoded as an array. [...] Granted that this is not a fully satisfactory approach to the endowment of a computer with an ability to manipulate fuzzy concepts, it is at least a step in the direction of enhancing the ability of machines to emulate human thought processes. It is quite possible, however, that truly significant advances in artificial intelligence will have to await the development of machines that can reason in fuzzy and non-quantitative terms in much the same manner as a human being." [108, p. 132][9]

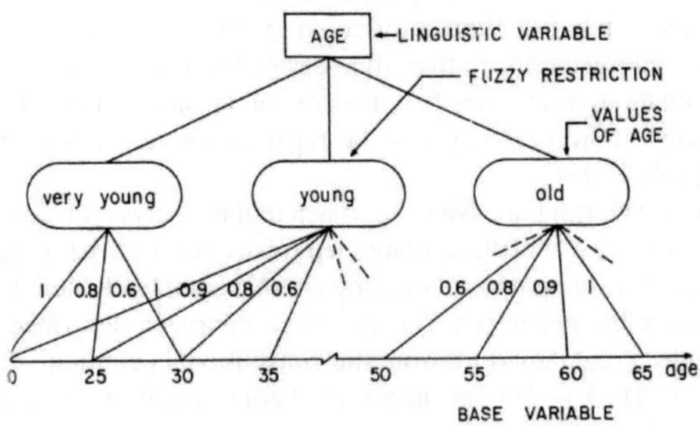

Fig. 3.5 Linguistic Variable Age

3.4 Fuzzy Sets and Systems in Medicine

Reasoning with unsharp concepts is standard practice in medical thinking. In 1926, the in chapter 3.1.1 already mentioned Polish physician and philosopher Ludwik Fleck expressed this fact in striking manner: "It is in medicine that one encounters a unique case: the worse the physician, the 'more logical' his therapy." Fleck said this in a lecture to the *Society of Lovers of the History of Medicine at Lvov* entitled "Some specific features of the medical way of thinking", which was published in 1927 (in Polish) [27]. Even though he was close to the Polish Lvov-Warsaw-School of logic, he opposed the view that medical diagnoses are the result of strong logical reasoning. He thought that medical symptoms and diseases are essentially indeterminate and that physicians rely on their intuition rather than on logical consequences to deduce a disease from a patient's symptoms. His lecture begins with the following sentence: "Medical science, whose range is as vast as its history is old, has led to

[9] For more details on the history of Fuzzy Sets and Systems see chapters IV - VI in [77].

the formation of a specific style in the grasping of its problems and of a specific way of treating medical phenomena, i.e. to a specific type of thinking." A few lines later, he exemplified this assumption: "Even the very subject of medical cognition differs in principle from that of scientific cognition. A scientist looks for typical, normal phenomena, while a medical man studies precisely the atypical, abnormal, morbid phenomena. And it is evident that he finds on this road a great wealth and range of individuality of these phenomena which form a great number without distinctly delimited units, and abounding in transitional, boundary states. There exists no strict boundary between what is healthy and what is diseased, and one never finds exactly the same clinical picture again. But this extremely rich wealth of forever different variants is to be surmounted mentally, for such is the cognitive task of medicine. How does one find a law for irregular phenomena?—This is the fundamental problem of medical thinking. In what way should they be grasped and what relations should be adopted between them in order to obtain a rational understanding?" Fleck emphasized two points:

- The first of these was the impact of the knowledge explosion in medical science. Accelerated progress in medical research had led to an enormous number of highly visible disease phenomena. Fleck argued that medical research has "to find in this primordial chaos, some laws, relationships, some types of higher order". He appreciated the vital role played by statistics in medicine, but he raised the objections that numerous observations "eliminate the individual character of the morbid element" and "the statistical observation itself does not create the fundamental concept of our knowledge,which is the concept of the clinical unit." Therefore "abnormal morbid phenomena are grouped round certain types, producing laws of higher order, because they aremore beautiful andmore general than the normal phenomena which suddenly become profoundly intelligible. These types, these ideal, fictitious pictures, known as morbid units, round which both the individual and the variable morbid phenomena are grouped, without, however, ever corresponding completely to them— are produced by the medical way of thinking, on the one hand by specific, far-reaching abstraction, by rejection of some observed data, and on the other hand, by the specific construction of hypotheses, i.e. by guessing of non observed relations." [27, p. 39f]
- The second point that concerned Fleck was the absence of sharp borders between these phenomena: "In practice one cannot do without such definitions as 'chill', 'rheumatic' or 'neuralgic' pain, which have nothing in common with this bookish rheumatism or neuralgia. There exist various morbid states and syndromes of subjective symptoms that up to now have failed to find a place and are likely not to find it at any time. This divergence between theory and practice is still more evident in therapy, and even more so in attempts to explain the action of drugs, where it leads to a peculiar pseudo-logic." [27, p. 42]

Clearly, it is very difficult to define sharp borders between various symptoms in the set of all symptoms and between various diseases in the set of diseases, respectively. On the contrary, we can observe smooth transitions from one entity to another and perhaps a very small variation might be the reason why a medical doctor diagnoses a patient with disease x instead of disease y.

Therefore Fleck stated that physicians use a specific style of thinking when they deliberate on attendant symptoms and the diseases patients suffer from. Of course, he could not have known anything about Fuzzy Sets and Systems, but he was a philosopher of vagueness in medical science. He contemplated a "space of phenomena of disease" and realized that there are no boundaries either in a continuum of phenomena of diseases or between what is diseased and what is healthy.

However, Sadegh-Zadeh arrived at another conclusion when I confronted him in an interview with Fleck's view: "From the inability of physicians to make explicit the tacit methods of their clinical decision-making, we should rather conclude the following imperative: Stop diagnostic-therapeutic decision-making without using any explicit logic and methodology because by conducting clinical judgment intuitively - i.e., without any explicit logical and methodological foundations – you produce too many errors of diagnosis and treatment!

Ludwik Fleck's works demonstrate that like other physicians, he didn't possess specific knowledge of logic. Therefore, his skepticism against logic and its application in clinical decision-making is unjustified. Obviously he has had the colloquial idea of 'logic' in mind. But such an idea is not a very useful one in science. I strongly believe that if Fleck had a deep understanding of logic, and more importantly, if he had been in the position to get to know fuzzy logic and its secrets, he would have judged otherwise." [72]

3.4.1 From Fuzzy Control to Fuzzy Medicine

"Medicine has been among the privileged areas to early recognize this revolution and to embrace the fuzzy theory in parallel with the seminal Mamdani and Assilian application in the engineering sciences and technology" wrote Sadegh-Zadeh at the beginning of his article "The Fuzzy Revolution: Goodbye to the Aristotelian Weltanschauung" [69]. In fact it was Zadeh's 1973-paper "Outline of a New Approach to the Analysis of Complex Systems and Decision Processes" [110] that Ebrahim H. Mamdani (1942-2010) read by shortly after he became professor of electrical engineering of the University of London. He then suggested to his doctoral student Sedrak Assilian that he devise a fuzzy algorithm to control a small model steam engine, as he mentioned in the article that he published together with Assilian:

> "The true antecedent of the work described here is an outstanding paper by Zadeh (1973) which lays the foundations of what we have termed linguistic synthesis [...] and which had also been described by Zadeh as Approximate Reasoning (AR). In the 1973 paper Zadeh shows how vague logical statements can be used to derive inferences (also vague) from vague data. The paper suggests that this method is useful in the treatment of complex humanistic systems. However, it was realized that this method could equally be applied to 'hard' systems such as industrial plant controllers." [46, p. 325].

With the success of Fuzzy Control in the 1980 the theory of Fuzzy Sets and Systems became more and more popular. This is often traced back to the implementations of the fuzzy control principles for products in the household appliance and entertainment industries. But there is another historical pathway of Fuzzy Sets and Systems that opened out into the medical sciences.

In 1969 Zadeh found that the field of medical sciences was a promising possible field of application for his new mathematical theory: "Specifically, from the point of view of fuzzy set theory, a human disease, e.g., diabetes may be regarded as a fuzzy set in the following sense. Let $X = x$ denote the collection of human beings. Then diabetes is a fuzzy set, say D, in X, characterized by a membership function $\mu_D(x)$ which associates with each human being x his grade of membership in the fuzzy set of diabetes" ([7], p. 205). He formulated these proposals very accurately and pointed: "In some cases, it may be more convenient to characterize a fuzzy set representing a disease not by its membership function but by its relation to various symptoms which in themselves are fuzzy in nature. For example, in the case of diabetes a fuzzy symptom may be, say, a hardening of the arteries. If this fuzzy set in X is denoted by A, then we can speak of the fuzzy inclusion relation between D and A and assign a number in the interval $[0,1]$ to represent the 'degree of containment' of A in D. In this way, we can provide a partial characterization of D by specifying the degrees of containment of various fuzzy symptoms $A_1,\ldots,A_k$ in D. When arranged in a tabular form, the degrees of containment constitute what might be called a containment table." ([107], p. 205)

Maybe the first scientific work on Fuzzy sets in Medicine was the dissertation *Fuzzy Sets and Their Applications to Medical Diagnosis and Pattern Recognition* [5] that Merle Anne Albin wrote already in 1975 under Berkeley mathematics professor Hans-Joachim Bremermann (1926-1996), a friend of Zadeh's. Unfortunatley its bibliography does not include any of the texts by Zadeh. Zadeh's aforementioned works with comments about possible applications of fuzzy sets in medicine likewise went unnoticed both by Harry Wechsler in his 1976 article "Applications of Fuzzy Logic to Medical Diagnosis" [91] and by Alonso Perez-Ojeda in his M.S. thesis *Medical Knowledge Network. A Database for Computer Aided Diagnosis* [54], led to his paper with Moon, Jordanov and Türksen [51]. Petre Tautu and Gustav Wagner, with their aforementioned review article [86], and Richard C. Elder and Augustine O. Esogbue also failed to mention them in the two parts of their paper [24, 25] from 1979 and 1980 about a fuzzy model for medical decision making processes, which traced back to Elder's M.S. thesis Fuzzy Systems Theory and Medical Decision Making. [23]

All of these works dealt with the application potential of Fuzzy Set Theory in the medical field without making any mention of Zadeh's explicit comments on this subject. They fuzzified medical laboratory findings that were classified either as normal or as pathological; they established continuous transitions, for instance, from shortened to normal to prolonged bleeding times or from slightly elevated to severely elevated cholesterol level corresponded more to a medical mindset. Using membership functions, values were established to state the degree to which the test results belonged to the respective fuzzy sets. [5, 24, 25, 51, 86] They suggested that the painfulness or severity of symptoms such as headaches or cyanosis could be represented by membership functions or by the degree of abnormality of a clinical or diagnostic test result [24, 51], or they proposed a nearly linear membership function for a fuzzy set abnormal cholesterol C, expressed in mg/100 ml of serum [24, 25], they used the modifiers Zadeh had introduced to calculate the degree of membership of a test result in a fuzzy set S_2 of the degree of membership of the test result in fuzzy set S_1 [51].

Also Philip Smets and his co-authors [80] emphasized the fuzziness of diagnostic terms such as arteriosclerosis or angina pectoris. Such diseases are not clearly or sharply defined, which is why it was often not possible to determine precisely the symptoms that clearly stand for a disease. However, diagnoses could also be defined as fuzzy sets whose elements are symptoms. These are assigned a membership value that indicates the intensity with which the symptom belongs to the fuzzy set representing the disease in question.

Moon, Jordanov, Perez-Ojeda and Türksen [51] had attempted to represent symptom combinations by means of logical conjunctions ($\wedge$ and $\vee$) of fuzzy sets.

A short time later Elie Sanchez chose for this purpose the concept of the fuzzy relation $R \subseteq S \times D$ between the symptom set S and the diagnosis set D. In doing so, he assumed that a doctor translates his knowledge and his experience into degrees of association between symptoms and diagnoses. This suggestion by Sanchez resulted in the successful application of Fuzzy Set Theory in the field of medical diagnosis.

3.4.2 Medical Decision-Making

Elie Sanchez considered relationships between symptoms and diseases mathematically and he intended to expand Zadeh's theory of fuzzy relations towards medical aspects. The shape this plan would take can be gleaned from his contributions *Compositions of Fuzzy Relations* [73] and *Medical Diagnosis and Composite Fuzzy Relations* [74] in a volume about advances in Fuzzy Set Theory and its applications, which was published in 1979. In these two papers, he demonstrated how the max-min composition rules Zadeh had introduced in his seminal article [103] could be used as a rule of inference, in particular in medical diagnostics.

He referred to the fact that medical diagnoses often had to be made without any precise analysis being possible. One or more illnesses then had to be inferred from a patient's symptoms, which most often be cannot be described in any exact way. In so doing, neither the set of diseases taken into consideration nor the conclusion about the disease(s) drawn from the symptoms can be precise. Sanchez introduced the relationships between the set of symptoms and the set of diseases as fuzzy relations.

“In a given pathology, we denote by S a set of symptoms, D a set of diagnosis and P a set of patients. What we call “medical knowledge” is a fuzzy relation, generally denoted by R, from S to D expressing associations between symptoms, or syndromes, and diagnosis, or groups of diagnosis. [74, p. 438]

The important new idea in Sanchez's work was his suggestion to use Zadeh's max-min composition rule as an inference rule to develop diagnoses. Given symptom and diagnosis sets S and D and an existing fuzzy relation $R \subseteq S \times D$ between them, the max-min composition can serve as an "inference rule", which makes it possible to deduce imprecise descriptions of a patient's illnesses (fuzzy sets of D) from imprecise symptom descriptions (fuzzy sets of S). With this inference rule, medical diagnoses D_j about a patient's disease can be derived by fuzzy logic from symptoms S_i with the help of the medical knowledge represented by the fuzzy relation R. The membership function is then computed as follows:

$$\mu_{D_i}(d) = max_{s \in S} \quad min\{\mu_{S_i}(s); \mu_R(s,d)\}, \qquad s \in S, \quad d \in D. \qquad (3.10)$$

By taking into account a set P of all patients considered and a fuzzy relation Q between P and the symptom set S, it was now possible with the aid of the max-min composition rule to obtain a fuzzy relation $T = Q \circ R$ with the membership function $T(p,d)$:

$$\mu_T(p,d) = max_{s \in S} \quad min\{\mu_Q(p,s); \mu_R(s,d)\}, \qquad s \in S, \quad d \in D, \quad p \in P. \ (3.11)$$

The membership function of the fuzzy relation R is denoted with $\mu_R(s,d)$. The fuzzy relation R can be expressed as a matrix, the entries of which can be made after interviewing doctors about their diagnostic experiences. This expert medical knowledge must additionally be translated into *degrees of association* between symptoms and diagnoses.

Sanchez interpreted this equation in this way: If the condition of a patient p is described with the help of a fuzzy set A of symptoms from S, then diagnoses from D can be associated with this patient p with the help of a fuzzy set B, specifically by means of the fuzzy relation R between S and D. Given fuzzy subsets A of S and B of D, the max-min composition $B = A \circ R$ describes the condition of the patient with respect to the symptoms he is experiencing and the diseases from which he may be suffering. The membership function below defined the fuzzy subset B in D.

$$\mu_B(d) = max_{s \in S}(\mu_A(s); \mu_R(s,d)), \qquad d \in D. \qquad (3.12)$$

Simultaneously studying an entire set P of patients p led Sanchez to the definition of the fuzzy relation $Q \subseteq P \times S$ to characterize the relationship between these patients and their possible symptoms. Finally, the newly composed fuzzy relation $TonP \times D$ can be composed from the fuzzy relations Q and $R : T = Q \circ R$ with the membership function

$$\mu_T(p,d) = max_{s \in S} \quad min\{\mu_Q(p,s); \mu_R(s,d)\}, \quad s \in S, \quad d \in D, \qquad p \in P. \ (3.13)$$

Zadeh had devised the max-min rule in 1965 as a composition rule for fuzzy relations and – as we said already – Assilian and Mamdani used it in 1972 to calculate inference rule relationships once they had implemented the fuzzy IF-THEN rules for their fuzzy algorithm to control their steam engine. Sanchez now interpreted it directly as a "fuzzy inference rule": $B = A \circ R$: IF A THEN B by R.

Using this inference rule, it is possible to logically infer medical diagnoses B of a patient's ailment from symptoms A with the aid of the medical knowledge represented as fuzzy relation R.[10]

3.4.3 Computer-Supported Medical Diagnostics

The rapid accumulation of data from medical research gave rise to the speculation that computers could be used to help in the field of medical diagnosis. Thus, shortly after the emergence of computers the first projects started when medical investigators used automatic data processing techniques to study correlations of signs and symptoms with diseases and to store medical knowledge in computer systems. One of the protagonists of computer assistance in medical diagnosis and decision-making was Lee Browning Lusted (1922-1994), a physician and mathematician who later was the founding editor of the journal *Medical Decision Making*. Some of his writings reflect the events of the times: "I felt that medical data could be processed by computer and that medical information could be made more useful to physicians by repacking it in a more usable form. I was not sure how this could be done but the idea of making information more useful by making it more usable stuck with me" [45].

Lusted and Robert Steven Ledley (1926-2012), a doctor of dentistry and electrical engineer who later became the founding president of the *National Biomedical Research Foundation* (NBRF), wrote the *Science* article, "Reasoning Foundations of Medical Diagnoses" that was published in the 1959 [42]. They introduced logical analysis in the medical diagnosis process and to open medical science for methods of decision-making and computer sciences. However, this "software thinking" is only a half of what was developed at the time; it was attended by "hardware ideas":

Also toward the end of the 1950s, the physician Martin Lipkin (born 1936) and his mentor James Daniel Hardy (1904-1985) began to wonder how the new computer technology could be used in medical research and within the scope of a doctor's activity. In the department of medicine of New York Hospital-Cornell Medical Center, Lipkin and Hardy sought ways to master the constantly growing flood of information. They were well aware of the developments in computer technology, thanks to the writings of Vannevar Bush but also from other publications reaching back to the 1940s and even the 1930s and touching upon "mechanical" computing and sorting machines that used cards and needles or punch cards. The idea arose of using machines of this type to build collections of data sets that were being accumulated during medical research, to carry out classifications and to develop interconnections among them. It was also thought that it might be possible to use this method to mechanically store data from patients' medical histories and to study whether this technology might be helpful in medical diagnostics. In 1958, Lipkin and Hardy reported on their project in the *Journal of the American Medical Association*, in which they sought to classify all of the diagnosis data from hematological

[10] For more details see chapter 7 in [77].

cases by means of a "mechanical apparatus" and to identify relationships between them. [43]

A brief description of this "first 'computer diagnosis' of disease, in this case hematology disorders" gives the biographical memoir on Hardy by Arthur B. Dubois: "The computer consisted of punched cards in a shoe box. Diagnostic criteria had been obtained from a hematology textbook and were wedge-punched at the edge of each of 26 cards to match the symptoms and laboratory findings of the 26 blood disorders. Knitting needles were run through the holes that corresponded to the symptoms and laboratory findings of each of 80 patients, matching those to the diagnostic criteria wedge-punched into the edges of the set of 26 hematology cards. Shaking the box made the card whose criteria matched those of the patient drop out of the shoe box to show the diagnosis printed on the hematology card." [22, p. 13f]

Following intensive collaboration between physicians, mathematicians and electrical engineers, medicine became, to a certain extent, a quantitative science. Various approaches to computerized diagnosis emerged in the 1960s and 1970s, using Bayes rule [90, 98], factor analysis [89], and decision analysis [42]. On the other hand, artificial intelligence approaches also came into use, e.g., DIALOG (Diagnostic Logic) [56] and PIP (Present Illness Program) [52]. These were programs to simulate the physician's reasoning in gathering information, as well as simulate the diagnosis using databases in the form of networks of symptoms and diagnoses.

As a next step we should mention the introduction of medical expert systems shortly after general non-fuzzy expert systems appeared in the 1970s. The first of these being MYCIN[11] [79], INTERNIST [50] and CASNET (Causal Associational Networks) [92, 93].

Revisiting the work of Ledley and Lusted [42] we notice how the authors considered also probabilitic concepts in the "Reasoning Foundations of Medical Diagnoses". They argued that in many cases our medical knowledge is not exact but in the form "If a patient has disease 2, then there is only a certain chance that he will have symptom 2 – that is, say, approximately 75 out of 100 patients will have symptom 2. [...] Since 'chance' or 'probabilities' enter into 'medical knowledge', then chance, or probabilities, enter into the diagnosis itself." [42, p. 13]

However, six years later, it seemed that Lusted had given up the program to use methods of exact mathematics in medicine; in his contribution to a volume on *Computers in Biomedical Research* [83] he was agreeing with a very new claim: "Research on medical diagnosis has served to emphasize the need for better methods of collecting and coding medical information and to demonstrate the inadequacy of conventional mathematical methods for dealing with biological problems. In a recent statement Professor L. A. Zadeh (1962) summed up the situation as follows: ..." ThenLusted quoted Zadeh's paragraph that we quoted already in chapter 3.3.1.

The first computer assisted system for medical diagnosis using the theory of fuzzy sets was the Viennese *C*omputer-*A*ssisted *Diag*nostic System CADIAG-II.

[11] MYCIN was written in Lisp as the subject of the doctoral dissertation of Edward Shortliffe (born 1947). This expert system identified bacteria causing severe infections and it recommended the dosage of antibiotics, depending from the patient's body weight. However, it was never used in practice.

Experts at the Department of Medical Computer Sciences, the University of Vienna Medical School, Vienna General Hospital, had proposed the development of a computer-assisted diagnostic system that did not use stochastic methods. "It was intended to develop a system which is not based on statistical assumptions like normal distribution, mutual independency of symptoms, constant probabilities of symptoms in different populations and at different observation times. There is no need for information about the frequency or lack of certain symptoms with the sick or the healthy. Therefore, rare complaints are considered as well as frequent diseases" ([1, p. 141]). To systemize and formalize medical knowledge and to store it in a suitable form, the head of the University Department of Medical Computer Sciences and simultaneously head of the University Clinic of Gastroenterology and Hepatologymedical Georg Grabner (1923-2006) and the IBM computer scientist Walter Spindelberger (1929-2011) started to use a computer for medical diagnosis in the late 1960s. Motivated by the work of Ledley and Lusted this was followed by intensive collaboration between physicians and mathematicians and engineers and in 1968 they constructed a first computer-assisted diagnostic system [82]. One year later Grabner and co-workers published their first experiences with this system for the differential diagnosis of hepatic diseases [30].

The second generation (called CADIAG-I) was developed in the 1970s on the basis of three-valued logic [2] and ten years later the "Fuzzy version" CADIAG-II appeared, based on the conjecture that "Fuzzy set theory with its capability of defining inexact medical entities as fuzzy sets, with its linguistic approach providing an excellent approximation to medical texts as well as its power of approximate reasoning, seems to be perfectly appropriate for designing and developing computer-assisted diagnostic, prognostic and treatment recommendation systems." ([3, p. 203]).

In the "fuzzy logical model", published by Klaus-Peter Adlassnig (born 1950) all symptoms $S_i \in S$ are considered to be fuzzy sets of X with membership functions $m_{S_i}(x)$, for all $x \in X$, indicating the strength of x's affiliation in S, and all diagnoses $D_j \in D$ are considered to be fuzzy sets in the set P of all patients under consideration with $m_{D_i}(p)$ assigning the patient p's membership to be subject to D_j. To describe "medical knowledge" as the relationship between symptom S_i, and diagnosis D_j, Adlassnig found two fuzzy relations, namely occurrence (How often does S_i, occur with D_j?) and confirmability (How strongly does S_i, confirm D_j?) ([3, p. 225]). These functions could be determined by (a) linguistic documentation by medical experts and (b) medical database evaluation by statistical means, or a combination of both. In both ways, to determine these fuzzy relations between symptoms and diagnoses, occurrence and confirmation, they have been defined as fuzzy sets. When physicians had to specify these relationships by the exclusive use of the terms *always*, *almost always*, *very often*, *often*, *unspecific*, *seldom*, *very seldom*, *almost never* and *never*, they choose fuzzy sets defined by Adlassnig's determination of their membership functions (see Fig. 3.6). In the case of medical databases the membership function's values of occurrence and confirmability could be defined as relative frequencies. CADIAG-II can infer all meaningful fuzzy relations between S, D, P, and their complements representing 'medical knowledge' by 'max-min composition'. By doing so, confirmed diagnoses, diagnostic hypotheses, and excluded diagnoses were determined. This diagnostic process was very successful in partial tests. For instance, in a study of 400 patients with rheumatic diseases, CADIAG-II yielded the correct diagnosis in 94.5% ([4, p. 264])

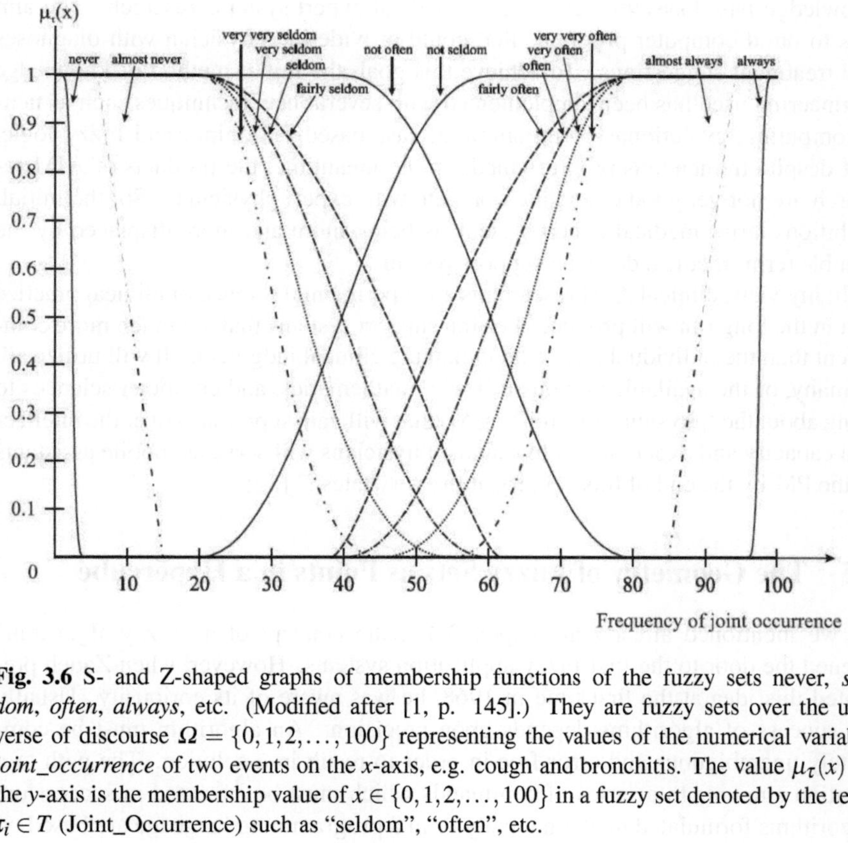

Fig. 3.6 S- and Z-shaped graphs of membership functions of the fuzzy sets never, *seldom*, *often*, *always*, etc. (Modified after [1, p. 145].) They are fuzzy sets over the universe of discourse $\Omega = \{0,1,2,\ldots,100\}$ representing the values of the numerical variable *joint_occurrence* of two events on the *x*-axis, e.g. cough and bronchitis. The value $\mu_T(x)$ on the *y*-axis is the membership value of $x \in \{0,1,2,\ldots,100\}$ in a fuzzy set denoted by the term $\tau_i \in T$ (Joint_Occurrence) such as "seldom", "often", etc.

When Sadegh-Zadeh had been asked about his view on the development of Computer and AI support in Medicine, his answer was surprising: "Ledley and Lusted in their seminal paper (1959), and Lusted in his subsequent book, gave rise to the emergence of the discipline Medical Decision-Making (MDM) that goes under the same name still today. They introduced probability theory, especially Bayes's Theorem, logic, and utility theory into medicine as a basis for clinical reasoning. In the meantime it has become a serious scientific field. But it has remained a theoretical field rather than a practical one. In the 1970s, the focus of research shifted from numerical-probabilistic approach to knowledge-based techniques that came to be known as (medical) expert systems or knowledge-based systems research. They were pioneered by early artificial intelligence systems such as DENDRAL, an expert system for identifying chemical structures from mass spectrograms; and MYCIN, an experimental expert system to assist in the selection of antibiotic therapy for patients with infectious diseases of blood and nervous system. A host of experimental medical expert systems such as CASNET, INTERNIST, PIP, and others followed. A new field of research and practice developed that has come to be known as Artificial Intelligence in Medicine (AIM), Medical Artificial Intelligence, medical knowledge-based systems research, or medical expert systems research. The aim was to build computer programs that could provide the physician with diagnoses and treatment suggestions. To achieve this goal, the initial method of knowledge engineering used has been supplemented with several new techniques such as neurocomputing, evolutionary programming, case-based reasoning, and fuzzy logic. But despite tremendous progress made in the meantime, the products of AIM research are not yet good enough to compete with expert physicians. So, the initial, ambitious term 'medical expert system' is being more and more displaced by the humble term 'medical decision support system'.

In my view, clinical AIM research is an experimental science of clinical practice that in the long run will produce decision support systems that are much more competent than the individual physician in making clinical judgments. It will utilize all, or many, of the available systems of logic, mathematics, and computer sciences to bring about the 'physician machine' (PM) that will gain supremacy over the intellectual capacity and expertise of physicians. Physicians will serve as mobile assistants of the PM by the end of this century at the very latest." [72]

3.5 The Geometry of Fuzzy Sets as Points in a Hypercube

As we mentioned already in chapter 3.4.1, the concept of a "fuzzy algorithm" opened the door to the first fuzzy application systems. However, when Zadeh presented this idea at the first time in 1968, he was aware of its coriousity. Usually the success of algorithms depends upon precision. An algorithm must be completely unambiguous and error-free in order to result in a solution. The path to a solution amounts to a series of commands which must be executed in succession. Algorithms formulated mathematically or in a programming language are based on classical set theory. Each constant and variable is precisely defined; every function and procedure has a definition set and a value set. Each command builds upon them. Successfully running a series of commands requires that each result (output) of the execution of a command lies in the definition range of the following command, that it is, in other words, an element of the input set for the series. Not even the smallest inaccuracies may occur when defining these coordinated definition and value ranges. But now, Zadeh saw "that in real life situations people think certain things. They thought like algorithms but not precisely defined algorithms." [106] Inspired by this idea, he wrote: "Essentially, its purpose is to introduce a basic concept which, though fuzzy rather than precise in nature, may eventually prove to be of use in a wide variety of problems relating to information processing, control, pattern recognition, system identification, artificial intelligence and, more generally, decision processes involving incomplete or uncertain data. The concept in question will be called fuzzy algorithm because it may be viewed as a generalization, through the process of fuzzification, of the conventional (nonfuzzy) conception of an algorithm. [106, p. 94] To illustrate, fuzzy algorithms may contain fuzzy instructions such as: (a) 'Set y approximately equal to 10 if x is approximately equal to 5,' or (b) 'If x is large, increase y by several units,' or (c) 'If x is large, increase y by several units; if x is small, decrease y by several units; otherwise keep y unchanged.' The sources of fuzziness in these instructions are fuzzy sets which are identified by their underlined names. [106, p. 94f] All people function according to fuzzy algorithms in their daily life, Zadeh wrote – they use recipes for cooking, consult the instruction manual to fix a TV, follow prescriptions to treat illnesses or heed the appropriate guidance to park a car. Even though activities like this are not normally called algorithms: "For our point of view, however, they may be regarded as very crude forms of fuzzy algorithms." [106, p. 95f]

One year later, in "Toward a Theory of Fuzzy Systems", written in 1969, Zadeh clarified "Roughly speaking, a fuzzy algorithm is an algorithm in which some of the instructions are fuzzy in nature. Examples of such instructions are:

(a) increase x slightly if y is slightly larger than 10;
(b) decrease u until it becomes much smaller than v;
(c) reduce speed if the road is slippery."

"More generally, we may view a fuzzy algorithm as a fuzzy system A characterized by equations of the form:

$$X^{t+1} = F(X^t, U^t), U^t = H(X), \tag{3.14}$$

where X^t is a fuzzy state of A at time t, U^t is a fuzzy input (representing a fuzzy instruction) at time t, and X^{t+1} is the fuzzy state at time $t+1$ resulting from the execution of the fuzzy instruction represented by U^t. .... The function F defines the dependence of the fuzzy state at time $t+1$ on the fuzzy state at time t and the fuzzy input at time t, whereas the function H describes the dependence of the fuzzy input at time t on the fuzzy state at time t.

To illustrate ..., we shall consider a very simple example. Suppose that X^t is a fuzzy subset of a finite set $X = \{\alpha_1, \alpha_2, \alpha_3, \alpha_4\}$ and U^t is a fuzzy subset of a finite set $U = \{\beta_1, \beta_2\}$. Since the membership functions of X^t and U^t are mappings from, respectively, X and U to the unit interval, these functions can be represented as points in unit hypercubes R^4 and R^2, which we shall denote for convenience by C^4 and C^2. Thus, F may be defined by a mapping from $C^4 \times C^2$ to C^4 and H by a mapping from C^4 to C^2. For example, if the membership function of X^t is represented by the vector $(0.5, 0.8, 1, 0.6)$ and that of U^t by the vector $(1, 0.2)$, then the membership function of $X^t + 1$ would be defined by F as a vector say $(0.2, 1, 0.8, 0.4)$ whereas that of U^t would be defined by H as a vector $(0.3, 1)$, say." ([109], p. 485f)

In Lotfi Zadeh's opus we don't find another remark on a connection of fuzzy sets and hypercubes even though he pointed out in 1969 that there exists a representation of fuzzy sets in the hypercube and there is no other paper on vector-valued variables to characterize a property of a system.

An important step in the history of the fuzzy mathematics is Bart Kosko's work on fuzzy sets as points in the hypercube. Kosko (Fig. 3.7 (a)) developed this theory in the 1980s during his graduate studies in electrical engineering of the University of California at Irvine and there he earned the Ph. D. in electrical engineering on the foundations of fuzzy systems in 1987.

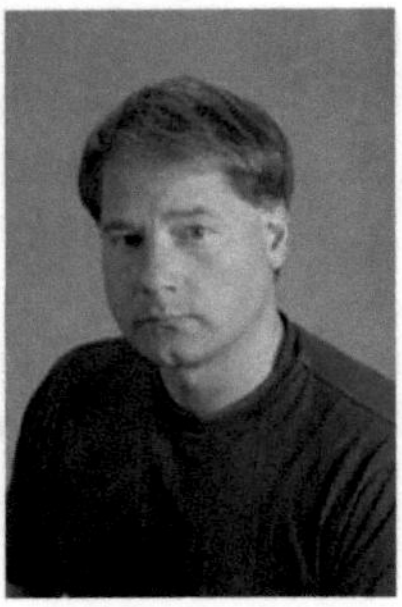

(a)

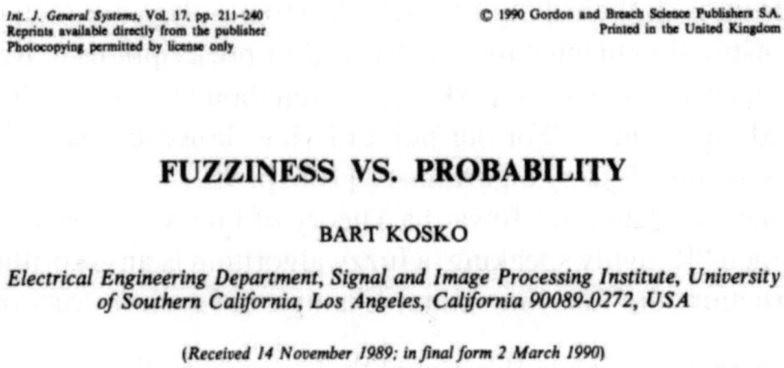

Int. J. General Systems, Vol. 17, pp. 211–240
Reprints available directly from the publisher
Photocopying permitted by license only

© 1990 Gordon and Breach Science Publishers S.A.
Printed in the United Kingdom

FUZZINESS VS. PROBABILITY

BART KOSKO

Electrical Engineering Department, Signal and Image Processing Institute, University of Southern California, Los Angeles, California 90089-0272, USA

(Received 14 November 1989; in final form 2 March 1990)

(b)

Fig. 3.7 (a): Bart Kosko in the 1990s.; (b) Headline of his article [35].

Therefore it took more than 15 years for this concept to became well-known when Kosko established the "geometry of fuzzy sets" in a hypercube. Already from the mid-eighties he wrote papers on his results and later he also published successful books on this subject and the article "Fuzziness vs. Probability" [35]. Kosko intended to ostensive oppose this concept of the fuzzy hypercube to Zadeh's "sets-as-functions definition of fuzzy sets" [35, p. 216]. He argued that the interpretation of "fuzzy sets as membership functions, mappings A from domain X to range $[0,1]$" is "hard to visualize. Membership functions are often pictured as two-dimensional graphs, with the domain X misleadingly represented as one-dimensional.

In his 1990-paper "Fuzziness vs. Probability" (Fig. 3.7 (b)), Kosko wrote: "It helps to see the geometry of fuzzy sets when discussing fuzziness. To date this visual property has been overlooked. The emphasis has instead been on interpreting fuzzy sets as membership functions, mappings A from domain X to range $[0,1]$. But functions are hard to visualize. Membership functions are often pictured as two-dimensional graphs, with the domain X misleadingly represented as one-dimensional. The geometry of fuzzy sets involves both the $domain X = \{x_1, \dots x_n\}$ and the $range[0,1]$ of mappings $\mu_A : X \to [0,1]$. The geometry of fuzzy sets is a great aid in understanding fuzziness, defining fuzzy concepts, and proving fuzzy theorems. Visualizing this geometry may by itself be the most powerful argument for fuzziness.

The geometry of fuzzy sets is revealed by asking an odd question: What does the fuzzy power set $F(2^X)$, the set of all fuzzy subsets of X, look like? Answer: A cube.

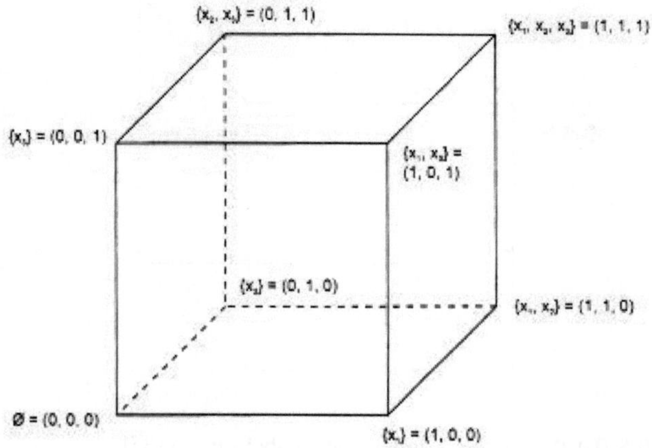

Fig. 3.8 The 3-dimensional cube I^3; Fig. in [35]

What does a fuzzy set look like? A point in a cube. The set of all fuzzy subsets is the unit hypercube $I^n = [0,1]^n$. A fuzzy set is a point in the cube I^n." [35, p. 216]

The set of all fuzzy subsets is the unit hypercube $I^n = [0,1]^n$. A fuzzy set is a point in the cube I^n." [35, p. 216] For illustrations see Figs 3.8 and 3.9. "Vertices of the cube I^n are nonfuzzy sets. So the ordinary power set 2^X, the set of all 2^n nonfuzzy subsets of X, is the Boolean n-cube $B^n : 2^X = B^n$. Fuzzy sets fill in the lattice B^n to produce the solid cube $I^n : F(2^X) = I^n$. Therefore, fuzzy set $A = \{(x_1,a_1),\ldots,(x_n,a_n)\}$ is represented by the n-dimensional vector (x_n,a_n) and all a_i are elements in $[0,1]$. Consequently, A is a point in the n-dimensional unit hypercube $[0,1]^n$.

3.5.1 The Fuzzy Hypercube and Structures

In 1989 Sadegh-Zadeh founded the international journal "Artificial Intelligence in Medicine" where he published in the following year his article "Advances in fuzzy theory" (Fig. 3.10 (a)) going back to Kosko's results. He pointed to the success of Zadeh's fuzzy concepts and methods in Medicine that already "have become standard in the application of fuzzy-theoretic tools to medical artificial intelligence subjects". However, by "Advances" he now turned to Kosko's new concepts of the fuzzy hypercube, fuzzy set inclusion, equality, and similarity that "are of high relevance to artificial intelligence in medicine research." [64, p. 309]

We will present these concepts in the vein of this article and before that we will reproduce Sadegh-Zadeh's definitions of *basic Zadeh structures*, *Zadeh structures* and *Zadeh spaces*. After that we will "complete" the fuzzy hypercube to be a *Zadeh space*:[12]

[12] Here, "iff" means "if and only if".

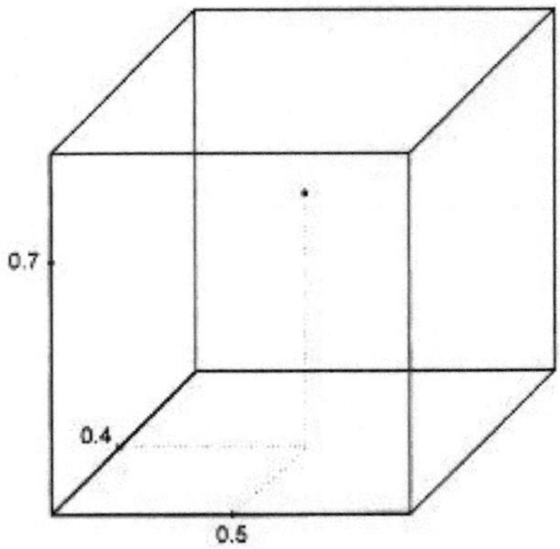

Fig. 3.9 Point $(0.5, 0.4, 0.7)$ in the 3-dimensional cube; Fig. in [35]

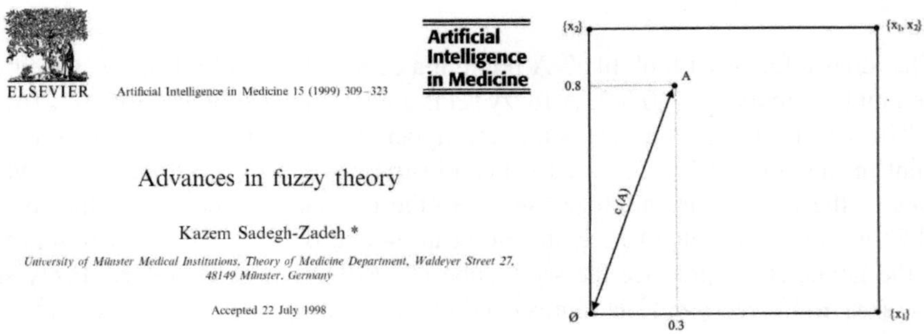
ELSEVIER Artificial Intelligence in Medicine 15 (1999) 309–323

Artificial Intelligence in Medicine

Advances in fuzzy theory

Kazem Sadegh-Zadeh *

University of Münster Medical Institutions, Theory of Medicine Department, Waldeyer Street 27, 48149 Münster, Germany

Accepted 22 July 1998

(a) (b)

Fig. 3.10 (a): Headline of Sadegh-Zadeh's article [64]; (b): Geometrical interpretation of the count of a fuzzy set A as the Hamming length of the vector drawn from the origin of the hypercube to the point A. In the present case we have $c(A) = (1.1)$ for $A = (0.3, 0.8)$. Fig. in [64, p. 315].

In his "Goodbye"-article Sadegh-Zadeh introduced the notion of the basic fuzzy structure to "shed some light" on Zadeh's creation of fuzzy sets. He emphasized that this was "a creation and not a discovery of a pre-existent entity."! Because the young history of the theory Fuzzy sets and Systems comprises so many controversies and misinterpretations concerning the question 'What is a fuzzy set?' Sadegh-Zadeh tried to resolve this problem by using a *structuralist approach*:[13] "the *definition* [of a fuzzy set] subsumes a particular kind of structure under the label 'fuzzy set', whether they be abstract or concrete, real or unreal, natural or artificial, subjective or objective, existent or non-existent." [69, pp. 17f] Therefore he defined the first structure as follows and following that he re-defined what is a fuzzy set:

[13] For more details on this approach in philosophy of science we refer to section 3.9.

Definition 4. ξ *is a* basic Zadeh structure *iff there are X, f, and A such that:*

1. $\xi = \langle X, f, A, \rangle$;
2. *X is a non-empty set;*
3. *f is a function such that* $f : X \to [0,1]$;
4. $A = \{(x, f(x)) \mid x \in X\}$.

Definition 5. *A is a fuzzy set iff there are X and f such that* $\xi = \langle X, f, A, \rangle$ *is a basic Zadeh structure.*

However, Sadegh-Zadeh refered here to the more general concept of a ('non-basic') *Zadeh structure* that he had already defined in the "Advances"-article. We notice that the following definitions of *Zadeh structures* and *Zadeh spaces* are generalizations of the *basic fuzzy structures*:[14]

Definition 6. ξ *is a* Zadeh structure *iff there are X, Y, and Z such that:*

1. $\xi = \langle X, Y, Z, \rangle$;
2. *X is a non-empty set;*
3. $Y = \{\mu_1, \mu_2, \dots\}$ *is a finite or infinte set of functions;*
4. $Z = \{A_1, A_2, \dots\}$ *is a finite or infinite family of sets;*
5. *Each* $\mu_i \in Y$ *maps X to the unit interval* $[0,1]$;
6. $A_i = \{(x, \mu_i(x)) \mid x \in X\}$ *for every* $A_i \in Z$ *with* $i \geq 1$.

To pass on to *Zadeh spaces* we need the concept of *metric spaces*:

Definition 7. *The pair* $\langle \Omega, d, \rangle$ is a metric space *iff there are* Ω, *and d such that:*

1. Ω *is a non-empty set;*
2. *d is a binary function from* $\Omega \times \Omega$ *to* $\mathbb{R}$ *such that for all* $x, y, z \in \Omega$:
   - $d(x,y) \geq 0$ *(non-negativity),*
   - $d(x,y) = 0$ *iff* $x = y$ *(identification property),*
   - $d(x,y) = d(y,x)$ *(symmetry),*
   - $d(x,y) + d(y,z) = d(x,z)$ *(triangel property),*

d is called a *metric* or a *distance function* over Ω and if, e.g., $\Omega = \mathbb{R}^n$, the set of all *n*-dimensional real vectors ($n \geq 1$), then we get the most well-known class of metrics, the

- *Minkowski metrics*: $l^p(x,y) = (\sum_{i=1}^n |a_i - b_i|^p)^{1/p}$ for $p \geq 1$

Special cases of this metrics class are the following distance functions:

- Hamming distance: $l^1(x,y) = \sum_{i=1}^n |a_i - b_i|$, $(p = 1)$.
- Euclidean distance: $l^2(x,y) = \left(\sum_{i=1}^n |a_i - b_i|^2\right)^{1/2}$, $(p = 2)$.

[14] Moreover, in Sadegh-Zadeh's own contribution to this book (chapter 2) we have a definition of his concept of a *fuzzy structure*.

Definition 8. ξ is a Zadeh space *iff there are X, Y, Z, and d such that:*

1. $\xi = \langle X, Y, Z, d \rangle$;
2. $\langle X, Y, Z, d \rangle$ *is a Zadeh structure,*
3. *d is metric over Z.*

To pass to identify the fuzzy hypercube as a particular Zadeh space, Sadegh-Zadeh defined some more concepts and – for simplicity's sake he also confined himself to finite sets only

Definition 9. *A set X with n elements has* 2^n *subsets. We name the set of all these subsets the* powerset of *X and it is denoted by* 2^X.

Definition 10. *The* fuzzy powerset of *X, is the set of all fuzzy subsets in X and it is denoted by* $F(2^X)$.

We emphasize that $F(2^X)$ is uncountably infinite and we have $F(2^X) \subseteq 2^X$. Particularly we mention that $F(2^X)$ is not a fuzzy set!

Definition 11. *A Zadeh structure* $\xi = \langle X, Y, Z, \rangle$ *is called* complete *if* $Z = F(2^X)$.

Finally, Sadegh-Zadeh brought it to the point: "In a complete Zadeh structure $\langle X, Y, F(2^X) \rangle$, the fuzzy powerset $F(2^X)$ forms a unit hypercube $[0,1]^n$. The singletons $\{x_i\}$ of $2^X \subseteq F(2^X)$ are the n coordinates of the cube. Thus, the 2^n members of the ordinary powerset 2^X inhabit the 2^n corners of the cube. The rest of the fuzzy powerset $F(2^X)$ fills in the lattice to produce the solid cube. The cube $[0,1]^n$ may therefore be termed a *fuzzy hypercube*." [64, p. 313]

Definition 12. *A Zadeh space with metric d is complete..*

Using Minkowski metrics in the fuzzy hypercubes, we can calculate distances between fuzzy sets. For that we define $c(A) = \sum_{i=1}^{n} \mu_A(x_i)$ as the sum of the membership values of the corresponding fuzzy set A (*fuzzy set cardinality* or *fuzzy set count*). However, this is the Hamming distance of a to the empty set $\emptyset$ at the origin of the hypercube:

$$c(A) = \sum_{i=1}^{n} \mu_A(x_i) = \sum_{i=1}^{n} |\mu_A(x_i) - 0| = \sum_{i=1}^{n} |\mu_A(x_i) - \mu_\emptyset(x_i)| = l^1(A, \emptyset) \qquad (3.15)$$

3.5.2 Fuzzy Entropy

"The amount of vagueness and indeterminacy a set carries within itself is referred to as its fuzziness or *fuzzy entropy*" Sadegh-Zadeh wrote starting the section "Fuzziness and clarity" in [64]. To the word "*fuzzy entropy*" he pinned a footnote saying "This terminology is due to relationsships between fuzziness and probabilistic Shannon entropy. The latter one is a special cse of fuzzy entropy" and then he referred to the works of Kosko that already have been cited, but first of all to a pioneering article by Aldo de Luca and Settimo Termini [21].

How fuzzy is a fuzzy set? – It could be worthwhile to attempt Italian physicists Settimo Termini and Aldo de Luca thought in the early 1970s it could have been worthwhile to attempt to "measure fuzziness". Termini recalled in an interview in 2010 "The very important thing was the truth functionality of fuzzy sets. It was very appealing that there was a way of approaching the representation of uncertainty in a truth functional way. In a single word, this appeared to me, simply: Wonderful! However, it was important having ways of controlling this uncertainty, and this should appear clearly by just looking to some properties of fuzzy sets. In a sense it should be something that each fuzzy set carries with it, independently from any other things." [87]

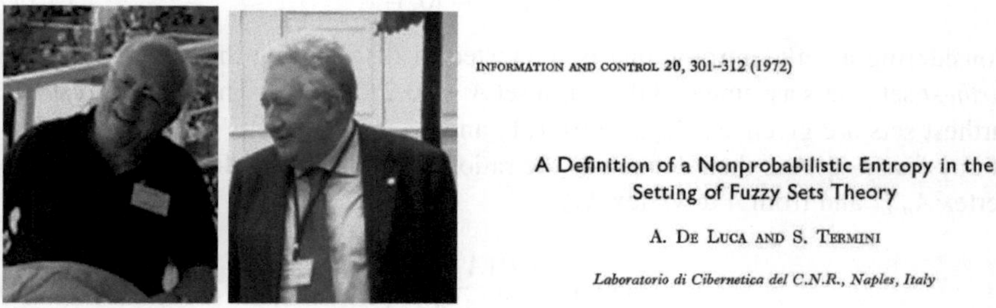
INFORMATION AND CONTROL 20, 301–312 (1972)

A Definition of a Nonprobabilistic Entropy in the Setting of Fuzzy Sets Theory

A. De Luca and S. Termini

Laboratorio di Cibernetica del C.N.R., Naples, Italy

(a) (b) (c)

Fig. 3.11 (a): Aldo de Luca; (b): Settimo Termini; (c): their article [21]

In 1972 the two proposed "the introduction of a 'measure of the degree of fuzziness' or 'entropy' of a generalized set" [21], "starting from the information provided by a fuzzy set, although all the tools of probability had been defined. We asked ourselves also what kind of properties (hoping to find strange things) this new concept should satisfy [...] at the same moment it was absolutely clear to us that these 'entropies' were 'measures of fuzziness', or, ways of measuring how much fuzzy a fuzzy set was. The central point of thus firm conviction was the introduction of the 'sharpened order'. It is this the central idea in which the theory of 'measures of fuzziness' is based, and in my view it corroborated the naive conviction that 'fuzziness' was not only an interesting concept but that it was really a *true new scientific concept*." [87]

When de Luca and Termini considered the entropy e of a fuzzy set of 2^X they beared in mind a measure that gives a value in the interval $[0,\infty]$ and that satisfies the following conditions:

- $e(A) = 0$ if A is a crisp set.
- $e(A)$ is maximal if A is the constant fuzzy set $A(x) = 1/2$ for all $x \in X$.
- $e(A) \geq e(B)$ if A is 'more fuzzy' than B by the *'sharpen' order* $\leq_S$.
- $e(A) = e(A^c)$.

where the *'sharpen' order* $\leq_S$ is defined as follows:

$$B \leq_S A \text{ if for any } x \in X : \begin{cases} \text{when A(x) } \leq 1/2 \text{ then } B(x) \leq A(x) \\ \text{when A(x) } \geq 1/2 \text{ then } B(x) \geq A(x). \end{cases} \quad (3.16)$$

Sadegh-Zadeh referred to this approach by de Luca and Termini when he wrote: "The amount of vagueness and indeterminacy a set carries within itself is referred to as its fuzziness or *fuzzy entropy*." In a footnote he then added: "This terminology is due to relationships between fuzziness and probabilistic Shannon entropy. The latter one is a special case of fuzyy entropy (see [21, 34, 35]). To measure the fuzziness of a Fuzzy set or its entropy he denoted the fuzzy entropy measure by *ent*,a map from the hypercube to the interval $[0,1]$:

$$\text{ent } : F(2^X) \rightarrow [0,1] \quad (3.17)$$

Considering a set's entropy, one is interested in determining the *nearest* and the *farthest* set. Let's assume that there is a set $A = (0.2, 0.8, 0.6)$. Then the nearest and farthest sets are given as: $A_{near} = (0,1,1)$ and $A_{far} = (1,0,0)$. The fuzzy entropy of any fuzzy set A is then defined as the ratio of the Hamming distances from A to vertex A_{near} and from A to vertex A_{far}:

$$\text{ent } (A) = \frac{l^1(A, A_{near})}{l^1(A, A_{far})}. \quad (3.18)$$

Sadegh-Zadeh defined then *clarity* of A, denoted as $clar(A)$, as the additive inverse of its fuzzy entropy:

$$\text{clar } (A) = 1 - \text{ent } (A) \quad (3.19)$$

At the vertices, $clar(A) = 1$ and in the centre of the hypercube $clar(A) = 0$.

3.5.3 Fuzzy Supersethood, Subsethood, Equality and Difference

Now, Sadegh-Zadeh continued with the special metric hypercube $\langle [0,1]^n, d\rangle$ that represents a complete Zadeh space $\langle X, Y, Z = F(2^X), d\rangle$. The 2-dimensional example $\langle X, Y, Z = F(2^X), l^1\rangle$, i.e. with the Hamming distance as metric shows some interesting properties that we present in the following.

In his seminal 1965 paper "Fuzzy sets" Zadeh had defined the properties of "containment" and "equality" for fuzzy sets as follows [103, p. 340]:

Definition 13. *"A is contained in B (or, equivalently, A is a subset of B, or A is smaller than or equal to B) if and only if* $f_A \leq f_B$. *In symbols*

$$A \subseteq B, \text{ if and only if } \mu_A(x) \leq \mu_B(x) \text{ for all } x \in X." \quad (3.20)$$

Definition 14. *"Two fuzzy sets A and B are equal, written* $A = B$, *if and only if* $f_A(x) = f_B(x)$ *for all* $x \in X$, *we shall write more simply* $f_A = f_B$.*)"*[103, 340]

As Sadegh-Zadeh emphasized, "Bart Kosko observed recently, however, this set inclusion is an all-or-none relationship" and also Zadeh's equality of fuzzy sets is

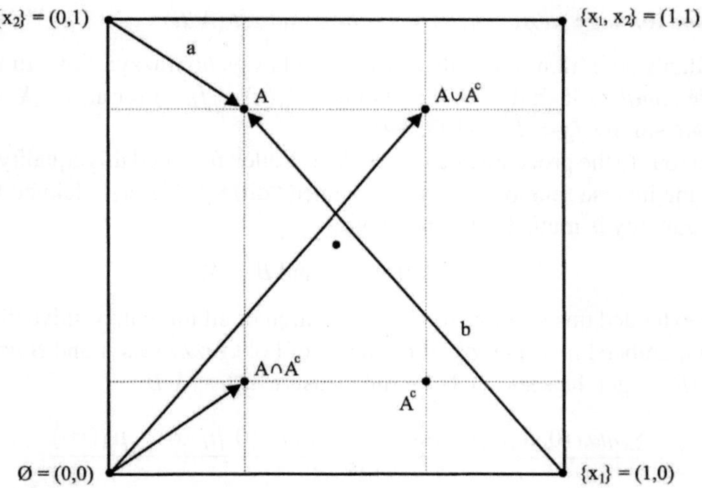

Fig. 3.12 Symmetrical position in the hypercube of the four sets A, A^c, $A \cap A^c$, and $A \cup A^c$. They are therefore equidistant from their vertex$_{near}$ and vertex$_{far}$. This is due to how complement, intersection, and union are defined in fuzzy theory. As these four set points move from periphery to the midpoint of the cube, they become more and more similar to one another until they equalize at the midpoint: $A = (0.5,\ldots,0.5) = A^c = (0.5,\ldots,0.5) = A \cap A^c = (0.5,\ldots,0.5) = A \cup A^c = (0.5,\ldots,0.5)$. We have therefore at the midpoint $ent(A) = ent(A^c) = ent(A \cap A^c) = ent(A \cup A^c) = 1$ and $clar(A) = clar(A^c) = clar(A \cap A^c) = clar(A \cup A^c) = 0$. For fuzzy set $A = (0.2, 0.8)$ with $ent(A) = 0.25$ we have $clar(A) = 1 - 0.25 = 0.75$.

nonfuzzy. For both relationships applies "It is therefore not a fuzzy relationship, but a crisp one [36, pp. 278ff]" [63, p. 318]. He reported Kosko's new concepts of set inclusion, equality, and similarity: "fuzzy subsethood" and "fuzzy equality" that is, as we will see now, the same as "fuzzy similarity".

To present these definitions, we start with their inverse relationships, i.e. "fuzzy supersethood" and "differ" between fuzzy sets A and B. Having these relations, we can define their inverse relations as "fuzzy subsethood" and "similarity", or "fuzzy equality", resp..

Starting with Zadeh's "crisp" *Definition* 13 it is clear that the relationship $\mu_A(x) \leq \mu_B(x)$ for all $x \in X$ is not longer valid if there is only one x_i with $\mu_A(x_i) > \mu_B(x_i) \Leftrightarrow \mu_A(x_i) - \mu_B(x_i) > 0$.

To obtain the concept of the "superset"-relation for A and B we will now count all positive differences of the membership values of all $x_i \in X$ to the sum $\sum_{i=1} max(0, \mu_A(x_i) - \mu_B(x_i))$. Then we normalize this measure by the count of A:

Definition 15. *fuzzy superset* $(A, B) = \frac{\sum_i max(0, \mu_A(x_i) - \mu_B(x_i))}{c(A)}$.

Analogous to the procedure before, Sadegh-Zadeh fuzzified this equality-relationship via the inverse relationship that he named "differ". He first claimed that ordinary set equality is mutual subsethood, i.e.:

Definition 16. *fuzzy subset* $(A,B) = 1-$ *fuzzy subset* (A,B).

Also Zadeh's definition of equality of fuzzy sets was nonfuzzy: "Two fuzzy sets A and B are *equal*, written $A = B$, if and only if $f_A(x) = f_B(x)$ for all $x \in X$, (we shall write more simply $f_A = f_B$.)"[103, 340]

Analogous to the procedure before, Sadegh-Zadeh fuzzified this equality-relationship via the inverse relationship that he named "differ". He first claimed that ordinary set equality is mutual subsethood, i.e.:

$$A = B \text{ iff } A \subseteq B \text{ and } B \subseteq A. \tag{3.21}$$

Then he extended this relationship by summation of all mutual, positive differences between membership-values of all members of boht fuzzy sets A and B normalized by $c(A \cup B)$ to get the scale $[0,1]$ for the measure *differ* (A,B):

$$\frac{\sum_i max\,(0, \mu_A(x_i) - \mu_B(x_i)) + \sum_i max\,(0, \mu_B(x_i) - \mu_A(x_i))}{c(A \cup B)}. \tag{3.22}$$

Thus, we can define the maps *differ* and *equal* or *similar*, resp.:

Definition 17. *differ:* $F(2^X) \times F(2^X) \to [0,1]$, *with*

$differ(A,B) = \frac{\sum_i max\,(0,\mu_A(x_i)-\mu_B(x_i))+\sum_i max\,(0,\mu_B(x_i)-\mu_A(x_i))}{c(A\cup B)}$.

Because the numerator of this fraction results in the Hamminc distance between A and B we have then:

Theorem: differ: $F(2^X) \times F(2^X) \to [0,1]$, with differ$(A,B) = \frac{l^1(A,B)}{c(A\cup B)}$.

As we already mentioned we can define the degree of equality, *equal*(A,B), as the additive inverse of the their difference:

Definition 18. *equal* $(A,B) = 1-$*differ* (A,B).

Therefore we also have:

Definition 19. *similar* $(A,B) =$ *equal* (A,B).

At the end of his "Advances in fuzzy theory" Sadegh-Zadeh gave a list of theorems:

Theorems

1. *similar* $(A,B) = 1 - l^1(A,B)/c(A \cup B)$
2. *similar* $(A,B) = c(A \cap B)/c(A \cup B)$
3. *similar* $(A,A^c) = c(A \cap A^c)/c(A \cup A^c) = ent(A)$
4. *similar* $(A,A) = 1$
5. *similar* $(A,B) = similar(B,A)$

With *Theorem* 3. we see that "the more similar a set A is with its complement, the fuzzier it is and vice versa. The maximum similarity $1 =$ equality with its own complement is exhibited by a set $A = (0,5,\ldots 0.5)$ at the hypercube midpoint. In contrast, a set $A \in 2^X$ residing at any of the 2^n corners of the hypercube is similar to its complement only to the extent 0." [63, p. 321]

3.6 Fuzzy Health, Patienthood, Illness and Diseases

Ever since the 1980's Sadegh-Zadeh discussed the nature of health, illness, malady, patienthood, and disease in medical sciences and philosophy and, and precociously combined his investigations with the theory of Fuzzy sets and systems. In the "Goodbye"-article he asserted that "Medicine is a healing profession, however, it is not a natural science discipline. It is concerned with health, illness, disease, therapy, life, and death of the *patient* as a human being, i.e., with something that is defined not by nature, but by human values, society, and culture." Moreover, he claimed that "medical thinking and practice has been concerned with this value-laden and action-theoretical subject [...] it has taken place in a methodological vacuum until now."

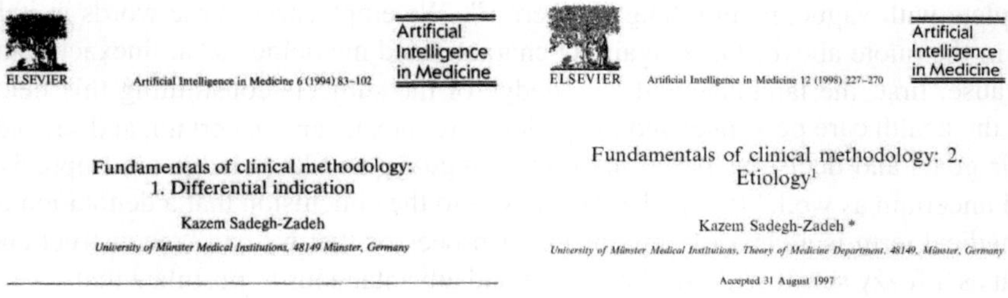
ELSEVIER Artificial Intelligence in Medicine 6 (1994) 83–102 Artificial Intelligence in Medicine

Fundamentals of clinical methodology: 1. Differential indication

Kazem Sadegh-Zadeh

University of Münster Medical Institutions, 48149 Münster, Germany

ELSEVIER Artificial Intelligence in Medicine 12 (1998) 227–270 Artificial Intelligence in Medicine

Fundamentals of clinical methodology: 2. Etiology[1]

Kazem Sadegh-Zadeh *

University of Münster Medical Institutions, Theory of Medicine Department, 48149, Münster, Germany

Accepted 31 August 1997

(a) (b)

Fig. 3.13 (a): Headline of article [61]; (b) Headline of article [62]

Already in the introduction to the first part of his quadripartite article "Fundamentals of clinical methodology" ([61], Fig. 3.13 (a)) he referred to "medicine's failure to recognize the need for, and to establish, a *Methodology of Clinical Practice* as a research and training branch. Medical students are not tought any algorithm or logic for their clinical problem-solving. every physician is thus left alone to rediscover the wheel of proficient practicing. And she carries it with herself into her grave. This is the entire (hi)story of clinical thinking." [61, p. 83]

In the "Goodbye"-article he declared expressly that "there is as yet no methodology in medicine" and he gave as a reason "the fact that medical language and knowledge are inherently and irremediably vague and, therefore, not amenable to traditional methodological approaches that rely on precisionism." [69, p. 19] As an example he quoted the following paragraph from a standard medical textbook [53, p. 18.28]:

> "In *adolescents* and *adults* the onset is *sudden* and may come 'out of the blue'; but *often* the patient has a *cold* or other upper respiratory infection and *rapidly* becomes *much more ill*, *perhaps* with an initial *rigor* but always with a sharp rise in temperature, usually to 101 – 103°F. Pleuritic pain *usually* develops over the affected lobe."

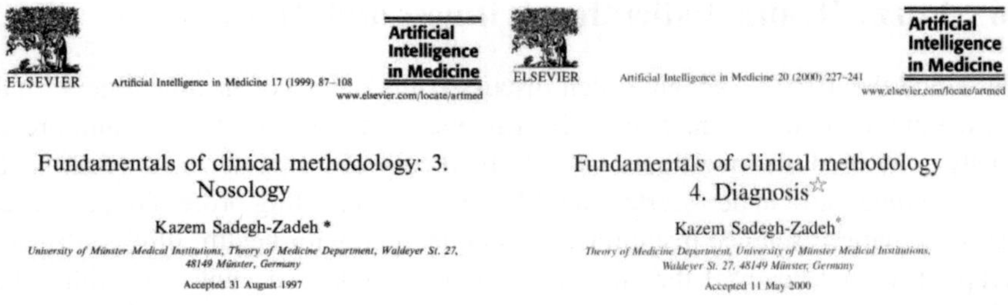

ELSEVIER Artificial Intelligence in Medicine 17 (1999) 87–108
Artificial Intelligence in Medicine
www.elsevier.com/locate/artmed

Fundamentals of clinical methodology: 3. Nosology

Kazem Sadegh-Zadeh *

University of Münster Medical Institutions, Theory of Medicine Department, Waldeyer St. 27, 48149 Münster, Germany

Accepted 31 August 1997

(a)

ELSEVIER Artificial Intelligence in Medicine 20 (2000) 227–241
Artificial Intelligence in Medicine
www.elsevier.com/locate/artmed

Fundamentals of clinical methodology 4. Diagnosis☆

Kazem Sadegh-Zadeh*

Theory of Medicine Department, University of Münster Medical Institutions, Waldeyer St. 27, 48149 Münster, Germany

Accepted 11 May 2000

(b)

Fig. 3.14 (a): Headline of article [63]; (b) Headline of article [65]

Sadegh-Zadeh argued that this passage, an archetypical example of medical text, is “replete with vague, natural language terms”. We emphasized these words in italics in the quote above. Once again he characterized medicine as “an inexact field, because, first, the language and knowledge of the subjects constituting this field, i.e. the health care personnel and the patient, are inexact and uncertain, and second, their goals and decisions based upon that language and knowledge are imprecise and uncertain as well.” [69, p. 19] He arrived to the conclusion that a denotation of a medical term is a class of any objects or processes that we can “reconstruct and treat as a fuzzy set. It will thus be correct and advantageous to postulate that

Everything in medicine is fuzzy.

rendering the entire medicine an application domain of fuzzy theory.” [69, p. 19]

In “Fuzzy Health, Illness, and Disease” ([66], Fig. 3.15), published in 2000, Sadegh-Zadeh claimed that the concepts “health”, “illness”, and “disease” “are not amenable to classical logic” and he rejected the conceptual opposition that an individual could simply be either healthy or ill. [66] Eight years later, in “The Prototype Resemblance Theory of Disease” ([70], Fig. 3.13) he clarified his position that “this traditional view is a semantic naivety.” He argued “that the opposite of health, that is ‘unhealth’, is not disease but *malady*. Malady is a broader category than disease. It comprises, besides disease as one of its subcategories, also many others such as injury, wound, lesion, defect, deformity, disorder, disability, and the like. An individual need not necessarily have a disease to lack health. [...] Based on these considerations, we may metalinguistically state that the antonym of the term ‘health’ is the term ‘malady’ and not the term ‘disease’. Every disease is a malady, but not vice versa.” [70, p. 107]

Early in the 1980s he created a fuzzy theoretic approach toward a novel theoretical framework of these concepts: “health is a matter of degree, illness is a matter of degree, and disease is a matter of degree” [60]. He introduced the concept of *patienthood* that means “being afflicted by a malady” [60] in the discussion “of which the notion of *health* will be the additive inverse in the following sense:

$$\text{Health} = 1 - \text{patienthood.”}$$

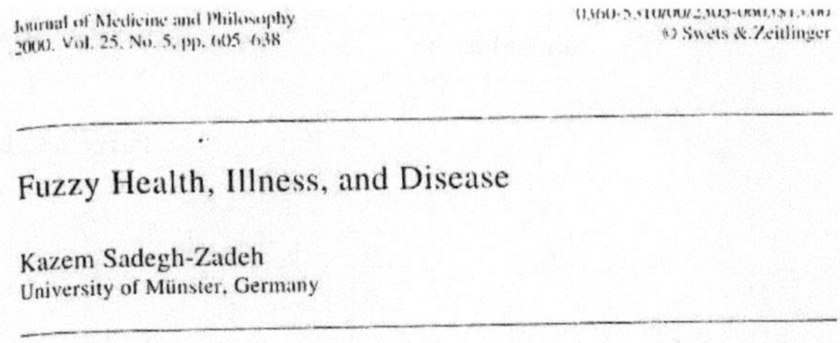
Journal of Medicine and Philosophy
2000, Vol. 25, No. 5, pp. 605–638

[illegible]
© Swets & Zeitlinger

Fuzzy Health, Illness, and Disease

Kazem Sadegh-Zadeh
University of Münster, Germany

Fig. 3.15 Headline of article [66]

3.6.1 The Fuzzification of the State of Health

In "Fuzzy Health, Illness, and Disease" Sadegh-Zadeh presented the following framework: "With Ω being the set of human beings at a particular time we have a fuzzy subset P (the set of patients) of Ω whose members are to various extents characterized by discomfort, pain, endogenously threatened life, loss of autonomy, loss of vitality, and loss of pleasure. The extent to which an individual is a member of this fuzzy set P is called the degree of patienthood." [66, p. 612] The membership function $\mu_P(x) \in [0,1]$ indicates the degree of patienthood of the individual $x \in \Omega$. H, the set of healthy people, is the complement of P. He continued:

$$\begin{aligned} \mu_p(x) &= \text{ degree of patienthood of } x, \\ \mu_h(x) &= \text{ degree of health of } x, \end{aligned} \tag{3.23}$$

by definition $\mu_h(x) = 1 - \mu_p(x)$, and $H = (x, \mu_h(x))|x \in \Omega$ is the fuzzy set *health*.

Basing on this view, "wellness" and "illness" are particular fuzzy states of health: ill health and well health –- and there are many others, because Sadegh-Zadeh defined the linguistic variable *state-of-health*, "whose term set may be conceived of as something like: $T_{\textit{state-of-health}} = \{$*well, not well, very well, very very well, extremely well, ill, not ill, more or less ill, very ill, very very ill, extremely ill, not well and not ill,* ... etc. ...$\}$" This *state-of-health* operates over the fuzzy set H (health) and it assigns to degrees of health, $\mu_H(x)$ values, elements of the term set $T_{\textit{state-of-health}}$ (see Fig. 3.16).

3.6.2 On Nosology – The Fuzzification of Diseases

"Despite all paradigm shifts in the last three millennia, no rational human bing since Hippocrates' times would deny that ther are instances of death caused by dramatic life events such as heart attack, stroke, and breast cancer, or would disagree with labeling such a real-life drama as a *dis*-ease = disease. That means that obviously there are some anthropological constants which all rational human beings would be prepared to label a 'disease' by pointing to them and declaring, 'look: this is a disease!'. Why not use such generally accepted, demonstrable prototypes as a point of departure?" Sadegh-Zadeh asked the readers of his article [66, p. 621] and then

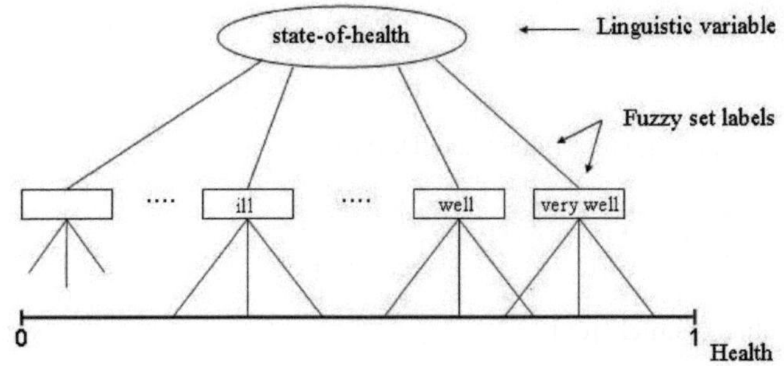

Fig. 3.16 Linguistic variable *State-of-health*

he introduced the term "disease" not as a linguistic but a social definition: There are complex human conditions "that in a human society are termed diseases", and he specifies potential candidates "like heart attack, stroke, breast cancer, etc." [66, p. 621] In his later article [70] he also mentioned 'myocarial inforction', 'gastric ulcer', 'diabetes mellitus', and 'AIDS'. In this article he referred to an estimation of approxmately 50,000 individual diseases or clinical entities. He named every phrase that denotes any of these huge amount of individual diseases a *nosological predicate*[15] that is used to predicate an individual disease attributed to a person.

Sadegh-Zadeh emphasized that all our definitions for many individual diseases do not give us a definition of the term "disease", "the general concept 'disease' that comprises all these 50,000 individual diseases and is thus, as a class, something different from each one of its 50,000 members." [70, p. 108] However, this may remind us of *Bertrand Russell's antinomy*[16] that usually is handled with a kind of "type theory" and Sadegh-Zadeh also proceeds with an example to the same tune: "The general category of birds as a class is not identical weith particyular bird species such as robin, sparrow, crow, ostrich, and so on. We must therefore not confuse a category with its members. Disease is the category. Individual diseases, or diseases for short, are its members." [70, p. 108]

3.6.3 Concepts, Categories, and Prototypes

In [70] Sadegh-Zadeh referred to the "classical, essentialist view" that reduces a category and concept to a finite number of defining features". This "view of *reductive*

[15] Nosology is the name of a branch of medicine that deals with classification of diseases. $\nu o \sigma o \varsigma$ (nosos) is an Ancient Greek word that means "disease", and $\lambda o \gamma \iota \alpha$ (logia) means "study of".

[16] "If *R* is the set of all sets that are not members of themselves. – Is *R* a member of itself? – If we say 'yes', then this contradicts the definition of *R* as a set containing all sets that are *not* members of themselves. On the other hand, if we say 'no', then we say that *R* is a set that is not a member of itself and that means that it belongs as a member to itself. Russell discovered this antinomy or – more generally – paradoxon in 1901.

definability of concepts says that something is a member of, say, category *C* if it possesses "a set of defining features to meet the nature or essence of C-hood." To distinguish *classical* and *nonclassical* concepts he gave the following definition:

Definition 20. *"A concept is said to be:*

1. *a reducible or classical one iff it denotes a reducible category [...] and*
2. *an irreducible or nonclassical one iff it denotes an irreducible category, for example our concept of disease [...]. " [70, 114]*

It is well-known that ancient philosophers characterized categories as reducible concepts and refering back to Bunge's *Iatrophilosophy* (see section 3.2.1) we notice that also his approach tried to define the concept of disease by a finite number of properties. However, Sadegh-Zadeh emphasizes that "nearly all real-world categories are irreducible ones and, according to our terminology introduced above, all concepts denoting such categories are nonclassical concepts."

Moreover, "in an irreducible category, there are no comon-to-all features because both regarding their number as well as their intensity the features are unequally distributed over the category members to the effect that some members appear more typical than other ones." [70, 119] Again using his favorite example he asked to "propose a defining set of features that are common-to-all members of the category *bird* embracing such diverse subcategoriesa as robin, sparrow, nightingale, crow, bird of paradise, bird of prey, albatros, ostrich, emu, penguin, etc. You will not succeed because these innumerable bird types do not share a birdhood-estblishing feature set such as, for instance, {has-feathers, has-a-beak, flies, chirps, lays-eggs, ...} that would uniformly recur in all of them to define the nature of birdhood. Rather they are characterized by only partially overlapping feature sets such as {A, B, C}, {B, C, D}, {C, D, E}, {D, E, F}, {E, F, G} and other ones in the folowing fashion:

Table 3.1 Some birds and their features

Robin	A	B	C				
crow		B	C	D			
eagle			C	D	E		
ostrich				D	E	F	
penguin					E	F	G
...					...		

Although neighboring bird types in this chain have something in common, two distant ones such as robin and penguin evidently have nothing in common. and most interestingly, there is nothing common to all." [70, 116]

It is understood that Sadegh-Zadeh linked these irreducible categories to Wittgenstein's concept of "familiy resemblances" that he suggested in the *Philosophical Investigations* finally writing that we:

> “can see how similarities crop up and disappear. And the result of this examination is: we see a complicated network of similarities overlapping and crisscrossing: sometimes overall similarities.”
> “I can think of no better expression to characterize these similarities than ‘family resemblances’; for the various resemblances betweenmembers of a family: build, features, colour of eyes, gait, temperament, etc. etc. overlap and crisscross in the same way.” [97, §§ 65, 66]

However, Sadegh-Zadeh pointed out that Wittgenstein’s expression of family resemblance is a metaphor and that we can not use it to define nonclassical categories and particularly the category of *disease*. Wittgenstein explained that some objects belong to the same family *because* of the resemblance between them, therefore we can not use his term “family” to explain nonclassical concepts. Rather, Sadegh-Zadeh linked Wittgenstein’s philosophical thinking to the experimental-psychological studies on categorization by Berkeley psychologist Eleanor Rosch “to construct the concept of a resembalnce structure that we wll use as our basic tool.” [70, 119]

In the 1970s, Rosch had developed the so-called *Prototype Theory* on the basis of empirical studies. This theory assumes that people perceive objects in the real world by comparing them to prototypes and then ordering them accordingly. [58]. Using his example of the category of birds Sadegh-Zadeh appleid this theory: “a robin seems to be a more birdlike, typical bird than a penguin. This was convincingly demonstrated by Eleanor Rosch who in experimental studies asked the subjects to rate on a scale from 1 to 7 the typicality of different kinds of birds. Robins were considered the best examples followed by doves, sparrows, and canaries. Owls, parrots, and toucans occupied a medium position. Ducks and peacocks were considered less good examples. Penguins and ostriches ranked lowest. Similar experiments were carried out for the categories furniture, fruit, and clothing [59]

Sadegh-Zadeh arrived to the conclusion that “a nonclassical theory of concepts is emerging according to which a concept determines a category not by identifying necessary and sufficient features of its members, but by exhibiting the relational structure of the category that is characterized by best examples, called prototypes, such that other category members resemble them to different extents.” [70, 119] E.g., concerning the category of birds we can compare various members of this category, e.g. robins and penguins, in table 3.2:

Table 3.2 Robins and penguins as birds

Bird	has feathers	has a beak	lays eggs	chirps	flies	...
Robins	yes	yes	yes	yes	yes	...
Penguins	yes	yes	yes	no	no	...

Thus, a robin is *more birdlike* than a penguin and in general: there are members of nonclassical categories that are a *more-typical-instance* than other members of this category. This relational feature “induces some kind of gradedness of membership in the category.” [70, p. 120] As we will see in the next section, Sadegh-Zadeh reconstructs this gradedness "as degrees of feature matching, that is similarity between less prototypical members of the category and its prototypes. Such a category we, therefore, call a prototype resemblance category", [70, 120] and to establish these kind of categories mathematically we need to use the concept of a fuzzy set.

3.6.4 Human Conditions

To clarify what is a "disease" we revisit the human conditions that we considered already in subsection 3.6.2. 12 years ago Sadegh-Zadeh wrote that such complex human conditions are not, and should not be, merely confined to biological states of the organism. They may be viewed and represented as large fuzzy sets which also contain parts that refer to the subjective, religious, transcendental and social world of the ill, such as pain, distress, feelings of loneliness, beliefs, behavioral disorders, etc." [66, p. 621] Thus, Sadegh-Zadeh's approach to philosophy of diseases is oriented to the actual lives, needs and interests of people in their communities and societies. Because these human conditions build the category where the term "disease" is applied. In 2008 he gave the following example of their "global feature space $\mathscr{H}^*$:[17]

$$\mathscr{H}^* = \{F_1, F_2, F_3, \ldots, F_n\}, \text{ whith the features } F_i,\ i \in \{1, \ldots, n\}, \text{ e.g.:}$$

$$\begin{aligned}\mathscr{H}^* = \{&\text{chest pain, elevated CPK concentration, tachycardia, vomiting,}\\ &\text{anorexia, epigastric pain, rash, Koplik's spots, cought, fever,}\\ &\text{increased whith blood count,bodily lesion, distress, discompfort,}\\ &\text{incapacity, dependency, premature death, dyspepsia, coma,}\\ &\text{bradycardia, elevated LDH, delusion, fear} \ldots \text{etc.} \ldots \text{etc.}\}\end{aligned}$$

With selections of features or criteria in $\mathscr{H}^*$ Sadegh-Zadeh represents human conditions as sets of members of this "global feature space", e.g.:

- heart_attack = {chest pain, elevated CPK concentration, tachycardia, ... etc. ... }
- measless = {rash, Koplik's spots, cough, fever, ... etc. ... }
- gastric_ulcer = {epigastric pain, anorexia, vomiting, ... etc. ... }
- alopecia areata = {hair loss on the scalp, ... etc. ... }
- being in love = {happy, sleepless nights, longing for the lover, ... etc. ... }

In analogy to the members of the category "birds' we can present members of the category "human conditions" as in a table 3.3 showing wich features they have and which features they not have:

We also can represent a human condition H by the pairs of all its features (taken from $\mathscr{H}^*$) and their respective membership indicator to be present as a feature in H or not, as Sadegh-Zadeh showed in [70, 125]: "A feature F_i from feature set $\mathscr{H}^*$

[17] CPK: creatine phosphokinase is an enzyme found mainly in the heart, brain, and skeletal muscle; LDH: lactate dehydrogenase (or lactic acid dehydrogenase) is an enzyme found in almost all body tissues.

Table 3.3 Human conditions

human condition	chest pain	elevated CPK	rash	Koplik's spots	...
heart attack	yes	yes	no	no	...
measles	no	no	yes	yes	...

that is present in H is written $(F_i, 1)$, whereas a feature F_j that is not present in H is written $(F_j, 0)$, for example:

$$\begin{aligned} \text{heart attack} &= \{(F_1,1),(F_2,1),(F_3,1),\ldots,(F_i,0)(F_j,0),(F_k,0)\ldots,\ \text{etc.},\ldots,\}, \\ \text{measles} &= \{(F_1,0),(F_2,0),(F_3,0),\ldots,(F_i,1)(F_j,1),(F_k,1)\ldots,\ \text{etc.},\ldots,\}, \end{aligned}$$

more specifically:

$$\begin{aligned} \text{heart attack} &= \{(\text{chest pain, } 1),(\text{elevated CPK, } 1),\ldots,(\text{rash, } 0),\ldots \\ &\quad \ldots,(\text{Koplik's spots, } 0),\ldots\ \text{etc.},\ldots\} \\ \text{measles} &= \{(\text{chest pain, } 0),(\text{elevated CPK, } 0),\ldots,(\text{rash, } 1),\ldots \\ &\quad \ldots,(\text{Koplik's spots, } 1),\ldots\ \text{etc.},\ldots\}. \end{aligned}$$

3.6.5 Fuzziness of Human Conditions

However, Sadegh-Zadeh fuzzified the representation of human conditions H as pairs of features that are present or not present in H, to model also real world human conditions where "a feature may not be definitely present or absent, but present to a particular extent different that 1 and 0. For example, someone may have

$$\{\text{mild chest pain , highly elevated CPK,} \ldots, \text{ severe tachycardia,} \ldots, \}$$

whereas someone else has:

$$\{\text{severe chest pain , slightly elevated CPK,} \ldots, \text{ moderate tachycardia,} \ldots, \}$$

and still another person has:

$$\{\text{very severe chest pain , slightly elevated CPK,} \ldots, \text{ mild tachycardia,} \ldots.\}.$$

We may therefore generalize the above-mentioned fuzziness of a human condition H thus:

$$H = \{(F_1, \mu_H(F_1)), (F_2, \mu_H(F_2)), \ldots, (F_n, \mu_H(F_n))\}, \tag{3.24}$$

where an F_i is a feature such as chest pain, levated CPK, etc. and $\mu_H(F_i)$ is a real number in the unit interval $[0,1]$ indicating the degree of its membership in the human condition H." [70, 126]

3.6.6 *Similarity of Diseases*

Why do we categorize a human condition H_i as disease but not human condition H_j? Sadegh-Zadeh named "menstruation, pregnancy, tax evasion, smoking, torture, terrorism" to clarify distinctly: "We do not mean that the latter examples are or have to be categorized as diseases. We only ask why they are *not* categorized as diseases. His answer is: "What is called a disease in medicine is representable as a fuzzy human condition of the form $H = \{(F_1, \mu_H(F_1)), (F_2, \mu_H(F_2)), \ldots, (F_n, \mu_H(F_n))\}$." as in equation 3.24. [70, 128]

Already in 2000 Sadegh-Zadeh established the following rules to determine when human conditions $\{D_1, D_2, \ldots, D_n\}$ are called diseases with respect to their corresponding features (or criteria) $\{C_1, C_2, \ldots, C_n\}$:

- Every element $D_i \in \{D_1, D_2, \ldots, D_n\}$ is a disease.
- Every element that is *similar* to a disease with respect to criteria $\{C_1, C_2, \ldots, C_n\}$ is a disease.

To define what is meant by *similar* diseases Sadegh-Zadeh used the map *differ*(A, B), i.e. the difference of two fuzzy sets A and B. As we mentioned in definitions 18 and 19 in subsection 3.5.3, the *similarity* of two fuzzy sets A, B is resulted from the inversion of their difference *differ*(A, B). To calculate *similarities* between fuzzy sets, we use Sadegh-Zadeh's theorem 2 in the list at the end of the subsection 3.5.3, i.e.

$$\textit{similar}\ (A, B) = \frac{c(A \cap B)}{c(A \cup B)}.$$

3.7 The Prototype Resemblance Theory of Diseases

Sadegh-Zadeh's line of argument (see subsection 3.6.3) shows that he was not interested in "similarity-in-general" but in "similarity-in-some-particulars". To declare his intent he provided, already in 2000, this example: "a human condition, such as a myocardial infarction, may be construed as a set consisting of a large number of attributes, such as myocardial ischemia, arrhythmia, abnormal EEG, elevation of LDH enzyme, chest pain, fear of death, ..., ... In comparision, another human condition, such as gastric ulcer, may be another set consisting of another large number of attributes. Although phenomena of these divers kinds are in principle comparable with one another, they are not easily comparable in their entirety." [66, p. 623]

To compare such phenomena not as a whole but "only with respect to a particular set of criteria, that is, with respect to a *comparable subset* of their attributes," Sadegh-Zadeh introduced the relationship of *partial similarity*. Thus, if we want to compare "two large, possibly incommensurable human condition sets D_i and D_j, we ask: *everything else left aside*, how similar are D_i and D_j with respect to the few criteria", say, $\{C_1, C_2, \ldots, C_m\}$ "they share to varying extends? This kind of similarity confined to particular criteria such as $\{C_1, C_2, \ldots, C_m\}$ is referred to as *partial similarity* with respect to this set of criteria." [66, p. 623] To define this relationship he introduced the following notation:

Definition 21. *If A is a fuzzy set of arbitrary length and if X is a part of A, then we write $A \setminus X$ to indicate that A is a fuzzy set with X being part of it.*

With this notation Sadegh-Zadeh arranged in [66] human conditions, like heart attack and stomach ulcer, "as *uniform fuzzy sets* with respect to their comparable criteria $\{C_1, C_2, \ldots, C_m\}$:

- myocardial_infarction $\setminus \{(C_1, a_1), (C_2, a_2), \ldots, (C_m, a_m)\}$
- gastric_ulcer $\setminus \{(C_1, b_1), (C_2, b_2), \ldots, (C_m, b_m)\}$

as, for example

- myocardial_infarction $\setminus$ {bodily_lesion, 1), (pain, 0.7), (distress, 0.8)}
- gastric_ulcer $\setminus$ {(bodily_lesion, 1), (pain, 0.3), (distress, 0.5)}

and to compare them with respect to their uniform, terminal criteria segments:

- $X = \{(C_1, a_1), (C_2, a_2), \ldots., (C_m, a_m)\}$
- $Y = \{(C_1, b_1), (C_2, b_2), \ldots, (C_m, b_m)\}$"

Obviously there are many other features that are not considered in these segments, e.g. blood pressure, bacterial infections etc. because they may not be comparable. Due to the fact that this arrangement allows just *partial* comparisions of human conditions Sadegh-Zadeh defined "partial similarity, symbolized by *p-similar* $(A \setminus X, B \setminus Y)$, according to the following definition [66, p. 623f.]:

Definition 22. *p-similar* $(A \setminus X, B \setminus Y) = r$, *if and only if similar* $(X, Y) = r$."

With this definition and [theorem 2 in the list at the end of the subsection 3.5.3] we can calculate the partial similarity of myocardial_infarction and gastric_ulcer in the example above as follows:

$$\textit{p-similar}\ (\text{myocardial\_infaction} \setminus X, \text{gastric\_ulcer} \setminus Y) = \frac{1+0.3+0.5}{1+0.7+0.8} = \frac{1.8}{2.5} = 0.72.$$

Let's assume that $\{D_1, D_2, \ldots, D_n\}$ would be a small set of human conditions, because of a set of criteria $\{C_1, C_2, \ldots, C_m\}$ which these conditions have in common. Each of these conditions is interpreted in a certain society as a disease. For this society there is an agreement of degree ε of partial similarity. This degree is "a pillar of the construction" [66, p. 623f.]:

Definition 23. *1. Any element of the base set $\{D_1, D_2, \ldots, D_n\}$ is a disease.*

2. A human condition $H \setminus X$ is a disease, if there is a disease $D_i \setminus Y \in \{D_1, \ldots, D_n\}$ and an $\varepsilon > 0$ such that p-similar $(H \setminus X, D_i \setminus Y) \geq \varepsilon$.

According to this definition a proper choice of ε is essential: The smaller the ε is chosen, the more diseases a society accepts and vice versa. However, the value of ε is not chosen by a physician but by society. Anyway, this notion of disease is a notion that can be comprised in binary logic, an explicit difference is made between

between states that are consistent with a disease and states that are not. Therefore, Sadegh-Zadeh expands this notion of disease to a notion of "disease to a certain degree":

Let's assume $\mathscr{H}$ to be a small set of human conditions. A fuzzy set $\mathscr{D}$ over $\mathscr{H}$ is considered as a set of diseases only if there is a subset $\{D_1, D_2, \ldots, D_n\}$ of $\mathscr{H}$ and there is a function $\mu_{\mathscr{D}}$ so that: $\mu_{\mathscr{D}} : \mathscr{H} \to [0,1]$ with

$$\mu_{\Delta}(H_i \setminus X) = \begin{cases} 1, & if H_i \setminus X \in \{D_1, D_2, \ldots, D_n\}, \\ & \text{called prototype disease.} \\ \varepsilon, & \text{if there is a prototype disease } H_j \setminus Y \\ & \text{with } \textit{p-similar}((H_i \setminus X, H_j \setminus Y) = \varepsilon \\ & \text{and no prototype disease } H_k \setminus Z \\ & \text{with } \textit{p-similar}((H_i \setminus X, H_k \setminus Z) > \varepsilon \\ & \text{and } \Delta = \{(H_i, \mu_{\Delta}(H_i)) \mid H_i \in \mathscr{H}\} \end{cases} . \tag{3.25}$$

In this expanded definition a fuzzy set of following kind is created:

$$\mathscr{D} = \{(D_1, \mu_{\mathscr{D}}(D_1)), \ldots, (D_q, \mu_{\mathscr{D}}(D_q))\}, \tag{3.26}$$

which consists of individual "prototypes" of diseases, which are all members of the set $\mathscr{D}$ to different degrees.

The membership degree $\mu_{\mathscr{D}}(Di)$ is of interval $[0,1]$. From this, we conclude that a person may have a disease to a certain degree and that this person may have no disease to a certain degree at the same time.

As already demonstrated, diseases can be classified by a set of symptoms. In medicine, the study of classification of diseases is called *nosology*. Conventional nosological systems classify a disease by cause (*etiology*), by genesis and developing of the disease (*pathogenesis*) or by the diseases' symptoms.

Today, the most common system is the *International Classification of Diseases* (ICD) that is also a billing system and classifies causes of death [33]. However, as Sadegh-Zadeh argues, those conventional nosological systems pose problems and need some improvements. He demands from nosological systems not only providing a database of classified diseases but also a clinical diagnosis. But due to the fact that diseases are sets of symptoms that often go along with uncertainty, a one-dimensional system isn't able to solve this problem as diseases with n-dimensional sets can't be compared in only one dimension. Here is the point where the fuzzy hypercube comes into play: Considering a disease with a set of criteria of length n, this disease may be converted into a vector of length n and therefore displayed in the hypercube [63].

Another disease with assimilable criteria can by displayed in the same hypercube and thus, these diseases are not only classified but also comparable through their distance. The fuzzy sets' Hamming and Euclidean distances can be easily determined. In doing so, one is able to make statements about relationships to other diseases and possible diagnosis. This could be also an advantage if a disease is unknown. Moreover, it is possible to display the developing of a disease in the hypercube. Every point in the hypercube would be the disease at a particular time, and achievements of therapies, for example, could be reproduced. [63]

Journal of Medicine and Philosophy, 33: 106–139, 2008
doi:10.1093/jmp/jhn004

The Prototype Resemblance Theory of Disease

KAZEM SADEGH-ZADEH
University of Münster, Münster, Germany

Fig. 3.17 Headline of article [70]

3.8 Prototype Resemblance Structures

In the last section we arrived at the definition of what is a disease in Sadegh-Zadeh's "Prototype Resemblance Theory of Disease". In this section we will briefly report the science-theoretical framework of this theory, i.e. the structures that build its bases. The first structure that Sadegh-Zadeh defined in [70] is the fuzzy prototype resemblance frame:

Definition 24. *ξ is a fuzzy prototype resemblance frame iff there are Ω, A_1, A_n, B,s, and f such that:*

1. $\xi = \langle \Omega, \{A_1, \dots, A_n\}, B, f, s \rangle$.
2. *Ω is a nonempty set referred to as the universe of discourse.*
3. *$\{A_1, \dots, A_n\}$ is a subset of Ω with $n >\geq 1$.*
4. *B is a fuzzy set in Ω.*
5. *f is a similarity function that maps pairs of Ω to $[0,1]$ as function similar in definition 19 in section 3.5.3.*
6. *s is a human society.*
7. *Each member of $\{A_1, \dots, A_n\}$ is a member of B to the extent 1 if it is considered a prototype in B by the society s.*
8. *A member X of Ω is a member of B to the event ε iff ε is the maximum degree of its similarity with the prototype in B, and $\varepsilon \neq 0$; that is iff there is a prototype A_i in B such that $f(X, A_i) = \varepsilon$, and there is no prototype A_j in B such that $f(X, A_j) > \varepsilon$*

To illustrate this structure Sadegh-Zadeh went back to his example of birds: Let us assume that

- Ω is the class of animals.
- $\{A_1, \dots, A_n\} = \{$robin, sparrow, blackbird, crow$\}$ with $n = 4$,
- B is the class of birds, i.e. a fuzzy set in Ω as we know from the last section.
- f is our similarity function *similar*.
- s is the society of West Europeans.

The animals in subset $\{A_1, \ldots, A_n\}$ = {robin, sparrow, blackbird, crow} of all animals (universe of discourse Ω) are considered prototype birds by West Europeans and therefore they are members of the class B of birds with membership value1.

Any other species X in Ω is to an extent $\varepsilon \neq 0$ a bird iff $similar\ (X, A_i) = \varepsilon$ is the maximum degree of this species' similarity to the four prototype birds. Therefore, $\langle$animals, {robbin, sparrow, blackbird, crow}, birds, *similar*, West Europeans$\rangle$ is a fuzzy prototype resemblance frame.

From definition 24 of a *fuzzy prototype resemblance frame* we can vice versa define what is a *fuzzy prototype resemblance category*:

Definition 25. *B is a fuzzy prototype resemblance category iff there are Ω, A_1, A_n, s, and f such that $\langle \Omega, \{A_1, \ldots, A_n\} B, f, s \rangle$ is a fuzzy prototype resemblance frame.*

Sadegh-Zadeh referred to the fact that these definitions are dependent from the society s as part of the fuzzy prototype resemblance frame: "For example, it may be that what Australians view as the category of birds, vegetables, fruits, furniture, or cloths is not identical with what Siberians do because the focal members of an Australian category differ from those of the Siberian category. an Australian category may partially overlap a Siberian one, though, they need not match completely." [70, p. 133]

With these structures we have now all requirements to get the goal of Sadegh-Zadeh's article [70]:

Hypothesis 1
The category of diseases in Western medicine, denoted $\mathscr{D}$, is a fuzzy prototype resemblance category.

To support this hypothesis he considered the following points:

1. $\mathscr{H}$, the class of all fuzzy human conditions, is the universe of discourse.
2. $\{D_1, \ldots, D_n\}$ is a subset of $\mathscr{H}$, that comprises e.g. D_i = heart attack, D_j = breast cancer, D_k = measles, D_r = small pox, etc. and some of these human conditions are prototype diseases in Western societies.
3. $\mathscr{D}$ is a family of fuzzy sets in $\mathscr{H}$.
4. s may be the human society of West Europeans.
5. f is the similarity function *similar*.

With these premises he came to the next hypothesis:

Hypothesis 2
$\langle \mathscr{H}, \{D_1, \ldots, D_n\}, \mathscr{H}, similar$, West Europeans$\rangle$ is a fuzzy prototype resemblance frame.

For every class $\mathscr{H}$ of all fuzzy human conditions holds:

If there exist $\langle \mathscr{H}, \{D_1, \ldots, D_n\}, \mathscr{H}, similar$ and West Europeans$\rangle$ **such that** the structure $\langle \mathscr{H}, \{D_1, \ldots, D_n\}, \mathscr{H}, similar,$ West Europeans$\rangle$ is a fuzzy prototype resemblance frame, **then** the family $\mathscr{D}$ of fuzzy sets in $\mathscr{H}$ is a fuzzy prototype resemblance category.

From this result and *Hypothesis 2* it follows *Hypothesis 1*!

3.9 Outlook: A Fuzzy Structuralist View on Scientific Theories

In order to give an introduction to Kazem Sadegh-Zadeh's work as a philosopher of medicine I have often and interchangeably employed the so-called "structuralist approach" or "Metastructuralism" to define important concepts in Analytical Philosophy of Medicine. In this vein I quoted already in section 3.5.1 Sadegh-Zadeh's definitions of a *(basic) fuzzy structure*, a *fuzzy structure*, a *metric space*, a *Zadeh structure* and a *Zadeh space* and in section and in section 3.8 I continued with the definitions of a *fuzzy prototype resemblance frame* and a *fuzzy prototype resemblance category*. The reader may have a look to the preface in this volume to have more details on the framework of this approach to philosophy of science!

With this "structuralist view" we are able to axiomatize scientific theories in a precise way without recurring to formal languages. This approach, also called nowadays "Metastructuralism", uses only informal logic and informal set theory. When I wrote my Ph.D thesis on "Probabilistic Structures in Quantum Mechanics" [75] using this structuralist approach, I already thought about the possibility of "fuzzifying" this approach. In the nineties I did not know that Kazem Sadegh-Zadeh, already a well-known philosopher of medicine then, used this structuralist approach, Later, when I started my work on history and philosophy of the theory of Fuzzy Sets, I also considered the developments of the first Fuzzy systems in medicine [76, 77].

In 2006 I visited Kazem Sadegh-Zadeh at home in Tecklenburg, Germany and during our discussions we also thought on the fuzzification of the "structuralist view" in philosophy of science into a "Fuzzy structuralism". We wondered why nobody ever used fuzzy sets and fuzzy relations instead of usual sets and set relations to reconstruct scientific theories! Then we started thinking on fuzzifications of (partial (potential)) models of scientific theory elements and some of Sadegh-Zadeh's considerations to this subject found their place in his *Handbook on Analytical Philosophy of Medicine* [71].

Acknowledgement. The author warmly thanks Prof. Dr. Kazem Sadegh-Zadeh and his wife Maria Klein for help during writing this chapter. He also thanks Marco Elio Tabacchi for discussions and valuable comments and for making figure 3.11 (a) available. Work leading to this paper was partially supported by the Foundation for the Advancement of Soft Computing Mieres, Asturias (Spain).

References

1. Adlassnig, K.-P.: A Fuzzy Logical Model of Computer-assisted Medical Diagnosis. Methods of Information in Medicine 19, 141–148 (1980)
2. Adlassnig, K.-P.: The Viennese Computer Assisted Diagnostic System, Its Principles and Values. Automedica 3, 141–150
3. Adlassnig, K.-P.: A Survey on Medical Diagnosis and Fuzzy Subsets. In: Gupta, M.M., Sanchez, E. (eds.) Approximate Reasoning in Decision Analysis, pp. 203–217. North-Holland Publ. Comp. (1982)
4. Adlassnig, K.-P.: Fuzzy Set Theory in Medical Diagnosis. IEEE Transactions on Systems, Man, and Cybernetics SMC-16(2), 260–265 (1986)
5. Albin, M.A.: Fuzzy Sets and Their Application to Medical Diagnosis and Pattern Recognition. Ph.D. Thesis, University of California Berkeley, California (1975)
6. Aristotle: The Metaphysics, Books I-IX, Engl. William Heinemann, London (1961); Engl. translation by Hugh Tredennick
7. Bellman, R.E., Kalaba, R., Zadeh, L.A.: Abstraction and Pattern Classification. Journal of Mathematical Analysis and Applications 13, 1–7 (1966)
8. von Bertalanffy, L.: Kritische Theorie der Formbildung (= Schaxels Abhandlungen, 27). Gebrüder Bornträger, Berlin (1928); English translation: Modern Theories of Development: An Introduction to Theoretical Biology. Oxford University Press, Harper, New York (1933)
9. von Bertalanffy, L.: Allgemeine Systemtheorie. Wege zu einer neuen Mathesis Universalis, Deutsche Universitätszeitung, vol. 5/6 (1957)
10. von Bertalanffy, L.: General System Theory. In: von Bertalanffy, L., Rapoport, A. (eds.) General Systems (= Yearbook of the Society for the Advancement of General Systems Theory), vol. I, pp. 1–10. Abacus Press, Tunbridge Wells (1965)
11. von Bertalanffy, L.: Vorläufer und Begründer der Systemtheorie. In: Kurzrock, R. (ed.) Systemtheorie (= Forschung and Information, Band 12), pp. 17–27. Colloquium Verlag, Berlin (1972)
12. Blackburn, S.: The Oxford Dictionary of Philosophy. Oxford University Press (2012), Read more:
`http://www.answers.com/library/Philosophy+Dictionary-letter-1W#ixzz29RyHgMc4`,
`http://www.answers.com/library/Philosophy+Dictionary-cid-2260782`
13. Bourbaki, N. (pseudo.): Elements of Mathematics: Theory of Sets. Addison-Wesley, Reading (1968)
14. Brentano, F.C.H.H.: Aristoteles und seine Weltanschauung. Quelle & Meyer, Leipzig (1911); 2nd ed., intr. by Rolf George. Meiner, Hamburg (1977); English translation: George, R., Chisholm, R.M. (trans.) Aristotle and His World View. University of California Press, Berkeley (1978)
15. Bunge, M.: Epistemología: ciencia de la ciencia. Ariel, Barcelona (1980)
16. Carnap, R.: Der Logische Aufbau der Welt. Felix Meiner Verlag, Leipzig (1967); English translation: George, R.A. (trans.) The Logical Structure of the World. Pseudoproblems in Philosophy. University of California Press, Berkeley (1967)
17. Carnap, R.: Die physikalische Sprache als Universalsprache der Wissenschaft. Erkenntnis 2, 432–465 (1931/1932)
18. Carnap, R.: The Unity of Science. Translated with an Introduction by Max Black. Kegan Paul, Trench, Trubner & Co., London (1934)

19. Carnap, R.: The Methodological Character of Theoretical Concepts. In: Feigl, H., Scriven, M. (eds.) Minnesota Studies in the Philosophy of Science. The Foundations of Science and the Concepts of Psychology and Psychoanalysis, vol. I, pp. 38–76. University of Minnesota Press, Minneapolis (1956)
20. Chang, C.-L.: Fuzzy Topological Spaces. Journal of Mathematical Analysis and Applications 24, 182–190 (1968)
21. de Luca, A., Settimo, T.: A Definition of a Nonprobabilistic Entropy in the Setting of Fuzzy Sets Theory. Information and Control 20(4), 301–312 (1972)
22. Dubois, A.B.: James Daniel Hardy 1904-1985. A Biographical Memoir, National Academy of Sciences, Biographical Memoirs 88 (2006)
23. Elder, R.C.: Fuzzy Systems theory and Medical Decision Making. M. S. Thesis. School of Industrial and Systems Engineering, Georgia Institute of Technology, Atlanta, Georgia (1976)
24. Esogbue, A.O., Elder, R.C.: Fuzzy Sets and the Modelling of Physician Decision Processes, Part I: The Initial Interview-Information Gathering Session. Fuzzy Sets and Systems 2, 279–291 (1979)
25. Esogbue, A.O., Elder, R.C.: Fuzzy Sets and the Modelling of Physician Decision Processes, Part II: Fuzzy Diagnosis Decision Models. Fuzzy Sets and Systems 3, 1–9 (1980)
26. Feyerabend, P.: Against Method: Outline of an Anarchistic Theory of Knowledge. Verso, London (1975); first edition in: Michael, R., Winokur, S. (eds.): Analyses of Theories and Methods of Physics and Psychology. University of Minnesota Press, Minneapolis (1970)
27. Fleck, L.: O niektórych swoistych cecach mys's'slekarskiego. Archiwum Historji i Filozofji Medycyny oraz Historji Nauk Przyrodniczych 6, 55–64 (1986); english Translation: Fleck, L.: Some specific features of the medical way of thinking. In: Cohen, R.S., Schnelle, T. (eds.), Cognition and Fact. Materials on Ludwik Fleck, pp. 39–46. D. Reidel Publ. Comp. Dordrecht (1986)
28. Fleck, L.: Entstehung und Entwicklung einer wissenschaftlichen Tatsache, Lwow (1935); english translation: Genesis and Development of a Scientific Fact (1979)
29. Fuller, S., Kuhn vs. Popper: The Struggle for the Soul of Science. Columbia University Press, New York (2005)
30. Gangl, A., Grabner, G., Bauer, P.: Erste Erfahrungen mit einem Computerprogramm zur Differentialdiagnose der Lebererkrankungen. Wiener Zeitschrift für Innere Medizin & IHRE Grenzgebiete 50, 553–586 (1969)
31. Haller, R.: Neopositivismus. Eine historische Einführung in die Philosophie des Wiener Kreises. Wissenschaftliche Buchgesellschaft, Darmstadt (1993)
32. Hempel, C.G.: The Theoretician's Dilemma. In: Feigl, H., Scriven, M., Maxwell, G. (eds.) Minnesota Studies in the Philosophy of Science. Concepts, Theories and the Mind-body Problem, vol. II, pp. 37–98. University of Minnesota Press, Minneapolis (1958)
33. International Classification of Diseases (ICD), `http://www.who.int/classifications/icd/en/`
34. Kosko, B.: Fuzzy Entropy and Conditioning. Information Sciences 40, 165–174 (1986)
35. Kosko, B.: Fuzziness vs. Probability. International Journal of General Systems 17, 211–240 (1990)
36. Kosko, B.: Networks and Fuzzy Systems. A Dynamical Systems Approach to Machine Intelligence. Prentice Hall, Engelwood Cliffs (1992)
37. Kuhn, T.S.: The Copernican Revolution. Harvard University Press, Cambridge (1957)

38. Kuhn, T.S.: The Structure of Scientific Revolutions, 1st edn. University of Chicago Press (1962)
39. Lakatos, I.: The Methodology of Scientific Research Programmes. Cambridge University Press, Cambridge (1978)
40. Laudan, L.: Progress and its Problems: Towards a Theory of Scientific Growth. The University of Chicago Press, Chicago (1977)
41. Laudan, L.: Beyond Positivism and Relativism. Westview Press, Boulder (1996)
42. Ledley, R.S., Lusted, L.B.: Reasoning Foundations of Medical Diagnosis. Science 130(3366), 9–21 (1959)
43. Lipkin, M., Hardy, J.D.: Mechanical Corellation of Data in Differential Diagnosis of Hematological Diseases. Journal of the American Medical Association 166, 113–125 (1958)
44. Lusted, L.B.: Computer Techniques in Medical Diagnosis. In: [83], pp. 319–338
45. Lusted, L.B.: Some roots of clinical decision making. In: Proceedings of the Association for Computing Machinery (= ACM, Conference on the History of Medical, Informatics, Conference, Papers Presented at the Conference, National Library of Medicine Bethesda, November 5-6), pp. 165–193. National Library of Medicine Bethesda, Maryland (1987)
46. Mamdani, E.H.: Advances in the Linguistic Synthesis of Fuzzy Controllers. International Journal of Man-Machine Studies 8, 669–678 (1976)
47. Mamdani, E.: Interview by Rudolf Seising on September 9, 1998 in Aachen, RWTH Aachen, at the margin of the European Congress on Intelligent Techniques and Soft Computing EUFIT 1988 (1998)
48. Mayr, E.: This is Biology. University Press, Harvard (1997)
49. Mesarović, M.D.: Views on General Systems Theory. In: Proceedings of the Second Systems Symposium at Case Institute of Technology, Robert E. Krieger Publ. Comp., Huntington (1964)
50. Miller, R.A., Pople, H.E., Myers, J.D.: Internist-I, An Experimental computer-based Diagnostic Consultant for General Internal Medicine. New England Journal of Medicine 307(8), 468–476 (1982)
51. Moon, R.E., Jordanov, S., Perez, A., Burhan Türksen, I.: Medical Diagnostic System with Human-Like Reasoning Capability. In: Shires, D.B., Wolf, H. (eds.) MEDINFO 1977. Proceedings of the Second World Conference on Medical Informatics, Toronto, August 8-12. IFIPWorld Conferences Series on Medical Informatics, vol. 2, pp. 115–119. North-Holland Publishing Comp., Amsterdam (1977)
52. Pauker, S.G., Gorry, G.A., Kassirer, J.P., Schwartz William, B.: Towards the Simulation of Clinical Cognition: Taking a Present Illness by Computer. American Journal of Medicine 60, 981–996 (1976)
53. Passmore, R., Robson, J.S.: A Companion to Medical Studies, vol. 3, part I. Blackwell, Oxford (1975)
54. Perez-Ojeda, A.: Medical Knowledge Network. A Database for Computer Aided Diagnosis. Master Thesis. Department of Industrial Engineering, University of Toronto (1976)
55. Philips, D.C.: System Theory — A Discredited Philosophy. Abacus (September 1969)
56. Pople Harry, E., Myers, J.D., Miller, R.A.: DIALOG: A Model of Diagnostic Logic for Internal Medicine. In: Forth International Joint Conference on Artificial Intelligence, September 3-8, pp. 848–855. USSR, Tblis (1975)
57. Popper, K.R.: Logik der Forschung. Mohr-Siebeck, Tübingen (1934/1935); English translation: The Logic of Scientific Discovery. Routledge, London (1959)

58. Rosch, E.: Natural Categories. Cognitive Psychology 4, 328–350 (1973)
59. Rosch, E.: Cognitibe Representations of Semantic Categories. Journal of Experimental Psychology: General 104, 192–233 (1975)
60. Sadegh-Zadeh, K.: Organism and Disease as Fuzzy Categories. Presented at the Conference on Medicine and Philosophy, July 2. Humboldt University of Berlin (1982)
61. Sadegh-Zadeh, K.: Fundamentals of Clinical Methodology: 1. Differential Indication. Artificial Intelligence in Medicine 6, 83–102 (1994)
62. Sadegh-Zadeh, K.: Fundamentals of Clinical Methodology: 2. Etiology. Artificial Intelligence in Medicine 12, 227–270 (1998)
63. Sadegh-Zadeh, K.: Fundamentals of Clinical Methodology: 3. Nosology. Artificial Intelligence in Medicine 17, 87–108 (1999)
64. Sadegh-Zadeh, K.: Advances in Fuzzy Theory. Artificial Intelligence in Medicine 15, 309–323 (1999)
65. Sadegh-Zadeh, K.: Fundamentals of Clinical Methodology: 4. Diagnosis. Artificial Intelligence in Medicine 20, 227–241 (2000)
66. Sadegh-Zadeh, K.: Fuzzy Health, Illness, and Disease. The Journal of Medicine and Philosophy 25, 605–638 (2000)
67. Sadegh-Zadeh, K.: Fuzzy Genomes. Artificial Intelligence in Medicine 18, 1–28 (2000)
68. Sadegh-Zadeh, K.: The Fuzzy Polynucleotide Space Revisited. Artificial Intelligence in Medicine 41, 69–90 (2007)
69. The Fuzzy Revolution: Goodbye to the Aristotelian Weltanschauung. Artificial Intelligence in Medicine 21, 1–25 (2001)
70. Sadegh-Zadeh, K.: The Prototype Resemblance Theory of Disease. The Journal of Medicine and Philosophy 33, 106–139 (2008)
71. Sadegh-Zadeh, K.: Handbook of Analytical Philosophy of Medicine. Philosophy and Medicine, vol. 113. Springer, Heidelberg (2012)
72. Sadegh-Zadeh, K.: Interview by R. Seising, in: Philosophy & Soft Computing Newsletter (to appear, 2013), forthcoming at: `http://docs.softcomputing.es/public/NewsletterPhilosophyAndSoftComputingNumber_7.pdf`
73. Sanchez, E.: Compositions of Fuzzy Relations. In: Gupta, M.M., Ragade, R.K., Yager, R.R. (eds.) Advances in Fuzzy Set Theory and Applications, pp. 421–433. North-Holland Publ. Comp., Amsterdam (1979)
74. Sanchez, E.: Medical Diagnosis and Composite Fuzzy Relations. In: Gupta, M.M., Ragade, R.K., Yager, R.R. (eds.) Advances in Fuzzy Set Theory and Applications, pp. 437–444. North-Holland Publ. Comp., Amsterdam (1979)
75. Seising, R.: Probabilistische Strukturen in der Quantenmechanik. Peter Lang Frankfurt am Main (Europ.äischen Hochschulschriften: Reihe 20, Philosophie Band 500) Zugl.: Ludwig-Maximilians-Universität München, Univ., Diss. (Institut für Philosophie, Wissenschaftstheorie und Statistik, 1995) (1996)
76. Seising, R.: From Vagueness in Medical Thought to the Foundations of Fuzzy Reasoning in Medical Diagnosis. Artificial Intelligence in Medicine 38, 237–256 (2006)
77. Seising, R.: The Fuzzification of Systems. The Origins of Fuzzy Set Theory and Its Initial Applications – Its Development to the 1970s. Springer, Berlin (2007)
78. Seising, R., González, V.S. (eds.): Soft Computing in Humanities and Social Sciences. STUDFUZZ, vol. 273. Springer, Heidelberg (2012)
79. Shortliffe, E.H.: Computer based medical consultations: MYCIN. Elsevier, New York (1976)

80. Smets, P., Vainsel, H., Bernard, R., Kornreich, F.: Bayesian Probability of Fuzzy Diagnosis. In: Shires, D.B., Wolf, H. (eds.) Proceedings of the Second World Conference on Medical Informatics, MEDINFO 1977, Toronto, August 8-12. IFIPWorld Conferences Series on Medical Informatics, vol. 2, pp. 121–122. North-Holland Publishing Comp., Amsterdam (1977)
81. Sneed, J.D.: The Logical Structure of Mathematical Physics. Reidel, Dordrecht (1971)
82. Walter, S., Grabner, G.: Ein Computerverfahren zur diagnostischen Hilfestellung. In: Fellinger, K. (ed.) Computer in der Medizin—-Probleme, Erfahrungen, Projekte, pp. 189–221. Verlag Brüder Hollinek, Wien (1968)
83. Stacy, R.W., Waxmann, B.D. (eds.): Computers in Biomedical Research, vol. I. Academic Press, New York (1965)
84. Stadler, F.: The Vienna Circle. Studies in the Origins, Development, and Influence of Logical Empiricism. Springer, Wien (2001); German original: Studien zum Wiener Kreis. Ursprung, Entwicklung und Wirkung des Logischen Empirismus im Kontext. Suhrkamp, Frankfurt am Main (1997)
85. Stegmüller, W.: The Structure and Dynamics of Theories. Springer, New York (1976)
86. Tautu, P., Wagner, G.: The Process of Medical Diagnosis: Routes of Mathematical Investigations. Methods of Information in Medicine 17(1), 1–10 (1978)
87. Termini, S.: Interview by R. Seising. Newsletter Philosophy and Soft Computing 2(2), 7–14 (2010)
88. Thews, G., Mutschler, E., Vaupel, P.: Anatomie, Physiologie, Pathophysiologie des Menschen, 5th edn. Wissenschaftliche Verlagsgesellschaft, Stuttgart (1999)
89. Überla, K.: Zur Verwendung der Faktorenanalyse in der medizinischen Diagnostik. Methods of Information in Medicine 4(2), 89–92 (1965)
90. Wardle Anthony, A., Wardle, L.: Computer Aided Diagnosis—–a Review of Research. Methods of Information in Medicine 17, 15–28 (1978)
91. Wechsler, H.: Applications of Fuzzy Logic to Medical Diagnosis. In: Proceedings of the 1975 International Symposium on Multiple-Valued Logic, vol. 75, CH 0959-7C. IEEE (1975)
92. Weiss, S.M., Kulikowski, C.A., Amarel, S., Safir, A.: A Model Based Method for Computer-aided Medical Decision-making. Artificail Intelligence 11, 145–172 (1978)
93. Weiss, S.M., Kulikowski, C.A., Safir, A.: Glaucoma Consultation by Computer. Computers in Biology and Medicine 8, 25–40 (1978)
94. World Health Organization: Preamble to the Constitution of the World Health Organization as adopted by the International Health Conference, New York, June 19-22, 1946, and entered into force on April 7, 1948, Parts: http://www.who.int/bulletin/bulletin_board/83/ustun11051/en/
95. World Health Organization: Regional Office for Europe and the International Diabetes Federation, Europe. Diabetes mellitus in Europe: a problem at all ages and in all countries. A model for prevention and self care. Meeting. Giorn Ital Diabetol 10(suppl.) (1990)
96. Wiener, N.: Cybernetics or Control and Communications in the Animal and the Machine. MIT Press, Cambridge (1948)
97. Wittgenstein, L.: Philosophical Investigations. Blackwell Publishing, Oxford (1953)
98. Woodbury, M.A.: The Inapplicabilities of Bayes Theorem to Diagnosis. In: Thomas, C.C. (ed.) Proceedings of the Fifth International Conference on Medical Electronics, Liege, Belgium, Springfield, Ill, pp. 860–868 (1963)
99. Zadeh, L.A.: System Theory. Columbia Engineering Quarterly 8, 16–19 (1954)

100. Zadeh, L.A.: What is optimal? IRE Transactions on Information Theory IT-4(1) (March 1958)
101. Zadeh, L.A.: From Circuit Theory to System Theory. Proceedings of the IRE 50, 856–865 (1962)
102. Zadeh, L.A.: Optimality and Non-Scalar-Valued Performance Criteria. IEEE Transactions on Automatic Control, Correspondence, 59f (1963)
103. Zadeh, L.A.: Fuzzy Sets. Information and Control 8, 338–353 (1965)
104. Zadeh, L.A.: Fuzzy Sets and Systems. In: Fox, J. (ed.) System Theory, Brooklyn. Microwave Research Institute Symp. Series XV, pp. 29–37. Polytechnic Press, New York (1965)
105. Zadeh, L.A.: Probability Measures of Fuzy Events. Journal of Mathematical Analysis and Applications 10, 421–427 (1968)
106. Zadeh, L.A.: Fuzzy Algorithms. Information and Control 12, 99–102 (1968)
107. Zadeh, L.A.: Biological Applications of the Theory of Fuzzy Sets and Systems. In: The Proceedings of the International Symposium on Biocybernetics of the Central Nervous System, pp. 199–206. Little, Brown and Company, Boston (1969)
108. Zadeh, L.A.: Fuzzy Languages and their Relation to Human and Machine Intelligence, Man and Computer. In: Proceedings of the International Conference, Bordeaux (1970)
109. Zadeh, L.A.: Towards a theory of fuzzy systems. In: Kalman, R.E., DeClaris, N. (eds.) Aspects of Network and System Theory, pp. 469–490. Holt, Rinehart and Winston, New York (1971)
110. Zadeh, L.A.: Outline a New Approach to the Analysis of Complex Systems and Decision Processes. IEEE Transactions on Systems Theory 3, 28–44 (1973)
111. Zadeh, L.A.: On the Analysis of Large-Scale Systems. Memorandum No. ERL-M418. Electronic Research Laboratory, College of Engineering, University of California, Berkeley (January 8, 1974)
112. Zadeh, L.A.: The Concept of a Linguistic Variable and its Application to Approximate Reasoning I, II, III. Information Science 8, 199–249, 301–357 (1975); 9, 43–80

4

Specificities and Vagaries of Medicine from the Viewpoint of Hard Sciences

Settimo Termini and Marco Elio Tabacchi

4.1 Introduction

The thought-provoking and encyclopedic *Handbook of Analytic Philosophy of Medicine* by Kazem Sadegh-Zadeh[3] poses many challenging questions of different types and nature. Even after just a quick skimming of the book, the reader will find himself entangled in a very long list of questions to be answered, of curiosities to be satisfied, and of problems to be further dissected and analyzed. This is a testimony to the importance of the punctual scrutiny and the general contributions provided by Sadegh-Zadeh's opus, and at the same time what makes almost impossible to limit the focus of a contribution about the book to just a small subset of all these questions and problems.

Another kind of reaction, generated by an overall impression of such a titanic enterprise so happily completed by the author calls for a move toward a completely different direction. And indeed there will be a time for deeper and closer looks at the details, there will be a time for painstakingly analyzing the structure and deeply searching a synthesis, a time for the criticism and a time for the replies, and yet a time for a hundred indecisions, and for a hundred visions and revisions, before finally arriving at some conclusive stage and more solid conclusions about such a hot topic, if a reference points and conclusive arguments do exist at all.

In our opinion, the best way of honoring the author in the immediate proximity of the book publication is briefly dealing with a number of very general remarks, independently of how and if the book has provided answers to them – and even if apparently it has not generally dealt with. An herculean task indeed, as the author has meticulously left no medical stone unturned in his quest for a rigorous, in-depth and exhaustive scrutiny of the topic.

4.2 Medicine as a Peculiar Science

The Italian linguist Tullio DeMauro – who comes from a family of physicians – in his book *La cultura degli Italiani*[2], reports the following episode:

R. Seising and M.E. Tabacchi (Eds.): *Fuzziness and Medicine*, STUDFUZZ 302, pp. 77–81.
DOI: 10.1007/978-3-642-36527-0_4

> Once upon a time, I happened to speak at the Faculty of Medicine of University "La Sapienza" in Rome, and I perceived a sort of astonishment written in the faces of my colleagues when I said that – not only in ancient times, but also in the contemporary world – medical practice is the mother of all sciences. They thought that my statement wanted just to capture their benevolence.

Without the pretense of a detailed exegesis of DeMauro's thought, we can certainly affirm that the his assertion is closely related to the author's conception of culture. In search of a definition is important not to isolate specific aspects of various and different components (artisanal, technical, applicative and theoretic, etc) but to consider the complex network created by all these viewpoints, in order to shed a more global light on the problem to be afforded. In this sense, the fine interplay between rigor and morality, measuring and experience that is Medicine poses unique and specific dilemmas, more complex than the ones of any other science: is this the intimate sense in which DeMauro's "medical practice" can be really considered so crucial.

Medicine, however, besides being "the mother of all sciences" is certainly also a science in its own right: but which kind of science? It is a science in the sense that it is just a definite version of applied biology (or, more specifically, the combination of applied biochemistry, applied genetics and the likes)? Can it be considered also as an *autonomous* science, instead of just an applied science? But if we shift our perspective toward this more independent stance, some challenging questions suddenly appear. Medicine is clearly a science that deals with classes and species, but it is also and foremost the science of a single individual – the patient. This approach shows medicine as something epistemologically more similar to Cosmology than to Physics, in the sense that it is the science of a *unicum*. To add a further complication, the cornerstone scientific notion of "repeatable experiment under controlled conditions" is in this instance quite difficult to apply. And this not just in one, but in two different senses: as for the first, it is clearly not possible to do any kind of proper experiment, as following the usual framework is not conceivable; furthermore even for the very limited class of experiments for which a sort of repetition is possible, it remains elusive to establish the same identical boundary conditions when the experiment is repeated. The *ceteris paribus* paradigm is foiled by complexity in both the exogenous (environment, medical personnel) and endogenous (conditions of the patient, interaction between processes and therapies) department. The latter aspect makes our situation, perhaps, also worse than the one existing in Cosmology: in our case we cannot fully isolate the different aspects. There is a very strong interaction between different levels (psychological, mental, genetic, functional, etc) besides the one between the individual and the environmental context.

4.3 Fuzziness and the Art and Science of Medicine

The context we have outlined in the previous section brings us to discuss the many-faceted concepts of precision (and lack thereof), numerical accuracy and more generally of uncertainty, their relationship with the concepts underlining Fuzzy Set Theory (FST) and the links with medicine. We have already discussed these aspects in a broader setting [5, 7], as well as in other domains [1, 6, 8] and the specific topic has been given an historically perspective treatment in [4]. We stipulate that in a setting where the classical scientific pillars of repeatability, accuracy and exact measures have to confront themselves with the much more vague concepts of moral, vagueness, feelings, etc. the introduction and heavy application of fuzziness becomes of paramount importance. Fuzziness, we claim, is the only scientific notion in mankind's history in the framework of which a tentative step to cross the border of all the received classification of disciplines has been made; and while even in this context we recognize the need for a sort of *precision*, fuzziness has differentiated itself by never superimposing the concept itself with the notion of *numerical accuracy*.

Sadegh-Zadeh acknowledges this beautifully in his book: he promotes FST among the basic instruments of logic for medical understanding (how true); highlights the importance of vagueness in the medical language and as an intrinsic property of medical epistemics; points out the clear advantages of a medical fuzzy taxonomy to get over the binary concepts of healthy/ill; advanced the idea of the organism as a fuzzy-causal system, representable through the schematics of a fuzzy machine; clearly states that self-consciousness is based on subjective mental states that are fuzzy in nature, and as a consequence their matching mental terms cannot be agreed upon; uses the concepts from FST as a tool to introduce both the notion of disease and the notion of similarity needed in analyzing the resemblance of individual diseases with prototypes; employes the bag of tools from FST to assess an explicatum of the notions of health, illness, and disease, and in the same fuzzy framework demonstrates their fuzzy character, and the fact that the concepts of health, illness, and disease turn out to be three completely different categories; gives a convincing description of a fuzzy etiology using fuzzy causal structures and fuzzy causal spaces; theorizes and details fuzzy counterparts for medical diagnosis, epistemology, concept formation, ontology and many other concepts. In synthesis Sadegh-Zadeh offers a significant contribution to systematization of FST in medicine, elevating fuzziness as a first class citizen among the foundational tools needed to define the analytic philosophy of medicine.

The consequences of this treatment are staggering, and will contribute to a change in the perception of what medicine is: all the people – the scientist, the physician, the patient, the philosopher of science – working in such a crucial field move, operate and reason in the *terra nullius* between what we would call *scientific medicine*, a facet of medical praxiology, and what in fact still remains, in a very specified and pregnant sense, an art: the *medical art*, which encompasses many of the factors of medical epistemology and deontic. The boundaries between those two modalities are, as always, not sharp at all, and sometimes the gap between them seem about to be filled, at least for some specific angle. But this is rarely the case, and maybe this chasm can be reduced to a slit, but never completely filled. Hopefully in the future, by acknowledging its existence and treating it with the tools offered by FST in the spirit of Sadegh-Zadeh's approach, the gap could become so thin as the one existing between Maxwell theory and electrical engineering, a situation so very different from the actual conditions.

4.4 Conclusions

Medicine, as viewed from a hard scientist perspective, assumes substantially the shape and features of a *monster*, and this in both the senses that this word carries from ancient times: medicine is at the same time *portentuous*, due to its continuous generation of questions that are always interesting, often crucial and in most of the instances too complex to master or difficult to formalize to produce a satisfactory answer in the general case – something which is bound to happen when we mix human nature and a pretense of exactness; and *abnormal* in its strict but necessary refusal to conform to the rules and established good practices of all sciences that aspire to a perfect end eternal repeatability under severe scrutiny. This change in perspective is never too late to come – as soon as what differentiates the scientist from the experimental subject is no more the capacity of introspection in actions, any standard application of rules guided by numerical precision becomes at best wishful thinking and in the worst cases too close to playing god for anyone's comfort. In order to navigate through the perilous sea of medical practice, our guide cannot be just a list of coordinates to attain and of close ports to call our owns: we must refer to a well balanced mix of empirical knowledge, a huge and well cultivated baggage of tacit knowledge that can only be build with experience and the practice of what we have already referred to as *art of medicine*, an aesthetic sense of morality. This does not exclude traditional methodologies culled from hard sciences: measuring is still of paramount importance, and most of the pieces that have been already solved in this great jigsaw of a science have already been dissected, examined and understood through methods and common practices that belongs to engineering, biology, physics, chemistry and the likes. But it is certain that focusing just on this side of the equation is not enough to develop medicine satisfactory as a science. Sadegh-Zadeh's handbook is clearly not just a very important contribution for filling this gap, but - by showing many of the possibilities offered for a different approach to a number of crucial questions - is also a fundamental tool for looking at what we need for reducing the gap.

References

1. Cardaci, M., Di Gesú, V., Petrou, M., Tabacchi, M.E.: On the Evaluation of Images Complexity: A Fuzzy Approach. In: Bloch, I., Petrosino, A., Tettamanzi, A.G.B. (eds.) WILF 2005. LNCS (LNAI), vol. 3849, pp. 305–311. Springer, Heidelberg (2006)
2. De Mauro, T.: La Cultura degli Italiani. Laterza, Bari (2010)
3. Sadegh-Zadeh, K.: Handbook of Analytic Philosophy of Medicine. Springer, Amsterdam (2012)
4. Seising, R.: On the Absence of Strict Boundaries — Vagueness, Haziness, and Fuzziness in Philosophy, Science, and Medicine. Applied Soft Computing 8, 1232–1242 (2008)

5. Tabacchi, M.E., Termini, S.: Varieties of Vagueness, Fuzziness and a Few Foundational (and Ontological) Questions. In: Proceedings of the 7th conference of the European Society for Fuzzy Logic and Technology (EUSFLAT-2011) and "Les Rencontres Francophones Sur La Logique Floue et Ses Applications" (LFA 2011): Advances in Intelligent Systems Research, Aix-les-Bains, France, pp. 578–583. Atlantis Press (memory stick) (2011)
6. Tabacchi, M., Termini, S.: Measures of Fuzziness and Information: Some Challenges from Reflections on Aesthetic Experience. In: Yager, R.R., Reformat, M.Z., Shahbazova, S.N., Ovchinnikov, S. (eds.) Proceedings of the World Conference on Soft Computing, May 23-26, San Francisco State University San Francisco (memory stick, paper no. 152) (2011)
7. Termini, S.: On Some Vagaries of Vagueness and Information. Annals of Mathematics and Artificial Intelligence 35, 343–355 (2002)
8. Pinna, B., Tabacchi, M.E.: A Fuzzy Approach to the Role of Symmetry in Shape Formation: The Illusion of the Scalene Triangle. In: Di Gesù, V., Pal, S.K., Petrosino, A. (eds.) WILF 2009. LNCS, vol. 5571, pp. 197–204. Springer, Heidelberg (2009)

Part II

Ethics, Philosophy, and Medicine

5

Medical Ethics, Fuzzy Logic and Shared Decision Making

Julia Inthorn

5.1 Introduction

Doctors especially those working in hospital surroundings characterize their everyday life as a continuity of decisions. Even routine examinations and treatments of patients who have a cold can be described as a succession of decisions starting with the first questions the patient is asked, ruling out severe illnesses with similar symptoms up to the medication chosen. Decisions have to be made on the use of diagnostic tools, the diagnosis itself as well as therapies. Decision-making processes usually have to take place under time pressure which may result in stress. Adding to the stress is the responsibility for a patient who is especially vulnerable in this situation. Patients trust in a doctor's ability to make correct decisions based on the latest standard of scientific knowledge. Various tools like guidelines and codes of conduct have been established to support doctors in their decisions for the patient.

But not only the medical, knowledge-based side of decisions is complex. Decisions should be based on medical knowledge while at the same time normative aspects like the respect for the autonomy of a patient should be taken into account. This leads to complex decision making processes where descriptive as well as normative reasons can come together.

In his book *Handbook of Analytic Philosophy of Medicine* Sadegh-Zadeh analyzes the dimensions and structure of medical knowledge and it's relation to decision making processes in diagnosis and therapy. By integrating the notion of fuzziness he can modify the notion of decision making processes in medical practice and describe decisions as based on fuzzy concepts. He shows the advantage of fuzzy logic to deal with decisions in medicine, especially medical practice. [11] His approach may lead to new ways of decisions better adapted to the structure of medical knowledge than current guide lines and check lists in medicine.

He also discusses the normative dimension of decisions by reconstructing medicine as a deontic discipline. The following chapter takes his thoughts on the normative dimension of decision making as a starting point. While Sadegh-Zadeh focuses on the structure of medical knowledge as a whole this chapter wants to have a closer

R. Seising and M.E. Tabacchi (Eds.): *Fuzziness and Medicine*, STUDFUZZ 302, pp. 85–95.
DOI: 10.1007/978-3-642-36527-0_5

look at individual decisions within the framework of doctor-patient relationships and wants to reflect on the possibilities and limits of the notion of fuzziness for those decisions from the perspective of medical ethics.

5.2 Ought-to-Do Rules and Medical Ethics

Sadegh-Zadeh reconstructs common morality as "a deontic-social institution constitutive of particular deontic-social practices." [11, p. 569] His analysis of morality starts from the practice of moral statements like ought to do rules or prohibitions. Examples for moral statements are sentences like "The autonomy of a patient ought to be respected" or "It is forbidden to sell organs". His analysis results in an understanding of morality as a set of sentences with a specific structure. The epistemic value of such sentences or the moral reasoning for specific rules or principles is not part of his analysis. Taking moral sentences as such his approach can be interpreted as a contribution to the formalization of descriptive ethics.

He distinguishes three types of normative rules: rules on what is obligatory, what is forbidden, and what is permitted. In the reconstruction of normative sentences he uses deontic operators in order to formalize those sentences. He limits normative rules to sentences about actions such as "A doctor is prescribing medicine" or "The patient refuses to take the medicine". This enables him to define deontic action sentences and deontic rules that base on a broad understanding of human actions [11, p. 564]. Sadegh-Zadeh describes normative sentences as action rules that are either unconditionally or in specially defined cases morally binding. Normative sentences derived from law have the same structure as normative sentences derived from ethics. By means of deontic logic he shows that all deontic rules can be described as ought to do rules (ibd., p. 565).

Taking these thoughts one step further Sadegh-Zadeh interprets medicine as a deontic endeavor where certain types of knowledge lead to moral obligations. He argues that medicine in itself has certain goals like trying to heal a person or providing treatment in order to reduce pain and suffering that have prescriptive character. Therefore, the knowledge of a diagnosis is not only a description of a person's physical or mental status but, according to Sadegh-Zadeh, in itself has deontic character. The general rule derived from the diagnosis is to provide treatment for the patient according to the state of medical knowledge. Thus medicine has descriptive as well as normative parts and their combination results in deontic rules such as "A person's high blood pressure ought to be treated with medication *xy*".

Sadegh-Zadeh derives the normative dimension of medicine by having a look into medical practice. By means of descriptive ethics he lays open what is considered as the right thing to do within the community of doctors. From an ethical point of view the normative practice cannot be left unquestioned but there need to be normative arguments to show that the rules in place are well justified and not only a contingent maybe even harmful practice. Different aspects need to be considered. Therefore, I will start with having a look at the currently most prominent approach in bioethics, the four principles of bioethics. This will secondly be embedded into more theoretical thoughts on the role of morality and ethics within culturally different medical practices. Thirdly the perspective of patients on and role within decision making processes will be sketched and the problem of shared decision making in medical contexts will be discussed.

5.3 Principle Based Bioethics

Sadegh-Zadeh already mentions the Principles of Bioethics by Beauchamp and Childress. [3] The approach which is also called principlism is based on four middle range principles and can currently be seen as one of the most prominent approaches in normative medical ethics [11, p. 558ff.]. Beauchamp and Childress suggest four principles as a starting point for normative medical ethics. The principles are autonomy, beneficience, non-maleficience, and justice.

Autonomy refers to liberal ideas of self determination and individual freedom of decisions. Especially decisions concerning one's own health and body and decisions of vulnerable persons have a high importance for the persons affected. Therefore, the person his/herself should be in charge of the decision. In medical practice this is put into practice by informed consent. Before a treatment a patient has to consent to it, otherwise is is illegal for the doctor to treat the patient or even do surgery. The principle of autonomy gives the patient a strong stand within medical decision making processes and is currently further strengthened by instruments such as living wills.

Beneficience highlights the idea that every treatment and also diagnosis should be for the benefit of the patient. It should add to his well-being and/or add to his chances of being cured. This principle gives a normative reason for Sadegh-Zadeh's descriptive approach of medicine as an deontic discipline. If a person is sick and a doctor can tell a diagnosis, then the doctor's work is not finished but should be followed by the suggestion of a helpful treatment. The principle of beneficience also tells that the treatment should have a positive outcome thus ruling out treatments with no or even negative outcome. In current medicine this is evaluated in clinical trails in the context of evidence based medicine.

Non-Maleficience puts the focus on not harming a patient. Harm may be forced on a patient by diagnostic tools that do not add to the knowledge of a patient's state but only provide a possibility for doctors to bill or add to legal security for a doctor. Treatment can be harmful if it is already futile and the patient still has to suffer from side effects or if it is otherwise not indicated. Since many diagnostic as well as therapeutic tools are invasive, involve a certain risk or can have side effects, the principle of non-maleficience usually cannot be seen or followed on it's own but has to be considered in connection with the principle of beneficience or other normative reasoning in order to weigh positive as well as negative effects of a proposed action.

Justice describes the necessity to have a closer look at the allocation and distribution of ressources in health care and to find a just solution to provide for all patients. Justice as a principle needs to be reflected with regard to the micro-, meso- and macro level of resources. Doctors and nurses have to decide how to divide their time between the patients in a unit. A hospital has to manage resources and political and legal regulations organize the allocation of ressources within the health care system.

At first sight the four principles seem to be highly plausible normative guidelines for decision making in a medical context that are easy to apply. Beauchamp and Childress argue that their four principles approach is more concrete and better applicable than abstract ethical theories on the one hand side. On the other hand side the four principles are open enough to be applied to different situations and in different contexts and do not need to be too detailed like complex rule systems. Another advantage of this approach can be seen in its simplicity. Ethical theory and meta ethics provide a vast variety of approaches and theoretical starting points. This leads to an ongoing debate about complex theoretical assumptions and ultimate justification of normative rules. It is unlikely that this plurality will dissolve in the near future, the debate will go on and thus commonly share rules like those based on human rights will not be derived from a commonly shared theoretical approach in ethics. Similar to the plurality (and disagreement) on the level of theories there is a plurality of positions on the level of evaluation of concrete actions such as abortion or stem cell research. Here it is also difficult to find commonly shared positions. In spite of the plurality on the level of theoretical approaches as well as concrete applicable rules there is a level of commonly shared principles within certain contexts. Beauchamp and Childress therefore suggest four principles of medical ethics that can be seen as commonly shared positions despite differences with regard to theory or concrete practice. On the intermediate level of mid-level norms they describe a normative position that can be seen as a least common denominator and shared starting point in medical ethics.[1]

The four principles in between theoretical reasoning on the one hand side and concrete rules on the other hand side also describe the position of ought to do rules derived from those principles within a system of deontic rules. Ought to do rules derived from the four principles provide ethical guidance and have a structure like "You should not harm the patient". The rules still need to be applied in concrete situations and principles can aim in different even conflicting directions when applied. Cutting someone during surgery could be understood as an act of bodily violence against the principle of non-maleficience while at the same time the surgery aims at the beneficience of the patient. A patient might wish for an unsecure treatment or refuse a necessary treatment and thus by following the principle of autonomy and respecting the patient's wish a doctor may harm the patient and act against the principle of non-maleficience. Providing care for one patient as good as possible may lead to neglecting and thus harming other patients bringing the principles of beneficience and justice into conflict. The examples show that the principles can conflict with each other and thus cannot be applied in a mechanistic simple way. The openness of the principlism, which is described as strength by Beauchamp and Childress, can thus be also seen as a central problem of this approach. As Feuerstein and Kollek point out, the principles are under-determined as well as over-determined

[1] Besides the wide use the principles have also been criticized from different sides. For a critique of the principles in different fields of application see the contributions in [8].

at the same time. They are under-determined because they need interpretation in concrete situations and these interpretations can vary widely. And they are also over-determined because in most situations more than one principle they can be applied which leads to the necessity to weigh the principles [7, p. 569]. In cases of conflicts between principles there need to be additional rules, norms or processes of deliberation in order to get to a good normative solution of the situation. These solutions cannot be provided by the principles themselves but they need further ethical reflection. Within a fuzzy logic-based system of rules the principles in the form of ought-to-do rules are over – and under-determined in the same way. Application of those rules – fuzzy or not – need further knowledge and interpretation of a situation as well as further ethical reflection in case of conflicting rules. This leads to the question how ethical theory might help in those situations.

5.4 Ethics as a Reflection on Morality

Within the systematic of ethics medical ethics are classified as applied ethics. This implies theoretical reflection and a foundation within ethical theory, especially meta ethics as well as reference to theoretical positions such as anthropological or other philosophical or theological theory. Thus medical ethics can be understood as part of philosophical or theological ethical theory and refers to theories for the foundation of norms from these disciplines [14, p. 12 ff.].

At the same time medical ethics is applied meaning that the academic debate is closely connected to decision making processes in clinical situations. Medical ethics in this understanding is a practical science like medicine and should provide concrete rules or conditions for decision making processes. For example the aims and scope of the Journal of Medical Ethics describe this twofold aim as follows: "The journal seeks to promote ethical reflection and conduct in scientific research and medical practice."[2] As already seen in the discussion of the bioethical principles within pluralistic societies there is a plurality of values and norms. It is difficult to find a general agreement on norms. Public debates on bioethical issues like stem cell research or active euthanasia show these difficulties and plurality of positions. The aim of the journal as cited therefore needs to be seen in a dialectic way. On the one hand side the plurality of different ethical positions and the reflection and deliberation of them is given room. On the other hand side the improvement of conduct needs a more rule based approach with a reduction of differentiations and different positions. This dialectic shows that neither the reflection on ethical problems nor the search for concrete solutions in concrete situations can be made obsolete.

Ethics as the reflection on morality takes this twofold task into account. On a theoretical level ethics can show if normative positions are non-self-contradictory or how norms can be derived from ethical theories. Ought-to-do rules based on the four principles approach as shortly introduced above thus can be analyzed in their relation to ethical theory as well as in concrete situation. Secondly the analysis of ethical decision making processes or ethical problems can help to structure problems

[2] `http://jme.bmj.com/site/about/`

and gain a better understanding of the factual as well as normative dimension of a decision. The four principle approach can thus not only be interpreted as a set of rules but also as a tool to analyze ethical decision making processes. The principles are shown to have great heuristic value in such situations. They can help to structure a problem and to start a multifold reflection of the problem guided by the principles. Ethical committees in their discussions of ethical problems in clinical situations for example use the four principles in this way [9].

The twofold aim of ethics between pluralistic theories and applicability implies a difficult balance between individual ethics, normative ethics and universal approaches. While legal regulation can be based on ethical as well as political deliberation and found through consensus, the expectation towards (universal) normative ethics is often to tell right from wrong. As already shown this is not easily possible for reasons shown above. The critique towards universal normative approaches can best be seen in the critique from the perspective of intercultural and cross-cultural bioethics. These perspectives strongly emphasize the cultural relativity of norms, values and ethical considerations. Momentarily the development of bioethics in international contexts such as the WHO or World Medical Association is strongly linked to Western approaches. These approaches mainly focus on normative questions of national and international regulations like regulation of clinical trials, rules for doctor-patient interactions or international organ trade. As the same time they take an individualized view point and strongly protect the autonomy of the patient. Bowman points at several limitations of western bioethics within intercultural settings [4]. He criticizes the concept of culture and religion in western bioethics where culture and religion are regarded as two factors among other factors that influence decisions. These factors are often reduced to stereotypical differences between cultures. He argues for a concept of decisions cannot be seen as embedded within a cultural framework that shapes these. In order to get a closer understanding of decision making processes culture needs to be conceptualized not only as one of many dimensions of a decision but as the specific framework that leads to a very specific understanding of a situation as a decision. The example Bowman provides is the culturally different understanding of health, disease and illness. In western understanding there is a dichotomy between health and illness that is one of the foundations of western understanding of medicine. In a western understanding a person is either healthy or sick. In other cultural discourses health and illness are seen as equilibrium and a person can be healthy and sick at the same time. These two fundamentally different perspectives lead to different perceptions of decisions with regard to health care.

This critique shows that not only questions of norms and values but also social, religious and cultural factors need to be taken into account when talking about ethical decision making. Ethics as an academic discipline can provide a better understanding of the intercultural differences between concepts such as health, disease and illness but also by conducting cross-cultural empirical research in order to better understand the framework of decisions and the embedment of norms. Taking the critique one step further this does not only apply to decisions in different cultures but – maybe to a lesser degree – also to the differences of decisions between persons. Due to social, religious and cultural factors individuals frame decisions on the basis of their personal experiences and life stories. This can lead to different understandings of situations and thus to different structures of the decisions – independent of the final outcome. Thus the "concept of culture serves as a reminder of local variations in understanding of health, illness, suffering, and death" [13, p. 308]. In order to take patients seriously these individual perspectives need to be taken into account for example when doctors seek informed consent from them. By integrating the notion of culture and religion into ethics the contingent as well as universally shared aspects of decisions can be investigated in depth.

5.5 Shared Decision Making: Patients' Perspectives

The discussions above can be brought together and made more concrete when analysing shared decision making processes between doctors and patients. The structure of informed consent as the typical model of shared decisions is described as a two pillar model. On the one hand side there is medical information. Doctors take all information about a patient as well as scientific knowledge into account in order to find out which therapies are medically indicated. The best option or maybe different options are presented to the patient. The patient on the other hand provides his or her consent to one of the options. Only if both conditions are fulfilled a therapy can start.

This ideally construed decision situation is much more complex in reality. This starts with the medical side. As already broadly discussed by Sadegh-Zadeh the medical diagnosis and indication are not easily at hand but needs to be understood as the result of numerous decisions. At the same time these medical decisions are not always sharp but based on many uncertainties and vagueness. Here fuzzy logic can help to restructure information and come to a conclusion – but this conclusion can only be part of the medical side of the decision. Bates and Young discuss how fuzzy logic could improve intensive care therapy. They see the advantage that decisions can be made rapidly "on the basis of a large and disparate array of information" [2, p. 948]. The alternative and current method in clinical practice is usually to take the knowledge at hand combined with experience, which can lead to results that may vary from person to person. For the authors one central aim of the use of fuzzy systems therefore can be to reduce unwanted variation in clinical practice and the automation of devices. But the authors also see critical aspects of relying on fuzzy systems within medical decisions. Since in medicine there are still lots of unknown interrelationships doctors rely on experience and rules of best practice. These needs to be integrated into fuzzy algorithms. They state: "Indeed, the performance of the fuzzy algorithm depends greatly on whose expertise it encapsules (i.e. who fuzzified the parameters and set up the rule tables). Thus, we would expect some disagreement even between different experts" (ibd., p. 951) This might lead to similar problems as with decisions based on personal experience in areas where no established algorithm is known: "A fuzzy logic algorithm operating in such an area is only as good as the expertise of the individual who defined its fuzzy sets and rule table entries." (ibd., p. 952). Statistically speaking this might not make any difference with regard to the quality of medical care. But with regard to trust it makes a difference whether the decision was made by an algorithm or a machine or whether it was made by a person. From the perspective of a patient, in a situation of vulnerability such as being ill decisions need to be trustworthy and there needs to be an instance that can be held responsible in case the decision was wrong. Usually it is difficult for patients to ascribe trust and responsibility to a machine but they would rather have a person like a doctor in between them and the algorithm. Thus the doctor would have the responsibility to guarantee the trustworthiness of the machine. If the doctor trusts the results then the patients can trust them as well because they trust the doctor. Thus the algorithm might support decision making processes on the level of processing information, but it cannot help with questions of responsibility of a doctor. The doctor and his or her diagnostic evaluation remain on pillar of informed consent.

Turning to the second pillar, the consent of patients, the picture gets even more complicated. For example there is an ongoing debate on how much information a patient should be given and to what he or she should give consent. Should the patient learn about different options and weigh them for him- or herself? Or is this a task of the doctor? Schwab discusses this problem with regard to risk-benefit assessment and asks in how far risk assessment and the possibility of failure of a treatment should be communicated openly to the patient. He argues for epistemic humility and that the patient should not only give his or her consent to a treatment but also to the risk-benefit ratio that comes along with it [12]. Following Schwab's idea would mean to communicate much more information to the patient. The evaluation of different therapeutic options would be a shared process between doctor and patient.

When patients are asked about participating in shared decision making processes with doctors and how much they want to be involved we see a different picture. Chung et al. asked patients at a general internal medical service in Chicago about their preference in decision making processes and gave them different ways of distributing responsibility within a decision as options. The empirical research shows that although most patients want to be asked their opinion (87% strongly agree) and want to be involved there is also a strong tendency to delegate the last decision about medical care to the doctor (34% strongly agree, 33% agree) [6]. So many but not all patients do not wish to decide about the therapy. They want to be involved but not fully responsible. In order to structure a decision making process a doctor needs to know in how far a patient wants to be involved in the process.

But the ability as well as the will to decide for oneself varies with the degree of illness. Strengthening the autonomy of a patient is the aim of various tools such as advance directives and living wills for cases when a patient cannot decide anymore. But still many situations occur where patients do not have a document transporting their wishes. Rid and Wendler therefore ask for alternatives in decision making processes when informed consent cannot be gained. They especially focus on Alzheimer patients who are incapacitated and cannot make decisions. They suggest integrating the patient's wishes into decision making processes as far as possible even when a patient cannot communicate his or her wishes anymore. They argue for surrogate decision making that is assisted by a preference predictor which suggests decisions based on factors such as age, gender, race and also most recent decisions [10]. The advantage is to have a broader basis for the decision by referring to different types of data. One disadvantage may be seen in the categorization of decisions along age, gender or race. Though there are statistical similarities the idea of individualized decisions that is strengthened by the idea of autonomy seems to be reduced. A preference predictor thus can be seen as helpful in situations where there is not enough knowledge about a patient and family or friends who might tell more about the patient are not available.

While in some situations the integration of patients' wishes is not wanted by patients or patients are incapacitated there are also situations in medical decision making where a patient wishes for a special treatment while medical indication points into another direction. Alt-Epping and Nauck discuss the role and significance of positive wishes for therapy by patients in clinical decisions on therapy. While the usual situation in clinical decision making is a therapeutic decision of a doctor based on an indication and an agreement to this therapy in the form of an informed consent by a patient this model mainly supports the right of a patient to refuse a treatment. This right is broadly discussed, legally secured and usually accepted by doctors but what about a situation where a patient wishes for a special treatment? Alt-Apping and Nauck discuss an example of divergent perspectives on risk and chances of a cancer treatment by doctor and patient and analyse different options how to integrate a patient's wish into medical decision making. The authors stress the point that even principles like beneficience and non-maleficience rely on subjective measures or criteria such as the individual therapeutic aim of a patient (or a doctor) [1, p. 21]. Terms like life quality, compliance, chances or risk show how the evaluation of the outcome of a treatment is based on subjective factors that may vary from patient to patient but also from doctor to doctor. While some patients and doctors may think that a 23% chance of curing is a good chance other patients might want to avoid side effects with regard to higher life quality instead. Empirical evidence shows that the assessment not only varies between patients but that patients change their mind during treatment as well [5]. The authors conclude that by taking the personal risk assessment of a patient seriously and thus understanding his or her approach to a special therapy can lead to a re-evaluation of the medical indication.

The three different examples of patients show how different patients want to get involved within medical decision making. All three lead to different decision situations and different forms of communication. Processing medical information is only one part of this decision making process that needs to be adapted to a patient's individual needs for information and involvement.

5.6 Conclusion

Decision making processes in medicine are a shared process between doctors and patients. Due to reasons of responsibility the participants cannot easily be replaced by machines, algorithms or even proxies. The question of trust and responsibility needs to be addressable throughout this process where patients are more vulnerable than doctors. The process of giving information for informed consent hereby has a twofold task. The first task is to enable the patient to make a decision based on all relevant facts. The second task is communication with the patient as a task in itself. Especially in situations where risks are high and decisions might mean decisions over live and death building a trust relationship is equally important for the patient. Though decisions might be based on fuzzy concepts and risks that are relevant for processing medical information the results – leaving the hospital cured or suffering from side effects or even being dead – are not fuzzy for the patient him/herself. From an ethical point of view the analysis shows that communication over a problem and structuring a decision making process together can be seen as part of a solution of an ethical problem already. Being listened to and the mutual understanding of different perspectives on a problem built the basis of deliberation and shared decisions. Therefore the application of fuzzy sets and algorithms can only be implemented within these structures but not instead of them.

References

1. Alt-Epping, B., Nauck, F.: Der Wunsch des Patienten – ein eigenständiger normativer Faktor in der klinischen Therapieentscheidung? Ethik in der Medizin 24, 19–28 (2011)
2. Bates, J.H.T., Young, M.P.: Applying Fuzzy Logic to Medical Decision Making in the Intensive Care Unit. American Journal of Respiratory and Critical Care Medicine 167, 948–952 (2003)
3. Beauchamp, T.L., Childress, J.F.: Principles of Biomedical Ethics, 5th edn. Oxford University Press (2001)
4. Bowman, K.: What are the Limits of Bioethics in a Culturally Pluralistic Society? Journal of Law, Medicine & Ethics 32(4), 664–669 (2004)
5. Chochinov, H.M., Tataryn, D.J., Clinch, J.J., Dungeon, D.: Will to live in the terminally ill. Lancet 354, 651–661 (1999)
6. Chung, G.S., Lawrence, R.E., Curlin, F.A., Arora, V., Meltzer, D.O.: Predictors of hospitalised patients' preferences for physician-directed medical decision making. Journal of Medical Ethics 38(2), 77–82 (2012)
7. Feuerstein, G., Kollek, R.: Flexibilisierung der Moral: Zum Verhältnis von biotechnischen Innovationen und ethischen Normen. In: Honnegger, C., Hradil, S., Traxler, F. (eds.) Grenzenlose Gesellschaft? Kongressband des Freiburger Kongresses der DGS, ÖGS und SGS, part 2, 1st edn., Opladen, pp. 559–574 (1999)
8. Inthorn, J. (ed.): Richtlinien, Ethikstandards und kritisches Korrektiv. Eine Topographie ethischen Nachdenkens im Kontext der Medizin, 1st edn. Edition Ruprecht (Edition Ethik Band 7), Göttingen (2010)
9. Marckmann, G., Mayer, F.: Ethische Fallbesprechungen in der Onkologie: Grundlagen einer prinzipienorientierten Falldiskussion. Der Onkologe 15(10), 980–988 (2009)
10. Rid, A., Wendler, D.: Can we improve Treatment Decision-Making for Incapacitated Patients? Hastings Center Report 40(5), 36–45 (2010)
11. Sadegh-Zadeh, K.: Handbook of Analytic Philosophy of Medicine. Springer, Dordrecht (2012)

12. Schwab, A.: Epistemic Humility and medical Practice: Translating Epistemic Categories into Ethical Obligations. Journal of Medicine and Philosophy 37, 28–48 (2012)
13. Turner, L.: From the Local to the Global: Bioethics and the Concept of Culture. Journal of Medicine and Philosophy 30, 305–320 (2005)
14. Vieth, A.: Einführung in die Angewandte Ethik. Wissenschaftliche Buchgesellschaft, Darmstadt (2006)

6 Health, Illness, and Disease – Adjusting the Coordinates

Lukas Kaelin

Abstract. "Medicine is not concerned with illness and disease, but with suffering human beings called patients." (148) Rather than understanding the patient from illness, Kazem Sadegh-Zadeh takes the inverse trajectory. A comprehensive theory of the patients sheds light on the concepts of health, illness, and disease. In such a perspective disease is not the opposite of health, and needs to be construed as a nonclassical concept based on a number of prototype diseases. Dwelling upon Wittgenstein's family resemblance theory and Eleanor Rosch's theory of categorization, Sadegh-Zadeh's theory of prototype diseases allows for gradual membership in the category of diseases. The boundary of diseases and non-diseases thus becomes blurry and is construed as a matter of social definition depending on the cultural context. Such a social construction of disease reorients the basic coordinates of the philosophy of medicine. This paper will track the way the coordinates are reoriented and test them from perspectives at the edge respectively critical to orthodox medicine such as Arthur Kleinman's medical anthropology and Michel Foucault's archeology of medical institutions.

6.1 Introduction

Kazem Sadegh-Zadeh's book attempts to provide nothing less than a comprehensive account of the philosophy of medicine in an analytic tradition. A titanic endeavor, which also takes titanic proportions. Starting point is the observation on the enduring high percentage of misdiagnosis with devastating effects. Why, one might ask, is the complex medical system not able to significantly reduce the problem of misdiagnosis including the incredible amount of suffering that follows? Why is medical progress unable to solve the problem of misdiagnosis? The starting point, thus, is a genuinely philosophical one – the naïve wondering at the world. The entire book can be read as an attempt to rectify the conceptual medical self-understanding. Part of the problem addressed is an inadequate understanding of the medical profession, a significant shortcoming of the philosophy of medicine. What is needed,

R. Seising and M.E. Tabacchi (Eds.): *Fuzziness and Medicine*, STUDFUZZ 302, pp. 97–108.
DOI: 10.1007/978-3-642-36527-0_6

then, is better grasp of the functioning of medicine as such – a proper philosophy of medicine. Here the insight of medicine as a deontic discipline, the account of disease and illness based on a theory of the patient as well as the close analysis of the clinical encounter are reframing the field of the philosophy of medicine. The adjustment of the coordinates in the title of this paper is referring to this conceptual shift.

Key to this change in emphasis in the philosophy of medicine is the inversion of the relation between patient and disease. Rather than understanding the patient from disease and illness, the suffering of the patient is taken as the starting point for the exploration of diseases. The first part of this paper is to explore the newly adjusted realm of health, illness and disease. The consequences of this readjustment get especially visible when read before the background of Arthur Kleinman' medical anthropology. This is the second part of this paper. The third part is reading this account of the clinical encounter based on the specific understanding of illness and disease in front of the background of Michel Foucault's archeology of medical knowledge.

Thus, my modest attempt in comparison with this titanic task is to read the "analytic philosophy of medicine" from the background of the margins of the medical system. From psychiatry and medical anthropology; one might say from the perspective of the psychic, social and cultural influences to medicine. But first let me start with an account of the shift of the concepts illness and disease suggested by Sadegh-Zadeh.

6.2 Mapping the Current Discourse on Health and Disease

Discussing illness, health and disease requires a philosophical foundation; a foundation that in many of the accounts in contemporary medical theory is missing. The theory of disease is founded in the concept of the patient, thus ultimately based on anthropology. Traditionally such definitions of the human being tend to be strongly normatively biased and thus might be challenged on ideological ground. Sadegh-Zadeh' understands the human being becomes a patient by virtue of his suffering. It is from there medicine as a whole gets its legitimacy. The human being in turn is defined as a bio-psycho-social agent, as an endopoietic system, i.e. a system capable of creating inner worlds (such as the psyche) but structured also through social discourses. The organization of these inner worlds, i.e. of the psyche, is conditioned by external discursive influences. Psychosomatic diseases thus turn out to be as much psychosocial in origin as they actually are psychosomatic [13, p. 314]. Already this brief account of the social factors of medicine enlarges the traditional account given of medicine.

The understanding of the suffering human being as a living body, which in turn is framed as a fuzzy system able to create inner worlds, serves as a background for the following discussion of the concepts of health and disease, which has been a main focus of the philosophy of medicine. Knowing the background of this discussion and the unsettled dispute sheds light on Sadegh-Zadeh's exploration of field. Large part of the discussion plays out between a *Biostatistical Theory of health* (BST), as presented by Christopher Boorse and the more encompassing *Holistic Theory of Health* (HTH) suggested by Lennard Nordenfeld. The opposition of these two theories is one between a naturalist and a normativist understanding of health and disease; Boorse understanding himself as an "unrepentant naturalist" [2, p. 5]. It is the simplicity, rather than the accuracy, of these two theories, which makes them an ideal point of departure. The brief outline of these positions serves as parameter to position the theory of disease suggested by Sadegh-Zadeh and to test it against the current discourse.

Roughly spoken, Boorse suggests in his classical and straightforward definition to understand disease as "a type of internal state which impairs health, i.e. reduces one or more functional abilities below typical efficiency" (Boorse 1977, 555). Such a definition has the benefits of referring – in theory – to objective empirical data allowing for drawing clear boundaries between health and disease. Healthy is someone without a reduction of the functional abilities necessary for life. The practice, however, turns out to deal with the challenging problem of having to define statistical normality, biological function and the frame of reference. Biological function is defined with reference to the causal conditions to suit the individuals and species survival. Reference class pertains to a specific "an age group of a sex of a species" [2, p. 7]. Abilities are relative to sex and age group, otherwise old age might generally be considered as a disease, a consequence that Boorse wants to avoid. This functional explanation of health is supposedly, as Boorse argues, a value free definition of disease and should therefore allow for a more or less clear delimitation between health and disease. Health in turn is defined as the absence of disease: "Health is the absence of disease" [2, p. 8]. Such binary logic is nicely embedded within the context of evolutionary biology. Serving somewhat of a standard model in the field of the philosophy of medicine (having a similar function as the four principles of Beauchamp and Childress in the bioethical discourse), a large number of challenges have been raised against Boorse's theory. Nevertheless, proofed wrong over and over again, due to its simplicity it has remained the standard theory, the default model as it were, of health and disease: "It is as if the health concepts debate got stuck in a loop. After each contribution it reboots to Boorse" [4, p. 19]. A prominent theory challenging Boorse's is the one of Nordenfelt. His account of health focuses more on the quality of life (or welfare) rather than on survival. "A is completely healthy if, and only if, A has the ability, given standard circumstances, to reach all of her vital goals." [10, p. 7] Optimum health is reached if the person is able on the biological as well as psychological level "to have the second-order ability to realize, given reasonable circumstances, all her or his vital goals." [8, p. 72] The qualifier "second-order ability" pertains to the fact that not the actual ability (e.g. of driving a bike) is necessary for being healthy but the potential ability (e.g. the ability of learning to drive a bike given a regular amount of exercise). Rather than some functional ability, health is understood teleologically as the ability "given standard circumstances, to reach all of her vital goals." [10, p. 7] Standard circumstances do not refer to statistical means or functional ability but rather to the social and cultural framework. Health is relative to the social expectation, too.

But health is not merely understood in biological terms, external influences can severely influence the well-being including "the physical topography of the country, cultural institutions, basic assets, and its economic conditions" [9, p. 109]. Ill health is not restricted to functional inability and might be produced by a wide range of external influences.

Rather than taking the empirical category of the disease as the starting point, Nordenfelt starts with the personal illness experience. Illness takes on epistemological primacy vis-à-vis disease. It is through the experience of ill health that people start looking for what is common to the different forms of these states. In this first phase illnesses are identified, recognized and communicated, without knowing the underlying disease causing the illness. In the second step, the sick are seeking experts for assistance. Communicating in the illness-language, they explain their ill health. The physicians in turn are then searching for the causes of the illnesses. Finally, the medical profession finds these causes and calls them "diseases". Such an account is applicable for the historical genesis of the medical profession and the understanding of the particular diseases; but they are repeated in each illness episode. It emphasizes the subjective suffering perspective vis-à-vis the objective empirical functional limitation.

From the perspective of this debate, health is thus understood on the one side as the function of an internal process, as Boorse does, or on the other side as the ability to reach vital goals in the case of Nordenfelt; it might be defined in biological and statistical terms, or with reference to personal and cultural norms. Finally, it might be the opposite of diseases or the two terms are not mutually exclusive. This unsettled dispute mirrors the debate whether medicine is an art or a science. This issue also touches upon the question of the place of natural science in medicine. Even the either-or-logic of these debates is refuted, questions still are raised about the localization of health and disease as key terms of medicine in the scientific coordinates.

The definition of health and disease is also relative to the perspective: Medicine and psychotherapy will provide different answers, but so will different disciplines within medicine. Palliative care, cardiology, psychiatry, and internal medicine will have different concepts of the human body and accordingly also different concepts of what it means to be healthy. This leads to the point of certain relativity inherent in the debate. "A definition of health cannot be false in the strong sense but merely inadequate to serve its purpose." [15, p. 12] Within the broad field stretched between these two authors, a large number of different definitions of health disease are placed.

6.3 The Readjustment of the Coordinates – Disease, Illness and Health

This controversy about the understanding of disease and the consequent lack of consistency in the medical ethical discussion about health and disease asks for conceptual clarity. It is "the source of a semantic chaos that has rendered the philosophy of health and disease an academic palaver preventing any progress" ([14], p. 112).

Whether progress is genuinely attainable in a discipline that spent the last two and a half millennia in assembling footnotes to the founder of the Western philosophical tradition, as the famous word of Alfred North Whitehead goes, might be arguable. However, conceptual clarity might nevertheless be an important goal to avoid misunderstanding and reach a genuine discourse worth its name.

Sadegh-Zadeh's epistemological starting point in the exploration of health, illness and disease is the last of these three terms. "Medicine is concerned with human suffering only if it is a facet of illness. Illness [...] may be engendered by a variety of causes. Among them is a cause of a particular type called disease." [13, p. 151] Disease is the crucial category because the knowledge of disease only enables the physician to provide his professional help. The explicit concern of Sadegh-Zadeh is to provide clarity in how the concept of the disease actually works. It is partly a Wittgensteinian task to show the confusion generated by an erroneous use of language – and to show "the fly the way out of the fly-bottle" [16, § 309]. His contribution to the existing discourse on the concept of health and disease can be summarized in three main points: First, a conceptual clarification to better grasp what we actually discuss with the term of disease; second, an account of the concept of disease with Wittgenstein grasping the concept of disease precisely in its fuzziness (the prototype resemblance theory of disease), and finally, a normative turn not only understanding disease as a deontic concept, but also medicine as a deontic discipline.

The conceptual clarification consists in a distinction of different understandings of disease - the general category often is confused with individual diseases and/or with the disease state of an individual patient. The approach differentiates on the one hand between the general category of disease and the particular types such as diabetes, alcoholism and ADHD. Token diseases in turn are disease state of a particular patient; while type diseases refer to particular diseases such as diabetes, heart attack or schizophrenia. Clarity is created if there is a clear boundary drawn between diagnostics on the one hand that deals with the particular disease of a concrete patient (token disease) and the nosology – serving as a background – which comes up with the classification of all types of disease. This first clarification is rather straightforward, although it has to be noted that these categories are sometimes confused in the literature.

However, the term disease is as most concepts not a simple straightforward concept. It is not a classical concept like a square. While instances of a classical concept have a common nature, a non-classical is fuzzy in nature. There is no clear set of features that serves as the distinguishing marker for all members of a non-classical concept. Examples are concepts like birds, vegetables or diseases, which do not share a common set of features, rather the features are partly overlapping. Wittgenstein's notion of the family resemblance serves as the model for this theory. In a famous paragraph of this Philosophical Investigations, Wittgenstein points out the working of concepts such as "game" – "board-games, card-games, ball-games, Olympic games, and so on." [16, §66] Wittgenstein reminds us not simply to assume that they must have something in common, but rather to observe the way these concepts work more closely. They have many things in common - but no single feature is shared by all members. It is like a family where one can see that the individual members are part of the same family however; they do not share a single feature.

The prototype resemblance theory of disease gives this Wittgensteinian framework a further twist. As well as some family members are more typical than others, so are some diseases more typical than others. Such as an orange is a more typical fruit than a coconut and a sparrow a more typical bird than a penguin, so is heart attack a more typical disease than hair loss. But how does the set of prototype diseases come into existence? Ultimately, the understanding of disease rests on democratic ground: "there are some anthropological constants which all rational human beings would be prepared to label a 'disease' by pointing to them and declaring, 'look: this is a disease!'" [12, p. 621]. The prototype theory of disease is thus grounded in the lifeworld in such a way that rational human beings cannot but recognize these states as diseases. Prototype diseases are thus baptized as such. Other human conditions can be called disease to the extent to which they resemble the prototype disease. More specifically: The more the symptoms of certain human conditions are similar to the ones of prototype disease, the more they can be classified as diseases. The boundary between non-disease and disease cannot be drawn clearly - this follows from the observation about of disease being a non-classical concept.

The reading of the text at this point is ambiguous: The prototype resemblance theory of disease might be understood in a Universalist, rationalistic vein in terms of all diseases classified as such by all rational human beings. But it also might be defined more cultural relativist as it is the case with concepts such as fruits or birds. In the same way as a coconut might be considered a more typical fruit than orange in some parts of the world, so the prototype diseases might be dependent on the cultural framework. In the *Handbook of Analytic Philosophy of Medicine* (*Handbook*, for short), Sadegh-Zadeh writes that disease "is a social construct in that it is a society-relative category whose prototypes are established by that society" [13, p. 565]. Depending on a universalist/rationalist or relativist/constructivist interpretation of the prototype resemblance theory the consequences are different. In the first case, there exists a set of diseases, which each rational being has to agree that this is a disease. In the second case, the qualification of disease is stronger dependent on the respective culture. Both interpretations are not without problem: The Universalist interpretation has to face the tough challenge that disease turns out to be a category beyond the social and cultural influences as the set of prototype disease must be the same at every moment in history. The constructivist interpretation leaves room diseases that might leave the door open for discriminatory uses of disease; like the branding of homosexuality as one.

The normative turn, lastly, is a reflection of the inherent normativity of the concept of disease. Having a disease – more specifically: being ill – serves as a call for others to provide assistance. Diseases "are action provoking." [14, p. 135] Defining diseases is not merely a descriptive endeavor but rather strongly value-laden one. If we call something a disease, we are called upon to assist in case of the medical profession or at least to relieve the sick person from his duties. That disease is a deontic concept makes medicine a deontic discipline like morality. As a consequence, the difference between morality and ethics (as a reflection of morality) is akin to the one between clinical practice and clinical research: "Clinical practice is practiced morality" and "clinical research is normative ethics" [13, p. 775]. The deontic character shifts the way we should think about medicine. It does not primarily pertain to truth, but rather to hypotheses and deontic rules. This clarification of the notion of disease lays the ground for then understanding illness and health in connection to it. Sadegh-Zadeh avoids simple opposition. The fuzzy notion of disease is not the opposite of health; nor of illness. The concept of health is constructed independently. One might be a patient without suffering a disease, without even being ill – for example in the case of consulting the physician because of an insect bite. If health has an opposed concept at all, it is the one of patienthood. Neither one of these concepts is classical. Patienthood can be characterized by "a particular degree of discomfort, pain, endogenously threatened life, loss of autonomy, loss of vitality, and loss of pleasure" [13, p. 184]. Finally, neither is illness opposed to health. Rather health is the umbrella term subsuming illness and wellbeing. Illness is one of many states of health, and it might exist to varying degree, not ill, more or less ill, ill, very ill, extremely ill, etc.

As briefly sketched out, such an account of disease can overcome the blockage between the different descriptivists and normativists by focusing on the very working of the concept of disease. Moreover, it does away with the false expectation to draw a clear boundary between disease and non-disease. By situating further the state of health on a meta-level and understanding illness compatible with health, this account further does away with unproductive opposition (be it the one between health and disease, or even between health and illness). The productivity of this account will further be critically examined against the background of the illness and disease understanding of medical anthropology as conceived by its doyen Arthur Kleinman.

6.4 Reading Disease and Illness in the Context of Medical Anthropology (Kleinman)

The implicit task of medical anthropology was to challenge the cultural oblivion of orthodox medicine and its epistemic framework on the basis of culture. The *Handbook* leaves implicitly room for cultural difference: Understanding diseases with reference to a certain frameworks especially shaped by linguistic framing leaves room for a factual plurality of disease-understandings. The framing of diseases through "socionomics" – and the power of discourse – is acknowledged. Culture, however, is almost exclusively used for the self-identification of the Western culture, which serves as the framework. What this Western culture exactly is, however, remains vague. The closing paragraphs about the evolution of medicine towards an engineering science or even anthropotechnology give an inkling about the classification of medicine as "Western".

Medical anthropology takes its starting point similarly in the paradoxical situation that in spite of progress in biomedicine there is increasing concern about maldistribution of care and moreover a crisis of trust in the health care sector [6, p. 140].

The issue of a lack of trust in the modern medical profession has been addressed from different perspectives; and the question indeed might be raised whether it is the complementary to the raise of autonomy as a bioethical principle ([11]). Kleinman raised the question already in the 1970s and linked it to the lack of the medical profession to take the illness narratives of the patients seriously. Without disregarding the importance of biomedical research, the solution to many of the current medical problems is not seen in further research into the causes of disease – but rather a better grasp of the clinical encounter especially the notion of illness experience. The distinction between illness and disease is crucial for the entire field of medical anthropology. In a constructivist vein, he states that disease and illness are two different explanatory models; as well as there are different partly conflicting explanatory models in medicine. The differences might be between different medical disciplines or even within one and the same [7, pp. 119ff]. Without disregarding the importance of the explanatory model of disease so successful in Western medicine, Kleinman puts his focus on the illness narrative: "Illness is shaped by cultural factors governing perception, labeling, explanation, and valuation of the discomforting experience, processes embedded in a complex family, social, and cultural nexus." [6, p. 141] Taking the cultural construction of the illness narrative serious, however, should not lead to a culturalization of illness as such. The reification of the cultural explanation can easily obstruct the clinical encounter, as Kleinman is well aware of ([5]). The cultural construction of the illness experience is acknowledged by Sadegh-Zadeh without falling into the trap of an essentialist concept of culture. He rightly points to linguistic framing of illness episodes and the way their experience is shaped. It makes a difference whether you understand it as "you are in pain" or "you are under demonic attack".

However, the disentanglement of illness and disease is taken one step further by the conceptual framework of medical anthropology. Illness and disease are two distinct explanatory models, taking on the phenomenon from different sides. One main problem of clinical practice, in Kleinman's perspective, is that the illness experience is disregarded in search of the disease; the reason being the tremendous progress in terms of technological intervention battling diseases. The consequences of such disregard of illness, however, are severe: Patient noncompliance, dissatisfaction with the medical treatment and insufficient medical care might follow. The exploration of the illness is in many cases tantamount for being able to bring about a successful treatment. There is strong communicative task at hand for the physician to negotiate towards a model of illness/disease shared by physician and patient. This leads to stark claims demanding for equal attention paid to both explanatory models: "Where only disease is treated, care will be less satisfactory to the patient and less clinically effective than where both disease and illness are treated together" [6, p. 146].

This communicative task towards the exploration of the illness is rather undervalued in the Sadegh-Zadeh's Handbook. This already becomes visible by the space given to the two concepts; disease takes ten times more space than illness in the Handbook. The paragraph discussing pathology vs. nosology in a historical perspective gets the closest to make space for the illness narrative as a complimentary understanding of medical phenomena – thus challenging the medical sovereignty of health, illness and disease interpretation. Furthermore, Martin Buber is rhetorically invoked with his emphatic notion of encounter [Begegnung] in the context of the physician-patient-interaction and trust is rightly stressed as a crucial component of the clinical encounter; however it quickly gets clear that above all stands the physicians ability to attain and structure information from the patient fitting into his disease-knowledge. Disease is what the physician is concerned with; the explanatory model of the patient can largely be ignored. The anamnesis and diagnostic processed as described with the fuzzy logic approach is primarily geared towards knowledge generation that fits into the disease categorization. Although such categorization is important for proper diagnosis, it runs the risk of objectifying the patient and not taking the patient's own illness narrative seriously enough. This emphasis on the analytical skill is at the same time an undervaluation of the illness experience.

The disease orientation (and illness ignorance) of orthodox medicine certainly is of good service in many clinical cases, especially the severe ones. The success of Western medicine and this system of diagnosis is all too evident; but the discontents of this medical system have equally to be acknowledged. The focus, therefore, has to be put on illness equally – not just for establishing trust but also for the simple reason that "50% of visits to the doctor are for complaints without ascertainable biological base" [6, p. 141]. Furthermore, about four out of five sickness episodes are treated without looking for professional help. It is thus of great importance to understand the way these sickness episodes are understood and interpreted, and to gather knowledge about the therapeutic strategies to deal with illness in popular medicine. An approach focusing exclusively on the underlying disease might lose the importance of the illness narrative out of sight.

In addition, there is an increasing medical pluralism, i.e. patients carefully choose between different medical traditions – Western, traditional Chinese, folk etc. Understanding this medical pluralism only as a transitory phenomenon would fail to grasp the desire of people to choose a medical approach which serves best there need. Medical pluralism should not be understood in terms of a deficiency of Western medicine to adequately diagnose diseases; rather it mirrors the inability to address adequately illness narratives. It seems to me at least very doubtful whether a further development of analytical skills would solve the trust issues that the medical profession has to deal with and dissolve the choice of people of different medical approaches. In this context, the popular medical treatments have to be stressed, which are able to cope with four out of five sickness episodes.

There are a number of convergences in the two accounts, Kleinman's and Sadegh-Zadeh's – compared. They both refute a simplistic opposition of health and disease, and differentiate between illness and disease in similar ways. Furthermore, the constructivist thrust is common to both; Kleinman understanding illness and disease as explanatory models rather than entities, Sadegh-Zadeh making it clear that the "patient's true state is a construct of medical knowledge" [13, p. 274]. However, they alter significantly in their focus. The examples in the preface of the Handbook illustrate already the disease focus attempting to avoid misdiagnosis, whereas

Kleinman's main interest is the withering of trust in the medical profession caused by an ignorance of the patient's illness narrative. From a perspective of medical anthropology, the right twist of Sadegh-Zadeh of understanding disease from the patient would need further deepening in terms of the significance of the illness narrative for the healing process.

6.5 Disease and Power – Concluding Remarks with Michel Foucault

At the end of this paper, I will take a last twist and read the *Handbook* in the light of the historical, even archeological, account of Michel Foucault. Rather than seeing modern medicine as the result of a humanitarian progress, Foucault is seeing in it yet another means of control. His *Birth of the Clinic* ([3], 1973) is analyzing the ways power is exerted in clinical practice – power in terms of control and knowledge. The patients in hospitals are not only cared for; their examination is also a method of control, which establishes a power structure. The physician's judgment is creating truths and setting a norm. The constant observation further creates a hierarchical structure; the patient becoming the object of the physicians manipulation. The suffering individual in the hospital setting is thus transformed in an object of knowledge; a transformation also making the patient one case among many to be medically treated but also controlled.

This Foucaultian perspective has well become part of academic knowledge. As arguable as it might be, it can help counteract academic naïveté of a too idealistic construction of the medical profession. Power and control (as exerted through medicine) are not part of the conceptual framework of the *Handbook*. The belief in the analytic tools of the physician, if correctly applied, leaves possible concerns about the power dimension of the generated knowledge unmentioned. Although there is partial mention of the wider clinical setting – the importance of family members of the patient and the staff of the physician in the framing of the clinical encounter – the physician's task is described "as if" it took place outside the regular interaction of society. This ideal construction of the clinical encounter allows putting medicine next to charity and beyond the systemic dynamics in the health care sector and real-world constraints. Such an ideal construction has its benefits but also its costs. On the benefits side, it allows for a clear grasp of the concepts involved; on the cost side, however, it leaves out important aspects of the clinical encounter. These aspects of control and the intertwinement of knowledge/power are not merely external to modern Western medicine, but part of its conceptual framework. The generation of knowledge as well as the increasing professional differentiation is an inherent part of modern medicine. The clinical view unveiled by Foucault points to the same one-sidedness of the Handbook as Kleinman's concern about inadequate care due to an overly focus on the category of diseases. The *Handbook* tends to strengthen this disease orientation of modern medicine.

Defending Sadegh-Zadeh's approach one might rightly point out at the different vantage points but also different scope and interests from Kleinman and Foucault;

a scope that lies beyond an analytic analysis of the field of medicine. Furthermore, both, Kleinman and Foucault are starting off a psychiatric vantage point and then move generalizing towards the whole of medicine. Incertitude about the correct diagnosis, stigmatization, the power of imposing normality and the political dimension of medical truths are more virulent in the psychiatric field than elsewhere in medicine. Sadegh-Zadeh acknowledges the special role of psychiatry in the field of medicine; and he points to a conceptual problem in psychiatry, which puts him in surprising proximity to Foucault, when he states that "something in the conceptual basis of psychiatry and psychosomatics must be defective." [13, p. 722] The psychiatric diseases are actually to be understood from the social rather than the psychic field: "The pathogenic forces come not from the psyche, but rather from the social structure and values of the group and community in which an individual interacts with others, as well as from the mode of their interaction." ([13], p. 732) Psychosomatic, so the argument goes, should be replaced by sociosomatics.

Such insights gained through an analytic approach to the philosophy of medicine can provide new avenues and a better understanding of the medical field. And looked at the Handbook from this vantage point, the differences seem smaller. It is such insights as well as the conceptual clarification of the concepts of health, illness and disease that provide an important contribution to the philosophy of medicine. Taking into account the perspective of medical anthropology of Kleinman and the critical stance of Foucault can then help to put modern medicine in a certain context and remind us of the importance of the subjective side of medicine. Taking the subjective side in terms of the patient's explanatory model of illness more serious might not only addresses the trust issue haunting modern medicine; it might actually be a remedy for the problem of misdiagnosis, too.

References

1. Boorse, C.: Health as a Theoretical Concept. Philosophy of Science 44(4), 542–573 (1977)
2. Boorse, C.: A Rebuttal on Health. In: Humber, J., Almeder, R. (eds.) What is Disease?, pp. 1–134. Humana Press, Totowa (1997)
3. Foucault, M.: The Birth of the Clinic. Pantheon Books, New York (1973)
4. Khushf, G.: An Agenda for Future Debate on Concepts of Health and Disease. Medicine, Health Care and Philosophy 10, 19–27 (2007)
5. Kleinman, A., Benson, P.: Anthropology in the Clinic: The Problem of Cultural Competency and How to Fix it. PLoS Medicine 3(10), 1673–1676 (2006)
6. Kleinman, A., et al.: Culture, Illness, and Care. Focus 4(1), 140–149 (2006)
7. Kleinman, A.: Patients and Healers in the Context of Culture. University of California Press, Berkeley (1980)
8. Nordenfelt, L.: Talking about Health. A Philosophical Dialogue, Stockholm (1997)
9. Nordenfelt, L.: Health, Science, and Ordinary Language. Edition Rodopi, Amsterdam (2001)
10. Nordenfelt, L.: The Concepts of Health and Illness Revisited. Medicine, Health Care and Philosophy 10, 5–10 (2007)
11. O'Neill, O.: Autonomy and Trust in Bioethics. CUP, Cambridge (2002)

12. Sadegh-Zadeh, K.: Fuzzy Health, Illness, and Disease. Journal of Medicine and Philosophy 25(5), 605–638 (2000)
13. Sadegh-Zadeh, K.: Handbook of Analytic Philosophy of Medicine. Springer, Dordrecht (2011)
14. Sadegh-Zadeh, K.: The Prototype Resemblance Theory of Disease. Journal of Medicine and Philosophy 33, 106–139 (2008)
15. Schramme, T.: A Qualified Defence of Naturalist Theory of Health. Medicine, Health Care and Philosophy 10, 11–17 (2007)
16. Wittgenstein, L.: Philosophical Investigations. Blackwell, Oxford (1953) (English & German)

7

What Does It Mean to Be an Individual? The Patient as a Vague Object in Medicine and Research

Karin Hutflötz

From the moment a human being is called a patient, an individual becomes an object for medical care or research. Medicine is concerned with his illness transforming it into a disease, actually not with herself as an individual person suffering in a unique way and in a non-reccurring situation.

If a person arrives at a hospital for example, or undergoes surgery as a patient, she has to give up exceedingly the availability of her own time and personal space, of her privacy and boundaries. Disrobement, different kinds of infantilization, and the necessity of invading another person's very own space are generally inherent to the system of medical practice. This explains why Sadegh-Zadeh's *Handbook* mentioned in the first sentence of its Preface the ambivalence of medicine as "a science and practice of intervention, manipulation and control"[1], although the ethical rule of thumb is taking the patients health and his dignity as a priority: "Medicine is not concerned with illness and disease, but with suffering human beings called patients. For this reason a theory of the patient ought to constitute its basis." (§12.2.4)

Objectifying the unique case in order to generalize and model it in a rational manner, this is the typical western form of the scientific way and medical methods we favored in our culture and time to increase the domination and possession of nature, above all the nature of man. But the formal goal of medicine, to intervene and to control arbitrarily, clashes with the main concern all further advancement in medicine is dedicated, namely "to develop a philosophy of medicine that will be tailored to the needs and interests of the patient."[2]

Therefore, the thesis I want to put forward in this paper is that we actually do not need a (new) "theory of the patient"[3], but some new tools and fuzzy set models to

[1] [5], the first sentence of the preface: "Medicine is a science and practice of intervention, manipulation and control – concerned with curing ills, caring for ills, preventing maladies and promoting health."

[2] [5], Preface, p. 3.

[3] [5], §12: "However, the subject of medicine is the patient with the ends being directed toward the relief and prevention of human suffering and saving life." Thus, "medicine needs a theory of the patient first of all."

R. Seising and M.E. Tabacchi (Eds.): *Fuzziness and Medicine*, STUDFUZZ 302, pp. 109–121.
DOI: 10.1007/978-3-642-36527-0_7

quantify his "needs and interests" in the situation of being a patient. So, this paper wants to show, why it is not as necessary to have "essential features to characterize human beings as individuals"[4], but to know *who* somebody is, rather than what he or she individually needs in the situation and interaction of medical care and research.

First of all, this paper wants to point out the problem of taking the patient generally as an object (Part 1), even if it is considered to be a vague object based on an individual and "fuzzy concept of person" (§12.2.3). The main idea of this paper – I will give reasons for in Part 2 – is the need for a renewed practice in medicine traced back to the first person's perspective, instead of a more precise theory of the concept of ‚person', Sadegh-Zadeh argued for. Finally, I want to give some hints at the application of fuzzy sets in medical diagnosis and therapy, especially in order to measure and formalize the patient's degree of illness and needs.

7.1 What Is the Problem of Taking the Patient as an Object in Medicine and Research?

7.1.1 A Loss of Self-respect and Privacy: Consequences of Being Treaten as an Object

Before asking "What should we do?" we have to ask "What do we *actually* do?" In the summary of §12, the chapter about "The patient", Sadegh-Zadeh points out what I mentioned above, that "medicine is not concerned with illness and disease, but with suffering human beings called patients." Beyond doubt that is a well intentioned approach of a general orientation, in order to enhance the confidence of the patients and to declare that the physicians do it for the best. But from the moment a human being changes into the status of being a patient, medicine – due to its methods – is not concerned with himself (as an individual human being suffering in an specific way), but with himself reduced on the fact of disease. Thus, he or she is systematically used to be treated as a more or less dysfunctional object for diagnostic and therapy. Why that?

[4] Accordingly to "the inevitable vagueness of the concept of a person" (§12.2.3), Sadegh-Zadeh [5] tried to identify the category of persons as a fuzzy set. In respect of this purpose he exposes an interesting and detailed "description of the person" – referring to the categories figured out by Eric Cassell [1], p. 36-41 – which includes several aspects as some essential features to characterize human beings as individuals. What is called personhood in individuals can be shown as an irreducible but gradually vague term or factor, although not a crisp property that one definitely has or lacks in sharp measures. Hence, 'personhood' is present in human beings to one degree or another. It begins and ceases gradually and it varies in a single individual at different periods of his life.

The question is, if this draft of a fuzzy concept of person also shows how the suffering of a patient in fact depends on these aspects, even if they are describable in terms of the fuzzy set theory. And to what extend the entirety of the individual "as a bio-psycho-social-agent" (§12.2.) is involved, so why suffering is not mere pain and unwellbeing said to be objectified as illness or disease.

Objectivation basically means to make no difference between a dead or living body, between a nonorganic mechanism and a human being – in the way you look at it or in the way you observe or examine it. Consequentially, if you are accepted as a 'patient' you will get less respect and you have to give up your privacy to a large extend – much more than in other situations. And persons although demand less respect and privacy, as soon as they accept themselves as being a patient.

Entering hospital or a surgery, first of all one has to give up to a large degree the disposal of one's time, of one's very personal space and boundaries – much more than in other commonplace situations we know. What makes the difference is the demand of disrobement for example, and a certain kind of infantilization in behaving towards a patient, more or less incapacitation, that takes place almost automatically in medical care. That happens to be a really common and accepted practice in the last decades, because of the demands of economization and efficiency, which became the top-level values also in the field of medicine and for the service and habits of doctors and nursing staff.

If you are a patient in a hospital e.g., it's suddenly 'normal' and sanctified to be treated as an object without will and autonomy, in a deeper sense also without being allowed to feel frightened or to be shamed. Compared to all other situations we are used to, that is a kind of strange social convention generating suppressed feelings. This is the price for the promise of health we have to pay as tribute for the high level ideal of objectivation in the technical world and society.

In any other situation, if one lies almost naked in bed, one would be horrified if an unknown person (nurse, doctors) came into his bedroom at any time, even without knocking at the door, or if a group of unknown people (as happening during the ward round) stands around an uncovered patient's body without asking and talking about him in the third person's perspective. But when you are a patient in hospital, it's said to be 'normal'. The fact that this kind of – strictly speaking – strange behavior and social interaction is accepted in our daily life as a matter of course, is perhaps only legitimated by an implicit believe and trust in medicine as an ultimate authority – morally and epistemologically. No other institution in society demands to occupy the moral high ground as unquestionable as medicine in science and practice does.

From our childhood we are trained to repress feelings of shame or abasement in medical practice or institutions. In some respect, it's necessary to act and behave as if you do not have boundaries or need for privacy. But the price of this social accepted methodological abasement is in fact a temporary reduction of self-esteem. And the only way to hold one's head up, is to train the disconnection between mind and body – in fact a good strategy to keep inner distance to the loss of respect, in order to account yourself also as an object. It is difficult to estimate, even more to measure the effect and consequences in terms of negative outcome on healing process and therapy. Thus it is an open question and it opens a wide field of future research about the role of negative and self-respect depressing feelings like shame and abasement on healing process and resistance to therapy.

7.1.2 *Reducing the Fact of Being Individual to Some Measurable Variables: The Problem of Misdiagnosis in Medicine*

On the other side, there could be a correlation between this usual way of starting situation and relationship between the patient and the physician and the huge rate of misdiagnosis, just because of the distance to the very own feelings, that involves a reduced body awareness in return to the self-objectivation of the person as a patient. The problem is, as Sadegh-Zadegh points to from the very beginning of his book: "There are still so many wrong diagnoses [about 38% misdiagnoses] and treatments, pains and physician-caused deaths. Why and how do they arise?"

He raises concern over the "surprising and even disturbing"[5] experience, that there are more often different diagnosis to one and the same illness of a patient, quiet a lot of differences between the views and judgments of medical experts faced with the individual case of disease. This problem cannot be solved from the physician's perspective alone, because his acting and observing depends on the individual patient and has to take care of her particular and most concrete, personally unique and singularly situation. The solution might not only be found in improving methods and measurement tools for diagnostics, but in changing the physician's attitude and perspective on the situation and patient.

The idea, that the huge number of misdiagnosis in medicine can decrease, if the physicians improve their methods and machines in diagnostics (e.g. with fuzzy sets theory), is based on a certain image of the physician as a repairing or healing expert dealing with the patients disease or physiology. But the relationship between physician and patient is always an intersubjective interplay between two individual persons, not a one-sided relationship between a technical expert and his object.

To be an individual means not only to be confronted at any time with a unique and singularly situation, but to be characterized as a "unique and singularly being"[6], so the philosopher Martin Heidegger figures out as a formal definition of human beings existing in Time.[7]

---

5 [5], Preface, p. 2.

6 [3], p. 29 ff: "jeweiliges und jemeiniges Dasein" (translated by K. H.)

7 This fundamental description of a person's structure of being and existing in Time can be understood in analogy to the physical description of an atomic particle (and his movement) in quantum mechanics. Any particle is assigned and can be defined by its position x and its momentum p at a certain time. The Heisenberg uncertainty principle between the position and the momentum (mass times velocity) of particles, such as an electron, means that the more precisely the position is determined, the less precisely the momentum is known in this instant, and vice versa. The uncertainty principle is any of a variety of mathematical inequalities asserting a fundamental limit to the precision with which certain pairs of physical properties of a particle, such as position x and momentum p, can be simultaneously known. This relation has profound implications for such fundamental notions as causality and the determination of the future behavior of a particle. Thus it can be called more descriptively the "principle of indeterminacy." To transfer this to the better understanding of individuals being unique in time and (inter)acting singularly in new situations, makes clear why it will be necessary to apply fuzzy set methods to life science and medicine. That would mean to accept vagueness not as a deficit but as a leading principle for dealing and interacting with person, at last because it is constitutive (ontologically essential) for the notion of freedom and autonomy human rights are mainly related to.

That is the reason why in reality it is not possible to achieve "a diagnosis and treatment *in general*" – nor to learn a kind like that as students in medicine. Therefore Sadegh-Zadeh says: "we had acquired nothing about how to search for a diagnosis and treatment *in general*, i.e. how to arrive at a clinical judgment ... My extensive search was disappointing. It revealed that there was no such methodology."[8]

Taking the individual patient as an object in medicine is strictly speaking a category mistake. The only thing to be in fact taken as an object is empirical data or a detailed description or a quantified model of a measurable symptom, not the patient as a whole, individual person can be objectively verifiable.

But even if there is no technique or distinct method to give in general for medical diagnostics, it nevertheless is possible to get *practical knowledge*, to increase the insight into the interplays of an organism by exercise. That is what happens in good medical education and that characterizes a physician with long term experience: to achieve an understanding of the patient as "a bio-physical-agent", to get the "eye" by training,[9] to train the intuition for judging and treating the patient as an individual taking him seriously as an expert in his own history and body.

7.1.3 Vague Decision If a Person Is a Patient or Not

As Sadegh-Zadeh shows (especially in §12), the advantage of introducing fuzzy logic into the field of medicine is to develop a philosophy of medicine that will be tailored to the needs and interests of the human being, therefore: "My starting point is *the patient*". But it is not so easy to decide, if a person *is* a patient or not. "The aim is to inquire into how medicine is engaged in shaping the human world by deciding who is a patient – to be subjected to diagnostics – and who is a non-patient."[10]

In general a 'patient' is a person, (a) who has a living body, (b) which develops a psyche as it grows and (c) which is always embedded in a surrounding world. Consequently Sadegh-Zadeh wants the 'patient' being understood and interpreted as "a bio-phsycho-social and moral agent" (§12.2). The next step will be to grasp what it means to say, that such an agent can be categorized as diseased. The question is: How can we notice or confirm that a person is a 'patient'? If there are observable

[8] [5], Preface, p. 2.

[9] In every profession dealing with a complex and changing subject, there is necessary to get "the eye" by exercise, theoretical know-how, increasing measure methods and modeling is not enough. Take for example the job of an editor or corrector of texts: To understand a language, to see the mistakes, hear what's wrong, to find a fast solution to express it better – that's similar to the physician's situation in face of the patient: he has to understand the structure of physiology, the language of the body, his task is to find "the mistake", to see what's going wrong, to find a solution. The professional role of a physician is much more comparable to an editor dealing with texts written in a natural grown and living language, not with a mechanic repairing machines.

[10] [5], Preface, p. 4.

or measureable data, symptoms, signs of dysfunctions: this will be the answer the medical practice is usually based on. But the problem with this very common answer is, that only the third person's position is taken serious, just the perspective of the medical expert on the biological process and physiology of the body. The thesis I will put forward, is to extend the definition of being a 'patient' accordingly to the threefold definition of 'person' as "a bio-psycho-social agent". Thus, the question how we can notice or confirm that a person is a 'patient', should be answered with the following disjunction: A person is called a patient, needs help and gets treatment in medical care, if either A or B is valid, that means:

(A) if a person is suffering or showing symptoms OR
(B) if a person generates suffering or induces symptoms in her surrounding.

If A, we should make a further distinction between (a) and (b) – both a function of the observer's point of view:

(A.a) if the suffering or symptoms are perceived from the person herself, i.e. experienced from the first person's point of view. So there is an expression and consciousness of suffering, pain or at least uneasiness by the person herself.
(A.b) if a symptom or anomaly is observable from outside, by monitoring from the third person's perspective.

It is pretty clear, that (a) does not presuppose (b), but it may be interesting to consider, that also (b) does not presuppose (a) – both kind of indications are independent from each other. Actually (a) could be valid but not (b). Take for example a person in pain without the finding of any measurable indications by medical diagnosis. And vice versa there are persons without any feelings of pain or being unhealthy, but for example the diagnosis of leukemia could be derived from an analysis of the blood.

The case of B often goes unnoted in the discussion about the question how to decide, whether a person is a patient or not. B is the case, if a person isn't able to feel herself ill or in pain, and there's also no bodily sign of illness or disease pattern observable from outside. But she could be called a patient, if she raises pain or suffering in her environment, acting in a destructive way to other people's health.

There are some examples to mention: a psychopathic or a homicidal maniac like the Norwegian Anders Breivik should be paradigmatically for this case B, but also e.g. an alcoholic surgeon making mistakes or causing an accident. They have in common a non-working (self-)consciousness of (mental) pain, even less for the pain of others; they usually have no feeling for themselves being ill or having problems in that situation, and there are no physical indications of disease. Although a person is accepted as "a patient" in the sense of B, than the consequences of her actions are forcing diagnosis and intervention of physicians in medical care and therapy.

7.2 "What Does It Mean to Say, That the Patient Ought to Be Treated as a Person?"[11]

7.2.1 The Person as a "Bio-psycho-social and Moral Agent": Understanding the Individual as a Dynamic and Social Embedded System

Taking the patient actually as a "bio-psycho-social agent" means to take for serious that you have to deal with a living body. So we take into account, that his physical actions and reactions are correlated with mind and *sensible* actions and reactions interacting with other things and perceptions in each moment of existing. That's the reason why Martin Heidegger defines the person as "Being-in-the-world"[12] and why Ludwig Wittgenstein remarked the game-character of language embedded in the structures of our social world. Without doubt, this is one of the main insights of 20th century philosophy, that individual acting – that emerges from permanent interaction between biological, mind and social processes – is always under-determined and it can't be a result of linear causation. That's the reason why from the perspective of Analytical Philosophy as well as from the point of view of Continental Philosophy, being of individual persons is only describable in notions and structures of process ontology ore game theory (e.g. Wittgenstein's idea of "family resemblance").

Also in medicine, as Sadegh-Zadeh mentioned in his Handbook, the human organism is regarded as a "poietic system" (§12.2.1.), that is always changing through adaption to the social environment, i.e., the human organism is a dynamic and interacting system, that is never the same in each moment of existing.[13] To live as a human organism means to interact in a creative and complex way, re-constituting the adaption on the surrounding as well as the unity as an organism and as *one* person in each moment of being. That's the reason why a living organism is basically not

[11] [5], §12.2.3.

[12] [2], p. 14: "An ontological inquiry into human being, then, will not look at the properties possessed by humans, but rather at the structures which make it possible to be human. One of Heidegger's most innovative and important insights is that the essence of the human mode of existence is found in our always already existing in a world... And our being is intimately and inextricably bound up with the world that we find ourselves in."

[13] The term "autopoiesis" literally means "self-creation" and expresses a fundamental dialectic among structure, mechanism and function. Introduced in 1972 by Chilean neurobiologists Humberto Maturana and Francisco Varela [4] the concept of "autopoiesis" was originally presented as a system description that was said to define and explain the nature of living systems, which are "organized (defined as a unity) as a network of processes of production (transformation and destruction) of components which: (i) through their interactions and transformations continuously regenerate and realize the network of processes (relations) that produced them; and (ii) constitute it (the organism) as a concrete unity in space in which they (the components) exist by specifying the topological domain of its realization as such a network." (p. 78) Autopoietic systems are "structurally coupled" with their medium, embedded in a dynamic of changes. "When we refer to our interactions with a concrete autopoietic system, however, we project this system on the space of our manipulations and make a description of this projection." (p. 89)

comparable with any man-made machine or computer. And in the last part of this paper I try to show why therefore no medical expert system could work not even in the future.

To be or to act as an individual patient *or* as a physician means to play a game of your own, although you are part of a social interplay, that always frames (but never totally determines) your thinking, feeling and acting in a certain situation and context, also your state of health and the very own reaction on therapy. It does not mean, to make 'the' game of your own, but to be involved in an open and uncertain game – of communication in between others, of responding and reacting to what happens – in an individual way.

7.2.2 The Integrity of an Individual in Conflict with the Primacy of the Third Person's Perspective

It is common sense to say, that the intactness or integrity of a person (physically or in a psychological sense) is a measure and criteria for being 'healthy' or not.[14] But 'integrity' of a person or its 'intactness' is not a distinct concept, even not for one and the same person. In fact it's a function of time and task, of the environment and of the individual estimation, so it cannot be evaluated from the third person's perspective.[15]

What the integrity of an individual means in a certain context and situation relies (i) on the persons self-perception, (ii) on the individually estimated special situation (the individual feelings and fears, thoughts and aims, dispositions and former experiences); and it depends also on (iii) the influence and impact of the environment and social affiliation.

But in medicine, just the non-functioning part of the individual is taken into account as far as it can be generalized and traced back to a supra-individual bench mark.

Let me take a self-experienced example: As I was five years old, I wanted to play the trumpet. The precondition to be allowed to take lessons was a medical checkup. The check-up found an above-average narrowing of the nose inside walls. As a consequence the physicians told my parents, that it would not be possible for me to play the trumpet. Even to have enough breath and power for doing any sports would be a problem. In consequence of this diagnosis they recommended a complex surgery to enhance and restructure the nose as a whole.

The other side was my own experience and my parent's point of view, that in fact I never have had a problem with breathing, nor with sports or running or swimming. So they decided to refuse this surgery, and I was not allowed to play the trumpet.

[14] In reference to part (7.1.3) of this paper it should be necessary to extend this criteria also on the person's environment!

[15] The 'intactness' depends on the task a person is dedicated to: Handicapped people e.g. without leg do not feel a lack of intactness if they read a book or playing an instrument. Only challenged by situations where they would need their leg, they are handicapped.

Some years later, I got the opportunity to learn playing the trumpet by chance – and it works perfectly.

I take this example to show, how much better it would be to include the first person's perspective next to the third person's perspective in medical diagnosis, prognosis and therapy – concerning what Sadegh-Zadeh mentioned on the very first pages of his book: "the subject of Medicine is *the patient*" and "their actions deal with the patient history" (§12).

Not only the notion of the person's dignity demands a serious consideration of the first person's perspective and its very own needs and history. Actually, in some way the physician always has to deal with the patient's history too and he has to decide if one is a "patient" or not, if he is intact or not. But the medical agent respects this 'subjective' and individually on context-dependent factors as the individuality of a person and his very own situation just in a heuristic sense of intuitive practice by doing. Although, there are no defined factors and formalized criteria used until now.

As Elaine Scarry describes in her book "The Body in Pain"[16], it is impossible to communicate pain in a full sense, therefore it cannot be formalized with distinct measures. Whereas the own personal pain is one of the most reliable cases of evidence for 'being certain', but to hear about the pain of the other is a prime example for 'being in doubt'. In her inquiry based on a well-founded analysis of Amnesty-International-files, Scarry argues, that the experience of pain hints to a kind of basic inseparability of knowledge and experience of a human being, therefore pain is enormously difficult to describe in words. So the pain felt and expressed by the other is not possible to conceptualize in an accessible way for understanding from the third person's perspective. But that doesn't matter for reliability, because we do understand and normally accept that one is in pain[17], it's just a kind of artificial problem in the technical bound medicine. But it shouldn't be, if the first person's perspective also counts as reliable in medicine. Why should the feelings of a person and her individual perceived signs of illness or deprivation be less trustworthy than a deficit or disease measured actually by another person (the physician) or by a measuring instrument or machine?

In the following I want to propose a helpful triad of criteria for medicine to take into account in every decision whether one is a 'patient' or not and to make less mistakes in diagnosis and therapy. Without doubt, all these three factors are 'subjective', but also measurable when taking fuzzy measures. So it would be possible to integrate the first person's perspective in a formalized way. That is necessary in order to consider *adequately* the real and special situation of the individual and his own experience.

---

16 [6], pp. 161ff.

17 [7], §293, 302, 303, 350: Here he discussed with a discerning eye the question of communicating and understanding the pain of the other.

7.2.3 Some Remarks on the Application of Fuzzy Sets – To Improve Diagnostics and Therapy for Individuals

The usual indicator factors for illness and intervention are quantifiable data of dysfunctions, physiological anomaly, non-standard incidents of the patient's body, etc. – all these moments we can take honestly from the third person's perspective. In addition to those, I would propose the following three indication marks to specify diagnostics and improve therapy for individuals.

This would allow integrating decisive and individual factors in diagnosis and therapy – not only from an ethical point of view, which would have more or less no impact on medical practice. But it would be possible to take in account as fuzzy sets the individual experienced und personal rated (1.) degree of pain or suffering: $d(p)$, (2.) also the degree of handicap or limitation: $d(h)$, and (3.) the degree of necessity of intervention: $d(n)$ – a measure resulting from subjective assigned factors like: individual purpose, estimated enhancement, improvement of living conditions, for example.

To explain how useful and significant for example these three indication points could be, let me go back to the nose-problem example. From an assumed objective point of view (from the third person's physician perspective) my nose seems to be dysfunctional structured.

But (1.) I was never adversely affected by this; (2.) I was not handicapped by this in real life; this would have been a limitation to me if I would ever have wanted to become a great trumpet player or diver. But (3.) I didn't target this kind of career. So there was no reason for the surgery and intervention.

A further example could shed light on this point. Especially significant for (2.) are some handicapped people e.g., who have almost no legs or arms by birth (contergan-child). Some of them are musicians or very successful in sports, but refuse artificial limbs, experiencing themselves not as harmed in their integrity, but entirely able to cope with their life and live their passions. Who should decide from the outside what another person fails or wants for?

Especially the importance of (1.) is actually a topic of discussion in medicine. Until this day, pain is not accepted as a sufficient indication for medical diagnosis and treatment. The feeling and suffering of pain does not count as a "disease", without measurable causation, it's no reason to take it serious enough in medical practice. Even if one suffers of chronic pain, much more than 20% of those patients don't get any treatment, about 40% of pain patients need to wait more than one year to get a therapy allotted.[18] This happens to be usual, just because feeling and suffering of pain is no accepted disease pattern in the health care sector. As a mere 'subjective' feeling and expression from the first person's perspective, it is not accepted neither in medical care practice nor in health insurance funds as an 'objective' sign of being ill and need for therapy. Things are slowly changing

[18] The official figures currently collected by a pan-European study, named "Pain Proposal", see: `http://www.efic.org` or `www.schmerzmessen.de`

through initiatives such as the "Initiative for measuring pain"[19] in Germany or the European Federation of IASP® Chapters who rally for the recognition of pain as a measurable indication and disease. But this can also be a good field of application for fuzzy set theory in future, perhaps more than the design and development of medical experts systems should be.

As Wittgenstein points out in his *Philosophical Investigations*, the first person's perspective (paradigmatically featured at the experience of pain) is not necessary less 'objectively' than the only assumed 'objective' third person's perspective. The patient's very subjective estimation of his own degree of (1.) pain, (2.) handicap or (3.) needed enhancement is also supported by the facts – but only from the very personal affected point of view. This point of reference is much closer to the empirical data of the ill body than an observer ever can get (even if he is an medical expert). Therefore no one, even not a physician, could perceive and decide as a substitute for the patient's first person's perspective.

The neutral observer's or third person's perspective in medicine, strictly speaking has the primacy only in the following case of a patient being (i) in the state of unconsciousness, or (ii) having at least no sensation, or (iii) having lost his ability to express sensations. That means, just in the case of a comatose patient (i) or in that of a severely handicapped or person in the state of shock (ii) or in the case of psychopathic person (iii) it will be required to decide exclusively from the external view of the third person's perspective on the patient's illness and the best treatment. These three cases have in common, that they point to three different ways of losing the connection to the social sphere. In these three possible cases an individual is actually isolated and no mind connected with others or social embedded in the world. In these cases, it needs the third person's perspective – precisely not as an 'objective' observer, but as a substitute for the first person's perspective, to represent the patient's probable own point of view in medical interaction. (If the person's own perspective is ignored, the interaction would be only an intervention.)

Hence, even in these cases the demand for the third person's view does not deny the primacy of the first person's point of view.

Another point to mention is, how artificial and highly questionable it would be to regard the physician as the embodied neutral observer. This might be a pre-assigned ideal, but at the same time it is presumably the most misrepresenting image in the dogmatism of institutional medicine. What the physician is doing in fact in every day practice, is coping with patients, which means interacting with living persons in individual situations. So each physician has to decide a lot of things in diagnosis and therapy from his own subjective point of view – by using his ability of empathy and intuition not as a vague, but as an experience based knowledge.

As a summary of our inquiry from an ethical point of view this paper wants also to give some hints in order "to develop a philosophy of medicine that will be tailored to the needs and interests of the patient" (§12.4), as Sadegh-Zadeh says.

[19] "Initiative Schmerz messen", a task group of physicians, which developed a fuzzy scale reading to make pain measureable individually – with a scale from 0 (no pain) to 10 (heaviest pain), see: `http://www.schmerzmessen.de/schmerz-messen/so-funkionierts.html`

To break new ground in treating patients as individuals it would be necessary to assign physicians to following duties:

- to show respect for the singularity of a person and its unique case, based on an attitude of acceptance of the primacy of the first person's perspective
- to take in account the "bio-psycho-social and moral"-factors and their interplay, that defines the patient as an individual, not to focus so much on the details and data mining that makes him countable for the models of medical disease
- to allocate more time to explore the patient's own narrative and trying to understand him in his own perspective of illness and hope
- to attach greater significance to the presence and continuity of the physicians in medical care
- at last it requests much more space and tolerance for self-defined privacy and retreat in hospital and rehabilitation.

7.3 Outlook: Why the Physician Basically Can't Be Replaced by a Medical Expert System. An Analogy

To assume, that – let us say – in some decades time, the physicians will be replaced by a medical expert system, is the same kind of assumption like: in about 50 years we'll be able to forecast a soccer game and its result. Such prophecies arise from the brief believe in the art and ability of computation, in order to render the whole complexity of such a interplay from the knowledge of the decisive data and all information we'll have about each player and therefore of the resulting game.

Even if we improve our measure methods and if we'll be able to quantify all 'information' (depending on language, context, method features) about each player – and even if we'll achieve to simulate a set of possible actions and interactions, it's basically not possible to forecast the real action neither the interaction and interplay of the whole participants that we'll happen in fact in a certain moment.

But in respect of a soccer game, no one believes seriously that it will be possible to forecast its result by computers at any time – and not many people really want to believe this. Why?

We know by intuition and by experience-based knowledge what a game is – and perhaps that's the reason, people love it, because of its underdetermined and just-open, thus 'future opened' character. Although in the case of medical expert systems, the wish to believe in calculating and forecast is much higher – refusing to see the analogy. The patient himself as "a bio-psycho-social agent" is also an each time individual and non-linear working system of high complexity. To be an individual and to be regarded as it in medical care situations, means a person to be taken as what it actually *is*: an open networking interplay of the organism parts which are in a permanent interaction and decision making situation with the psychological and social interactions one person is permanently involved. Therefore it won't be possible to render it and decide about diagnosis and therapy by computing in 'medical expert systems'.

References

1. Cassell, E.J.: The Nature of Suffering and the Goals of Medicine. Oxford Univ. Press, New York (2003)
2. Dreyfus, H.L.: Being-in-the-World: A Commentary on Heidegger's Being and Time. MIT Press, London (1991)
3. Heidegger, M.: Grundprobleme der Phänomenologie. In: Gander, H.-H. (ed.) Gesamtausgabe, 2. Abteilung: Vorlesungen 1919-1949, Band 58, 1992. 2. Verlag Vittorio Klostermann, Durchgesehene Auflage, Frankfurt a. M. (2010)
4. Maturana, H., Varela, F.: Autopoiesis and Cognition: The Realization of the Living. Boston Studies in the Philosophy of Science, vol. 42 (1980)
5. Sadegh-Zadeh, K.: Handbook of Analytic Philosophy of Medicine. Springer, Dordrecht (2011)
6. Scarry, E.: The Body in Pain. Oxford University Press, New York (1985)
7. Wittgenstein, L.: Philosophical Investigations, 3rd Revised edn. Blackwell Publishers, Cambridge (1963); translated by Gertrude Elizabeth Margareth Anscombe

8

Epistemology of Medical Knowledge

Clara Barroso

> "For, equally with the rest of science, therapeutics is based exclusively on its own facts, which must be observed and investigated for themselves, and judged on their own merits; and which can rarely be predicated at all, never with certainty, in advance of experience. We must, it is true, first find out what is wrong with exactness, before we can rectify that wrong."
>
> C. Radcliffe Hall: President's Address. British Medical Journal, 1860.

8.1 Introduction

There have been many attempts to define the limits between science and art within Medicine ever since it was established as a socially acknowledged, specialised practice. Despite these attempts, the questions regarding the epistemological statute of this discipline are not completely resolved, which presents an added difficulty when proposing how to develop computer models and applications capable of representing this area of knowledge. The appearance of an evidence-based practice (EBP) model which can guide new conceptions of Medicine and its practice has sparked further discussion on what kind of knowledge constitutes Medicine. ([1], also [6].)

This article reviews some of the historical milestones in the field of Medicine in order to discover what kind of knowledge constitutes the discipline and proposes a systemic interpretation of Medicine as an epistemological resource to justify and understand the different kinds of knowledge that, in our opinion, constitute the body of expert knowledge in this field.

The way Medicine is approached in this work is not linked to every cultural background; it reviews the milestones that have given rise to the knowledge recognised as 'medicine' in our cultural background, obviating contributions that in other cultures and in other periods of development have given rise to therapeutic practices, some of which are still used today. In other words, this article analyses knowledge that, in the development of 'science', has given rise to what is denominated Medicine in our culture.

R. Seising and M.E. Tabacchi (Eds.): *Fuzziness and Medicine*, STUDFUZZ 302, pp. 123–132.
DOI: 10.1007/978-3-642-36527-0_8

Finally, Professor Karem Sadegh-Zadeh's book is a stimulus and an opportunity to reflect upon the epistemological statute of medical knowledge and its impact on the analysis and development of medical knowledge engineering.

8.2 Science and Medicine

Like other scientific areas, Medicine began its development from a fundamentally mechanistic tradition that depended on the subjectively observable world. In this stage of development, Medicine included contingency as an argument of causality. The studies on puerperal fever carried out by Doctors Wendell-Holmes, Ignaz Semmelweis and Etienne Stéphane Tarnier are examples of this kind of argumentation. Their work in favour of hygiene during child birth is not justified by rational arguments, but rather an accumulation of evidence led them to induce that there is a relation between maternal mortality and the type of medical practice. The trial and error method which prevailed during the early stages of modern Medicine is the consequence of this inductive knowledge. The next stage in the construction of knowledge that constitutes Medicine is linked to the appearance of causal reasoning which, in contrast to the contingency reasoning, strives to explain the relationship between certain facts and the consequences that could be derived from them. Induction was replaced by deductive processes which allow consequences beyond the specific cases being studied to be explained. This stage of development coincides with the appearance of what would become basic knowledge in Medicine, guided by the principles of Positivism. Next, the first interpretative models appeared: the model based on the idea that disease stems from 'injuries' (clinical, anatomical); the model based on the belief that disease was caused by corrupted processes in the functioning of the organism (physiopathological); and the aetiological model which seeks the causes of the disease outside of the organism. Regardless of the implications of each model for medical practice, for the first time a scientific corpus was established regarding what is 'normal' and what is 'pathological'; as a result, Medicine was transformed into expert knowledge on what is normal and what is pathological. At the same time, these models sustained two principles:

- medical knowledge is based on Biology and
- only that which can be observed, measured and quantified is worthy of being considered when explaining the causes of an illness.

"In innumerable areas, medicine has succeeded by imposing the rigid and positivist model on those ideas that it accepts as true. But it has also ruled out as being deviant ideas that have later proved to be important in understanding a given problem" [4], p. 734.) In other words, Medicine took a positivist approach to knowledge that only considers knowledge certain if it is based on information that is not subject to interpretation. The later development of Biochemistry, Bacteriology, Genetics, linked to Biogenetics, and Biology, Microbiology and Histology, gave a new impulse to the kind of knowledge that would be acknowledged as the scientific fundamentals of what is called Experimental Medicine [2].

8.3 Valid Knowledge and Medicine

Positivist science tried to build reliable knowledge models, free from doubt; to develop theories founded on indisputably objective explanations. However, as a consequence to the contributions of epistemologists such as K.R. Popper (1959), and T.S. Kuhn (1962) positivist principles, which seek to provide science with criteria for truth, objectivity and neutrality, have been questioned. In opposition to the model proposed by epistemological positivism, another proposal arose defending the idea that science is knowledge that allows problems to be defined and searches for solutions to them through conventions in the scientific community using the criteria of validity. In this approach scientific knowledge is that which is valid to be used to analyse and resolve problems and whose cognitive consequences (theories) must be inter-subjectively confirmed to establish said validity. As a consequence it is accepted that:

- Knowledge is produced by perceiving areas of reality that break with previously held cognitive expectations; the search for answers to the questions that arise from this rupture is what stimulates the advance of scientific knowledge.
- Scientific knowledge is not only focused on developing knowledge, it is also concerned with answering questions that have social and human interest.

As a consequence of this new model, today science seeks to develop knowledge that is valid in terms of solving problems and which is not exclusively based on scientific neutrality and objectivity. Therefore:

- Valid knowledge is geared toward the comprehension and satisfactory resolution of problems relevant to society in a specific socio-historic moment.
- Validity is based on accepting that the knowledge used to resolve problems has varying degrees of verisimilitude; furthermore, the scientific community acknowledges that not everything is knowable but that there can be agreements on what is considered valid at a given time.
- Reality is complex and cannot be understood exclusively through the unavoidably partial processes which analyse data about reality.
- Factors which may not be taken into consideration in the initial approach to an issue could be relevant in later analyses of the problem being studied.
- There is a social component in the development of scientific knowledge that should not be underestimated when carrying out an epistemological analysis of that knowledge.

8.4 The Social Construction of Knowledge and Its Consequences for the Discipline of Medicine

In the area of Medicine, the 'valid knowledge' model recognises that purely 'objective' data interact with other cognitive realities, such as the historical and social contexts in which experts live and work. Thus, what is considered to be valid in the development of knowledge in Medicine not only varies with new advances in 'objective' medical science but also as a consequence of the interaction of this objective knowledge with other cognitive realities. This explains the existence of what Lorber and Moore described as the social construction of illness [9] in their work revealing how what is considered normal and what is considered pathological is socially constructed. Not considering medical knowledge as external from social values and interests, etc., is not new in the debate surrounding the constitution of scientific knowledge. Kuhn (already pointed out that all scientific knowledge is permeated by what he denominates 'the cognitive expectations of the ruling paradigm' and, as expert knowledge, Medicine is no exception. In every society and historical moment there are cognitive expectations that will determine how disease is conceived and its consequent diagnostics and treatments.

"We have, thus far, pointed out the requirement that the physician listen to the narrative of the particular patient and that she must have a database of reliable and accessibly organized medical case stories. What must happen next is that the highly subjective patient narrative must be heavily edited. Some features of the story will be identified by the physician as medically important. On what grounds those decisions are made are, to a significant extent, matters decided by the social construction of medicine." ([13], p. 223.)

One example of the social influence on how disease is defined can be found in the symptoms associated with 'Multiple Chemical Sensitivity' (MCS). Individuals who display certain kinds of dysfunctions are stimulating research on the existence of this syndrome and the study of possible treatments. This pathology can be interpreted as allergic reactions, toxic events or corrupted processes in the genetic, neurological or psychological area [5]. The current lack of definition for this new illness can be summed up in this 2010 study by the Spanish Ministry of Health, Social Policy and Equality, in which the experts reviewing the available scientific documentation conclude:

"The most methodologically rigorous research has found results that either put in doubt the relation between causal factors and the illness, or conclude that the relation cannot be demonstrated. In one line of research no relation was found between chemical substances and the symptoms reported by patients, neither did they find evidence of a possible initial exposure, nor any later exposures that could have brought on the illness. In a double-blind, controlled provocation study in which no differences between the groups was found, the authors concluded that it was necessary to doubt the veracity of the MCS symptoms in the majority of cases and instead consider other physical and psychiatric pathologies".

To acknowledge that Medicine, as a discipline, is not independent from society does not mean that its area of knowledge is arbitrary. In this sense, the normative role of the World Health Organisation (WHO) must be pointed out; it is similar to the role of the scientific community when it carries out inter-subjective tests on the theories and methodologies of scientific research. This normative role is similar to what in Kuhnian terms would be called the construction of the disciplinary matrix: the definition of exemplars (typical cases that describe and define an illness), correspondence rules (protocols that standardise a methodology, allowing these exemplars to be compared with specific cases) and symbolic generalizations (definition of aetiology, pandemic, epidemic, etc.) [8].

Two 'exemplar' cases we can cite are Chronic Fatigue Syndrome (CFS) and fibromyalgia. CFS had not been recognised as a physical disease (it was considered to be a psychological disorder) in the past, but now the WHO has included it as a disease in ICD-10, classifying it with the G93.3 code. Similarly, until fibromyalgia was recognised by the WHO in 1992, it had been considered 'neurasthenia'; that is, a mental and behavioural disorder and not a physical problem.

It must be pointed out that, parallel to the function exercised by the WHO (generally recognised as a valid source of knowledge), there is social and ideological pressure which influences what is and is not considered to be an illness. A good example would be the consideration of homosexuality as an disease. Despite the fact that in 1973 the American Psychiatric Association rejected the idea that it was a mental illness and in 1990 the WHO followed suit, in certain social and medical circles it is still considered to be "*a mental disorder which alters behaviour*".

Finally, experts also participate in the social construction of the conception of disease through the diffusion of information. This was starkly illustrated by the repercussion of the study by Dr. Wakefield published in *The Lancet*, [12], in which a link was established between the MMR vaccine and autism. The social alarm generated by this study provoked further research on the matter. Those later studies produced evidence that refuted Wakefield's findings and exposed his study to be scientifically unsound. However, despite the scientific community's rejection of his work due to its numerous methodological and ethical irregularities and despite the retraction by the researchers who initially supported the results of that study, there is still a sector of society that continues to accept his hypothesis. As a consequence, a fraction of experts continue to sustain the validity of this study. With this in mind, it is clear that how we conceive of what is and what is not a disease is socially constructed, and this fact reveals that subjectivity and uncertainty are indeed incorporated into the field of Medicine.

"If we obscure or discount aspects of the reality in which we engage ourselves, we are guilty of falsifying not a theory but a problem and, not surprisingly, we tend to find that the solutions we propose are infected by that falsity." ([4], p. 737.)

8.5 Experience, Perception and Uncertainty

In practice, a doctor is like an investigator who works to clarify what kind of problem they are dealing with and discover what its solution might be. In this process physicians use both objective cognitive components (knowledge of the basic sciences used in Medicine) and subjective components provided by their personal 'experience' and 'perception', the latter mediating how 'objective' medical knowledge is put into practice. Just like scientific researchers, physicians use certain theories to analyse the data and facts they are presented with. However, unlike scientific researchers, their analyses also incorporate their prior professional experiences and information related to what they are working on, factors which can also mediate how the problem is perceived and diagnosed.

For example, it would be unlikely for a first world physician to diagnose that a regular patient had a tropical disease like leprosy because it would be highly unusual for an individual from the first world to contract it and, therefore, the doctor would tend to discard it in an initial diagnosis. During the time of year when there is a great deal of pollen in the air it is easy to see why a physician could mistakenly attribute rhinitis caused by a viral or bacterial infection to an allergic reaction. When a significant number of patients are suffering from an outbreak of gastroenteritis, it is possible that a case of appendicitis could be misdiagnosed, as the symptoms are very similar to gastroenteritis. These are not examples of malpractice, but rather simple examples of how perception and prior experience mediate the way experts apply their knowledge, which is related to their ability to consider previous clinical histories as relevant.

"Once we understand why the originally simple relation between representation and the world is problematic and notice that a concept like 'signification' may offer insights in clinical practice, we begin to see the force of the pragmatist's claim that knowledge is tied to praxis-doing things. Ways of signifying serve certain ways of acting and obscure others." ([4], p. 730.) On the other hand, in addition to the data that can be obtained from blood tests, x-rays and other analyses, which allow a diagnosis to be put forth based on objective data, there is an accumulation of imprecise information with which physicians must work. The initial source of information on which a diagnosis is based comes from the perceptions that patients themselves have on their condition. However, it must be pointed out that what exactly a patient means when claiming to feel a 'strong pain' cannot be understood in an objective manner because the perception of pain is constructed subjectively and depends on the threshold for pain that an individual possesses. Similarly, information like 'discomfort' cannot be considered objectively because its meaning depends on what an individual considers to be 'normal' in daily life and the degree of variation that they understand to an altered state. At the same time, this initial source of information must be 'translated' by the physician according to previous experiences in order to identify a possible physical disorder and its aetiology. In other words, beyond the objective evidence presented by the symptoms (skin rashes, fevers, muscle pain, fatigue, etc.), the patient transmits information that must be interpreted by the physician, who then evaluates what must be considered, what could be considered and what can be directly discarded in order to make a diagnosis. This process includes uncertain factors that must be taken into account when considering the epistemological statute of Medicine.

8.6 Expert Knowledge in Medicine: A Case of Systemic Knowledge

In light of what has been described, this study proposes that Medicine constitutes expert knowledge.[1] It is emerging systemic knowledge in which different components of the discipline, with different levels of uncertainty associated to them, help to resolve the problem of how to construct valid knowledge to define disease and propose solutions in the areas of treatment and prevention. This study proposes the systemic model of building valid knowledge as a basis to justify that Medicine is expert knowledge which must consider different cognitive components in its construction. Some components come from the basic knowledge of science that it incorporates (Microbiology, Biochemistry, Biology, Genetics, etc.) and therefore share the characteristics of inter-subjective validation of these basic sciences. At the same time this basic knowledge interacts with cognitive components (experience, perception) whose validity is not established inter-subjectively. In consequence, the expert knowledge of medicine, in epistemological terms, is multiple and incorporates aspects that cannot be precisely measured.

More important than considerations on how scientific Medicine is, this study defends that different sources of (objective and subjective) information are necessary and important for the construction of expert knowledge. Consequently, Medicine is considered to be expert knowledge linked to the ability to construct systemic knowledge that emerges from the interaction between different types of information used by experts in their professional work. The occupation of experts is characterised by the development of heuristic abilities that will guide how they investigate and construct knowledge. According to the basic principles of the systemic model, this expert knowledge does not arise from an accumulation of objective information that is managed by each expert: it is the ability to self-organise the (subjective and objective) information that is considered in each case, along with the ability to assign meaning to the information, that guides the expert in his process of investigation and development of knowledge. Consequently, this field of knowledge is not free of subjectivity or uncertainty, although there are inter-subjective confirmation processes to the degree in which the validity of certain knowledge and practices is recognised by the medical community (represented institutionally by the WHO).

On the other hand, the systemic model allows the study of disease to be approached holistically. The WHO incorporates biological, psychological and social aspects in its definition of disease/health because it considers that, in addition to the aetiology of a disease, social and environmental factors that affect sick people should also be taken into consideration when investigating a disease. In this sense,

[1] In this text we will use the Systems Theory concept of "emergence". This idea supposes that interaction between components of a system causes new properties to appear in the system that do not belong to any of its components. Therefore, if the relations between the components are eliminated the emergent properties will disappear. In this work knowledge in Medicine is considered to need different components, all of which interact to create an "emergent expert knowledge in Medicine". Vid. [3].

the systemic model allows a knowledge model to be elaborated which takes into consideration different ideas, including:

- Disease and health affect an organism, not isolated organs.
- What is normal and pathological cannot be defined by universal parameters that are external to the social and environmental conditions in which they act. The organisms of patients interact with their physical and social environment and occasionally a disease cannot be separated from the physical environment in which it appears. At the same time, the perception of when an individual is considered to be sick (and therefore consults an expert on the state of their health) depends on the social context of their daily life.

From the point of view of constructing the discipline, the systemic model allows the incorporation of different areas of knowledge (identified throughout this work, regarding the different disciplines used in Medicine, as well as the objective and subjective knowledge used in medical practice) to be understood, as well as their relevance in the development of Medicine. From the point of view of working in the profession, the systemic model allows the abilities of experts in the process of constructing their field to be represented. Finally, it allows the criteria of validity linked to the resolution of problems to be incorporated, as well as uncertainty, not as a limitation of the available knowledge, but rather as an epistemological characteristic of the problems studied in the field of Medicine.

8.7 The Representation of Expert Knowledge in Medicine

There are no universal rules in the expert knowledge of Medicine, there are perspectives on how to analyse and resolve problems. From this it can be deduced that medical knowledge cannot be represented using unequivocal rules that connect evidence and standardised protocols. Until relatively recently, few defended the idea that medical knowledge could be modelled in 'expert programmes' that allowed rules to be defined with associated degrees of uncertainty[11]; however our analysis creates a new situation that is represented in the following concept map (see figure 8.1).

This representation highlights how the information that medical experts work with have different typologies. Some information is precise (laboratory tests) others are fuzzy (symptomology, subjective information provided by the patient, the subjective perception of the doctor, placement of the information provided by the patient in categories of contemporary medical knowledge, the subjective interpretation of the existence of disorders). In addition, the heuristic reasoning of the expert incorporates probability and possibility. In the case of making a diagnosis based on probability, the expert uses statistical estimation when studying cases. In the case of making a diagnosis using the criteria of possibility, the intuition of the expert intervenes. Thus, contemplating what is possible appears as a consequence of having evaluated and discarded what is probable. A possibilistic diagnosis is based on knowledge of studies and research that has been carried out on exceptional cases,

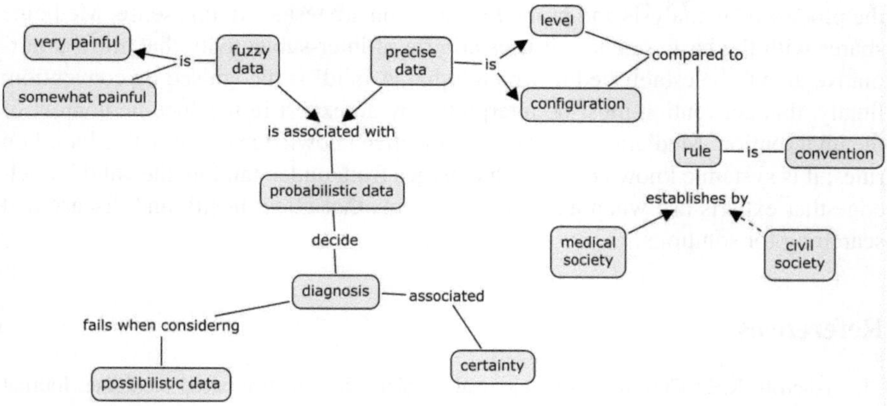

Fig. 8.1 Expert Knowledge of Medicine. Concept Map representation.

and the assumption that they are relevant to the case being considered. In other words, a diagnosis based on possibilities requires a broad understanding of exemplars and also a deep understanding of the comparative methodology that allows the correspondence rules to be used. Consequently, the representation of expert knowledge in Medicine should model reasoning based on the consideration of objective and subjective data, each with very different degrees of certainty; it should represent probabilistic and possibilistic reasoning and model the expert knowledge that emerges as a result of the interaction of all these factors. All of this is beyond the capacity of classic representation models in the area of applied informatics. As Zadeh points out, we must think about how we can represent perceptions.[15]

8.8 Conclusion

The History of Medicine reveals that there is no linear pattern of evolution of knowledge. Practices, facts and data that might have been rejected in certain moments could later emerge in different contexts and be meaningful in the development of new valid practices. The positivist model of knowledge, heavily involved in the definition of what is denominated 'experimental Medicine', does not reflect how medical knowledge and practice is really constructed. The positivist model only uses part of the knowledge necessary to understand and advance the comparison and verification of knowledge on health and disease, treatment and prevention, in the search for objectivity and certainty. Medicine is expert knowledge dealing with the resolution and prevention of health problems. The search for certainty and objectivity, just as in any other scientific field, is a goal to be strived for, but that does not mean that we must underestimate the value of knowledge and procedures that are significantly uncertain or subjective when elaborating and developing expert knowledge in Medicine. The validity of knowledge in Medicine is not indicated by objectivity, but rather by the ability to establish areas of inter-subjective comparison in which the processes of analysis and problem resolution are tested. In this sense, Medicine shares with the basic sciences it uses criteria of inter-subjectivity that allow a normative area to be established in which 'what is valid' is recognised by convention; finally, this convention must be interpreted by an expert in the specific context of the intervention. Medicine is more than objective knowledge or a practice based on rules, it is systemic knowledge which emerges from understanding the valid knowledge that experts use when analysing problems that affect health and disease and searching for solutions.

References

1. Ashcroft, R.E.: Current epistemological problems in evidence based medicine. Journal of Medical Ethics 30, 131–135 (2004)
2. Bernard, C., Greene, H.C., Henderson, L.J.: An Introduction to the Study of Experimental Medicine. Dover Publications, New York (1927) (reprinted in 1957)
3. von Bertalanffy, L.: General System Theory. Foundations, Development, Aplications. George Braziler, New York (1968)
4. Gillett, G.: Clinical Medicine and the Quest for Certainty. Social Science and Medicine 58, 727–738 (2004)
5. Simon, G.E., Daniell, W., Stockbridge, H., Claypoole, K., Rosenstock, L.: Immunologic, Psychological, and Neuropsychological Factors in Multiple Chemical Sensitivity: A Controlled Study. Annals of Internal Medicine 119, 97–103 (1993)
6. Jenicek, M.: The Hard Art of Soft Science: Evidence-Based Medicine, Reasoned Medicine or both? Journal of Evaluation in Clinical Practice 12, 410–419 (2006)
7. Kuhn, T.S.: The Structure of Scientific Revolutions. University of Chicago Press, Chicago (1962)
8. Kuhn, T.S.: Second Thoughts on Paradigms in the Structure of Scientific Theories. In: Suppe, F. (ed.) The Structure of Scientific Theories, pp. 459–482. Urbana University of Illinois Press, Urbana IL (1974)
9. Lorber, J., Moore, L.J.: Gender and the Social Construction of Illness, 2nd edn. AltaMira Press, Rowman & Littlefield Publishers, Inc. (2002)
10. Popper, K.R.: The Logic of Scientific Discovery. Hutchinson, London (1959)
11. Peter, S., Gibbon, G., Villanueva, H., Falconer, J.: Causal Reasoning in a Medical Knowledge Based System. In: Baets, W. (ed.) Proceedings of the Sixth European Conference on Information Systems, ECIS 1998, Euro-Arab Management School, Aix-en-Provence, France, pp. 1154–1165 (1998)
12. Wakefield, A.J., Murch, S.H., Anthony, A., et al.: Ileal-lymphoid-nodular Hyperplasia, Non-specific Colitis, and Pervasive Developmental Disorder in Children. Lancet 351, 637–641 (1998)
13. Currently Retracted Article, `http://www.thelancet.com/journals/lancet/article/PIIS0140673697110960/fulltext`
14. Waymack, M.H.: Yearning for Certainty and the Critique of Medicine as "science". Theoretical Medicine and Bioethics 30, 215–229 (2009)
15. Zadeh, L.A.: From Computing with Numbers to Computing with Words – From Manipulation of Measurements to Manipulation of Perceptions. IEEE Transactions on Circuits and Systems 45(1) (1999)

9

A Fuzzy-Logic Approach to Bioethics

Txetxu Ausín

"To be or not to be: that is the question. Rather, that is one question, since to be more or to be less is also a significant question."

Vásconez y Peña, "What is a Gradual Ontology?", 1996.

9.1 Bioethics

In a broad sense, Bioethics is the study of ethical controversies brought about by the advances in biology and medicine. It could be understood as a kind of "third culture", attending to the classical C.P. Snow's distinction of two cultures, between the humanities and the hard sciences. In that way, Bioethics represents a "bridge" between these two cultures, a sort of "survival science" in terms of V. R. Potter.

Anyway, Bioethics is an interdisciplinary activity, similarly to other applied ethics, since it deals with questions arising from the interactions among life sciences, biotechnology, medicine, politics, law, and philosophy.

Bioethics involves polemic issues such as euthanasia, abortion, embryonic research, human enhancement, the role of personhood and rational thinking in conferring rights and duties, or animal experimentation.

We find in the bioethical debate questions about facts (states of affairs), about definitions (categories), about reasons (arguments), and about norms (values). And it is usual to cope with them from a dichotomyzed point of view, from an "all-or-nothing" approach.

In this article we are going to argue that a fuzzy-logic approach to Bioethics is particularly fruitful in order to analyze the facts, definitions, and norms in Bioethics.

9.2 The Issue of Facts and Definitions in Bioethics

In order to defend a fuzzy-logic approach to Bioethics, I'll stand a strong ontological assumption but very reasonable from a commonsense viewpoint; that is, the gradualism of reality: Any fact, any property, any definition or category, or any state of

R. Seising and M.E. Tabacchi (Eds.): *Fuzziness and Medicine*, STUDFUZZ 302, pp. 133–143.
DOI: 10.1007/978-3-642-36527-0_9

affairs involved in bioethical debate (as in everyday life and in most sciences) is likely to have fuzzy edges and as regards borderline cases, without precise lines of demarcation [19]. This is the case to face life and death (related to euthanasia, abortion, and organ transplantation), personhood (abortion, embryonic research, hybrids, animal experimentation), health and illness,[1] ordinary treatments versus extraordinary ones, etc. etc.

In this vein, Sadegh-Zadeh [15] has remarked that most ethical rules depend on some factual circumstances which are vague states of affairs and admit of degrees to the effect that there is gradualness between their presence and absence.

> For instance, a patient's life may be endangered slightly, moderately, or severely. Similarly, the pneumonia of a patient may be slight, moderate, or severe. The lower the degree of existence of such a state of affairs X, the higher that of its complement not-X, and vice versa. X and not-X co-exist to particular extents. This brings with it that if under the circumstance X an action Y is obligatory (forbidden, or permitted) to a particular extent r, then it is not obligatory (not forbidden, not permitted) to the extent $1 - r$, respectively. Thus, an action may be obligatory (forbidden, or permitted) and not obligatory (not forbidden, not permitted) at the same time, respectively. ([15], pp. 153-154).

Remember that a property or a set is fuzzy in the sense that there are degrees of possession thereof or belonging to such a set -so that the relationship of a member belonging to a group varies in different degrees, in the same way as a property may possess it or lack it in various amounts.

This gradualism of reality is reflected in two kinds of linguistic expressions: Adverbs of intensity and decay: pretty, little, a lot, entirely, somewhat, ...; and, comparative constructions: healthier, more or less, so and so, likeness, similar, close, etc.

In the case of life and death, for example, are undoubtedly gradual (fuzzy) processes, not discrete phenomena that happen in one moment and don't happen in the next one. The issue is that we learn to recognize life (to live) and death (to die) better than to define them in a precise way. So, following Wittgenstein, recognition precedes and goes before definition and has a gradual character since we speak about "more or less life" and "more or less death", including not only the mere biological sense of life but also its biographical and narrative sense. In some languages, as Spanish, it is usual the expression "she is more dead than alive".

Another example refers to the status of personhood, about what or who is a person. We could consider two separate viewpoints: a) A person is every entity or being (material) belonging to the *homo sapiens* kind (species). b) A person is every thinking living being with reason, reflection, memory, and self-consciousness (as Locke said). The former puts at the same level any material with human DNA

[1] Health and illness are typical relational concepts or categories, with a triple dimension: empirical, psychological, and social. Sadegh-Zadeh [16] develops a theory of prototype diseases that allows for gradual membership in the category of diseases. See about this issue the contribution of Lukas Kaelin in this volume.

(like embryos) and other human and non-human entities capable of intentional psychological properties and skills (desires, interests, feelings, etc.). The latter is too restrictive since it does not recognize any privileged status of personhood to many beings that do not satisfy completely the required conditions (for example, children, disabled people, people who lost their memory, other primates, etc.). As an alternative, what is called 'personhood' in individuals can be seen as a gradual term or factor; it is not a crisp property.

In fact, as we have pointed out, what prevails in Bioethics about facts and definitions is a dichotomyzed approach which divides sets into two, separately or exclusively, as wholly or fully possessing or not a particular property. Thus, there is a profound disagreement between a continuous and a gradual reality, riddled with nuances and transitions, a reality in gray, and a logic (an analysis and description of it) bivalent, between sheer truth and complete falsehood, in "all-or-nothing" terms, black or white.

This leads us towards a critical analysis of some relevant dichotomies in Bioethics [3]. On the one hand, the issue of actions and omissions: Doing and not doing have a very different moral consideration in Bioethics. For example, in the euthanasia debate, usually it is banned active euthanasia (killing) but it is allowed passive euthanasia (letting die). Obviously, it is not the same to kill than to let die. If they were equivalent, then we would be just as (morally) responsible of the deaths that we cause as of the deaths that we do not prevent; it would be the same not to help the starved in Africa and to send them poisoned food ([7], pp. 161-162). However, the distinction between actions and omissions is more a matter of degree as it is the responsibilities they carry out. Omissions, as actions do, cause changes in the status quo and, therefore, have consequences. So, omissions are not radically different from actions and some scholars have analyzed them as a sort of 'negative actions' ([12], pp. 113-114). Thus, omissions should also be morally evaluated since omissions are not morally neutral. See, for example, the legal punishment of aid refusal; or cases of medical carelessness or negligence; or some parents who don't give food to their children. In euthanasia debate, someone as Helga Kushe [11] has defended that to kill is not always worse, and sometimes better, than to let die (in some circumstances, doctors assume that death is, from the patient's viewpoint, a benefit rather than a harm - for example, when giving up a breathing tube without deep sedation).

On the other hand, the issue of ordinary means versus extraordinary means (proportionate treatments versus disproportionate ones): A treatment will be proportionate if it offers a reasonable hope of benefit to the patient, and disproportionate if not -what is called "therapeutic obstinacy" (cruelty, futility). Related to the refusal of (burdensome) treatment, Catholic Church accepts "the right to die peacefully with human and Christian dignity" and says the following in its Declaration on Euthanasia (Sacred Congregation for the Doctrine of the Faith, 1980):

> When inevitable death is imminent in spite of the means used, it is permitted in conscience to take the decision to refuse forms of treatment that would only secure a precarious and burdensome prolongation of life.

But this distinction, which is considered morally significant, is not an abstract distinction on the different treatments; it is, rather, a distinction on the proportion of the benefits that treatment can offer, which will depend on the patient's situation. The key element is the 'degree' of benefit and welfare which may be provided with such an action or omission.

In short, facts, states of affairs, and categories in Bioethics are fuzzy and, therefore, should be treated in a fuzzy way. As Sadegh-Zadeh [14] says, "everything in medicine is fuzzy". In the case analyzed before, that on euthanasia, all other relevant features involved in it, apart from actions and omissions, and ordinary and extraordinary means, come in degrees too: terminalness, painfulness, unbearableness, and so on.

9.3 The Issue of Reasons and Argumentation in Bioethics

As we have said, Bioethics involves polemic issues and controversies since its starting point is the pluralism of society about preferences, interests, doctrines, and diverse conceptions of goodness. The other element involved in Bioethics is uncertainty, the issue of how to manage risks. The answer is clear: by means of discussion, by the public debate and the exercise of public reason, which imply a strong argumentative exchange.

Argumentation in Bioethics includes two main kinds of argumentative schemes that have a fuzzy and gradual character: Analogies and Slippery Slope Arguments. Let's see them in detail.

9.3.1 Analogies in Bioethics

Analogy has its root in the Greek word 'analogia', which means understanding as proportion, correspondence, and resemblance. It is the process of transferring information from a particular subject (the analogue or source) to another particular subject (the target). Thus, an analogy establishes an interrelation between two different spheres or domains; it enables us to see aspects of a particular domain in the light of another domain. In short, we can define analogy as similarity in some respects between things that are otherwise dissimilar; or as a comparison based on such similarity.

Analogies have two main functions, interconnected: a) Epistemic: An explanatory function, to shape our perceptions and conceptualizations (comprehension) of phenomena. b) Moral: An argumentative function, to guide us in our handling of phenomena, to argue how things should be, by comparison with others. This double sense of analogies is patent in Bioethics. Let's present some examples. In the case of abortion, there are some very well known analogies used in the debate [10]. The Violinist Analogy is one of those examples:

> You wake up in the morning and find yourself back to back in bed with an unconscious violinist. He has been found to have a fatal kidney ailment, and the Society of Music Lovers has canvassed all the available medical records and found you alone have the right blood type to help. They have therefore kidnapped you, and last night the violinist's circulation system was plugged into yours, so that your kidneys can be used to extract poisons from his blood as well as your own. The director of the hospital now tells you, "Look, we're sorry the Society of Music Lovers did this to you -we would never have permitted it if we had known. But still, they did it, and the violinist now is plugged into you. To unplug you would be to kill him. But never mind, it's only for nine months. By then he will have recovered from his ailment, and can safely be unplugged from you.

The rationale here is: A woman who carries in her womb an unwanted child is like a person who is forced to remain connected to the circulatory system (body) of another unconscious person in order to keep her alive. This analogy refers to the possibility of abortion in case of pregnancy against own will (for example, in the case of rape).[2]

Another realm in Bioethics where the use of analogies is relevant concerns the moral status of non-human animals:

> It may come one day to be recognized, that the number of legs, the villosity of the skin, or the termination of the os sacrum, are reasons equally insufficient for abandoning a sensitive being to the same fate. What else is it that should trace the insuperable line? Is it the faculty of reason, or perhaps, the faculty for discourse?...the question is not, Can they reason? nor, Can they talk? but, Can they suffer? Why should the law refuse its protection to any sensitive being?... The time will come when humanity will extend its mantle over everything which breathes...[3]

The issue is that most of the no-human animals -at least those who are closer to us in evolutionary terms (for example, apes)- have similar, analogous interests, preferences, and sensations (pain, fear) than humans do. However, their moral status is radically different.

---

[2] Another example related to the moral justification of abortion is the following:

Suppose you find yourself trapped in a tiny house with a growing child. I mean a very tiny house, and a rapidly growing child -you are already up against the wall of the house and in a few minutes you'll be crushed to death. The child on the other hand won't be crushed to death; if nothing is done to stop him from growing, he'll be hurt but in the end he'll simply burst open the house and walk out a free man. ... However innocent the child may be, you do not have to wait passively while it crushes you to death. Perhaps a pregnant woman is vaguely felt to have the status of house, to which we don't allow the right to self-defence. But if the woman houses the child, it should be remembered that she is a person who houses it.

[3] Jeremy Bentham (1748-1832), *Introduction to the Principles of Morals and Legislation*.

> We must fight against the spirit of unconscious cruelty with which we treat the animals. Animals suffer as much as we do. True humanity does not allow us to impose such sufferings on them. It is our duty to make the whole world recognize it. Until we extend our circle of compassion to all living things, humanity will not find peace.[4]

In analogies we use comparative expressions such as more or less, so and so, likeness, similar, near, close,... which have and undoubtedly gradual and fuzzy character. In fact, the degree of similarity between the analogue and the target gives weight to the analogy.[5]

9.3.2 Slippery Slope Arguments

Another example of fuzziness in bioethical argumentation is the case of slippery slope arguments. This kind of argumentation resembles the old Arabian proverb: If the camel once gets his nose in the tent, his body will soon follow. Slippery slope arguments state that a relatively small first step inevitably leads to a chain of related events culminating in some significant impact, much like an object given a small push over the edge of a slope sliding all the way to the bottom. That is, taking certain step may be fraught with indirect results which could eventually turn out disastrous -not as an unavoidable outcome, but as a quite possible upshot. Slippery slope arguments could be understood as a kind of presumption: Once that certain step has been taken, there is a presumption that some kind of pressure towards further steps may quite possibly be hard to resist, the thus triggered process yielding a bleak result.

Slippery slope arguments are far from being necessarily fallacious. What alone is fallacious with some slippery slope arguments is wording them as if they were conclusive, non-defeasible or deductively valid reasoning allowing a strong rejection of the proposal and thus closing the discussion [20]. In Bioethics, slippery slope arguments operate as a kind of 'precautionary principle': Caution in advance, a measure taken beforehand against possible danger or failure (risk).[6]

For example, a typical slippery slope argumentation in the euthanasia debate is the following:

---

[4] Albert Schweitzer (1875-1965), *The Philosophy of Civilization.*

[5] A deep study about the use of analogies in Bioethics is devoted to the case of biobanks [6].

[6] Precautionary principle has two main elements: 1.- An expression of a need by decision-makers to anticipate harm before it occurs. Within this element lies an implicit reversal of the onus of proof: under the precautionary principle it is the responsibility of an activity proponent to establish that the proposed activity will not (or is very unlikely to) result in significant harm. 2.- The establishment of an obligation, if the level of harm may be high, for action to prevent or minimise such harm even when the absence of certainty makes it difficult to predict the likelihood of harm occurring, or the level of harm should it occur. The need for control measures increases with both the level of possible harm and the degree of uncertainty. The problem with precautionary principle is the spreading of a culture of fear.

> A person apparently hopeless ill may be allowed to take his own life. Then he may be permitted to deputize other to do it for him should he no longer be able to act. The judgment of others then becomes the ruling factor. Already at this point euthanasia is not personal and voluntary, for others are acting "on behalf of" the patient as they see fit. This may will incline them to act on behalf of others patients who have not authorized them to exercise their judgment. It is only a short step, them, from voluntary euthanasia (self-inflicted or authorized), to directed euthanasia administered to a patient who has given no authorization, to involuntary euthanasia conducted as a part of a social policy. ... The dangers of euthanasia are too great to all to run the risk of approving it any form. The first slippery step may well lead to a serious and harmful fall.[7].

It is usual to identify the sorites (paradox of the heap) type of slippery slope arguments with the vagueness of key concepts or terms. In the discussion on euthanasia, Walton [20] says that slippery slope argument is due to the vagueness of expressions such as 'letting die', 'actively causing the death', 'complying with patient's willingness', and so on. However, such phrases can be used in a vague manner, but they can also be used with no vagueness. But, yet all of them denote properties which admit degrees. As we have pointed out before, all relevant features involved in euthanasia come in degrees: action, omission, terminal illness, painfulness, proportionate means, unbearableness, life, and death.

9.4 The Issue of Norms and Values in Bioethics

One of the most important issues in Bioethics is the one referring to the norms and values involved in the guidance of action. As we have seen before, controversies and hard cases are the core of Bioethics. Moral conflicts and dilemmas constitute the touchstone of Bioethics. Some have tried to minimize, or even deny, the existence of genuine moral dilemmas – in many occasions in order to avoid the acknowledgment of contradictions in the normative domain, especially among analytic philosophers of law. However, ethical pluralism, the protection of conflicting interests, the diversity of sources of obligations, casuistry itself, or even psychological answers, such as remorse or guilt, seem to incline us to accept the existence of normative conflicts [9]. So, weighing and balancing are the essential elements for rational argumentation in a contingent domain like Bioethics.[8]

In relation to bioethical dilemmas, or conflicts, given certain circumstances (with specific particular elements, with different agents involved), the choice in a particular moment of one particular precept, norm, or value over another does not cancel the one rejected. Even if it weakens it, the now rejected norm can be adopted under different circumstances. In other words, the non-applied norm still holds a degree

[7] J. Gay-Williams, [8].

[8] Leibniz coined the metaphor of "scales of reason", rooted in Aristotle's *phronesis*, to refer to this issue [2]. That concept of weighing is clearly inspired in the activities of jurists, particularly, in their 'juris-prudential' doings.

of normativity that will fade only insofar as it is not being used or in dialectical relation with its use or lack of use in ethical practice. This is especially contemplated in the case of legal norms, in which the jurist's interpretation in favor of a norm and against incompatible one does not eliminate conflict, since it does not necessarily cause its revision or derogation.

This way of normative reasoning would provide reasonable justified 'inclinations' in favor of one of the pans of the scale or one of the points of view at stake. This amounts to an inclination that is consistently non-definitive, non-conclusive, and revisable (*incliner sans necessiter*, in Leibniz' words).

All the previous invite us to a gradualist and fuzzy analysis of normative qualifications, values, and principles. The sense is a sort of 'modest' reason, typical in Bioethics, where moral reasoning should be related to circumstances and situations, against the oversimplification of the moral realm and against the 'tyranny of principles' [17]. The goal is 'practical wisdom', rejecting 'moral geometry' in the line of a new casuistry, which does not offer 'prescriptions' or 'recipes' but upholds the necessity of the analysis, weighing and evaluation of circumstances; it is, basically, 'prudent'.

As a result is that deontic qualifications are a matter of degree: Licitness, prohibition, and duty should be treated as gradual notions. From this perspective, a particular action can have a more or less degree of licitness and to the extent that it is not completely licit, it will have some degree of illicitness. In words of Sadegh-Zadeh [15], [16] it is usual and possible to compare the deontic strenght of different norms (on the basis of fuzzy deontic sets). This comparative notion of obligation would be based upon a fuzzy concept of obligation (permission, forbiddance). By fuzzifying deontic qualifications, norms may be ranked according to the degree of normativeness (obligatoriness, permission, prohibition) of what they prescribe. This approach, Sadegh-Zadeh says:

> [It] also enables a method by which (i) to interpret and reconstruct situations concerning the superiority of one legally protected interest over another by introducing a rank order of norms that are relevant in a given circumstance, and (ii) to introduce a comparative relation of performance order for diagnostic-therapeutic actions in clinical medicine. ([15], p. 153).

The core of our type of analysis is the principle of graduation, according to which, when two facts are similar, their deontic treatment must also be similar. The principle of graduation concerning norms leads to the rejection of the idea that rights, duties, and prohibitions, that is, moral or juridical matters (bioethical issues), are "all-or-nothing" issues. This entails an anti-absolutist approach to human rights and duties, which are unconditional but not absolute. Graduation leaves room for flexibility and adaptability when dealing with particular and contingent circumstances in the bioethical debate, and it gives an important role to prudence -understood as reasonableness- in the bioethical domain. From a normative point of view, this gradualist approach brings in an ingredient of malleability and flexibility, which rehabilitates, in some ways, a certain spirit closer to Anglo-Saxon common law. This leads us to develop a soft deontic logic based on transitive logic, a fuzzy-paraconsistent nonconservative extension of Anderson & Belnap's relevant logic E [5], [1]. Moreover, our approach to deontic realm is fact-sensitive. Norms and facts are partly interdependent - despite Hume's and Moore's qualms and strictures. What norms are in operation is not an issue entirely independent of what facts happen in the world. And the other way round. There is certain solidarity between facts and norms. Facts can abolish norms. So, we reject the sharp dichotomy between facts and norms [13]: Many duties and permissions are contingent on facts, that is, they arise only because (to the extent that) certain facts or circumstances exist. Otherwise, there would be no such duty or permission (whether moral or legal) [4].

9.5 Conclusion

There is a profound disagreement between a continuous and gradual reality [deontic and ontological], riddled with nuances and transitions (a reality in gray), and a logic (an analysis and description of it) bivalent, between sheer truth and complete falsehood, in "all-or-nothing" terms, black or white, without any gray area.

As an alternative to the 'principle of bivalence' that permeates the standard approach to reality in general, and Bioethics in particular, we maintain the 'principle of gradualism', which argues that everything is a matter of degree and therefore a fuzzy-logic approach is an appropriate theoretical method in Bioethics. However, gradualness is not the same as vagueness or lack of precision. It is not "indifference" about truth-value, but determination of a different kind: by degrees, neither exhaustive nor strong, with transitions and edges more or less blurred. Moreover, the fuzzy approach to the world is much more precise than that offered by their sharp and drastic correlates -which yield a simpler and more simplistic view. Otherwise, speech that uses fuzzy terms brings us closer and better to reality with adverbs of intensity and decay and comparative constructions.

Nevertheless, fuzzy logic does not benefit relativism (moral or epistemological) in any way, it highlights truth's relational character. Thereby the opposition between 'truth' and 'opinion', which has been a matter of concern in Western thought since pre-Socratic times, is rejected as irrelevant and confusing ([18], p. 40). In a fuzzy calculus, propositions take their truth-value in the interval $[0,1]$. Consequently, the notion of 'truth' can be 'modulated', as it happens in ordinary experience and argumentation, so that 'true' and 'false' have lost their static and abstract character.[9]

The notions of weighing (norms and values) as well as those of comparison and similarity (analogies) take place in a gradual manner, by means of transitions instead of leaps or breaks. So, the fuzzy approach to Bioethics entitles us to soften the sharp dichotomies usually stated about bioethical issues, as the well-known ones mentioned above (actions vs. omissions; ordinary means vs. extraordinary ones; proportionate vs. disproportionate).

[9] The relational notion of truth is closely similar to the ontological and moral views of Dewey's pragmatism.

The main consequence of the fuzzy approach to Bioethics is that it allows us to cope with thousands of dilemmas that arise in our discipline in a way less wrenching, traumatic, and arbitrary than the "all-or-nothing" approach. For example, it allows us rethinking about ethical and legal debates on the limits or boundaries of life (abortion, euthanasia) that presuppose a sharp and clear definition of the beginning and end of life and, thus, a sharp, clear, and absolutely different normative qualifications (and punishments) for very close, complex, and similar facts and situations. Consequently, similar behaviours and situations can receive a similar normative (ethical and legal) treatment, in the sense of the elementary principles of fairness and proportionality.

Acknowledgement. This work has been carried out within the project "The Limits of Precautionary Principle in Contemporary Ethical and Legal Praxis" (FFI2011-24414) funded by the Spanish Ministry of Economy and Competitiveness.

References

1. Anderson, A.R., Belnap Jr., N.D.: Entailment. The Logic of Relevance and Necessity. Princeton University Press, Princeton (1975)
2. Ausín, T.: Weighing and gradualism in Leibniz as instruments for the analysis of normative conflicts. Studia Leibnitiana XXXVII(1), 99–111 (2005)
3. Ausín, T., Peña, L.: Derecho a la vida y eutanasia: Acortar la vida o acortar la muerte? Anuario de Filosofía del Derecho XV, 13–30 (1998)
4. Ausín, T., Peña, L.: Arguing from Facts to Duties (and Conversely). In: van Eemeren, F., et al. (eds.) Proceedings of the Fifth Conference of the International Society for the Study of Argumentation, Sic Sat, Amsterdam, pp. 45–47 (2003)
5. Ausín, T., Peña, L.: Soft Deontic Logic. In: Seising, R., Sanz González, V. (eds.) Soft Computing in Humanities and Social Sciences. STUDFUZZ, vol. 273, pp. 163–178. Springer, Heidelberg (2012)
6. Bermejo-Luque, L., da Rocha, A.C.: Antonio Casado da Rocha: Bancos, bibliotecas y cementerios: Usos de las analogías en el razonamiento sobre biotecnologías. Theoria 71, 195–212 (2011)
7. Foot, P.: The Problem of Abortion and the Doctrine of Double Effect. In: Steinbock, B., Norcross, A. (eds.) Killing and Letting Die. Prentice-Hall, NJ (1980)
8. Gay-Williams, J.: The Wrongfulness of Euthanasia. In: Munson, R. (ed.) Intervention and Reflection: Basic Issues in Medical Ethics. Wadsworth, Belmont CA (1979)
9. Gowans, C.W.: Moral Dilemmas. Oxford University Press, Oxford (1987)
10. Jarvis Thompson, J.: A Defence of Abortion. Philosophy & Public Affairs 1(1), 47–66 (1971)
11. Kushe, H.: Why Killing is not Always Worse – and Sometimes Better – Than Letting Die. Cambridge Quarterly of Healthcare Ethics 7(4), 371–374 (1998)
12. Meyer, J.-J.C.: A Different Approach to Deontic Logic: Deontic Logic Viewed as a Variant of Dynamic Logic. Notre Dame Journal of Formal Logic 29(1), 109–136 (1988)
13. Putnam, H.: On the Collapse of Fact/Value Dichotomy and Other Essays. Harvard University Press, Cambridge (2002)
14. Sadegh-Zadeh, K.: The Fuzzy Revolution: Goodbye to the Aristotelian Weltanschauung. Artificial Intelligence in Medicine 21, 1–25 (2001)

15. Sadegh-Zadeh, K.: Fuzzy Deontics. In: Seising, R., Sanz, V. (eds.) Soft Computing in Humanities and Social Sciences. STUDFUZZ, vol. 273, pp. 141–156. Springer, Heidelberg (2012)
16. Sadegh-Zadeh, K.: Handbook of Analytic Philosophy of Medicine. Springer, Dordrecht (2012)
17. Toulmin, S.: The Tyranny of Principles. The Hastings Center Report 6, 31–39 (1981)
18. Trillas, E., Alsina, C., Terricabras, J.M.: Introducción a la lógica borrosa. Ariel, Barcelona (1995)
19. Vásconez, M., Peña, L.: Qué es una ontología gradual? Ágora 15(2), 29–48 (1996)
20. Walton, D.: Slippery Slope Arguments. Clarendon Press, Oxford (1992)

10

A Philosophical Anthropology of Medicine: The Split Subject

José Lázaro and Juan C. Hernández-Clemente

10.1 Introduction

Sadegh-Zadeh's magnificent *Handbook of Analytic Philosophy of Medicine* is designed in such a way that even those who are not specialists in logic and analytical philosophy can advance through its pages finding, on every one, all the theoretical resources needed to understand those that follow. This chapter tries to pose some issues belonging to our own intellectual world that fall outside the bounds of Sadegh-Zadeh's book but that, in our opinion, radically affect the essence of the problems he is dealing with.

The most distinguished philosopher of medicine we have had in Spain, Pedro Laín Entralgo (1908-2001), conceived in his youth a grand intellectual project, which he did not succeed in putting into practice directly, but which indirectly made sense of all the impressive work he carried out in the course of his long life. [6] This project consisted in creating a Philosophical Anthropology applied to Medicine. [5]

His goal was to construct a grand theory of the human being in sickness and in health. This philosophical concept of the human individual would form the basis of reflection on the theoretical foundations of language, rationality, ethics and technique with which one group of humans (medical doctors) try to help the rest to keep their health and fight illness. Laín Entralgo's philosophical references, mainly German and Spanish, were pure examples of what the Anglo Saxons call "continental philosophy": Dilthey, Scheler, Heidegger, Ortega y Gasset, Eugenio d'Ors, Zubiri. citecit:Entralgo1984

In the "Introduction" to Sadegh-Zadeh's book, he lists the kind of questions he is going to be dealing with: "conceptual, logical, linguistic, methodological, epistemological, moral and metaphysical issues". He naturally makes no mention of philosophical anthropology, a branch of the purest continental philosophy that lies at the furthest reaches of analytical philosophy.

Our speciality is not philosophical anthropology either, but medical humanities. In fact, we consider ourselves two modest specialist in building bridges between

R. Seising and M.E. Tabacchi (Eds.): *Fuzziness and Medicine*, STUDFUZZ 302, pp. 145–153.
DOI: 10.1007/978-3-642-36527-0_10

different specialisms: medicine, psychology, psychopathology, psychoanalysis, history, social sciences, continental philosophy, linguistics and, above all, the one we believe best links and relates them all: theoretical and practical narrative, literature.

All we are going to do, therefore, is suggest a hypothesis concerning the concept of "rationality", based on three texts by great authors of the 19th and 20th Centuries: George Frazer, grandfather of anthropology, novelist Marcel Proust and linguist Roman Jakobson.

The thesis we shall put forward can be summed up in three points:

1. In analyzing human thinking we come first to what can be described as "classical rationality", which respects the classical principles of identity and lack of contradiction.
2. But there is a set of linguistic phenomena (psychotic delirium; the discourse of dreams; the incipient language of infants; magical thinking; poetry...) that do not respect those basic principles of classical rationality. It is nevertheless possible to see reason in them by analyzing (as well as the classical rationality they partly contain) the mechanisms of metaphorical and metonymical association to be found in their structure. We shall call the dynamic governing this other component of much communication "poetic or associative rationality".
3. The human conversations that can be observed in every day life are an expression (in varying proportions) of classical and poetic (associative) rationality. It is not possible to account for all the different forms of our thought and our language without including this double component of what, together, could be called "human rationality" or "generalized rationality".

The underlying idea is that the history of western culture offers us two very different models of the human subject. The first is whole, open, natural, clear and distinct, simple, spontaneous, rational, sincere, transparent to him or herself, the Cartesian subject.

The second model is that of the split subject, dark, artificial, paradoxical, complex, repressed, multiple, contradictory, ironic, emotional, suspecting he or she is constantly playing tricks and having tricks played on him or herself. This second model (result of the slow digestion by European philosophy throughout the 20th Century of the triple impact of Marx, Nietzsche and Freud) is the subject of what has been called the "philosophy of suspicion". This is the one that interests us and that this chapter will discuss.

We shall mention two real situations, taken from every day life.

1. A doctor talks, in a hospital corridor, with the son of one of his patients. Although he has not said so openly, he already knows that she is gravely ill with a malignant tumor. Showing her son a piece of paper he has in his hand, the doctor says: "We've just received the results of your mother's autop... biopsy".
2. A lecturer in History of Medicine writes on the blackboard the title of the class on ergotism, a terrifying medieval illness that present day doctors are lucky not to have to see. He notices smiles and whispers among the pupils, a little unusual. He continues with his explanations but the stir among the pupils grows. When

he gets annoyed and asks the students to respect the tragic tale he is telling, one of them puts his hand up and points to the board: "Sir, it's that you've written 'eroticism'".

The mechanism of these lapses (one tragic, the other comic) is obvious: the doctor and teacher consciously wish to transmit a particular message and go about choosing the logically appropriate words and arranging them in the right order. At a certain point in their speech an unforeseen slip brings catastrophe. One of the words they want to pronounce is suddenly replaced by another that they had not summoned up deliberately.

There is a very clear phonetic analogy between the dropped word and the one that suddenly appears: biopsy-autopsy (in Spanish *biopsia-autopsia*), ergotism-eroticism (in Spanish even closer: *ergotismo-erotismo*). But the tiny difference between two similar signifiers produces a radical change in meaning: what the individual consciously wanted to say is supplanted by something else that he says unintentionally. And this something else is so authentic, so indiscreetly sincere, that both the person speaking and anyone listening are immediately and simultaneously convinced that what was said involuntarily is much closer to the truth than what was intended.

The mechanism by which it has been said is the brusque substitution of one signifier by another, similar but with a very different meaning from that foreseen. This happens in the middle of a perfectly well thought out speech that was meant to follow a plan of *classical rationality*, the kind that allows you to say what you consciously want to say. But the desired speech is suddenly ambushed by an another kind of rationality: a *rationality of wild association* which has the effect of making you say what you didn't consciously want, however true it may be.

Human rationality is the result of the interaction between *classical rationality* and *associative rationality*.

10.2 Delirious Thought

In one of his works, the Spanish psychiatrist Manuel Cabaleiro Goas records the story of a patient who, as he entered the doorway of his home, found a broken bottle in a puddle of red wine. His mind lit up and "everything became perfectly clear to him". He understood, without any doubt, that the bottle proved he was going to be killed and his blood spilled. "What I had just seen in the doorway revealed everything to me. In a few seconds all was explained to me, without any room for doubt". ([1], p. 977)

If someone enters the doorway of their home and finds a broken bottle in the middle of a red-coloured, alcoholic smelling stain, the most likely thing for him to say is: "a neighbor has dropped a bottle of wine and it has stained the doorway". This is a logical application of classical rationality.

But if he has a sudden illumination, the dazzling and certain revelation that the bottle and the stain prove his life will be destroyed and his blood shed, he has left classical rationality behind, made an arbitrary interpretation, gone mad. Classic psychopathology, represented by authors such as Kurt Schneider, [10] regards this kind of phenomena as delirious perceptions.

There are other forms of rationality that cannot strictly be considered classical either but that do not go as far as to be psychotic: the discourse of dreams, of certain literary works (such as the surreal) or of magical thinking.

Then there is the famous Shakespeare line: "*Though this be madness, yet there is method in it.*" (*Hamlet*, act II, scene II). To say that there is method in madness is like saying that there is a certain coherent structure to it, a certain rationality. Though it may not be classical. Though it may be poetic, that is to say associative.

Poets are not mad. At least not all of them. But between poetic and psychotic discourse there is a common element: they are two different ways of applying associative rationality. It is known that in the early days of 1889, as he sank into the madness from which he would not return, Nietzsche wrote a series of letters signed "The Crucified", but also "Dionysius", in which he identified with various famous figures (including God himself) and claimed to have attended his own funeral twice. ([8], pp. 173-176.) A few days later Nietzsche entered the asylum. He had lost his sanity through wanting to be both Nietzsche and God, through trying to be both alive and dead at the same time. It is clear that Nietzsche had gone mad but it could also be said that there was method in his madness, that his delirium could be regarded as the product of another kind of rationality and analyzed in terms of this. ([4], pp. 197-201.)

There is nothing strange in itself about the structure of the thought of Cabalerio's patient (or that of Nietzsche, who collapsed in Turin): the leap from a broken bottle to one's own life being broken or from a wine stain to a blood stain is nothing more than an association of ideas based on a relation of analogy.

We could regard them as two simple metaphors, if it were not for a series of accompanying circumstances (the absolute certainty with which the meaning imposes itself, its imperviousness to any kind of reasoning, its extravagance, its idiosyncratic nature) that lead to the conclusion that there is something more behind these metaphorical analogies.

The patient was a psychotic because, unlike what would have happened with his neighbors, the broken bottle did not merely symbolise but was his broken life and the wine stain was not a metaphor for a blood stain but rather the identities of the wine and the blood were confused. For him the wine was the same as the blood, it absolutely was blood, and this confusion of two distinct identities is what allows us to state that he was not creating a metaphor but suffering delirium. In his madness he has lost control over the mechanisms of analogical association, but they still have a certain coherence that makes them intelligible, a coherence that arranges the relationships between signifiers (image of broken bottle, image of red liquid) and significances (destroyed life, spilt blood).

It is possible that, if the madness progresses, the coherence and relative complexity of this structure may fall apart to leave only a simple association of signifiers without any comprehensible significance, signifiers that would continue to stem from a mechanism of analogical association but would now be nothing more than a series of similar sounds.

Psychotic language offers us an extreme example of a kind of rationality that has left logic behind and taken on other, associative mechanisms. But it is not the only case offered by clinical medicine of oscillation between classical and poetic rationality.

10.3 The Rationality of Magical Thinking

Medicine, as an experimental science, tries to work with classical rationality, whose rules allow ideas to be communicated clearly, coherently and unequivocally. But it is constantly being interfered with by the other kind of rationality, which uses the association of ideas by analogy (metaphor) and contiguity (metonym) in a very lax way: associative or poetic rationality.

Both in clinical practice and in other areas of daily life there are many examples (not as extreme as delirium) of association by analogy or contiguity bursting in on reasoning, sabotaging its logic with wild associations. This is the case with many beliefs in folk medicine, rooted in what has traditionally been called "magical thinking".

In his classic work *The Golden Bough*, first published in 1890, James George Frazer described this magical thinking, which he considered an erroneous mechanism of arbitrary association of ideas, typical of primitive mentalities. [3] His openly scornful tone towards these mentalities has earned him deserved reproach. But the description he offers is still of interest. According to Frazer, there are two sorts of what he called "sympathetic magic", each based on a type of association.

Firstly there is what he calls "homeopathic or imitative magic", based on the law of similarity by which "like produces like"; it can be deduced (arbitrarily), from the fact that two things are analogous, that one is cause and the other effect and that it is therefore possible to act on something simply by imitating it. This gave rise to the widespread belief that it is possible to harm an enemy by working on a wax doll in his or her likeness, pinching the doll's eyes to blind the enemy, piercing its heart to provoke a heart attack, afterwards shrouding it as though it were a corpse and giving it a ritual burial to be rid of it once and for all.

Then there is another kind of link, that of contiguity, that gives rise to another kind of magic: "contaminating or contagious magic". This is based on the principle that things that have once been in contact can continue to act on each other afterwards, so that an object can be manipulated to cause an effect on a person or animal that has previously been in contact with it. The groom who, when he sees that a horse has hurt its hoof on a nail, picks up the nail, cleans it and greases it for several days to prevent the foot from festering, is working on this principle. ([3], p. 68)

Amongst the enormous amount of casuistry collected by Frazer there are plenty of therapeutic applications of magical thinking. One of his examples even shows the combined use of the two basic types of association of ideas: analogy and contiguity:

"A cure for a tumor, based on the principle of homoeopathic magic, is prescribed by Marcellus of Bordeaux, court physician to Theodosius the First, in his curious work on medicine. It is as follows. Take a root of vervain, cut it across, and hang one end of it round the patient's neck, and the other in the smoke of the fire [so the two pieces are alike but have also been in direct contact]. As the vervain dries up in the smoke, so the tumor will also dry up and disappear."

This most interesting technique also guarantees that the doctor will collect his fee, as the prescription ends by saying:

"If the patient should afterwards prove ungrateful to the good physician, the man of skill can avenge himself very easily by throwing the vervain into water; for as the root absorbs the moisture once more, the tumor will return." ([3], p. 40)

Wittgenstein noted in his Observations on Frazer's 'Golden Bough': "When I read Frazer I'm always wanting to say: 'all these processes, these changes in meaning, we still have them before us in our spoken language'". ([12], pp. 69-70.) But Frazer himself had already pointed out that the "reasonings" he had described are "two different and mistaken applications of the association of ideas" and that "the order to be found in magic is only a generalization or extension by false analogy of the order in which ideas present themselves to our minds". ([3]p. 797.)

10.4 The Two Levels of Human Rationality

The associative mechanisms set off in psychotic delirium or magical thinking are also to be found, to a lesser extent, in many psychic processes that no one regards as pathological, such as the curiously winding paths of memory.

To demonstrate this we have only to recall the well-worn cliché of Proust's famous madeleine, the starting point for the long chain of associations we know as *In Search of Lost Time*. In the opening pages of part one Proust shows how language is an unfurling of memory. This begins when a perception of the present awakens the evocation of certain perceptions of the past. Proust's narrator, now an adult, is one day given a cup of tea with a madeleine by his mother. And when the taste of the madeleine, soaked in the cup of tea, reaches his mouth, a delicious pleasure invades him, dissolving his everyday cares and turning him inwards. The process of evocation has begun. A string of his soul has been plucked. The taste of the madeleine soaked in tea has acted as a trigger, unleashing a whole chain of associations. His soul turns in on itself because "that, which he seeks, is also the dark land through which he must search". ([9], p. 61.)

And the narrator does not fail to point out that this search is also an act of creation, in which the taste of the present madeleine revives the mnemic trace of other madeleines, the ones his Aunt Leonie used to give him when he was a child in Combray. This memory brings with it that of "the old grey house upon the street, where her room was" (...) "and with the house the town, from morning to night and in all weathers, the square where I was sent before lunch, the streets along which I used to run errands, the country roads we took when it was fine".

Once you succeed in unfurling the language of memory a great many things can come from the taste of a madeleine soaked in a cup of tea. The words fit together one after the other, the images contained in them calling up other images, and the discourse grows and grows until, in our chosen example, it fills seven impressive volumes.

Analogy and contiguity seem, therefore, to be the ties that bind the things whose representations are associated in the process of evocation. A taste leads to another similar taste, which in turn leads to the image of the place where it was tasted, and that image leads to a person known in that same place and then to an experience with that person, and so on, image after image, word after word, until the end of the text.

Analogy in shape or background, contiguity in time or space: these seem to be two fundamental mechanisms of human thought and language, at least when we devote ourselves to poetic evocation rather than exercises in formal logic.

The associative structures of memory (like those of magical thinking) have much in common with other kinds of everyday rationality. [11] If Proust's language backs up this hypothesis from the field of literary fiction, other discourses, taken from clinical observation (specifically of aphasias), point in the same direction.

Roman Jakobson's theory, [2] according to which speech consists of two basic and simultaneous operations, can be seen in this context. The first operation is to *select* the vocabulary: among all the more or less *similar* terms offered by the language, one is chosen (automatically discarding others), to be placed at a certain point in the speech. The second operation is to *combine* the chosen elements of language, putting them one after the other to form the line of argument.

These two operations correspond to the two chief axes which Jakobson finds in language: the paradigmatic (that of selection) and the syntagmatic (that of combination). According to this theory, aphasic disorders can be classified in two groups: those in which the capacity to associate analogous terms (and so substitute them for each other) is damaged and others in which the disorder affects the capacity to associate syntagmas by contiguity (and so combine them in the chain of speech). In the first case the patient would be incapable of metaphor, in the second of metonym.

Jakobson's theory (here summed up very briefly) confirms for us that relations of association by analogy or contiguity, found in Frazer's observations on the phenomena of magical thinking and Proust's literary evocations, are not peculiar to this kind of discourse but could become the basis for a general theory of language.

The mechanisms of metaphor (in which one term is replaced by another, similar one) and of metonym (in which it is replaced by a contiguous one), would no longer be the exclusive property of the poet or the shaman, but be integrated into our everyday language. They are not only rhetorical ornaments but foundations of its structure, so much so that they sometimes pass unnoticed, so automatically are they decoded.

So, while a teacher explains Jakobson's theory, one of his pupils may be thinking: "I hope he soon stops droning on and I can go for a pint". To do this he doesn't need to stop and analyze the metaphorical analogy between a monotonous hum and a metalinguistic lecture, nor the relationship of metonymic contiguity that allows him to call the liquid, generally alcoholic, served in this measure, "a pint".

The more or less arbitrary associations between images related by analogy or contiguity are therefore, far from being a characteristic peculiar to psychotic or magical thinking, at the very heart of human language. Every day when we speak we are in an unstable equilibrium between the two types of rationality that make up our mental processes - and with them our linguistic processes.

When we make the effort to compose a clear, distinct argument, to formalize it, even to make it mathematical, we are leaning towards one of the faces of our language, that of classical rationality. When we surrender ourselves to poetic evocation, dreamy or drunken fantasy, when we are possessed by obsessive rumination or delirium, we veer to the other side.

Whether fascinating or terrifying, this is obviously deeper, the one that lies behind, the one that was there before. But when we aim for all round intelligibility (and in particular an all round intelligibility of what the words are saying) we have to pay equal attention to both levels of rationality, integrating them into a genuinely human rationality, a generalized rationality.

Every speech has to be understood by evaluating its balance between both kinds of rationality and, from the rationality that allows us logical understanding, we have to enter as far as possible into poetic rationality and interpret it, if we want also to hear what unreason is trying to say, or at least listen to it as far as it is intelligible.

We shall be able to do this much better, the more open we are to rational understanding of the dual rationality of language. The dual rationality that allows us to grasp Pythagoras' Theorem but also a poem by Baudelaire. The dual rationality that allowed Descartes to write (and us to enjoy) the *Discourse on the Method*, but that also allowed the Spanish film maker Luis Buñuel to conceive (and us to "understand") the cinematic game of free association entitled *The Phantom of Liberty*.

Acknowledgement. This paper is included in the research project FFI-2008-03599.

References

1. Cabaleiro Goas, M.: Temas psiquiátricos, vol. II. Paz Montalvo, Madrid (1966)
2. Jakobson, R.: Dos aspectos del lenguaje y dos tipos de trastornos afásicos. In: Jakobson, R., Halle, M. (eds.) Fundamentos del Lenguaje, 2nd edn., Madrid, Ayuso (1973)
3. Frazer, J.G.: La rama dorada, 12 reimp. Fondo de Cultura Económica, Madrid (1989) (1st edn. 1890)
4. Berrios, G.E., de Diego, F.F.: Delirios y enunciados: la 'doble articulación lógico-retórica'. In: Delirio. Historia, Clínica, Metateoría, Trotta, Madrid (1996)
5. Laín Entralgo, P.: El autor habla de sí mismo. In: Obras. Editorial Plenitud, Madrid (1965)
6. Laín Entralgo, P.: Descargo de conciencia (1930-1960). Barral Editores, Barcelona (1976)
7. Laín Entralgo, P.: Antropología médica. Salvat, Barcelona (1984)
8. Nietzsche, F.: Correspondencia. Labor, Barcelona (1974)
9. Proust, M.: En busca del tiempo perdido. 1. Por el camino de Swann, 5 edn. Alianza, Madrid (1975)

10. Schneider, K.: Psicopatología clínica. Fundación Archivos de Neurobiología, Madrid (1997)
11. Trías, E.: Metodología del pensamiento mágico. In: Teoría de las Ideologías y Otros Textos Afines, pp. 109–221. Península, Barcelona (1970)
12. Wittgenstein, L.: Observaciones a La Rama Dorada de Frazer. Tecnos, Madrid (1992)

Part III

Models, Methods, and Representation

11

Automatic Linguistic Report on the Quality of the Gait of a Person

Alberto Alvarez-Alvarez and Gracian Triviño

Abstract. Gait analysis has been explored thoroughly during the last decade as a behavioral biometric measurement. Some areas of application include: access control, surveillance, activity monitoring and clinical analysis. Our work aims to contribute to the field of human gait modeling by providing a solution based on the computational theory of perceptions. Our model differs significantly from others, e.g., based on machine learning techniques, because we use a linguistic model to represent the subjective designer's perceptions of the human gait process. This model is easily understood and provides good results. Using accelerometers included in a smart phone, we propose a method for producing a linguistic report about the quality of the gait in terms of homogeneity and symmetry. This type of reports could be used to analyze the evolution of the human gait after a recovery treatment and also for preventing falls in elderly people.

11.1 Introduction

Human gait is a quasi-periodic phenomenon which is defined as the interval between two successive events of the same foot. Its analysis has been explored thoroughly during the last decade as a behavioral biometric measurement. Some areas of application include: access control, surveillance, activity monitoring and clinical analysis. Moreover, since the gait is a complex integrated task which requires precise coordination of the mental and musculoskeletal system, its analysis can help in the diagnosis and treatment of walking and moving disorders, identification of balance factors and assessment of clinical gait interventions and rehabilitation programs.

Our work aims to contribute to the field of human gait modeling by providing a solution based on the computational theory of perceptions. Our model differs significantly from others, e.g., based on machine learning techniques, because we use a linguistic model to represent the subjective designer's perceptions of the human gait process. This model is easily understood and provides good results. Using accelerometers included in a smart phone, we propose a method for producing a

R. Seising and M.E. Tabacchi (Eds.): *Fuzziness and Medicine*, STUDFUZZ 302, pp. 157–171.
DOI: 10.1007/978-3-642-36527-0_11

linguistic report about the quality of the gait in terms of homogeneity and symmetry. This type of reports could be used to analyze the evolution of the human gait after a recovery treatment and also for preventing falls in elderly people.

The remainder of this work is organized as follows. Section 11.2 presents the human gait modeling problem and our proposal for tackle it. Section 11.3 describes how to automatically generate a linguistic report on the quality of the gait based on the features obtained by our modeling system. Finally, Section 11.4 draws some conclusions and introduces some future directions in this research line.

11.2 Gait Modeling

11.2.1 Proposal

Human gait modeling consists of studying the biomechanics of this human movement aimed at quantifying factors governing the functionality of the lower extremities. Gait is a complex integrated task which requires precise coordination of the neural and musculoskeletal system to ensure correct skeletal dynamics [15]. Therefore, its analysis can help in the diagnosis and treatment of walking and movement disorders, identification of balance factors, and assessment of clinical gait interventions and rehabilitation programs [8, 11].

The gait cycle is a periodical phenomenon which is defined as the interval between two successive events (usually heel contact) of the same foot [5]. It is characterized by a stance phase (60% of the total gait cycle), where at least one foot is in contact with the ground, and a swing phase (40% of the total gait cycle), during which one limb swings through the next heel contact (see Fig. 11.1). These phases can be quite different between individuals but when normalized to a percentage of the gait cycle they maintain close similarity, indicating the absence of disorders [12].

We base on the accelerations produced during the human gait cycle. We use a expert knowledge based fuzzy finite state machine (FFSM) as a modeling tool, which has also been used to extract relevant features for the authentication purpose [14]. The main advantage of using this tool is its flexibility when dealing with the variations in both amplitude and states time span. The fuzziness of the model allows us to handle imprecise and uncertain data which is inherent to real world phenomena in the form of fuzzy if-then rules. Moreover, the use of linguistic terms makes easier its interpretation and does not require high computational cost thanks to the lack of a learning process. Nevertheless, there exists the possibility of making use of an automatic machine learning technique to design the main elements of the FFSM as explained in [1].

We attached a smartphone equipped with a three-axial accelerometer to a belt, centered in the back of the subject. The smartphone executes an application which provide us with the dorso-ventral acceleration (a_x), the medio-lateral acceleration (a_y), and the antero-posterior acceleration (a_z) at each instant of time. In this contribution, we only use a_x and a_y because a_z has to do with the walking speed and this speed can vary for the same person. Therefore, every record contained the three accelerations and a timestamp. Fig. 11.1 shows three different synchronized pictures. The first one (at the top) illustrates the dorso-ventral acceleration (a_x) and the medio-lateral acceleration (a_y) obtained from the three-axial accelerometer. The middle picture plots a sketch of a person representing the different phases of the gait with the right limb boldfaced. Finally, the picture at the bottom represents the time period from one event (usually initial contact) of one foot to the subsequent occurrence of initial contact of the same foot.

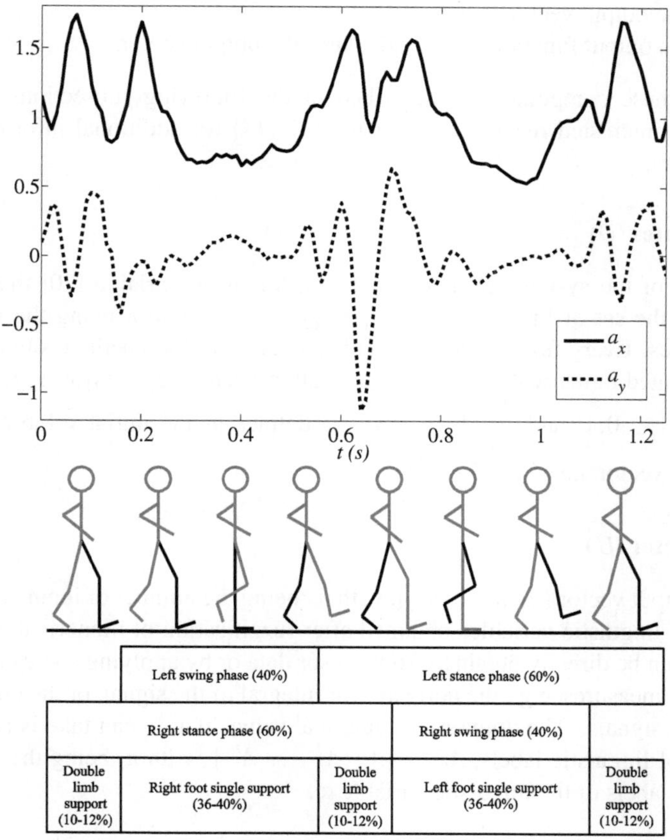

Fig. 11.1 One gait cycle illustrating the various phases and events and the dorso-ventral (a_x) and medio-lateral (a_y) accelerations

11.2.2 Fuzzy Finite State Machines

As said, we will consider a FFSM to deal with the human gait modeling problem. The theoretical basics of FFSMs were established by [13] and later developed by [6, 10, 18]. The model of FFSM presented is inspired by the concepts of fuzzy state and fuzzy system developed by Zadeh [19, 22]. More specifically, it can be considered an implementation of the input-output fuzzy models of dynamic systems proposed by Yager [17].

Here, we introduce the main concepts and elements of our paradigm for system modeling allowing experts to build comprehensible fuzzy linguistic models in an easier way. In our framework, a FFSM is a tuple $\{Q, U, f, Y, g\}$, where:

- Q is the state of the system.
- U is the input vector of the system.
- f is the transition function which calculates the state of the system.
- Y is the output vector of the system.
- g is the output function which calculates the output vector.

Each of these components is described in the following subsections. Furthermore, the interested reader can refer to [1–3, 14] for additional information and applications.

Fuzzy States (Q)

The state of the system (Q) is defined as a linguistic variable [20] that takes its values in the set of linguistic labels $\{q_1, q_2, \ldots, q_n\}$, with n being the number of fuzzy states. Every fuzzy state represents the pattern of a repetitive situation and it is represented numerically by a state activation vector $S[t] = (s_1[t], s_2[t], \ldots, s_n[t])$, where $s_i[t] \in [0,1]$ and $\sum_{i=1}^{n} s_i[t] = 1$. S_0 is defined as the initial value of the state activation vector, i.e., $S_0 = S[t=0]$.

Input Vector (U)

U is the input vector $(u_1, u_2, ..., u_{n_u})$, with n_u being the number of input variables. U is a set of linguistic variables obtained after fuzzification of numerical data. Typically, u_i can be directly obtained from sensor data or by applying some calculations to the raw measures, e.g., the derivative or integral of the signal, or the combination of several signals. The domain of numerical values that u_i can take is represented by a set of linguistic labels, $A_{u_i} = \{A^1_{u_i}, A^2_{u_i}, \ldots, A^{n_i}_{u_i}\}$, with n_i being the number of linguistic labels of the linguistic variable u_i.

Transition Function (f)

The transition function (f) calculates, at each time instant, the next value of the state activation vector: $S[t+1] = f(U[t], S[t])$. It is implemented by means of a fuzzy rule-based system (FRBS). Once the expert has identified the relevant states in the model, she/he must define the allowed transitions among states. There are rules R_{ii} to remain in a state q_i, and rules R_{ij} to change from state q_i to state q_j. If a transition is forbidden in the FFSM, it will have no fuzzy rules associated.

The generic expression of a rule to remain in a state q_i (R_{ii}) is formulated as follows: IF ($S[t]$ is q_i) $\vee$ (u_1 is $\widetilde{A}_{u_1}$) $\vee \ldots \vee$ (u_{n_u} is $\widetilde{A}_{u_{nu}}$) $\vee$ (d_i is T_{stay_i}) THEN $S[t+1]$ is q_i, where:

- The antecedent ($S[t]$ is q_i) calculates the degree of activation of the state q_i in the instant of time t, i.e., $s_i(t)$. Note that the FFSM cannot remain in the state q_i if it is not in this state previously.
- The antecedents (u_1 is $\widetilde{A}_{u_1}$) ,..., (u_{n_u} is $\widetilde{A}_{u_{nu}}$) are the constraints over the input variables to remain in the state q_i. Each $\widetilde{A}_{u_i}$ is a set of linguistic terms whose members are joined by a disjunctive operator, e.g., $\widetilde{A}_{u_1} = A^2_{u_1} \vee A^3_{u_1}$.
- The antecedent (d_i is T_{stay_i}) is a temporal constraint that calculates the membership degree of the duration of the state q_i (d_i, which is defined as the time that $s_i > 0$) to the linguistic label T_{stay_i}, which is the maximum time that the system is expected to remain in state q_i. In Fig. 11.2, can be seen an example of this linguistic label.
- Finally, the consequent of the rule is the next value of the state activation vector $S[t+1]$. It consists of a vector with a zero in all of its components except in s_i, where it has a one.

The generic expression of a rule to change form state q_i to the state q_j (R_{ij}) is formulated as follows: IF ($S[t]$ is q_i) $\wedge$ (u_1 is $\widetilde{A}_{u_1}$) $\wedge \ldots \wedge$ (u_{n_u} is $\widetilde{A}_{u_{nu}}$) $\wedge$ (d_i is T_{change_i}) THEN $S[t+1]$ is q_j, where:

- The antecedent ($S[t]$ is q_i) calculates the degree of activation of the state q_i in the instant of time t, i.e., $s_i(t)$. Note that the FFSM cannot change from the state q_i to the state q_j if it is not in this state previously.
- The antecedents (u_1 is $\widetilde{A}_{u_1}$) ,..., (u_{n_u} is $\widetilde{A}_{u_{nu}}$) are the constraints over the input variables to change from state q_i to the state q_j. Each $\widetilde{A}_{u_i}$ is a set of linguistic terms whose members are joined by a disjunctive operator, e.g., $\widetilde{A}_{u_1} = A^1_{u_1} \vee A^2_{u_1}$.
- The antecedent (d_i is T_{change_i}) is a the temporal constraint which calculates the membership degree of the duration of the state q_i (d_i, which is defined as the time that $s_i > 0$) to the linguistic label T_{change_i}, which is the minimum time that the signal is expected to remain in the state q_i before changing to the state q_j. In Fig. 11.2, can be seen an example of this linguistic label.
- Finally, the consequent of the rule is the next value of the state activation vector $S[t+1]$. It consists of a vector with a zero in all of its components except in s_j, where it has a one.

To calculate the next value of the state activation vector ($S[t+1]$), a weighted average using the firing degree of each rule k (ω_k) is computed as defined in Eq. 11.1:

$$S[t+1] = \begin{cases} \dfrac{\sum_{k=1}^{\#Rules} \omega_k \cdot (s_1,\ldots,s_n)_k}{\sum_{k=1}^{\#Rules} \omega_k} & \text{if } \sum_{k=1}^{\#Rules} \omega_k \neq 0 \\ S[t] & \text{if } \sum_{k=1}^{\#Rules} \omega_k = 0 \end{cases} \tag{11.1}$$

where (ω_k) is calculated using the minimum for the AND operator ($\wedge$) and the maximum for the OR operator ($\vee$). We used $\vee$ in R_{ii} to make more difficult the change of state, which makes the FFSM more robust against spurious in the input. Moreover, we used $\wedge$ in R_{ij} to define the conditions to change more sharply.

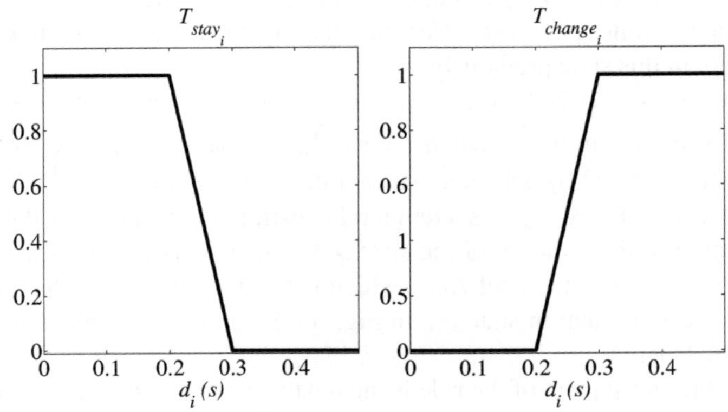

Fig. 11.2 Temporal conditions for the state q_i

Output Vector (Y)

Y is the output vector: $(y_1, y_2, ..., y_{n_y})$, with n_y being the number of output variables. Y is a summary of the characteristics of the system evolution that are relevant for the application.

Output Function (g)

The output function (g) calculates, at each time instant, the next value of the output vector: $Y[t] = f(U[t], S[t])$.

11.2.3 Fuzzy Finite State Machine for Gait Modeling

This section presents the design of the main elements needed to build a FFSM to model the human gait.

Fuzzy States (Q)

As stated in Section 11.2.2, every state represents the pattern of a repetitive situation. According to the diagram at the bottom of Fig. 11.1 and using our own knowledge about the process, we define four different fuzzy states which explain when double limb support, right limb single support, or left limb single support are produced. Therefore, we easily define the possible set of fuzzy states as follows:

- $q_1 \rightarrow$ The right foot is in stance phase and the left foot is in stance phase (double limb support).
- $q_2 \rightarrow$ The right foot is in stance phase and the left foot is in swing phase (right limb single support).

- $q_3 \rightarrow$ The right foot is in stance phase and the left foot is in stance phase (double limb support but different of q_1 because the feet position).
- $q_4 \rightarrow$ The right foot is in swing phase and the left foot is in stance phase (left limb single support).

Input Vector (U)

As we have explained, we only use two of the three available accelerations, which are a_x and a_y. Therefore, the set of input variables is: $U = \{a_x, a_y\}$. Each of these input variables will have only three associated linguistic labels because, as we will show in the experimental results, they are enough to achieve a good accuracy keeping a high interpretability of the model. The linguistic labels for each linguistic variable are: $\{S_{a_x}, M_{a_x}, B_{a_x}\}$ and $\{S_{a_y}, M_{a_y}, B_{a_y}\}$, where S, M and B are linguistic terms representing small, medium, and big, respectively.

As an initial step, we normalized the signals. First, we subtracted the average making them to be centered on zero. Then, we rescaled them in the range given by their standard deviations. This allowed us to perform the analysis at the scale that gives us more information about the signal changes.

Transition Function (f)

As showed in Section 11.2.2, the only thing required to determine the structure of the FRBS is the definition of which transitions are allowed and which are not. This is easily represented by means of a state diagram. Fig. 11.3 shows the proposed state diagram of the FFSM for the human gait cycle. This state diagram is very simple because the accelerations produced during the human gait are quasi-periodic, i.e., they are repeated with approximately similar values and periods. Moreover, all the states are correlative, i.e., they always follow the same activation order. Therefore, it is rather easy to define the allowed transitions and the forbidden ones.

From the state diagram represented in Fig. 11.3 it can be recognized that there are 8 fuzzy rules in total in the system, 4 rules to remain in each state and other 4 to change between states. In contrast to machine learning techniques, we derived the rules from the designer's perceptions about the human gait acceleration signals. We chose q_1 as the initial state, i.e., $S_0 = (1,0,0,0)$. The FFSM is able to synchronize without the need of doing previous segmentation of the signal when the conditions of q_1 are fulfilled. We defined the conditions of amplitude to remain in a state or to change between states by combining the information obtained from the sensors and the available expert knowledge about the human gait. We applied self-correlation analysis to the vertical acceleration to obtain an approximation of the signal period T. In agreement with our knowledge about the typical human gait cycle, we assigned to each state a duration according to its percentage of the period T. Fig. 11.2 shows a generic example of the linguistic labels T_{stay} and T_{change} used to define the temporal constraints.

R_{11}: IF $(S[t]$ is $q_1) \vee (a_x$ is $B_{a_x}) \vee (a_y$ is $B_{a_y}) \vee (d_1$ is $T_{stay_1})$ THEN $S[t+1]$ is q_1
R_{22}: IF $(S[t]$ is $q_2) \vee (a_x$ is $S_{a_x}) \vee (a_y$ is $M_{a_y}) \vee (d_2$ is $T_{stay_2})$ THEN $S[t+1]$ is q_2
R_{33}: IF $(S[t]$ is $q_3) \vee (a_x$ is $B_{a_x}) \vee (a_y$ is $S_{a_y}) \vee (d_3$ is $T_{stay_3})$ THEN $S[t+1]$ is q_3
R_{44}: IF $(S[t]$ is $q_4) \vee (a_x$ is $S_{a_x}) \vee (a_y$ is $M_{a_y}) \vee (d_4$ is $T_{stay_4})$ THEN $S[t+1]$ is q_4
R_{12}: IF $(S[t]$ is $q_1) \vee (a_x$ is $S_{a_x}) \vee (a_y$ is $M_{a_y}) \vee (d_1$ is $T_{change_1})$ THEN $S[t+1]$ is q_2
R_{23}: IF $(S[t]$ is $q_2) \vee (a_x$ is $B_{a_x}) \vee (a_y$ is $S_{a_y}) \vee (d_2$ is $T_{change_2})$ THEN $S[t+1]$ is q_3
R_{34}: IF $(S[t]$ is $q_3) \vee (a_x$ is $S_{a_x}) \vee (a_y$ is $M_{a_y}) \vee (d_3$ is $T_{change_3})$ THEN $S[t+1]$ is q_4
R_{41}: IF $(S[t]$ is $q_4) \vee (a_x$ is $B_{a_x}) \vee (a_y$ is $B_{a_y}) \vee (d_4$ is $T_{change_4})$ THEN $S[t+1]$ is q_1

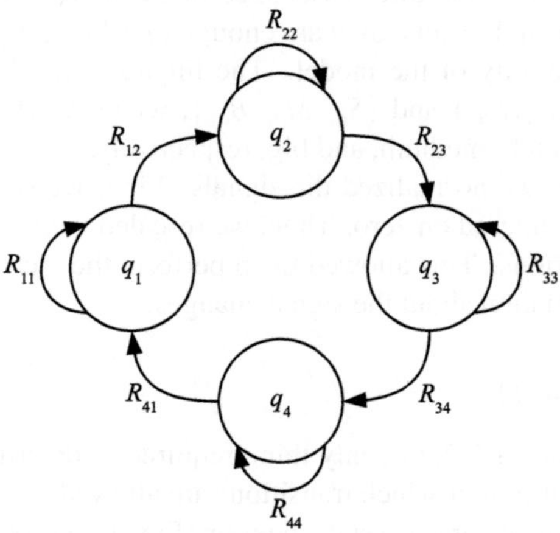

Fig. 11.3 State diagram of the FFSM for the human gait cycle

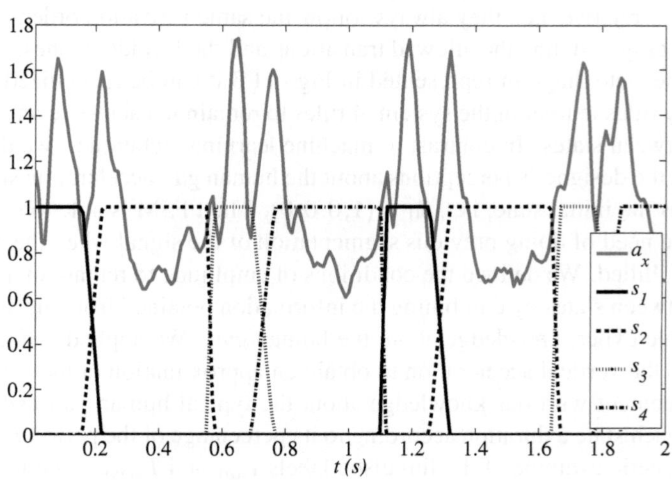

Fig. 11.4 Graphical representation of the state activation vector ($S[t]$) of the four states together with the evolution of dorso-ventral acceleration (a_x)

As an example of the performance of our proposal for human gait modeling, Fig. 11.4 represents the state activation vector ($S[t]$) of the four states together with the evolution of dorso-ventral acceleration (a_x). It shows how this set of fuzzy rules is able to model the four phases of the human gait.

Output Vector (Y) and Output Function (g)

Once identified the four phases in the signal, we focused on the characteristics of the vertical acceleration a_x, which provides sufficient information for our purpose. Fig. 11.5 shows the evolution of a_x along the four phases. The rectangles are the output of the FFSM and are calculated for each state within a complete gait cycle of duration T. Therefore, the output vector of the FFSM will be $Y = (y_1, y_2, y_3, y_4)$.

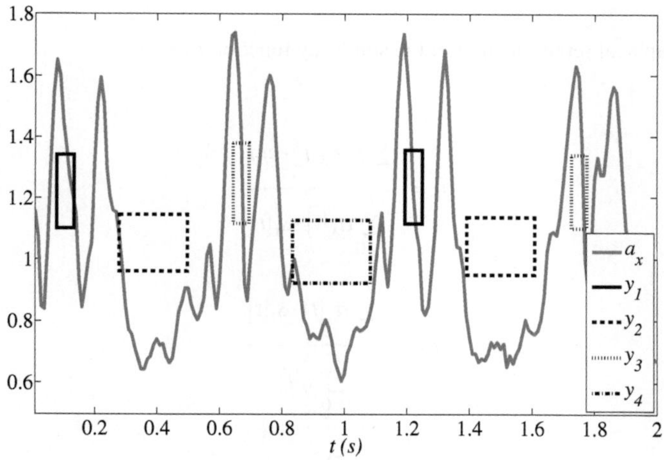

Fig. 11.5 Graphical representation of the dorso-ventral acceleration (a_x) and the rectangles that form the output of the FFSM

The dimensions of every rectangle summarize the values of the dorso-ventral acceleration (a_x) while staying in each state. The horizontal coordinate of the center of each rectangle ($\overline{t_i}$) is the temporal "center of mass" of a_x in the state q_i. Note that the "mass" in every instant t is calculated as the value of $a_x[t]$ weighted by the degree of activation $s_i[t]$ of the state q_i as shown in Eq. 11.2. The vertical coordinate of the center of each rectangle ($\overline{a_i}$) is the average of the dorso-ventral acceleration during the state q_i, which is calculated using Eq. 11.3. The width of each rectangle ($\sigma_{t_i}^2$) is the standard deviation of the temporal distribution of the dorso-ventral acceleration weighted by the degree of activation $s_i[t]$ of the state q_i as shown in Eq. 11.4. The height of each rectangle ($\sigma_{a_i}^2$) is the standard deviation of the dorso-ventral acceleration during the state q_i calculated using Eq. 11.5.

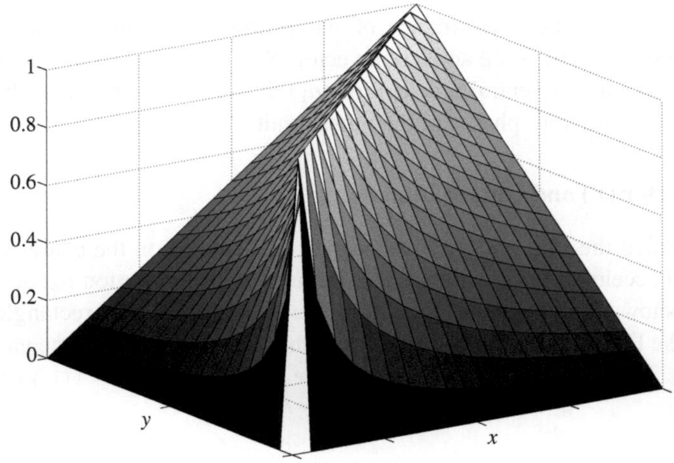

Fig. 11.6 Graphical representation of the similarity function $F(x,y)$

$$\overline{t_i} = \frac{\sum_{t=0}^{T} t \cdot a_x[t] \cdot s_i[t]}{\sum_{t=0}^{T} a_x[t] \cdot s_i[t]} \tag{11.2}$$

$$\overline{a_i} = \frac{\sum_{t=0}^{T} a_x[t] \cdot s_i[t]}{\sum_{t=0}^{T} s_i[t]} \tag{11.3}$$

$$\sigma_{t_i}^2 = \frac{\sum_{t=0}^{T} (t - \overline{t_i})^2 \cdot a_x[t] \cdot s_i[t]}{\sum_{t=0}^{T} a_x[t] \cdot s_i[t]} \tag{11.4}$$

$$\sigma_{a_i}^2 = \frac{\sum_{t=0}^{T} (a_x[t] - \overline{a_i})^2 \cdot s_i[t]}{\sum_{t=0}^{T} s_i[t]} \tag{11.5}$$

11.3 Quality of the Gait

Based on the areas of the rectangles (A^1, A^2, A^3, A^4) which summarize the values of the dorso-ventral acceleration (a_x), we have defined two parameters to measure the quality of a human gait, namely homogeneity ($\mathscr{H}$) and symmetry ($\mathscr{S}$).

Both homogeneity and symmetry are calculated using a similarity function $F(x,y)$, which is defined using Eq. 11.6 and provide values in the interval $(0,1]$. In Fig. 11.6, can be seen the shape of this function.

$$F(x,y) = \begin{cases} \frac{y}{x} & \text{if } x \geq y > 0 \\ \frac{x}{y} & \text{if } 0 < x < y \end{cases} \tag{11.6}$$

11.3.1 Homogeneity ($\mathscr{H}$)

The homogeneity ($\mathscr{H}$) is obtained by comparing a gait with itself and it is calculated for every state using two cycles. Therefore, a gait will be homogeneous for a state q_i in the cycle j if the area of its rectangle in this cycle (A^i_j) is similar to the area of its rectangle in the next cycle $j+1$ (A^i_{j+1}) as shown in Eq. 11.7. The total homogeneity for each cycle j ($\mathscr{H}_j$) is calculated as the average value of the homogeneities of the four states as shown in Eq. 11.8.

$$\mathscr{H}^i_j = F(A^i_j, A^i_{j+1}) \tag{11.7}$$

$$\mathscr{H}_j = \frac{1}{4} \sum_{i=1}^{4} \mathscr{H}^i_j \tag{11.8}$$

11.3.2 Symmetry ($\mathscr{S}$)

The symmetry ($\mathscr{S}$) is obtained by comparing the movement of both legs. Symmetry is based on comparing the areas of the rectangles which summarize the states q_1 and q_2 (stance and swing phase of the reference foot) versus the areas of the rectangles which summarize the states q_3 and q_4 (stance and swing phase of the opposite foot). A gait will be symmetric if the areas of the states q_1 and q_2 are similar to the areas of the states q_3 and q_4. The Symmetry in a cycle j ($\mathscr{S}_j$) is calculated using the similarity function $F(x,y)$ as can be seen in Eq. 11.9, where A^1_j, A^2_j, A^3_j, A^4_j are the areas of the rectangles corresponding to states q_1, q_2, q_3, and q_4 in the cycle j.

$$\mathscr{S}_j = F(A^1_j + A^2_j, A^3_j + A^4_j) \tag{11.9}$$

11.3.3 Linguistic Report

To automatically generate a linguistic report on the quality of the gait of a person, we will use the methodology proposed by Yager [16] and developed also by Kacprzyk [7], which is based in the concept of fuzzy cardinalities introduced by Zadeh [21].

The idea is to produce a set of natural language (NL) sentences of the type: "Most times the homogeneity is low" or "Few times the symmetry is high". First of all, we have to fuzzify the values of the homogeneity and the symmetry within the set

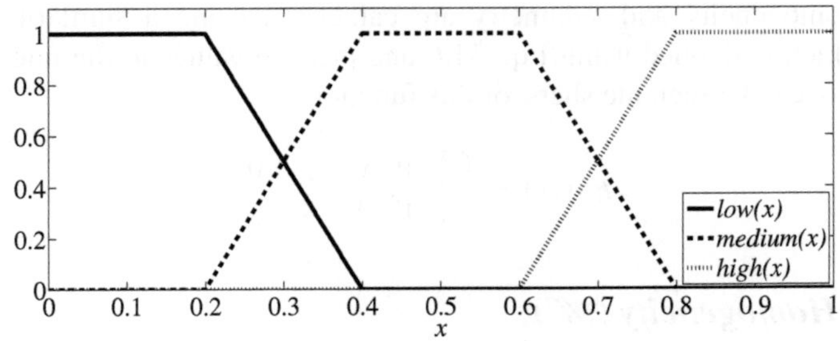

Fig. 11.7 Trapezoidal linguistic labels which fuzzify the values of the homogeneity and the symmetry

of linguistic labels represented in Fig. 11.7. Therefore, for each cycle, we will have the following set of possible NL sentences:

- "The homogeneity in the cycle j is { low | medium | high }", with validity degrees $low(\mathscr{H}_j)$, $medium(\mathscr{H}_j)$, and $high(\mathscr{H}_j)$ respectively.
- "The symmetry in the cycle j is { low | medium | high }", with validity degrees $low(\mathscr{S}_j)$, $medium(\mathscr{S}_j)$, and $high(\mathscr{S}_j)$ respectively.

Once we have fuzzified the homogeneity and the symmetry for each cycle j, we can calculate the frequency of the linguistic variables that describe the homogeneity and the symmetry along a complete gait of J cycles using the general expression of cardinality (Card) defined in Eq. 11.10. The cardinality of a fuzzy set provides us with a value in the interval $[0,1]$ than indicates how frequent is this fuzzy set. We can associate a new set of linguistic terms, which are represented in Fig. 11.8, to these values that lead us to the desired expressions such as "Most times the homogeneity is low" or "Few times the symmetry is high" whose validity degrees are $most\left[\mathrm{Card}\left(low(\mathscr{H})\right)\right]$ and $few\left[\mathrm{Card}\left(high(\mathscr{S})\right)\right]$ respectively.

$$\mathrm{Card}(x) = \frac{1}{J} \cdot \sum_{j=1}^{J} x_j \tag{11.10}$$

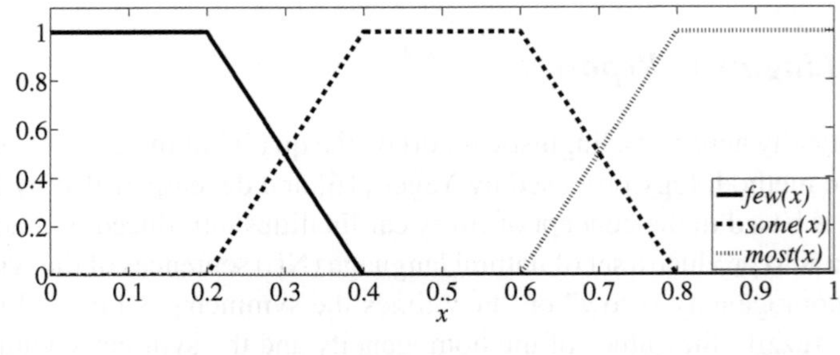

Fig. 11.8 Trapezoidal linguistic labels which fuzzify the values of the cardinality

In order to define the quality of a gait based on the validity of the NL propositions calculated previously, we have designed a FRBS which captures the expert knowledge thanks to its semantic expressiveness, using linguistic variables [20] and rules [9]. Thanks this FL formalism, when designing the fuzzy rules and linguistic labels, we can deal with isolated events of lack of symmetry or homogeneity due to turns, steps or stumbles. However, the existence of repetitive lacks of symmetry and homogeneity represents the presence of gait disorders that must be identified by the system. Therefore, the following set of fuzzy rules is aimed at qualifying the gait of a person by taking into account these issues:

R_1: If most times the homogeneity is low and most times the symmetry is low, then the quality is low.
R_2: If most times the homogeneity is medium and most times the symmetry is medium, then the quality is medium.
R_3: If most times the homogeneity is high and most times the symmetry is high, then the quality is high.
R_4: If few times the homogeneity is high and few times the symmetry is high, then the quality is low.
R_5: If few times the homogeneity is low and few times the symmetry is low, then the quality is high.
R_6: If some times the homogeneity is low and some times the symmetry is low, then the quality is medium.
R_7: If some times the homogeneity is high and some times the symmetry is high, then the quality is medium.

The output of the FRBS is calculated as a weighted average of the individual rules. The weight of each rule is calculated from its firing degree. To calculate this firing degree, we use the minimum for the *and* between the two antecedents, e.g., if the NL propositions “most times the homogeneity is low” and “most times the symmetry is low” have a validity degrees of 0.75 and 0.5 respectively, the firing degree of R_1 will be 0.5. Therefore, thanks to use of the FL formalism, we can express together with the total output the reasons of why this output is obtained.

As a practical example, consider the validity degrees of the NL propositions displayed in Table 11.1 which were obtained during 20 complete cycles for a certain person. With these values, only rules R_3, R_5, and R_7 are fired with firing degrees of

Table 11.1 Example of the validity degrees of the set of NL propositions

	few times	some times	most times
homogeneity is low	1	0	0
homogeneity is medium	0.62	0.38	0
homogeneity is high	0	0.38	0.62
symmetry is low	1	0	0
symmetry is medium	0.06	0.94	0
symmetry is high	0	0.94	0.06

0.06, 1 and 0.38 respectively. Therefore, the FRBS will conclude that the quality of the gait is medium with a validity degree of 0.26 and high with a validity degree of 0.74. Moreover, thanks to the hierarchical design of our system, we can pick up the rule with the maximum firing degree (R_5) to build the linguistic report as follows: "The quality of the gait during these 20 cycles is high because few times the homogeneity is low and few times the symmetry is low".

11.4 Concluding Remarks

This work is part of our research in the field of human gait modeling. Using accelerometers, we can obtain many information that must be interpreted in order to obtain useful conclusions about gait characteristics.

Here, we describe a quite simple and intuitive model that allows us to extract relevant features about the gait of a person. We show how the homogeneity and the symmetry of the human gait can be used to create a simple but useful model capable of describing the quality of the gait.

In collaboration with orthopedics and physiotherapist, we believe that this work opens possibilities of exploring relevant features of human gait, by combining relevant variables within the FL formalism. Moreover, the help of these specialists will allow us to refine our proposed system with the incorporation of their useful knowledge.

Acknowledgement. This work has been funded by the Spanish Government (MICINN) under project TIN2008-06890-C02-01.

References

1. Alvarez-Alvarez, A., Trivino, G., Cordón, O.: Body Posture Recognition By Means of a Genetic Fuzzy Finite State Machine. In: Proceedings of the 5th IEEE International Workshop on Genetic and Evolutionary Fuzzy Systems (GEFS), Paris, France, pp. 60–65 (2011)
2. Alvarez-Alvarez, A., Alonso, J.M., Trivino, G., Hernández, N., Herranz, F., Llamazares, A., OCaña, M.: Human Activity Recognition Applying Computational Intelligence Techniques for Fusing Information Related to WiFi Positioning and Body Posture. In: Proceedings of the 2010 IEEE International Conference on Fuzzy Systems (FUZZ-IEEE), Barcelona, July 18-23, pp. 1881–1885 (2010)
3. Alvarez-Alvarez, A., Trivino, G.: Comprehensible Model of a Quasi-periodic Signal. In: Proceedings of the 9th International Conference on Intelligent Systems Design and Applications (ISDA), pp. 450–455. IEEE Computer Society, Los Alamitos (2009)
4. lvarez-Alvarez, A., Trivino, G., Cordón, O.: Human Gait Modeling using a Genetic Fuzzy Finite State Machine. European Centre for Soft Computing Research Report: AFE 2010-2008, CGC 2010-01, Mieres, Spain (2010) (submitted)
5. Begg, R., Lai, D.T.H., Palaniswami, M.: Computational Intelligence in Biomedical Engineering. CRC Press, Boca Raton (2007)

6. Cao, Y., Ying, M., Chen, G.: Retraction and Generalized Extension of Computing with Words. IEEE Transactions on Fuzzy Systems 15(6), 1238–1250 (2007)
7. Kacprzyk, J., Yager, R.R.: Linguistic Summaries of Data using Fuzzy Logic. International Journal of General Systems 30, 133–154 (2001)
8. Lai, D.T.H., Begg, R.K., Palaniswami, M.: Computational Intelligence in Gait Research: A Perspective on Current Applications and Future Challenges. IEEE Transactions on Information Technology in Biomedicine 13(5), 687–702 (2009)
9. Mamdani, E.H.: Application of Fuzzy Logic to Approximate Reasoning using Linguistic Systems. IEEE Transactions on Computers 26(12), 1182–1191 (1977)
10. Mordeson, J.N., Malik, D.S.: Fuzzy Automata and Languages: Theory and Applications (Computational Mathematics). Chapman & Hall/CRC (2002)
11. Moustakidis, S.P., Theocharis, J.B., Giakas, G.: A fuzzy Decision Tree-based svm Classifier for Assessing Osteoarthritis Severity using Ground Reaction Force Measurements. Medical Engineering & Physics 32(10), 1145–1160 (2010)
12. Perry, J.: Gait Analysis: Normal and Pathological Function. Slack Incorporated (1992)
13. Santos, E.S.: Maxmin Automata. Information and Control 13, 363–377 (1968)
14. Trivino, G., Alvarez-Alvarez, A., Bailador, G.: Application of the Computational Theory of Perceptions to Human Gait Pattern Recognition. Pattern Recognition 43(7), 2572–2581 (2010)
15. Winter, D.A.: Biomechanics and Motor Control of Human Movement. Wiley-Interscience (1990)
16. Yager, R.R.: Fuzzy Summaries in Database Mining. In: Proceedings of the 11th Conference on Artificial Intelligence for Applications, pp. 265–269. IEEE Computer Society, Washington, DC (1995)
17. Yager, R.R., Filev, D.P.: Essentials of Fuzzy Modeling and Control. Wiley-Interscience, New York (1994)
18. Ying, M.: A Formal Model of Computing with Words. IEEE Transactions on Fuzzy Systems 10(5), 640–652 (2002)
19. Zadeh, L.A.: From Circuit Theory to System Theory. Proceedings of the Institute of Radio Engineers 50, 856–865 (1962)
20. Zadeh, L.A.: The Concept of a Linguistic Variable and its Application to Approximate Reasoning. Parts I, II, and III. Information Sciences 8, 9, 199–249, 301–357, 43–80 (1975)
21. Zadeh, L.A.: A computational approach to fuzzy quantifiers in natural languages. Computers and Mathematics 9, 149–184 (1983)
22. Zadeh, L.A.: Towards a Theory of Fuzzy Systems. In: Yuan, B., Klir, G.J. (eds.) Fuzzy Sets, Fuzzy Logic, and Fuzzy Systems: Selected Papers by Lotfi A. Zadeh, pp. 83–104. World Scientific Publishing Co., River Edge (1996)

12

Fuzziness in Medical Image Processing: Representation and Models

Miguel Pagola, Aranzazu Jurio, Daniel Paternain, and Humberto Bustince

12.1 Introduction

This chapter discusses Fuzziness in Medical Image Processing. We start summarizing different techniques of medical image acquisition and their main features. Fuzzy techniques have been widely used in the processing of all these medical images. Examining the specialized literature, we discuss the fuzziness present in these images, including:

- Fuzziness in pixel information. All medical images have a significant amount of noise, so the information of every pixel is uncertain.
- Fuzziness in model representation. Some properties of body organs, as for example size, location or shape, vary depending on each person, so it is not possible to determine an exact model of them.

One the most studied topics is the segmentation of medical images. This process is used as a previous step when creating a human body model or in the diagnosis of diseases (tumors, mental illness, ...). In this chapter we present a review of the most popular fuzzy techniques for medical image segmentation:

- Fuzzy cluster means
- Fuzzy connectedness
- Fuzzy rule based systems
- Fuzzy measures of uncertainty

Finally, we give to the reader a deeper view of the last technique of this list by presenting an example of the use of ignorance functions to segment ultrasound images.

12.2 Medical Imaging

Technical advances have allowed visualization of structures and their functions in the living human body. The interpretation of these images plays a prominent role

R. Seising and M.E. Tabacchi (Eds.): *Fuzziness and Medicine*, STUDFUZZ 302, pp. 173–190.
DOI: 10.1007/978-3-642-36527-0_12

in diagnostic and therapeutic decisions. A common definition of medical imaging is: The technique and process used to create images of the human body for clinical purposes (medical procedures seeking to reveal, diagnose or examine disease) or medical science (including the study of normal anatomy and physiology).

With the increasing size and number of medical images, the use of computers for processing and analyzing these images has become necessary. In particular, as a task of delineating anatomical structures and other regions of interest, image segmentation algorithms play a vital role in numerous biomedical imaging applications such as the quantification of tissue volumes, diagnosis, study of anatomical structure, and computer-integrated surgery. Classically, image segmentation is defined as the partitioning of an image into nonoverlapping regions which are homogeneous with respect to some characteristics such as intensity or texture.

An accurate segmentation of a medical image is necessary to determine the correct shape of a tumor or to make a 3D reconstruction of body organs. For this reason, this work focuses on fuzzy techniques for medical image segmentation. However, these techniques can also be used in denoising, superresolution or reduction of medical images.

Medical image segmentation can be tackled in very different ways due to the wide range of acquisition technologies of these images. The most used include:

- Radiography
- Magnetic resonance imaging (MRI)
- Nuclear medicine
- Tomography
- Ultrasound

Other acquisition techniques are not mentioned here, either because there are not many works in the literature related to them such us Photo acoustic imaging and Breast Thermography or because are not primarily designed to produce images but which produce data susceptible to be represented as maps (i.e. containing positional information) such as electroencephalography (EEG), magnetoencephalography (MEG) or electrocardiography (EKG).

12.2.1 Imaging Technologies

In this subsection we present a brief review of medical image acquisition technologies. An in depth study can be found in [33].

Radiography: This imaging modality utilizes a wide beam of x-rays for image acquisition and it is the first imaging technique available in modern medicine. Projectional radiographs, more commonly known as x-rays, are often used to determine the type and extent of a fracture as well as for detecting pathological changes in the lungs (see Fig. 12.1). With the use of radio-opaque contrast media, such as barium, they can also be used to visualize the structure of the stomach and intestines.

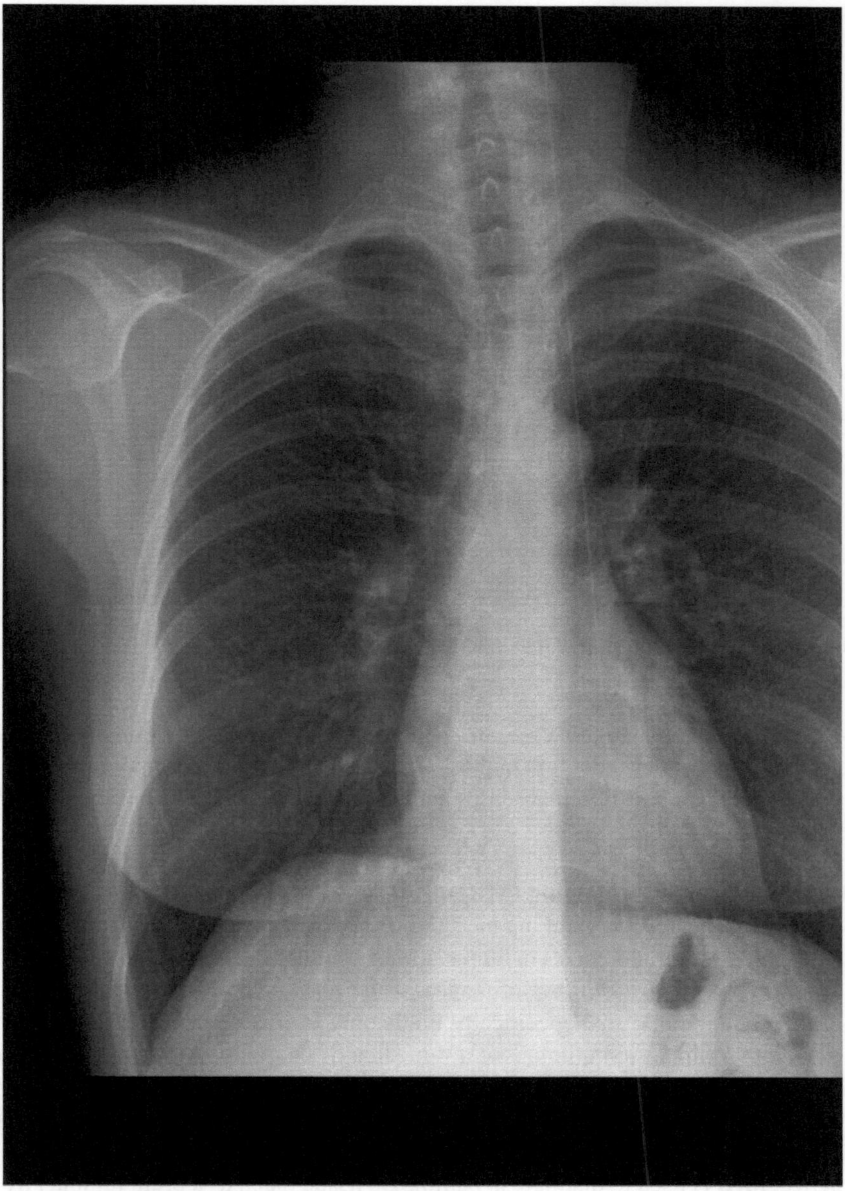

Fig. 12.1 Radiography image of the chest

Tomography: Computed Tomography (CT), or Computed Axial Tomography, is a helical tomography, which traditionally produces a 2D image of the structures in a thin section of the body. It uses x-rays. It has a greater ionizing radiation dose burden than projection radiography. CT is based on the same principles as

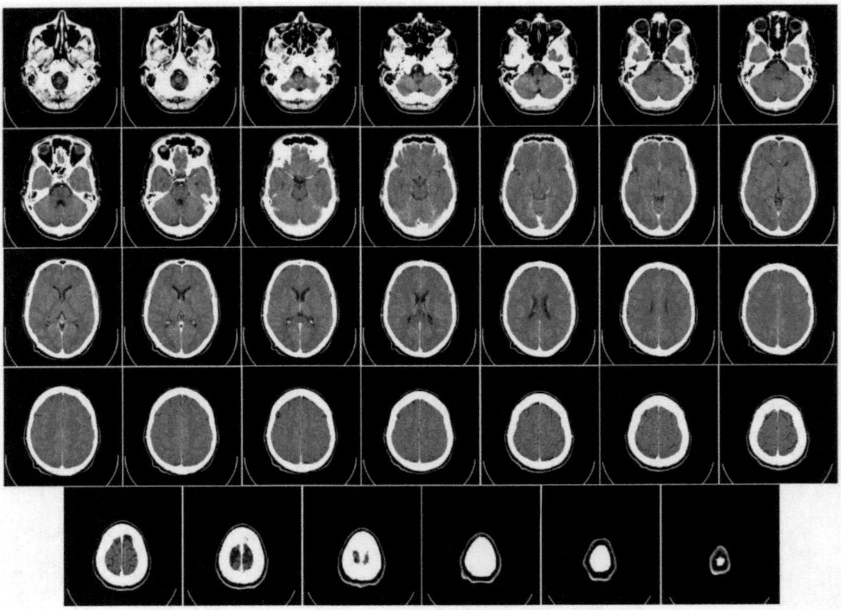

Fig. 12.2 Complete tomography image series of a brain

x-ray projections but in this case, the patient is enclosed in a surrounding ring of detectors. Since its introduction in the 1970s, CT has become an important tool and it is used to diagnose different diseases in the head (see Fig. 12.2), bones, lung, heart vessels, etc.

Magnetic Resonance Imaging (MRI): A magnetic resonance imaging instrument (MRI scanner), uses powerful magnets to polarise and excite hydrogen nuclei (single proton) in water molecules in human tissue, producing a detectable signal which is spatially encoded, resulting in images of the body. The MRI machine emits a radio frequency pulse that specifically binds only to hydrogen. MRI traditionally creates a two dimensional image of a thin slice of the body. Modern MRI instruments are capable of producing images in the form of 3D blocks, which may be considered a generalisation of the single-slice, tomographic, concept. MRI is sensitive to different tissue properties and has an excellent soft-tissue contrast. In clinical practice, MRI is used to distinguish pathologic tissue (such as a brain tumour) from normal tissue in every part of the body. MRI is an important research tool to map normal human brain (see Fig. 12.3).

Nuclear Medicine: Nuclear medicine encompasses both diagnostic imaging and treatment of diseases, and may also be referred to as molecular medicine or molecular imaging and therapeutics. Nuclear medicine uses certain properties of isotopes and the energetic particles emitted from radioactive material to diagnose or treat various pathologies. Gamma cameras are used in e.g. scintigraphy, SPECT and PET to detect regions of biologic activity that may be associated with disease. Relatively short lived isotope, such as Technetium 99mTC, Iodine 123I, Gallium 67Ga or 18F is administered to the patient. Isotopes are often preferentially absorbed by biologically active tissue in the body, and can be used to identify tumours or fracture points in bone. Images are acquired after collimated photons are detected by a crystal that gives off a light signal, which is in turn amplified and converted into an image. It is used heavily in clinical oncology (medical imaging of tumours and the search for metastases), and for clinical diagnosis of certain diffuse brain diseases such as those causing various types of dementias. PET is also an important research tool to map normal human brain (see Fig. 12.4) and heart function.

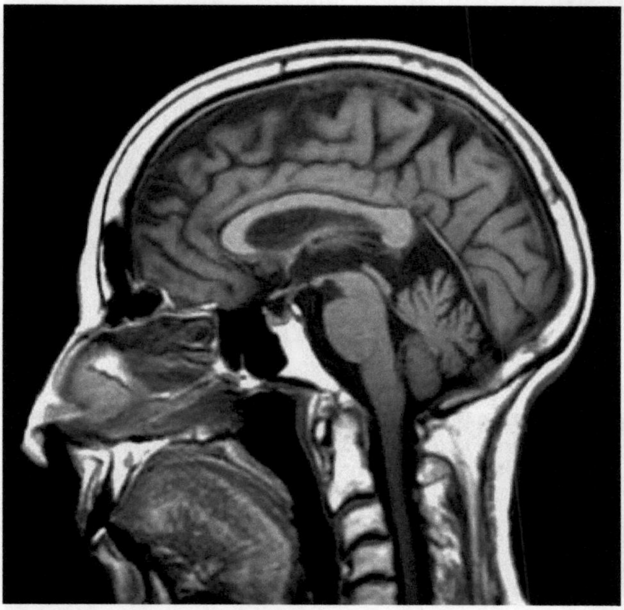

Fig. 12.3 MRI image slice of a head

Ultrasound: The ultrasound image is the result of reflection, refraction and deflection of ultrasound waves in the megahertz range, from different types of tissues with different acoustic impedance (see Fig. 12.5). Usually, the contrast in ultrasound images is very low and boundaries between region of interest and background are fuzzy. The sound wave is partially reflected from the layers between different tissues. Specifically, sound is reflected anywhere there are density changes in the body: e.g. blood cells in blood plasma, small structures in organs, etc. This is commonly associated with imaging the fetus in pregnant women. Uses of ultrasound are much broader, however. Other important uses include imaging the abdominal organs, heart, breast, muscles, tendons, arteries and veins.

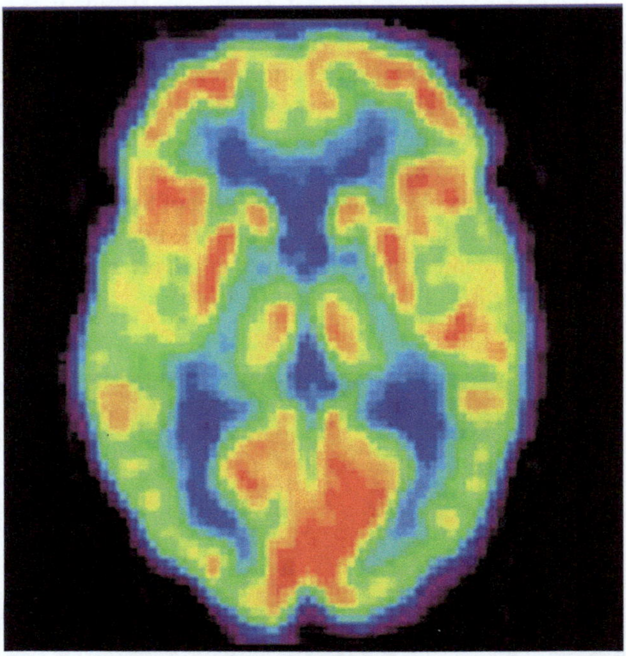

Fig. 12.4 Typical PET image slice of a brain

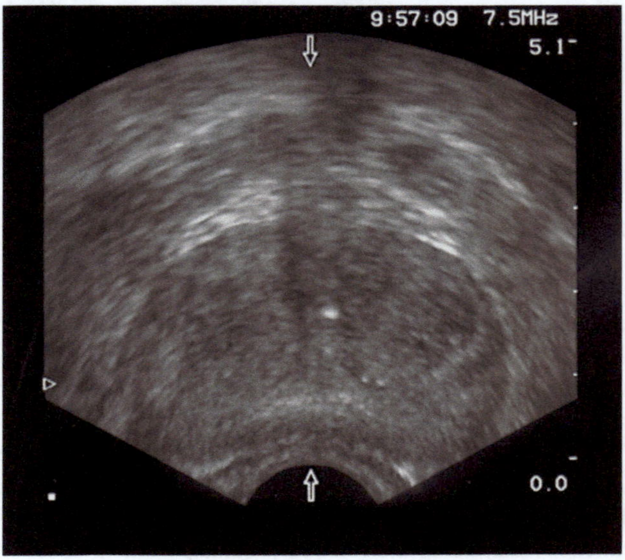

Fig. 12.5 Ultrasound image of a prostate

12.3 Fuzzy Images: Sources of Uncertainty

Despite of the variety of acquisition technologies, medical images suffer from low quality in contrast with conventional photography, that produces relatively noise-free images except where the grain of the film becomes visible. The main problems of medical images are noise and partial volume effect. These phenomena suggest to interpret them as fuzzy images.

12.3.1 Noise

All medical images contain some visual noise. The presence of noise gives an image a mottled, grainy, textured, or snowy appearance. Image noise comes from a variety of sources. No imaging method is free of noise, but noise is much more prevalent in certain types of imaging procedures than in others.

Ultrasound imaging and nuclear images (PET, SPET) are generally the most noisy. Noise is also significant in MRI, CT. In comparison to these, radiography produces images with the least noise.

- The noise in the PET image is mainly caused by attenuation of annihilation photons inside the body. Noise in photon counts are due to scattering and detection of false positive coincidendes. Also the noise in PET images is highly dependent on the reconstruction algorithm used.
- In all imaging procedures using x-ray like CT, most of the image noise is produced by the random manner in which the photons are distributed within the image. This is generally designated quantum noise. Recall that each individual photon is a quantum (specific quantity) of energy. It is the quantum structure of an x-ray beam that creates quantum noise.
- In MRI the main source of noise in the image is the patient's body (radio frecuency emission due to thermal motion). The whole measurement chain of the MR scanner (coils, electronics...) also contributes to the noise. This noise corrupts the signal coming from the transverse magnetization variations of the intentionally excited spins.
- The noise presented in ultrasound images is due to the variation in the detector sensitivity, environmental variations, the discrete nature of radiation, transmission or quantization errors, etc. This produces speckle noise and weak edges which makes difficult to identify the regions of interest.

12.3.2 Partial Volume Effect

The term partial volume effect (PVE) actually refers to 2 distinct phenomena that make intensity values in medical images differ from what they ideally should be [32].

The first effect is the 3-dimensional image blurring introduced by the finite spatial resolution of the imaging system. For example, the spatial resolution in PET images is limited by the detector design and by the reconstruction process. The resulting 3D blurring causes overlapping between regions. Because of the finite spatial resolution, the image of a small source is a larger but dimmer source. Part of the signal from the source spills out and hence is seen outside the actual source. Mathematically speaking, the finite resolution effect is described by a 3D convolution operation.

The second phenomenon causing PVE is image sampling. In PET, the radiotracer distribution is sampled on a voxel grid. Obviously, the contours of the voxels do not match the actual contours of the tracer distribution. Most voxels therefore include different types of tissues. This phenomenon is often called the tissue fraction effect. The signal intensity in each voxel is the mean of the signal intensities of the underlying tissues included in that voxel. Note that even if the imaging system had perfect spatial resolution, there would still be some PVE because of image sampling. This phenomenon is why PVE not only is an issue in PET, which has poor spatial resolution compared with other imaging modalities, but also is of concern in high-resolution imaging, such as MRI or CT.

12.4 Fuzzy Set Theory for Medical Image Segmentation

The variety of medical imagining techniques, with each own advantages and disadvantage, would make a global processing very inefficient. That is, it is not possible to develop an optimal algorithm to deal with all kind of images at the same time. However, when considering medical images as fuzzy images, we can use fuzzy techniques for image processing developed in last decades.

In this section we show a short review of fuzzy techniques most commonly used for medical image segmentation. Finally we study in depth an algorithm of image segmentation based on uncertainty measures using ignorance functions.

12.4.1 Fuzzy Cluster Means

One of the most used algorithms for medical image segmentation in the last decades is fuzzy cluster means (FCM). As we have explained in the previous section, the uncertainty present in images does not allow to know the correct intensity of each pixel. In this sense, FCM has been used to assign a membership degree of each pixel to every area (object) of the image. Besides, this is a non supervised method, so it is very useful for being used by medical staff non specialized in medical imaging.

FCM has been used for the majority of medical images and for multiple applications. A typical example is [18] where fuzzy c-means is used for segmenting breast cancer on MRI. Also it has been used in single-photon emission tomography SPET images [1] to detect dynamic neuroreceptors. Moreover it has been adapted to typical noisy and low resolution oncological PET images [6]. From retinal images [35] it has been used for the extraction of blood vessels. Among the applications, in [28] FCM has been used for automated detection of white matter changes of the brain in an elderly population or in [20] has been devoted to identify breast tissue regions judged abnormal .

Besides, FCM has been combined with other segmentation techniques as dynamic contours [2] for the segmentation of thalamus from brain in MRI. FCM has been also mixed with the FHCE frequency histogram of connected elements in mamogrphic microcalcification detection [7] and combined with Markov Random Fields for the detection of brain activation regions in Functional Magnetic Resonance Imaging (fMRI) [17].

The fact that in the standard fuzzy c-means no spatial context information is taken into account makes it sensitive to noise. Therefore there are a lot of proposals that try to solve this problem such as [30]. Other works modify the effective objective function of fuzzy c-means by replacing the Euclidean distance with kernel-induced distance [21] or with a robust kernel-induced distance [19] for clustering a corrupted dataset of breast and brain medical images. In [38] a spatial penalty on the membership functions and a kernel-induced distance metric for MRI segmentation are proposed.

12.4.2 Fuzzy Connectedness

The notion of fuzzy connectedness assigns a strength of connectedness to every possible path between every possible pair of image elements. This concept leads to powerful image segmentation algorithms [41], [34].

This methodolgy has been extensively used in medical image segmentation, for example [39] present a method to extract abdominal organs using a presegmented atlas. Another application was presented in [27] to segment phantom images, MRI, computed tomography, and infrared data. Fuzzy connectedness was combined with and edge detection for knee tissues in CT image and segmentation of brain tissues in MRI image [24].

Fuzzy conectedness has also been extended to combine methods with the concept of membership connectedness [16].

12.4.3 Fuzzy Rule Based Systems

Fuzzy rule based systems have been used to model the relations between body organs or other regions of interest by rules.

Identifying multiple abdominal organs or brain regions from medical image series is necessary for the diagnosis. To address the issue of high variations in organ position, shape and consecutive organ region overlap constraints, spatial fuzzy rules and fuzzy descriptors have been adopted in several papers [23]. Sometimes, the necessity of detecting a set of organs is called model based structural pattern recognition. In these techniques, models and data structures are based on the use of fuzzy restrictions. In [31] is presented a segmentation method of the coronary artery tree in x-ray angiographic images, based on a fuzzy structure pattern inferring. In [14] the role of the fuzzy logic is to fuse the voxel intensity information from the time of flight angiography with the corresponding vesselness information based on a designed rule base.

Application for the segmentation of brain structures in MRI and CT images, based both on atlas and real data are presented in [11]. In [22] it is proposed a method for segmenting cerebrospinal fluid and cerebral ventricles from MRI images. This method segments the cerebral ventricles by using a fuzzy If-Then rules that can implement physicians' knowledge on the ventricles, which can represent their abstract shape and position.

Another nuclear images as bone scintigraphy have been used as in [36] for the diagnosis of bone diseases with a small-sized rule base such that the resulting fuzzy rules can be easily understood by radiologists. Also the visualization of nerve fibers where investigated in [4] using fuzzy logic methods that allow better comprehension of the human brain.

Finally, hybrid techniques as a fuzzy-neural system have been developed for classifying kidney categories [29].

12.4.4 Fuzzy Measures of Uncertainty

The representation of medical images by means of fuzzy images (or fuzzy sets) allows to face segmentation problem by minimizing uncertainty measures. In this way, the result obtained with minimum uncertainty is asociated with the most accurate solution solution. For example, the main idea presented in [5] is to define the averages of a given fuzzy set by using different definitions of the mean of a random compact set. In particular, the average distance of Baddeley-Molchanov and the mean of Vorob'ev have been used. A medical image application of retinal vessel detection was performed. The Local fuzzy fractal dimension (LFFD) is proposed to extract Local fractal features of medical images [40]. The definition of LFFD is an extension of the pixel-covering method by incorporating fuzzy sets. For the segmentation of breast tumors in mammograms some measures of inhomogeneity where presented in [15]. They are computed from the pixels present in a suitably defined fuzzy ribbon and have indicated potential use in classifying the masses and tumors as benign or malignant .

Based on the idea of measures of uncertainty some authors have used extensions of fuzzy sets to represent this uncertainty. An intuitionistic fuzzy image was constructed using Sugeno type intuitionistic fuzzy generator and then a local thresholding is applied to segment medical images in [10]. Also in [12] intuitionistic fuzzy sets have been used in the segmentation of infrared images.

Next, we explain in detail how the concept of ignorance function is used as a measure of uncertainty for the segmentation of ultrasound images [9].

12.4.5 Ignorance Functions in Ultrasound Images

Ultrasound imaging is a widely used technology for prostate biopsy and brachytherapy. The accurate detection of the prostate boundaries in ultrasound images is crucial for clinical applications, such as the accurate placement of the needles during the biopsy, accurate prostate volume measurement from multiple frames, constructing anatomical models used in treatment planning and estimation of tumor border. However, the contrast in ultrasound images is usually low and the boundaries between the prostate and background are noise-corrupted and fuzzy. Speckle noise and weak edges make the ultrasound images inherently difficult to segment.

Due to the challenging nature of ultrasound images, all methods proposed in the literature are completely customized and incorporate specifically designed and tuned pre-processing techniques to prepare the image for the segmentation (generally thresholding).

The reader should bear in mind that an acceptable level of accuracy for these type of images can only be achieved by a proper developed processing chain, incorporating specifically designed and tuned pre-processing and post-processing techniques.

In Fig. 12.6 we show 10 prostate ultrasound images and their manual segmentation.

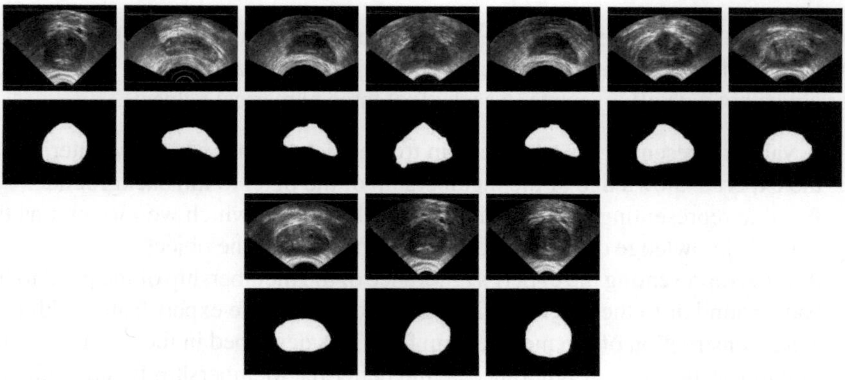

Fig. 12.6 Set of Ultrasound prostate images with their ideal segmentation made by an expert radiologist

In this study we have asked the expert to provide a point at the center of the prostate, making object detection/extraction easier. The image has been then filtered via median filter with 5×5 neighborhoods. Further, selective contrast enhancement as described in [3] has been applied to increase the image quality.

The objective of this work is to study the influence of the lack of knowledge (ignorance) of the experts with respect to the process of image segmentation. In classical fuzzy thresholding algorithms, the expert uses a single membership function to represent the whole image (see [8, 13, 25, 26, 37]). In our proposal, the expert should pick two different functions, one representing the background and another one representing the object. This representation allows the expert to better model the pixels for which he is not sure if they belong to the object or the background.

In Fig. 12.7 we show the histogram of an image and two membership functions, one to represent the background and the other to represent the object. From these fuzzy sets, in our proposal we introduce the concept of *ignorance function* G_u. Such

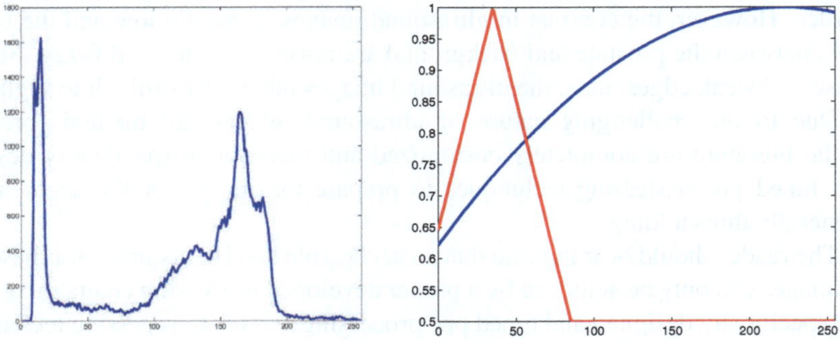

Fig. 12.7 Histogram of an image and two different membership functions to represent the background and the object

functions are a way to represent the user's ignorance in choosing the two membership functions used to represent the image (object and background). Therefore, in our algorithm we will associate to each pixel three numerical values:

- A value representing its membership to the background, which we interpret as the expert's knowledge of the membership of the pixel to the background.
- A value representing its belongingness to the object, which we interpret as the expert's knowledge of the membership of the pixel to the object.
- A value representing the expert's ignorance of the membership of the pixel to the background or to the object. This ignorance hinders the expert from making an exact construction of the membership functions described in the first two items. The lower the value of ignorance is, the better the membership function chosen to represent the membership of that pixel to the background and the one chosen to represent the membership to the object will be. Evidently, there will be pixels of the image for which the expert will know exactly their membership to the background or to the object but there will also be pixels for which the expert is not able to determine if they belong to the background or to the object.

Under these conditions, if the value of the ignorance function (G_u) for a certain pixel is zero, it means that the expert is positively sure about the belongingness of the pixel to the background or to the object. However, if the expert does not know at all whether the pixel belongs to the background or to the object he must represent its membership to both with the value 0.5, and under these conditions we can say that the expert has *total* ignorance regarding the membership of the pixel to the background and the membership of the same pixel to the object.

In [9] ignorance functions are defined in the following way:

Definition 26. *A function* $G_u : [0,1]^2 \to [0,1]$ *is called an ignorance function, if it satisfies the following conditions:*

(G_u1) $G_u(x,y) = G_u(y,x)$ *for all* $x, y \in [0,1]$*;*
(G_u2) $G_u(x,y) = 0$ *if and only if* $x = 1$ *or* $y = 1$*;*

(G_u3) *If* $x = 0.5$ *and* $y = 0.5$, *then* $G_u(x,y) = 1$;
(G_u4) G_u *is decreasing in* $[0.5,1]^2$;
(G_u5) G_u *is increasing in* $[0,0.5]^2$.

In this work a construction method of ignorance functions using t-norms and automorphisms is also presented. For example:

Example 1. Using the t-norm minimum

$$G_u(x,y) = \begin{cases} 2 \cdot min(1-x,1-y) \text{ if } min(1-x,1-y) \leq 0.5 \\ \frac{1}{2 \cdot min(1-x,1-y)} \text{ otherwise} \end{cases}$$

Example 2. Using the automorphism $\varphi(x) = \sqrt{x}$ for all $x \in [0,1]$

$$G_u(x,y) = \begin{cases} 2\sqrt{(1-x)\cdot(1-y)} \text{ if } (1-x)\cdot(1-y) \leq 0.25 \\ \frac{1}{2\sqrt{(1-x)\cdot(1-y)}} \text{ otherwise} \end{cases}$$

We call I_G the total ignorance of the image

$$I_G = \frac{1}{\sum_{q=0}^{L-1} h(q)} \sum_{q=0}^{L-1} G_u(\mu_{\tilde{Q}_B}(q), \mu_{\tilde{Q}_O}(q)) \cdot h(q) \qquad (12.1)$$

where L is the number of gray levels of the image and $h(q)$ is the number of pixels with intensity q. I_G represents the total influence of the ignorance in the construction of fuzzy sets Q_{Bt} and Q_{Ot}.

When I_G tends to zero, then

$$G_u(\mu_{Q_{Bt}}(q), \mu_{Q_{Ot}}(q)) \rightarrow 0 \text{ for all } q \in \{0,\cdots,L-1\}.$$

By the property (G_u2) we have $\mu_{Q_{Bt}}(q) \rightarrow 1$ or $\mu_{Q_{Ot}}(q) \rightarrow 1$. Therefore:

1. If $\mu_{Q_{Bt}}(q) \rightarrow 1$, then the pixels with intensity q are such that their intensity is very close to the average intensity of the pixels that represent the background. This fact enables us to assure that the pixel in question belongs to the background.
2. If $\mu_{Q_{Ot}}(q) \rightarrow 1$, then the pixels with intensity q are such that their intensity is very close to the average intensity of the pixels that represent the object. This fact enables us to assure that the pixel in question belongs to the object.

Experiment

In this experiment we compare the results of a classical fuzzy algorithm with respect to the algorithm that minimizes ignorance functions. The development tries to show that ignorance functions outperforms the results when the expert choose membership functions that do not fit the problem correctly.

We take 8 different membership functions to model the background and the object, following the expression $\mu(q) = 1 - |q - m_z(t)|^{\lambda}$ with $\lambda = 0.1, 0.3, 0.8, 1, 1.3, 2, 6, 15$, where z could denote the object or the background. For all the ultrasound images, we execute the Generalized fuzzy algorithm with two membership functions taken from the possible combinations of the membership functions (there are $8^2 = 64$ combinations). Then we execute the ignorance based algorithm using the expression given in Example 2 for all the cases, so we obtain 64 different solutions.

To interpret the results of this experiment we study the graphic in Fig. 12.8. This graphic is obtained in the following way:

1. We arrange all the cases from the smallest to the biggest percentage of badly classified pixels (error) in the solution of the fuzzy algorithm.
2. For each pair of membership functions, we calculate the error obtained with the ignorance based algorithm.

The crosses represents the error we get with the ignorance based algorithm, and the dotted line, the error we get with the fuzzy algorithm. (If the dots are under the cross, it means that for that pair of membership functions the error of the ignorance based algorithm is smaller than the error of the fuzzy algorithm). Observe that:

1. For the combinations of membership functions such that the fuzzy algorithm solution is good (small error), the ignorance based algorithm does not provide better results.
2. If the error we get with the fuzzy algorithm increases (i.e., if we have used bad-chosen membership functions), then the result of the ignorance based algorithm improves the fuzzy algorithm.

We observe that with the solutions obtained by the fuzzy algorithm, around 40% of possible combinations of membership functions do not represent correctly areas of the image and a very high error is obtained. However, the ignorance based algorithm gets good solutions for almost all the cases.

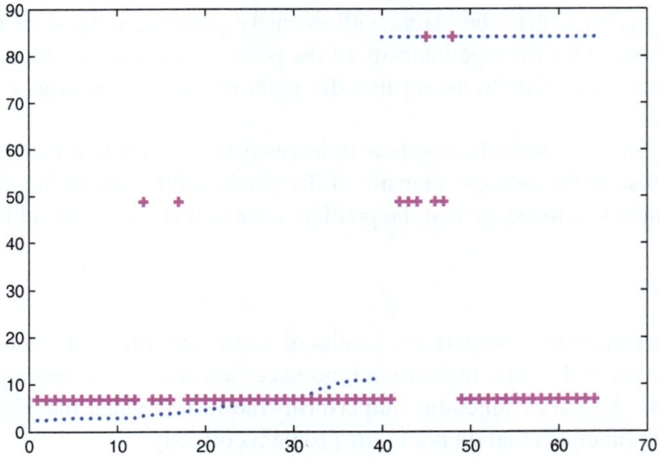

Fig. 12.8 Percentage of error in all cases of first prostate ultrasound image in Fig. 7 with ignorance function using the geometric mean

In seven of the ten studied images the ignorance based algorithm obtain better results than fuzzy algorithm. With these results, we can conclude that for real ultrasound images, ignorance based algorithm has a total mean error lower than the fuzzy algorithm.

12.5 Conclusions

In this chapter we have reviewed the use of fuzzy sets in medical image processing, mainly in the task of image segmentation.

There exist a large number of successful applications that prove that fuzzy set theory is a quality tool to handle the fuzziness present in medical images. But an extensive comparison with classical and new methods of standard image processing is needed.

Among fuzzy techniques, FCM is a well known and extensively method used in medical image processing. However, there are other techniques not widely used by the medical image processing community. For example fuzzy rule based modeling of organs, which is one of the best advantages of fuzzy set theory has not been exploited to its full potential. Indeed, fuzzy rule based systems can include knowledge from physicians and radiologists in the algorithms.

On the other side the definition of new measures of uncertainty or fuzziness, and their use to minimize fuzziness is a promising topic. These measures can be defined ad-hoc to each problem so they can represent the fuzziness from their acquisition.

Acknowledgement. This research was partially supported by grants TIN2010-15505 and TIN2011-29520 from the Government of Spain.

References

1. Acton, P.D., Pilowsky, L.S., Kung, H.F., Ell, P.J.: Automatic Segmentation of Dynamic Neuroreceptor Single-photon Emission Tomography Images Using Fuzzy Clustering. European Journal of Nuclear Medicine 26(6), 581–590 (1999)
2. Amini, L., Soltanian-Zadeh, H., Lucas, C., Gity, M.: Automatic Segmentation of Thalamus from Brain MRI Integrating Fuzzy Clustering and Dynamic Contours. IEEE Transactions on Biomedical Engineering 51(5), 800–811 (2004)
3. Awad, J.G.E., Abdel-Galil, T., Salama, M.M.A., Tizhoosh, H.R., Fenster, A., Rizkalla, K., Downey, D.B.: Prostate's Boundary Detection in Transrectal Ultrasound Images Using Scanning Technique. In: Olivier, G., Pierre, S., Sood, V.K. (eds.) 15th IEEE Canadian Conference on Electrical and Computer Engineering CCECE 2003: Canadian Conference on Electrical and Computer Engineering, Montreal, Canada, May 04-07. Proceedings: Toards a Caring and Humane Technology, pp. 1199–1202. IEEE, IEEE Canada, IEEE Eastern Canada Council, IEEE Montreal, St Maurice & Quebec Sect, Ecole Polytech Montreal, Manitoba HVDC Res. Ctr., Cooperat Etudiante Ecole Polytech, John Wiley & Sons Canada, McGraw Hill Ryerson Ltd. Cheneliere McGraw Hill, Oxford Univ. Press, Presses Int. Polytech (2003)

4. Axer, H., Jantzen, J., von Keyserlingk, D.G., Berks, G.: The Application of Fuzzy-based Methods to Central Nerve Fiber Imaging. Artificial Intelligence in Medicine 29(3), 225–239 (2003)
5. Ayala, G., Leon, T., Zapater, V.: Different Averages of a Fuzzy Set with an Application to Vessel Segmentation. IEEE Transactions on Fuzzy Systems 13(3), 384–393 (2005)
6. Belhassen, S., Zaidi, H.: A Novel Fuzzy C-means Algorithm for Unsupervised Heterogeneous Tumor Quantification in PET. Medical Physics 37(3), 1309–1324 (2010)
7. Bougioukos, P., Glotsos, D., Kostopoulos, S., Daskalakis, A., Kalatzis, I., Dimitropoulos, N., Nikiforidis, G., Cavouras, D.: Fuzzy C-means-driven FHCE Contextual Segmentation Method for Mammographic Microcalcification Detection. Imaging Science Journal 58(3), 146–154 (2010)
8. Bustince, H., Barrenechea, E., Pagola, M.: Image Thresholding using Restricted Equivalence Functions and Maximizing the Measures of Similarity. Fuzzy Sets and Systems 158(5), 496–516 (2007)
9. Bustince, H., Pagola, M., Barrenechea, E., Fernandez, J., Melo-Pinto, P., Couto, P., Tizhoosh, H.R., Montero, J.: Ignorance Functions. An application to the Calculation of the Threshold in Prostate Ultrasound Images. Fuzzy Sets and Systems 161(1), 20–36 (2010)
10. Chaira, T.: Intuitionistic Fuzzy Segmentation of Medical Images. IEEE Transactions on Biomedical Engineering 57(6), 1430–1436 (2010)
11. Costin, H., Rotariu, C.: Medical Image Analysis and Representation Using a Fuzzy and Rule-based Hybrid Approach. International Journal of Computers, Communications & Control 1(suppl. S), 156–162 (2006)
12. Couto, P., Filipe, V., Melo-Pinto, P., Bustince, H., Barrenechea, E.: A A-IFSs Based Image Segmentation Methodology for Gait Analysis. In: 2009 9th International Conference on Intelligent Systems, Design, and Applications, pp. 1318–1323. Machine Intelligence Res Lab., IEEE Syst. Man & Cybernetics Soc., Int Fuzzy Syst Assoc., European Neural Network Soc., European Soc. Fuzzy Log. & Technol., World Fed. Soft. Comp,
13. Di Zenzo, S., Cinque, L., Levialdi, S.: Image Thresholding using Fuzzy Entropies. IEEE Transactions on Systems, Man, and Cybernetics PART B-Cybernetics 28(1), 15–23 (1998)
14. Forkert, N.D., Schmidt-Richberg, A., Fiehler, J., Illies, T., Moeller, D., Handels, H., Saering, D.: Fuzzy-based Vascular Structure Enhancement in Time-of-Flight MRA Images for Improved Segmentation. Methods of Information in Medicine 50(1), 74–83 (2011)
15. Guliato, D., Rangayyan, R.M., Carnielli, W.A., Zuffo, J.A., Leo Desautels, J.E.: Segmentation of Breast Tumors in Mammograms Using Fuzzy Sets. Journal of Electronic Imaging 12(3), 369–378 (2003)
16. Hasanzadeh, M., Kasaei, S.: Fuzzy Image Segmentation Using Membership Connectedness. Eurasip Journal on Advances in Signal Processing (November 2008)
17. He, L., Greenshields, I.R.: An MRF Spatial Fuzzy Clustering Method for fMRI SPMs. Biomedical Signal Processing and Control 3(4), 327–333 (2008)
18. Kannan, S., Ramathilagam, S., Devi, R., Sathya, A.: Robust Kernel FCM in Segmentation of Breast Medical Images. Expert Systems with Applications 38(4), 4382–4389 (2011)
19. Kannan, S., Ramathilagam, S., Sathya, A., Devi, R.: Effective Fuzzy c-means Based Kernel Function in Segmenting Medical Images. Computers in Biology and Medicine 40(6), 572–579 (2010)

20. Kannan, S., Sathya, A., Devi, R.: Effective Fuzzy Clustering Techniques for Segmentation of Breast MRI. Soft Computing 15(3, Sp. Iss. SI), 483–491 (2011)
21. Kannan, S., Sathya, A., Ramathilagam, S., Devi, R.: Novel Segmentation Algorithm in Segmenting Medical Images. Journal of Systems and Software 83(12, Sp. Iss. SI), 2487–2495 (2010)
22. Kobashi, S., Kondo, K., Hata, Y.: Fully Automated Segmentation of Cerebral Ventricles from 3-D SPGR MR Images Using Fuzzy Representative Line. Soft Computing 10(12), 1181–1191 (2006)
23. Lee, C.-C., Chung, P.-C., Tsai, H.-M.: Identifying Multiple Abdominal Organs from CT Image series Using a Multimodule Contextual Neural Network and Spatial Fuzzy Rules. IEEE Tranactions on Information Technology in Biomedicine 7(3), 208–217 (2003)
24. Lin, Y., Tian, J., He, H.: Image Segmentation via Fuzzy Object Extraction and Edge Detection and its Medical Application. Journal of X-ray Science and Technology 10(1-2), 95–106 (2001)
25. Pal, S.K., Ghosh, A., Uma Shankar, B.: Segmentation of Remotely Sensed Images with Fuzzy Thresholding, and Quantitative Evaluation. International Journal of Remote Sensing 21(11), 2269–2300 (2000)
26. Pal, S.K., Rosenfeld, A.: Image Age-Enhancement and Thresholding by Optimization of Fuzzy Compactness. Pattern Recognition Letters 7(2), 77–86 (1988)
27. Pednekar, A.S., Kakadiaris, I.A.: Image Segmentation Based on Fuzzy Connectedness Using Dynamic Weights. IEEE Transactions on Image Processing 15(6), 1555–1562 (2006)
28. Pham, T.D., Berger, K.: Automated Detection of White Matter Changes in Elderly People Using Fuzzy, Geostatistical, and Information Combining Models. IEEE Transactions on Information Technology and Biomedicine 15(2), 242–250 (2011)
29. Bommanna Raja, K., Madheswaran, M., Thyagarajah, K.: A Hybrid Fuzzy-neural System for Computer-aided Diagnosis of Ultrasound Kidney Images Using Prominent Features. Journal of Medical Systems 32(1), 65–83 (2008)
30. Ramathilagam, S., Pandiyarajan, R., Sathya, A., Devi, R., Kannan, S.R.: Modified Fuzzy c-means Algorithm for Segmentation of T1-T2-weighted Brain MRI. Journal of Computational and Applied Mathematics 235(6), 1578–1586 (2011)
31. Shoujun, Z., Jian, Y., Yongtian, W., Wufan, C.: Automatic Segmentation of Coronary Angiograms Based on Fuzzy Inferring and Probabilistic Tracking. Biomedical Engineering Online 9 (2010)
32. Soret, M., Bacharach, S.L., Buvat, I.: Partial-volume effect in PET tumor imaging. Journal of Nuclear Medicine 48(6), 932–945 (2007)
33. Suetens, P.: Fundamentals of Medical Imaging, Cambridge University Press (2009)
34. Udupa, J.K., Saha, P.K., Lotufo, R.A.: Relative Fuzzy Connectedness and Object Definition: Theory, Algorithms, and Applications in Image Segmentation. IEEE Transactions on Pattern Analysis and Machine Intelligence 24(11), 1485–1500 (2002)
35. Yang, Y., Huang, S., Rao, N.: An Automatic Hybrid Method for Retinal Blood Vessel Extraction. International Journal of Applied Matehmatics and Computer Science 18(3), 399–407 (2008)
36. Yin, T.-K., Chiu, N.-T.: A Computer-aided Diagnosis for Locating Abnormalities in Bone Scintigraphy by a Fuzzy System with a Three-step Minimization Approach. IEEE Transactions on Medical Imaging 23(5), 639–654 (2004)
37. Emin, Y.M., Borlu, M.: Accurate Segmentation of Dermoscopic Images by Image Thresholding Based on Type-2 Fuzzy Logic. IEEE Transactions on Fuzzy Systems 17(4), 976–982 (2009)

38. Zhang, D., Chen, S.: A Novel Kernelized Fuzzy C-means Algorithm with Application in Medical Image Segmentation. Artificial Intelligence in Medicine 32(1), 37–50 (2004)
39. Zhou, Y., Bai, J.: Multiple Abdominal Organ Segmentation: An Atlas-based Fuzzy Connectedness Approach. IEEE Transactions on Information Technology and Biomedicine 11(3), 348–352 (2007)
40. Zhuang, X., Meng, Q.: Local Fuzzy Fractal Dimension and its Application in Medical Image Processing. Artificial Intelligence in Medicine 32(1), 29–36 (2004)
41. Zhuge, Y., Udupa, J.K., Saha, P.K.: Vectorial Scale-based Fuzzy-connected Image Segmentation. Computer Vision and Image Understanding 101(3), 177–193 (2006)

13

Medical Concept Representation and Data Mining

Mila Kwiatkowska and Najib T. Ayas

Abstract. Medical data stored in clinical files and databases, such as patient histories and medical records, as well as research data collected for various clinical studies, are invaluable sources of medical knowledge. The computer-based data-mining techniques provide a tremendous opportunity for discovering patterns, relationships, trends, typical cases, and irregularities in these large volumes of data. The patterns discovered from data can be used to stimulate further research, as well as to create practical guidelines for diagnosis, prognosis, and treatment. Thus, a successful data-mining process may result in a significant improvement in the quality and efficiency of both medical research and health care services. Many studies have already demonstrated the practical values of data-mining techniques in various fields. However, in contrast with more traditional areas of data mining, such as mining of financial data or mining of purchasing records, medical data-mining presents greater challenges. These challenges arise not only from the complexity of the medical data, but more fundamentally from the difficulty of linking the medical data to medical concepts or rather medical concepts to medical data. Thus, although computerized medical equipment allows us to store increasingly large volumes of data, the problem lies in defining the meaning of the data and even more so in defining the medical concepts themselves.

This paper will address issues specific to medical data and medical data mining in the context of Dr. Kazem Sadegh-Zadeh's discussion of the typology of medical concepts. In his *Handbook of Analytic Philosophy of Medicine*, Dr. Sadegh-Zadeh outlines four main classes of medical concepts: individual, qualitative (classificatory), comparative, and quantitative. Moreover, he introduces a novel distinction between classical and non-classical concepts. We will explain how his typology can be utilized for conceptual modelling of medical data. Specifically we will illustrate how this typology can pertain to data used in the diagnosis and treatment of sleep disorders.

R. Seising and M.E. Tabacchi (Eds.): *Fuzziness and Medicine*, STUDFUZZ 302, pp. 191–203.
DOI: 10.1007/978-3-642-36527-0_13

13.1 Introduction

Medical data stored in clinical files and databases, such as patient histories and medical records, as well as research data collected for various clinical studies, are invaluable sources of medical knowledge. The rapidly increasing number of electronically stored patients' data provides a tremendous opportunity for data mining, the process of automatically discovering useful information (discovering knowledge) in large data repositories [4]. Data-mining techniques allow for discovering patterns, relationships, trends, typical cases, and irregularities in these large volumes of data. These newly discovered information and knowledge can be used to stimulate further research, as well as to create practical guidelines for diagnosis, prognosis, and treatment. Thus, a successful data-mining process may result in a significant improvement in the quality and efficiency of both medical research and health care services. Many studies have already demonstrated the practical values of data mining in various fields. However, in contrast with more traditional areas of data mining, such as mining of financial data or mining of purchasing records, medical data-mining presents greater challenges. These challenges arise not only from the complexity of the medical data, but more fundamentally from the difficulty of defining medical concepts. Medical concepts must be clearly defined in order to build appropriate data models in the data-mining process. Thus, although computers allow us to store and process increasingly large volumes of data, the problem lies in the creation of the suitable conceptual models for the data. These models should be unambiguously defined, and they should be explicitly connected with the related medical concepts. Evidently, the quality of the data-mining process depends on the quality of the conceptual data models and the quality of the data.

This paper addresses issues specific to conceptual modeling of medical data in the data-mining process. We will situate our discussion in the context of Dr. Kazem Sadegh-Zadeh's typology of medical concepts [17]. In his *Handbook of Analytic Philosophy of Medicine*, Dr. Sadegh-Zadeh outlines four main classes of medical concepts: individual, qualitative (classificatory), comparative, and quantitative. Furthermore, Dr. Sadegh-Zadeh divides medical concepts into classical concepts and non-classical concepts. We demonstrate how Dr. Sadegh-Zadeh's typology can be utilized for conceptual modeling of medical data. Specifically we illustrate how this typology pertains to concepts and data used in the diagnosis and treatment of sleep disorders. The paper is structured as follows. Section 13.2 defines the key issues in modeling of medical concepts: definition of a concept, characteristics of medical concepts, and computational representation. Section 13.3 describes the fundamental issues in medical data mining and provides the example of operational definition for obstructive sleep apnea. Section 13.4 presents the semiotic approach to conceptual modeling. The final section, Section 13.5, provides the conclusions and future work.

13.2 Modeling of Medical Concepts

In this section, we discuss the notion of a natural concept and the creation of computational models for natural concepts. First, we describe natural concepts and place our description in the context of Dr. Sadegh-Zadeh's categorization of "classical concepts." Second, we discuss concept modeling in the context of knowledge representation. Next, we focus on medical concepts and their characteristics such as context-dependency, changeability and imprecision.

Since our ultimate goal is to create computational data models for data mining, we approach the "concept" definition from a representational perspective. Accordingly, we view "concept" as a principle of classification. Furthermore, we approach the concept definition from a cognitive perspective. First, we ask two fundamental questions: "How do people classify objects into categories?" and "How do people mentally represent categories?" The answers to these questions are fundamental for the creation of computational models. The findings from cognitive psychology about human categorization have demonstrated that category learning and classification in the real world are different from the creation and classification of artificial categories (e.g., mathematical categories) [1, 14, 15]. Furthermore, cognitive psychology describes three approaches to the mental representation of natural categories: *classical*, *prototype*, and *exemplar* [12, 14]. These three categories are described below since the distinction between them is critical for the creation of appropriate computational models in data mining.

- **Classical Approach.** In the classical approach, objects are grouped based on their properties. Objects are either a member of a category or not, and all objects have equal membership in a category. A category can be represented by a set of rules, which can be evaluated as true (object belongs to the category) or false (object does not belong to the category).

- **Prototype Approach.** In the prototype approach, the members are more or less typical of the category; in other words, they belong to the category to a certain degree. The prototype of the category usually represents the central tendency of the category and may be defined as the "average" of all the members of the category. Thus, in the prototype approach, a category is based on a "prototype," which exists as an ideal member of a category, and the other members of the same category may share some of the features with the ideal member [1].

- **Exemplar Approach.** In the exemplar approach, all exemplars of a category are stored in memory, and a new instance is classified based on its similarity to all prior exemplars [10]. This representation requires specification of a similarity measure, as well as storage and retrieval of multiple exemplars. In the exemplar-based representation, the category is defined by all exemplars belonging to a given category.

These three approaches to natural concepts can be mapped into Dr. Sadegh-Zadeh's *classical* and *non-classical* concepts. Dr. Sadegh-Zadeh defines the classical concepts as classes "characterized by the 'common nature' of its members, that is, by a number of properties that are common to all of them." Dr. Sadegh-Zadeh refers to this quality of the classical concepts as the "common-to-all postulate." Thus, a concept is categorized as classical "if it denotes a category that obeys the common-to-all postulate." Dr. Sadegh-Zadeh uses the concept of a square as an example of a classical concept. The concept of a square is characterized by four properties: closed figure, four straight sides, all sides equal in length, and equal angles. In the traditional distinction between artificial and natural concepts, the concept of a square is classified as an artificial concept since the properties have defining nature. Accordingly, all members of the class "square" must meet the four conditions. In contrast, a natural concept has characteristic features rather than defining features. Dr. Sadegh-Zadeh uses the concept of disease as an example of a non-classical concept. The concept of disease "does not denote a category whose members obey the common-to-all postulate."

In general, natural concepts (categories) have two fundamental characteristics: (1) The members of a natural category do not have to share all features; a natural category may have some attributes which are common to many members, and some attributes which may be shared by only a few members; and (2) The members of a natural category may not be equally representative for a category; thus, the members may vary in their typicality.

Most medical concepts can be classified as natural concepts rather than classical concepts. Medical concepts reflect the rapidly expanding and evolving nature of medical knowledge. They are characterized by a high level of changeability, context-dependency, and imprecision. Our discussion on the nature of medical concepts has an introductory character, and merely highlights some major issues in the context of the conceptual models in data mining. Our discussion has also a practical nature, and it presents an operational definition of obstructive sleep apnea.

13.3 Data Mining and Modeling of Medical Concepts

Data mining is based on a secondary use of existing medical data. Thus, the data are not purposely collected for data mining, and the meaning of the data should be interpreted in the context of the original task. In most cases, medical data are collected for three distinct reasons: for an individual patient's care, for medical research, and for patient administration. For the first reason, the data acquisition method is driven by the diagnostic, prognostic, or treatment process and the data are successively obtained, stored, and used by the healthcare practitioners. Since the intended use of the data is the patient's care, the data are often incomplete and have varied granularity. For medical research, data are prospectively acquired through purposely designed clinical trials, epidemiological studies, or studies of healthy populations. These data sets are collected by the researchers to answer specific clinical questions and afterwards are analysed using statistical methods for confirmation or negation of a particular medical hypothesis. For patient administration, data are collected and used for accounting and planning [6]. As a result, data mining uses heterogeneous data and multiple meanings. Integration of these diverse data and metadata requires creation of a unified conceptual data model. This task is complicated by the fact that data are collected using diverse collecting methods, inclusion criteria, sampling methods, sample sizes, types and numbers of measurements, and definitions of outcomes. Therefore, conceptual data modeling for data mining must address the problems related to the secondary use of the data, which means that the data were originally collected for other purposes and may have more or less explicitly defined meaning (metadata).

In his *Handbook of Analytic Philosophy of Medicine*, Dr. Sadegh-Zadeh outlines four main classes of medical concepts: individual, qualitative (classificatory), comparative, and quantitative. Individual concepts denote specific individual objects. For example, John Davey denotes specific patient. Qualitative or classificatory concepts are "either unary predicates or non-comparative, many-place predicates." For example, John Davey has excessive daytime sleepiness, EDS. Comparative concepts express relationship between two or more objects. For example, John Davey has higher EDS than John Smith. Quantitative concepts specify the magnitude of an attribute using a numerical function. For example, John Davey's sleepiness can be "measured" using the Epworth Sleepiness Scale (the standard questionnaire used in sleep clinics). Thus, we can say that John Davey has sleepiness of 20, and John Smith has sleepiness of 15. Dr. Sadegh-Zadeh defines quantitative concepts as "a homomorphism f from a particular empirical, i.e., experiential, structure $\langle R, \geq \rangle$ into a numerical structure R such that R is, usually, the set of positive real numbers, and $\geq$ is the 'is greater than or equals' relation." The quantification f is also called measurement and the homomorphism is referred to as a scale. Quantitative concepts are particularly important in medical diagnosis and treatment evaluation. We will discuss them further in context of the operational definition of concept.

Additionally, Dr. Sadegh-Zadeh discusses the notion of an attribute, and describes two types of attributes: categorical and dispositional. Categorical attributes are permanently present, for example, John Smith's weight. The specific value for weight may change with time, but weight is measurable under all circumstances. On the other hand, dispositional attributes may manifest only under certain circumstances, for example, John Smith's daytime sleepiness. Daytime sleepiness can be observed during day (assuming that John Smith is not a nightshift worker).

13.3.1 Operational Definition of a Concept

Operational definition is based on the notions of conceptualization and operationalization. Conceptualization defines the concept in the context of its use, for example, excessive sleepiness in the context of the clinical diagnosis of a specific sleep disorder. Operationalization states that a concept is defined in terms of the operations by which its referent is measured. For example, sleepiness is "measured" by a subjective measure [16]. The Epworth Sleepiness Scale (ESS) is a self-administered questionnaire composed of eight questions to measure the general level of daytime sleepiness in terms of the probability of falling asleep during daily activities: (1) sitting and reading, (2) watching TV, (3) sitting inactive in public place (e.g. a theatre or a meeting), (4) riding as a passenger in a car for an hour without a break, (5) lying down to rest in the afternoon when circumstances permit, (6) sitting and talking to someone, (7) sitting quietly after lunch without alcohol, and (8) sitting in a car, while stopped for a few minutes in traffic. Each item has a score between $0-3$. The answers are never, slight chance, moderate chance, and high chance. The maximum score is 24. Typically a score of 11 and above is recognized as excessive daytime sleepiness (EDS). Thus, the operational definition of daytime sleepiness allows for a mapping of the concept of sleepiness (in particular context) into an interval between 0 and 24. EDS is defined as a score of ESS ≥ 11. These definitions are essential for standardization of meanings and data integration in medical data mining. However, interpretation of the meaning of a particular ESS value requires thorough contextual analysis. We describe the main issues of the contextual interpretation in the next subsection.

13.3.2 Contextual Interpretation of Excessive Daytime Sleepiness

The symptom of sleepiness, although extensively used in screening and diagnosis, is not easy to describe and, moreover, to quantify. Sleepiness can be measured only indirectly – there is not yet a single laboratory test to identify 'sleepy' individuals. However, excessive daytime sleepiness (somnolence) is one of the most important symptoms of *OSA* used for screening, evaluation, and classification of the severity of *OSA* [3]. Sleepiness is a typical complaint of *OSA* patients (or their family members). But sleepiness is not a universal symptom; about 10% patients with *OSA* do not display excessive sleepiness. Moreover, reported sleepiness may be related to many other problems. Figure 13.1 illustrates the complex dependencies between Excessive Daytime Sleepiness (EDS) and shift work, sleep deprivation, circadian rhythm disruption (CRD), depression, insomnia, and presence of other sleep disorders such as periodic limb movement (PLM) or restless legs syndrome (RLS). The arrows represent possible causal relationships between the factors. For example, depression may increase insomnia and, vice versa, insomnia may increase the feeling of depression.

13.3.3 Operationalization of Obstructive Sleep Apnea

In the case of medical concepts, their meanings are a result of many possible interpretations depending on their context, their specific use, and the particular time of use. Therefore, modeling of medical concepts must be based on the following four premises: (1) only some clinical concepts have clearly defined boundaries; most concepts are fuzzy; (2) clinical concepts are used in specific contexts and are subject to various interpretations; (3) clinical concepts are created and used for specific

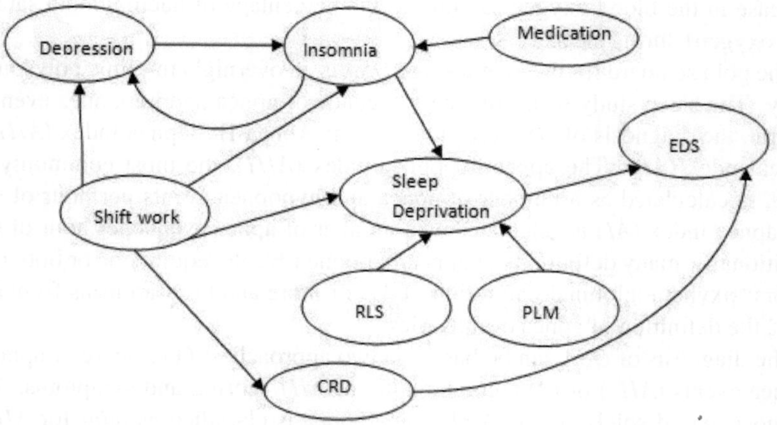

Fig. 13.1 Dependencies between the Excessive Daytime Sleepiness (EDS) and other factors. Daytime sleepiness is closely related to the length of sleep and pattern of sleep/awake hours, and, therefore, cannot be analysed without two additional important factors: duration of sleep and timing of sleep (circadian rhythm disruption).

purposes and must be interpreted in the context of these purposes; and (4) clinical concepts evolve over time.

We describe operationalization in more details using as an example of a particular diagnostic process for obstructive sleep apnea. In our discussion, we use the generic name obstructive sleep apnea (*OSA*) to indicate Obstructive Sleep Apnea Syndrome (*OSAS*) and Obstructive Sleep Apnea/Hypopnea Syndrome (*OSAHS*). *OSA* is a common, serious respiratory disorder afflicting, according to conservative studies, $2-4\%$ of the adult population. The differences in reported *OSA* prevalence values result from different diagnostic methods and varied definitions of *OSA*. "Apnea" means "without breath," and *OSA* occurs only during sleep, and is, therefore, a condition that might go unnoticed for years. *OSA* is caused by collapse of the soft tissues in the throat as the result of the natural relaxation of muscles during sleep. The soft tissue blocks the air passage and the sleeping person literally stops breathing (apnea event) or experiences a partial obstruction (hypopnea event). The apnea event in adult is defined as at least 10 second breathing pause (complete cessation of air flow) and the hypopnea event is defined as at least 10 second event with reduced air flow by at least 50%.

Although sleep apnea is not a new condition and has been mentioned sporadically in literature (e.g., Charles Dickens provided a description of Joe the fat boy), it was discovered and described only in 1965. Since then, it has been recognized as a serious respiratory disorder. One of the most important daytime symptoms of *OSA* is excessive daytime sleepiness (EDS). One of the important night symptoms is a decrease in the blood oxygen saturation (the percentage of haemoglobin saturated with oxygen) during sleep.

The gold standard for the diagnosis of *OSA* is an overnight in-clinic polysomnography. The sleep study measures the frequency of apnea and hypopnea events. In general, the diagnosis of *OSA* uses two scores: Apnea-Hypopnea Index (*AHI*) and Apnea Index (*AI*). The apnea-hypopnea index (*AHI*), the most commonly used score, is calculated as a number of apnea and hypopnea events per hour of sleep; The apnea index (*AI*) is calculated as a number of apnea events per hour of sleep. Additionally, many definitions of apnea/hypopnea events require one or both of two factors: oxyhemoglobin desaturation of 4% or more and brief arousals from sleep. Thus, the definition of apnea event varies.

The diagnosis of *OSA* can be based on two approaches: (1) a score of apnea/hypopnea events (*AHI*) or (2) a combination of *AHI* scoring and symptoms. In the diagnosis based solely on the *AHI* index, apnea is classified as *mild* for *AHI* between 5 and 14.9, *moderate* for *AHI* between 15 and 29.9, and *severe* for $AHI \geq 30$. The International Classification of Sleep Disorders (ICSD) [16] defines the severity of *OSA* in terms of the frequency of apnea events, the degree of oxygen desaturation, and the severity of daytime sleepiness.

The differences between the scoring and definitions of apnea have important implications for the conceptual data modeling in data mining. Most published medical research studies base the diagnosis of *OSA* on *AHI* or a combination of apnea index (*AI*) and *AHI* obtained from overnight in-clinic PSG. For example, the authors of two articles on craniofacial predictors [9] and [5] define respectively two criteria: (1) *OSA* defined as $AHI \geq 5$ and (2) *OSA* defined as $AI > 5$ or $AHI > 10$. To illustrate the difference between diagnostic criteria based on *AHI* and a combination of *AI* and *AHI*, we applied these two criteria to 233 records from the data set obtained from the authors of the first publication [3]. Figure 13.2 shows the number of records classified into *OSA* and non-*OSA* using two diagnostic criteria: *OSA* defined by $AHI \geq 5$ (column to the left) and *OSA* defined by $AH > 5$ OR $AHI > 10$ (column to the right). The second criterion is more restrictive and excludes 26 records (26/233) from the *OSA* group and classifies them as a non-*OSA*.

The definition of *OSA* is fuzzy. Different studies use different cut-off values to indicate *OSA*, for example $AHI \geq 5$, $AHI \geq 10$, $AHI \geq 15$. To illustrate the differences in prevalence of *OSA*, we applied three cut-off values to 795 records obtained from a sleep clinic [7, 8]. Figure 13.3 shows the changing proportions between non-*OSA* and *OSA* records for $AHI \geq 5$, $AHI \geq 10$, and $AHI \geq 15$.

OSA is operationalized using diverse methods. Thus, the conceptual model for data must define precisely the scoring criteria. The use of *AHI* or *AI* and three cut-off values can result in significant differences in classification of the patients (non-*OSA*, *OSA*), especially for patients with low *AHI* scores [13]. Furthermore, the difficulty with the scoring of *AHI* is compounded by the natural night-to-night variability in the severity of apnea and the differences in diagnostic equipment.

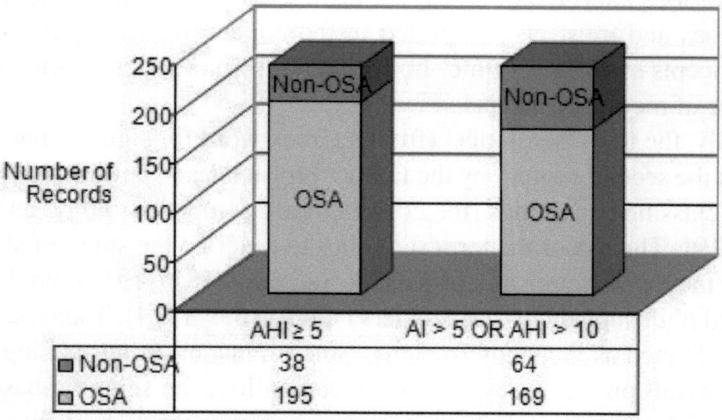

Fig. 13.2 *OSA* prevalence using diagnostic criteria based on two diagnostic criteria

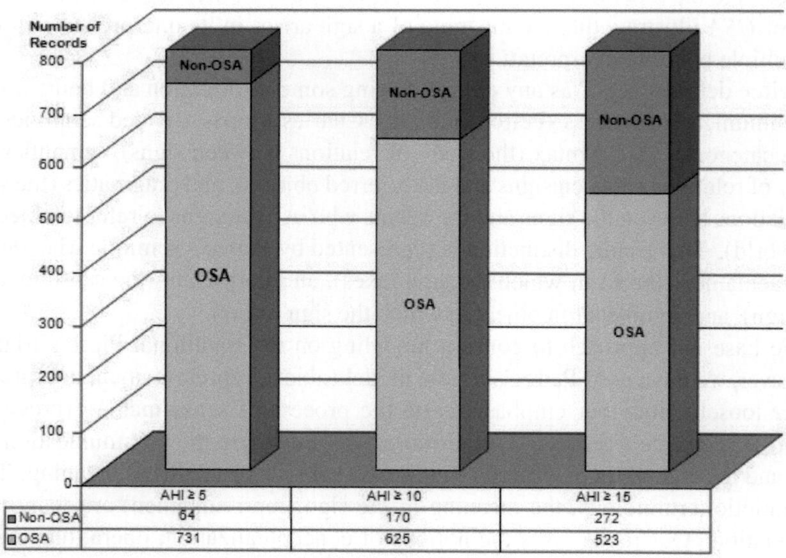

Fig. 13.3 *OSA* prevalence for three levels of *AHI* cut-off values: $AHI \geq 5, 10, 15$

13.4 Semiotic Approach to Concept Modeling

In the case of medical concepts, their meanings are a result of many possible interpretations depending on their context, their specific use, and the particular time of use. Therefore, in most cases, the interpretation is based on the following four premises: (1) only some clinical concepts have clearly defined boundaries; most concepts are fuzzy; (2) clinical concepts are used in specific contexts and are subject to various interpretations; (3) clinical concepts are created and used for specific purposes and must be interpreted in the context of these purposes; and (4) clinical concepts evolve over time. In this section, we describe a semiotic approach to modeling of medical concepts.

Originally, the term 'semiotics' (from a Greek word for sign "semaion") was introduced in the second century by the famous physician and philosopher Galen (129-199), who classified semiotics (the contemporary symptomatology) as a branch of medicine [19]. The use of the term semiotics to describe the study of signs was developed by the Swiss linguist, Ferdinand de Saussure (1857-1913) and the American logician and philosopher Charles Sanders Peirce (1839-1914). Today, semiotics can be broadly defined as the study of signs. Since signs, meaning-making, and representations are all present in every part of human life, the semiotic-based methods have been used in many disciplines, from mathematics through literary studies and library studies to information sciences. A semiotic paradigm is associated with different traditions and with a variety of empirical methodologies. Our intention in this paper is to define the basic terminology needed to present the need for the semiotic approach to the modeling of medical concepts. The examples of the operationalization of *OSA* illustrate that the meaning of a sign arises in its interpretation or even in multiple possible interpretations.

Peirce defined "sign" as any entity carrying some information and being used in a communication process. Peirce, and later Charles Morris, divided semiotics into three categories [2] : syntax (the study of relations between signs), semantics (the study of relations between signs and the referred objects), and pragmatics (the study of relations between the signs and the agents who use the signs to refer to objects in the world). This triadic distinction is represented by Peirce's semiotic triangle: the representamen (the form which the sign takes), an interpretant (the sense made of the sign), and an object (an object to which the sign refers).

We base our approach to concept modeling on the traditional Piece's triangle. However, we have used Peirce's triadic model (object, representamen, interpretant) rather loosely since our emphasis is on the process of sense-making (process of semiosis in Peirce's theory). Furthermore, we emphasize the communication process and the role of the interpreter in the creation (construction) of meaning. Thus, in semiotic terminology, the meaning of the sign (representamen) arises in its interpretation. Our model uses the notions of conceptualization, operationalization, and utilization. The notions of conceptualization and operationalization have their roots in social sciences. The notion of utilization of measures has been added by us to model the pragmatic aspects. We introduce a triplet for the representation of the concept and use the terms: conceptualization (what to measure), operationalization (how to measure), and utilization (how to use the measure). We observe a strong parallelism between the semiotic triangle (object, representamen, interpretant) and the triplet: conceptualization, operationalization, and utilization. In many ways, the semiotic approach presented here is oversimplified and does not reflect the richness of multiple semiotic traditions. However, we believe that a semiotic approach allows for modeling of complex medical concepts. We focus on the pragmatic aspects (utilization) of the models. Therefore, we have introduced a notion of "pragmatic modifiers," which represent the notion of "interpretant" or utilization. This notion focuses on the role of interpretation (interpreter) in the creation of meaning. We called them modifiers since in a way, they "modify" the meaning. We identified four groups of modifiers (this is not an exhaustive list of possible modifiers): goals (e.g., diagnosis, assessment, treatment evaluation), agents (e.g., patients, health professionals, medical sensors, computer systems), perspectives (e.g., health care costs, accessibility, ethics), and views (e.g., variations in the diagnostic criteria used by different experts or clinics). The names of the modifiers are used here in an arbitrary fashion, and they are introduced here to indicate various sources of modifications. For example, the important modifiers are health-care costs and accessibility of specialists.

The modeling of the concept of *OSA* in the context of various goals involves three aspects: conceptualization (what to measure), operationalization (how to measure), and utilization (how the measure is applied). We mapped these aspects using the semiotic triangle, shown in Figure 13.4.

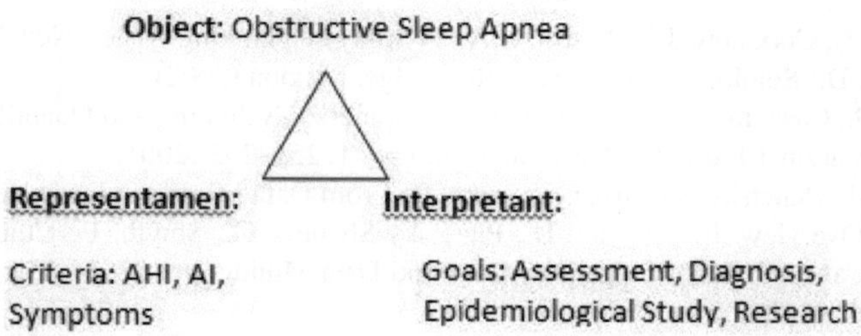

Fig. 13.4 Peircean semiotic triangle for contextual modeling of *OSA*

The multiplicity of diagnostic criteria and ongoing modifications clearly indicate the need for a flexible computational representation, which must model the various criteria and approaches to the diagnosis, assessment, and treatment of *OSA* (and other sleep disorders).

13.5 Conclusions and Future Work

In this paper, we have discussed the typology of medical concepts introduced by Dr. Kazem Sadegh-Zadeh in his *Handbook of Analytic Philosophy of Medicine*. Specifically, we have concentrated on three issues: non-classical concepts, qualitative concepts, and operational definition of concepts. We have used an example of obstructive sleep apnea to demonstrate that (1) medical concepts are created and used for specific purposes and must be interpreted in the context of these purposes; (2) medical concepts rarely have clearly defined boundaries; most concepts are fuzzy; (3) clinical concepts are used in specific contexts and are subject to various interpretations; and (4) clinical concepts evolve over time. To address these issues, we have used a semiotic approach to modeling of medical concepts. Semiotics provides the modeling constructs for the description of the concept, its representation, interpretation, and utilization. Furthermore, we have observed that (1) data mining requires explicit conceptual models based on operational definitions of medical concepts; and (2) the quality of the data-mining process depends on the quality of the conceptual data models and the quality of the data.

We are planning to further expand the proposed framework and to build a comprehensive computational model for the medical concept of obstructive sleep apnea and its symptoms. We will apply this model in a clinical decision support system for the diagnosis and treatment of *OSA*, as well as in a support system for the treatment of sleep disorders. Furthermore, we plan to utilize the proposed computational model for the analysis of patients' data from clinics which use diverse diagnostic criteria. The explicit modeling will allow us to compare treatment results from various clinics.

References

1. Bruner, J.S., Goodnow, J.J., Austin, G.A.: A Study of Thinking. Wiley, New York (1956)
2. Chandler, D.: Semiotics: The Basics. Routledge, London (2002)
3. Curcio, G., Casagrande, M., Bertini, M.: Sleepiness: Evaluating and Quantifying Methods. International Journal of Psychophysiology 41, 251–263 (2001)
4. Fayyad, U., Piatetsky-Shapiro, G., Smyth, P.: From Data Mining to Knowledge Discovery: An Overview. In: Fayyad, U., Piatetsky-Shapiro, G., Smyth, P., Uthurusamy, R. (eds.) Advances in Knowledge Discovery and Data Mining, pp. 37–54. The MIT Press, Menlo Park (1996)
5. Ferguson, K.A., Ono, T., Lowe, A.A., Ryan, C.F., Fleetham, J.A.: The Relationship Between Obesity and Craniofacial Structure in Obstructive Sleep Apnea. Chest 108(2), 375–381 (1995)
6. Goble, C.A., Glowinski, A.J., Nowlan, W.A., Rector, A.L.: A Descriptive Semantic Formalism for Medicine. In: Proceedings of the Ninth International Conference on Data Engineering, pp. 624–631 (1993)
7. Kwiatkowska, M., Ayas, N.T., Ryan, C.F.: Evaluation of Clinical Prediction Rules Using a Convergence of Knowledge-driven and Data-driven Methods: A Semio-fuzzy Approach. In: Zanasi, A., Brebbia, C.A., Ebecken, N.F.F. (eds.) Data Mining VI: Data Mining, Text Mining and their Business Applications, pp. 411–420. WIT Press, Southampton (2005)
8. Kwiatkowska, M., Atkins, M.S., Rollans, S., Ryan, C.F., Ayas, N.T.: Decision Tree Induction in the Creation of Prediction Models for Obstructive Sleep Apnea (*OSA*): A Pilot Study (Abstract). In: International Conference of American Thoracic Society, San Diego (2006)
9. Lam, B., Ip, M.S.M., Tench, E., Frank Ryan, C.: Craniofacial Profile in Asian and white Subjects with Obstructive Sleep Apnea. Thorax 60(6), 504–510 (2005)
10. Medin, D.L., Marguerite, M., Medin, D.L., Schaffer, M.M.: Context Theory of Classification Learning. Psychological Review 85, 207–238 (1978)
11. Minda, J.P., David Smith, J.: The Effects of Category Size, Category Structure and Stimulus Complexity. Journal of Experimental Psychology: Learning, Memory and Cognition 27, 755–799 (2001)

12. Nosofsky, R.M.: Exemplars, Prototypes, and Similarity Rules. In: Healy, A.F., Kosslyn, S.M., Shiffrin, R.M. (eds.) From Learning Theory to Connectionist Theory: Essays in Honour of William K. Estes, vol. 1. Erlbaum, Hillsdale (1992)
13. Redline, S., Kapur, V.K., Sanders, M.H., Quan, S.F., Gottlieb, D.J., Rapoport, D.M., Bonekat, W.H., Smith, P.L., Kiley, J.P., Iber, C.: Effects of Varying Approaches for Identifying Respiratory Disturbances on Sleep Apnea Assessment. American Journal of Respiratory and Critical Care Medicine 161, 369–374 (2000)
14. Reed, S.K.: Cognition. Theory and Applications, 4th edn. Brooks/Cole Publishing, Pacific Grove (1996)
15. Rosch, E., Mervis, C.B.: Family Resemblances: Studies in the Internal Structure of Categories. Cognitive Psychology 7, 573–605 (1975)
16. Rosenberg, R.S., Mickelson, S.A.: Obstructive Sleep Apnea: Evaluation by History and Polysomnography. In: Fairbanks, D.N.F., Mickelson, S.A., Tucker Woodson, B. (eds.) Snoring and Obstructive Sleep Apnea, 3rd edn. Lippincott Williams & Wilkins, Philadelphia (2003)
17. Sadegh-Zadeh, K.: Handbook of Analytic Philosophy of Medicine. Springer, Dordrecht (2012)
18. Sebeok, T.A., Danesi, M.: The Forms of Meaning: Modeling Systems Theory and Semiotic Analysis. Mounton de Gruyter, Berlin (2000)
19. Sebeok, T.A.: Signs: An Introduction to Semiotics. University of Toronto Press, Toronto (1999)

14

Application of Knowledge-Engineering Methods in Medical Knowledge Management

von Krzysztof Michalik, Mila Kwiatkowska, and Krzysztof Kielan

Abstract. This paper deals with Knowledge Engineering (KE), Clinical Decision Support Systems (CDSS), and Expert Systems (ES) as essential methods and tools supporting the Knowledge Management (KM) process in medicine. Specifically, we focus on the main component of the CDSS, knowledge base (KB). We demonstrate a hybrid approach to the creation, modification, verification, and validation of KB, which combines a fuzzy rule system with data mining. We describe the design and implementation of KB for two CDSS systems. The first system, which supports the evaluation of clinical depression, uses a combination of three methods: (1) creation of fuzzy rules based on expert clinicians' knowledge and standard guidelines, (2) construction of Artificial Neural Networks (ANN) based on patients' data, and (3) implementation of a CAKE (Computer Aided Knowledge Engineering) tool. The second system, which supports the diagnosis of obstructive sleep apnea, uses a combination of two methods: (1) creation of fuzzy rules derived from the medical literature and the expert clinicians' knowledge and (2) induction of decision trees from large clinical data sets. Based on these two clinical studies, we demonstrate that KE methods should be regarded as valuable methods and tools which can be successfully used in medical KM for the creation, validation, and maintenance of KB.

14.1 Introduction

Knowledge Management (KM) and Knowledge Engineering (KE) are two related disciplines that share several methods and tools. Most importantly, these two disciplines have the same subject – knowledge. On the other hand, KE and KM have diverse origins, and often use different definitions of the term "knowledge."

Knowledge Engineering (KE) is an engineering discipline, which is concerned with the development of knowledge-based information systems, and, thus, it is closely related to software engineering and Artificial Intelligence (AI). KE creates computational methods, languages, and tools for knowledge representation and problem solving by computers. The focus of KE has changed from "knowledge

R. Seising and M.E. Tabacchi (Eds.): *Fuzziness and Medicine*, STUDFUZZ 302, pp. 205–214.
DOI: 10.1007/978-3-642-36527-0_14

transfer" (eliciting knowledge from human experts and transferring elicited knowledge into knowledge-based systems) in the early eighties to "knowledge modeling" (creating computer models to solve particular problems in the area of interest) more recently. In the model-oriented KE methodology, the knowledge and problem solving techniques of the domain experts are explicitly modeled. This modeling process requires a specification of *what* the system should do, a plan describing *how* the system should solve specific problems, and an explanation *why* the system solves the problem in a particular way.

Knowledge Management (KM), on the other hand, is often defined as an area of business administration. Thus, KM views knowledge as a key asset and resource in an organization. KM concentrates on three aspects: people who create and communicate knowledge (*who*), knowledge communication process (*how*, *where*, *when*), and knowledge itself (*what*). KM is concerned with the entire KM process in the context of business enterprise. Thus, KM encompasses knowledge creation, acquisition, validation, presentation, distribution, and application. KM in medicine and healthcare faces many additional challenges such as extreme complexity of biomedical systems, high costs of errors, and fast-growing body of knowledge [9].

In broader context, KE and KM address all fundamental questions regarding knowledge: who, what, how, when, where and why. These questions are answered by various types of knowledge: declarative (what), procedural (how), causal (why), and organizational (when, where, who). One of the specific areas of interest for both disciplines is decision making. However, KE and KM have, to some extent, dissimilar approaches to decision making. Whereas KE has a long history of a practical approach to constructing computerized decision support systems, KM has been concerned more with organizational aspects of decision making. In spite of historical differences, both disciplines are closely interrelated and could benefit from collaboration. This need for interdisciplinary approach is especially visible in knowledge-rich applications, such as medicine, in which KE is strongly intertwined with each step of the KM process: knowledge acquisition, creation, validation, presentation, distribution, and application. Specifically, computer-based systems, which support clinical decisions, such as clinical decision support systems (CDSS), must explicitly represent the knowledge and its source, maintain the currency of the knowledge, and create guidelines for the application of knowledge in specific clinical settings [2].

The rest of the paper is structured as follows. Section 14.2 defines the key terms: expert system, decision support system, and clinical decision support system. Section 14.3 describes the Knowledge Base (KB), the most important component of CDSS. Furthermore, it lists user requirements regarding the medical KB. Section 14.4 discusses the verification and validation of KB using the data warehousing and data mining approach. Section 14.5 provides the conclusions and future work.

14.2 Decision Support Systems in Medicine

This section describes the Clinical Decision Support Systems (CDDS) in the context of Expert Systems (ES) and decision support systems (DSS). We define ES, DSS, and CDSS systems, and discuss the similarities and differences between these three terms. Specifically, we focus on the difference between ES and DSS systems in terms of the users' requirements.

Expert System (ES) can be defined as a software system which uses knowledge and intelligent reasoning for complex problem solving in, often, highly specialised areas of expertise. ES systems are often viewed as a subject of the AI research [1, 12, 15]. ESs have four characteristics which differentiate them from other information systems [15]: (1) explicit representation of knowledge; (2) ability to explain problem solution (how explanations) and ability to give explicit reasons for using particular solution (why explanations); (3) utilization of logical reasoning, as opposed to mostly imperative algorithmic approach used in information systems; and (4) processing based primarily on a symbolic approach.

Decision support system (DSS) has been defined in different ways by many ES and DSS researchers [5, 10]. In our research, we use a broad DSS definition given by Finlay [5], who describes DSS as "a computer-based system that aids the process of decision making". We view DSS as a wide-ranging category, which includes various subtypes identified by Power [10]: data-driven, model-driven, communication-driven, document-driven and knowledge-driven. We focus here on the knowledge-driven DSS systems, which use explicit knowledge representation and, therefore, are closely associated with the construction of ES systems.

Clinical Decision Support System (CDSS) can be defined as a specialized knowledge-based DSS used in medicine. Berner and La Lande [2] define CDSS as "a computer system designed to impact clinician decision making about individual patients at the point in time that these decisions are made." In general, the knowledge-based CDSS have three main components: the knowledge base (KB), the inference or reasoning engine, and the input/output mechanism to communicate with the users [2]. CDSS have been incorporated in medical systems for a long time, and they vary in the type of support they may offer. For example, CDSS differ in whether they are stand-alone or embedded in other systems such as, for example, electronic medical records (EMR). Also, CDSS differ in whether they provide general or speciality-based information and which clinical tasks they support. For example, many successful CDSS systems support laboratory test ordering [11] and provide computerized physician order entry (CPOE), which alert the users to possible interactions between prescribed medications [8]. One of the well-known classes of CDSS is clinical Diagnostic Decision Support System (DDSS). DDSS are defined by Miller and Geissbuhler [8] as "a computer-based algorithm that assists a clinician with one or more component steps of the diagnostic process."

Most CDDS arose out of earlier expert systems research; however, the intent of CDDS is not to simulate an expert's decision making, but to assist the clinicians in their decision making process. As stated by Berner and La Lande [2], "the role of the computer should be to enhance and support the human who is ultimately responsible for the clinical decision." The users of the CDSS actively interact with the system. They expect the CDDS system to provide deep explanation of suggested decisions. The users of CDDS want to be able to follow the reasoning, filter the information, discard useless information, utilize the useful information, and make the final decision based on their own clinical judgment. Furthermore, the users of CDDS expect the main component of CDSS, KB (1) to be transparent, i.e., human-readable; (2) to be updatable; (3) to be adaptable to local sites; and (4) to be able to learn from experience, i.e., from existing "solved" cases [3] .

14.3 Knowledge Base in CDDS

The two main tasks of KE are building and maintaining knowledge bases. These tasks require knowledge acquisition, verification, and validation. Knowledge acquisition is one of the well-known "bottlenecks" in the development of CDSS. However, medical knowledge acquisition is not the only problem of CDSS. Once KB has been created, it requires continuous maintenance. As pointed out by Spooner [14] : "Maintaining the knowledge base in such systems is the most significant bottleneck in the maintenance of such systems, since the knowledge base needs to be expanded and updated as medical knowledge grows." KB requires regular updates and verification that the newly introduced rules do not interfere with the existing set of rules.

In this paper, we concentrate on the verification and validation (V&V) of KB in CDDS. We argue that the V&V process should be explicitly incorporated in the design and implementation of the CDSS. Moreover, the knowledge representation used for KB and the V&V process should meet the four requirements of the CDDS users: transparency, updatability, adaptability, and learnability.

Transparency of KB: The users of CDSS expect to be able to review the KB and follow the reasoning apparatus. Thus, the KB representation should be human-readable. To fulfill the transparency requirement, we have used a rule-based knowledge representation. We have chosen this specific representation for two reasons. First, rules are common in medicine, and medical practitioners use rules such as Clinical Prediction Rules (CPR) in their daily practice. The prediction rules simplify the assessment process, expedite diagnosis and treatment for serious cases, and limit unnecessary tests for low-probability cases. Second, rule-based systems have been the prevailing representation for medical expert system since the 1970's, when Shortliffe created a well-known rule-based expert system, MYCIN [13].

Updateability of KB: The users of CDSS expect to be able to update the existing KB. To provide for updateability of the KB, we have utilized the KE tools such as knowledge editors. The updates of the KB rules must be verified, so the new rules or modified rules are not changing the rule-based inference system in an unintended way. We discuss the verification of the updates in the next section. Also, updateability is interrelated with the learning-from-experience process, which may necessitate modification of the existing rules.

Adaptability of KB: The users of CDSS expect to be able to adapt particular KB to their own clinical settings. This requirement is essential since (1) clinics must operate using their particular guidelines and procedures, (2) many clinical rules must be modified to be applicable to specific groups of patients, and (3) some clinical rules must be simplified to eliminate unavailable test results. To provide for the adaptability of KB, we have added a few adaptation rules. However, this aspect of the KB maintenance relies mostly on the user-driven updates to the rules, and has not been fully automated.

Learnability of KB: The users of CDSS expect the KB to be able to learn from the experience. To provide for the learnability of KB, we have used two components: data warehouse of medical cases and data mining tools. Since both of these components are also used to support the V&V process, we describe them in the next section.

14.4 Verification and Validation of the KB

In this section, we discuss verification and validation of the knowledge bases for CDDS. First, we differentiate between verification and validation. Second, we describe verification and validation process using examples from two CDDS, which support diagnostic tasks in two medical fields: psychiatry and sleep medicine. Both CDDS systems are based on fuzzy rules, and both support relatively narrow diagnostic tasks. The first system, which supports diagnosis of clinical depression, uses expert knowledge and clinical guidelines for the creation of the KB. The second system, which supports the diagnosis of obstructive sleep apnea, uses a combination of the medical literature and clinical experts' knowledge for the creation of the KB. We use these two systems to demonstrate the built-in support for verification and validation.

14.4.1 Verification vs. Validation

In software engineering, verification means checking if the software system is built according to the specification. On the other hand, validation means that the built software system is "valid" in the context of the user problem. Verification is a process which controls the quality and is used to determine whether the software system meets the expected standards. In contrast to this, validation is a process which assures the quality. It gives an assurance that the software system is successful in accomplishing what it is intended to do (solves the user problem).

The verification and validation (V&V) of the knowledge base is different from the V&V process for a typical information system. For example, in a rule-based system, verification is the process of checking the "syntactical" correctness of the rules, whereas validation is the process of checking the "semantic" and "pragmatic" correctness of the rules. A rule is semantically correct, if it is clinically valid. For example, a clinical prediction rule or diagnostic criteria must be validated through a number of research studies and approved by medical associations. A rule is pragmatically valid, if it is useful in a particular clinical setting. For example, a rule requiring complex laboratory tests may not be suitable for use in a clinic not equipped with a highly specialized laboratory equipment. In many cases, the verification process can be automated; the validation process must be performed by the users. However, the users can be assisted by a computerized analysis of data.

14.4.2 Rule-Based Representation for KB

Our examples are based on two CDSS systems, in which rules have three functions: descriptive, prescriptive, and predictive. In the descriptive sense, rules characterize the subpopulations of patients with higher or lower risks for the disease. In the prescriptive sense, rules define the typical (normative) values for specific predictors. In the predictive sense, rules assess the probability of a new patient belonging to one of the classes. The hypothetical quality of the rule is defined by the certainty factor (CF), a degree of belief ranging from -1.0 (absolute disbelief) to $+1.0$ (absolute belief), assigned to the rule by medical experts based on their clinical experience. Similarity to MYCIN, we use certainty factors (CF) to represent uncertainty characteristic to medical application. Furthermore, we use a fuzzy-logic approach to represent impression. Thus, the rules can be crisp and fuzzy.

The rule is comprised of two parts: a premise and a consequent. The premise of the rule uses predefined predictors, for example, age, gender, or snoring. A proposition is a logical expression composed of a predictor variable, the relational operator ($<, \leq, >, \geq, =$), and a value; for example, age > 65, habitual snoring $=$ yes. The rules are in the conjunctive propositional form, for example, age > 65 AND gender $=$ female. The conclusion of the rule includes the class label. The following two rules are simplified examples of diagnostic rules used in the screening for obstructive sleep apnea (OSA):

R1: IF habitual snoring = yes THEN OSA = yes (CF = 0.4)

R2: IF habitual snoring = yes AND age = older THEN OSA = yes (CF = 0.5)

The first rule, R1, has one binary predictor: habitual snoring (yes/no). Habitual snoring is one of the most important predictors of OSA. However, there are cases of OSA without snoring, as well as there are patient who habitually snore and do not have OSA. Studies have shown [4] that approximately 50% of habitual snorers have some degree of sleep-disordered breathing. Therefore, R1 has certainty factor of 0.4. The second rule, R2, has an additional predictor: age. Age is a linguistic variable. Older age increases the chances of having OSA. On the other hand, older age increases the chances of snoring. Therefore, R2 has certainty factor of 0.5.

14.4.3 Verification of KB

Knowledge bases for medical applications, even for narrowly specialized DSSs, are large and complex. Therefore, on-going verification of such systems requires automated tools. To support verification of a rule-based system, we have constructed Computer Aided Knowledge Engineering (CAKE) system for the management of knowledge base. CAKE system provides automatic detection of the following problems [7]:

Redundant Rules
Two rules are redundant if $R_i \leftarrow W_{i1} \wedge \ldots \wedge W_{in}$ and $R_j \leftarrow W_{j1} \wedge \ldots \wedge W_{jn}$, where R is conclusion, W are conditions and $i \neq j$, holds: $\{W_{i1} \ldots Win\} = \{W_{j1} \ldots Wjn\}$.

Subsuming Rules
If for two different rules: $R_i \leftarrow W_{i1} \wedge \ldots \wedge W_{im}$ and $R_j \leftarrow W_{i1} \wedge \ldots \wedge W_{in}$, holds $\{W_{il} \wedge \ldots \wedge W_{im}\} \subseteq \{W_{il} \wedge \ldots \wedge W_{in}\}$, then we say that rule R_i subsumes rule R_j.

Contradictory Rules
Two rules are contradictory if $R_i \leftarrow W_{i1} \wedge \ldots \wedge W_{in}$ and $\neg R_j \leftarrow W_1 \wedge \ldots \wedge W_n$, where $i \neq j$.

Inconsistent Rules
Two rules are inconsistent if $R_i \leftarrow W_1 \wedge \ldots \wedge W_n$ and $R_j \leftarrow W_1 \wedge \ldots \wedge W_n$, where $i \neq j$ and $R_i \neq R_j$.

Incompleteness of Rules (Missing Rules)
It is assumed that a knowledge base is complete when the rules include all possible combinations of the attributes and their allowable values in the rule antecedents (conditions) and the rule consequents (conclusions). It is important to notice that in practice most knowledge bases are incomplete, which is a normal situation.

Unused Attributes and Values
System checks if there exist attributes or values which are never used in the rules in KB.

14.4.4 Validation of KB

Validation of KB is supported by two components: data warehousing and data mining.

Data Warehousing
Most of the clinical data are already stored in a digital form, with some clinics using electronic patient records. The electronic storage of medical data provides a unique opportunity for a computer-assisted creation, validation, and modification of KB. In our research, we have used two databases: records of diagnosed depression cases and a large repository of diagnosed patient records provided by sleep disorders clinics. The data warehouse of diagnosed cases can be used in two ways: (1) to run the KB rules for each case and compare its results with the clinicians' diagnosis and

(2) to induce a predictive model from the data and compare the induced model with the model used in CDSS. The evaluation of the KB rules against the data warehouse of diagnosed cases provides the measurements for the validity of the KB in terms of its accuracy (sensitivity and specificity). The comparison of the existing KB rules and the induced rules provides a modification (refinement) mechanism for the rules.

Data Mining

Based on the data from the data warehouse, data mining (machine learning) techniques can be used to automatically induce descriptive and predictive models. In our research, we have used artificial neural networks (ANN), classification rule induction, and decision tree induction. The ANN methods were used in the CDSS system for the evaluation of clinical depression. The ANN model has been used as a part of a hybrid expert system. In case of the CDSS for the diagnosis of OSA, the clinicians require that the induced models should be comprehensible by humans; therefore, we have utilized the rule induction and the decision tree induction methods. In our study, we compared the rules in the existing KB with the automatically induced rules from the data warehouse. Three scenarios for the induced rules are possible: (1) they confirm the existing KB rules, (2) they contradict the existing KB rules (provide contradictory examples), or (3) they identify new insights (contribute new rules to KB).

To demonstrate how the data mining techniques can be used for the modification of KB rules, we present two examples from our studies.

Example 1

The following KB rule, R3, specifies low OSA risks for young female patients with normal weight. Normal weight is represented by the Body Mass Index (BMI) less than 25.

R3: IF BMI $<$ 25 AND age $=$ young AND gender $=$ female
THEN OSA $=$ no (CF $= 0.9$)

R3 is partially contradicted by the rule induced from data, I1, which additionally includes hypertension (HTN).

I1: IF BMI $<$ 26 AND age $=$ young AND gender $=$ female
AND HTN $=$ yes THEN OSA $=$ yes

Since hypertension is one of the important predictors of OSA, Rule 3 could be modified and it could include HTN $=$ no.

Example 2

The following two rules, I2 and I3, were derived from an induced decision tree:

I2: IF BMI ≤ 26.8 AND HTN $=$ no AND gender $=$ female
AND age ≤ 56 THEN OSA $=$ no

I3: IF BMI < 26.8 AND HTN $=$ no AND gender $=$ female AND age > 56 THEN OSA $=$ yes

These two rules provide a new KB insight. The induced decision tree divides female patients with normal blood pressure (HTN = no) and normal BMI (or slightly overweight) into two age groups: age ≤ 56 and age > 56. This specific age-based division could be associated with an increased risk of OSA among postmenopausal women. Thus, the existing rules for female patients can be modified to reflect the higher postmenopausal risk for OSA.

14.5 Conclusions

In this paper, we examined the KE methods and their roles in the KM process in medicine. We focused on the CDSS and its most important component – knowledge base (KB). We discussed verification and validation of the medical KB in the context of the user requirements. The CDSS users expect the KB component to be transparent (human-readable), updatable (users should be able to modify KB), adaptable (user should have support to adapt KB to their local clinical requirements), and learnable (KB should be able to learn from experience). To address these issues, we used a rule-based representation for KB. We built two highly specialized KBs for small sets of diagnostic rules, which are used in two domains: (1) psychiatry, for the diagnosis of clinical depression and (2) sleep medicine for the diagnosis of obstructive sleep apnea. To represent the vagueness of medical concepts and data, we used a combination of crisp and fuzzy rules. To represent the inherent uncertainty of clinical prediction rules, we used the certainty factors. Furthermore, we created two data warehouses, one for the data from the psychiatric clinic and the other one for the data from the sleep disorders clinics. We used these warehouses for the machine learning (data mining) tasks. We experimented with two main data mining techniques: the "black-box" approach (artificial neural networks) and the "transparent-box" approach (classification rule and decision tree induction).

In this paper, we argued that KB should include (1) an explicit mechanism for self-verification, (2) an automated mechanism for learning from experience, and (3) a built-in data warehouse (repository) of diagnosed cases. We demonstrated that the data warehouse of diagnosed cases could be used for the validation of KB. Furthermore, we used a machine-learning approach to demonstrate how the CDSS can learn from experience, which is represented by diagnosed cases stored in a data warehouse. We presented two examples of OSA diagnostic rules to illustrate how the induced rules could be used for KB modification. We are planning to integrate and formalize the proposed framework for the verification and validation of KB. We will expand the fuzzy-logic based rules and the fuzzy inference mechanism. Furthermore, we intend to create KB rules for other well-known predictors of obstructive sleep apnea such as diabetes, large neck, and excessive daytime sleepiness. Also, we will expand the rule system for the diagnostic criteria for clinical depression.

References

1. Beardon, C. (ed.): Artificial Intelligence Terminology - A Reference Guide, p. 86. Wiley, New York (1989)
2. Berner, E.S., La Lande, T.J.: Overview of Clinical Decision Support Systems. In: Berner Eta, S. (ed.) Clinical Decision Support Systems. Theory and Practice. Health Information Series, pp. 3–22 (2007)
3. Carter, J.H.: Design and Implementation Issues. In: Berner Eta, S. (ed.) Clinical Decision Support Systems. Theory and Practice. Health Information Series, pp. 64–98 (2007)
4. Collop, N.A., Cassell, D.K.: Snoring and Sleep-disordered Breathing. In: Lee-Chiong, T., Sateia, M., Carskadon, M.A. (eds.) Sleep Medicine, pp. 349–355. Hanley & Belfus, Inc., Philadelphia (2002)
5. Finlay, P.N.: Introducing Decision Support Systems. Blackwell Publishers, Blackwell (1994)
6. Kaushal, R., Shojania, K.G., Bates, D.W.: Effects of Computerized Physician Order Entry and Clinical Decision Support Systems on Medication Safety: A systematic Review. Archives of Internal Medicine 163, 1409–1416 (2003)
7. von Michalik, K.: Selected Aspects of Multi-Level Hybrid AI Environment for Decision Support. Journal of Artificial Intelligence Studies (Special Issue) 1(2(24)) (2004); Proceedings of VI International Conference on Artificial Intelligence AI (2004)
8. Miller, R.A., Geissbuhler, A.: Diagnostic Decision Support Systems. In: Berner Eta, S. (ed.) Clinical Decision Support Systems. Theory and Practice. Health Information Series, pp. 99–125 (2007)
9. El Morr, C., Subercaze, J.: Knowledge Management in Health Care. In: Cruz-Cunha, M.M., Tavares, A.J., Simões, R.J. (eds.) Handbook of Research on Developments in e-Health and Telemedicine: Technological and Social Perspectives, pp. 490–510. Medical Information Science Reference, IGI Global, Hershey, PA (2010)
10. Power, D.J.: Decision Support Systems: Concepts and Resources for Managers. Quorum Books, Westport (2002)
11. Shabot, M.M., LoBue, M., Chen, J.: Wireless Clinical Alerts for Physiologic, Laboratory and Medication Data, Proceedings – AMIA Symposium. In: Journal of the American Medical Informatics Association, pp. 789–793 (2000)
12. Shapiro, S.C. (ed.): Encyclopedia of Artificial Intelligence, vol. 1, p. 287. Wiley, New York (1990)
13. Shortliffe, E.H.: Computer-Based Medical Consultations: MYCIN. Elsevier/North-Holland, Amsterdam, London (1976)
14. Spooner, S.A.: Mathematical Foundations of Decision Support Systems. In: Berner Eta, S. (ed.) Clinical Decision Support Systems. Theory and Practice. Health Information Series, pp. 23–43 (2007)
15. Waterman, D.A.: A Guide to Expert Systems, pp. 4–5. Addison-Wesley, Reading (1985)

Part IV

Questioning and Reasoning in Medicine

15

A Layperson Reflection on Sorites

Enric Trillas and Itziar García-Honrado

15.1 Introduction

Concerning the so-called 'Sorites Paradox' there are dozens of papers, mainly of a philosophical character, in which the concept of 'heap' is viewed as only depending on the number of grains in each heap, but avoiding any consideration on its three-dimensional shape [9], [3]. Such a radical simplification can actually be surprising for a layperson who, interested in Philosophy has, at least, some perceptive experience on heaps.

In any case, heap is a word or linguistic term that refers to a particular instance of physical objects, whose meaning is captured through its common perceptive use in language and requires some kind of distinction between what is and what is not a heap. That is, to understand the statement 'h is a heap' it should also be understood when 'h^* is not a heap' ,to perceptually recognize if a physical object constituted by grains of sand is, or is not, a heap. On the contrary, any set of grains could simultaneously be a heap and a not-heap without the possibility of recognizing what it is actually.

All that is not to mention the actual lack of any antonym or opposite of the term heap, like it could be the non existent term 'unheap'. Only the term 'flat' referring to some set of grains of sand could tentatively be used as an opposite of heap.

In those philosophical papers, a heap appears as a theoretical construct not actually different from the finite subset of natural numbers denoting which is the number of grains in the heap, something that is absolutelly not in the layperson's perceptive use of the term. Hence, philosophical papers on the Sorites type of reasoning cannot be included in commonsense reasoning. In addition, their conclusions are reached by repeatedly using the scheme of Modus Ponens that, as it is well known, is a typical way of performing deductive reasoning. Consequently, Sorites deserves to be reconsidered from the point of view of everyday or commonsense reasonig, by distinguishing between the heap, and the set of the grains of sand in it.

The so-called paradox is often presented by saying that if a heap, denoted by $h(p)$, has p grains of sand, also when removing a single grain is $h(p-1)$ a heap, and $h(p-2),...,h(p-n),...,$ and after $p-1$ steps is $h(1)$ a heap, against the common

R. Seising and M.E. Tabacchi (Eds.): *Fuzziness and Medicine*, STUDFUZZ 302, pp. 217–231.
DOI: 10.1007/978-3-642-36527-0_15

perception of what is a heap. Hence, in the same classical paradox it appears a perceptive view of what is not a heap, since in the identification between heap and set of grains, there is no any paradox as far as $h(1)$ is a set. What is not clear at all is which is the first number p such that $h(p)$ is not a heap. In a perceptive-based view the only that perhaps could be known is some interval $(p-i, p+k)$ to which p belongs to.

From a flat three-dimensional set of grains to, for instance, a cone of them, there are many, many possibilities for having a heap in such a way that the statements 'h is a heap' are up to some degree. For instance, figure (a) in section 15.4.2 shows a heap up to a degree like 0.9, figure (b) up to a degree 0.1, and figure (c) up to a degree 0.4. Nevertheless, these degrees do be fixed in the most reasonable way than possible, that is, it should be specified by a clearly expresable point of view allowing such quantification through a comparative process.

Remark 1. The term 'heap' appears as gradable to the layperson by, at least, their different shapes with different basis in the floor, and the different heights they show, but not by their number of grains that nobody is actually going to count. What is not clear at all is if the 'degree up to which h is a heap' is, or is not always a number, and to which universe of discourse X heaps do belong to have the possibility of representing the numerical degrees (provided they exist) by means of a 'fuzzy set' in X. In any case, and if it is possible, what they can be considered to be are *indices* of 'heapness'.

Remark 2. As it will be shown in what follows, the comments made on 'heap' are applicable to other imprecise terms like, for instance, 'small' in a numerical universe of discourse and once a membership function according with its use in the corresponding context has been designed ([7]). In the field of medicine, that is full of imprecise technical concepts, the Sorites' process presented in this paper, could be useful to determine if a medical concept (C) can be specified, or not, by a classical set. In the negative case, it is not possible to conduct reasonings involving the concept in the classical 'boolean' way. For instance, if 'diabetes'(D) and 'high blood preassure'(B) are interpreted as fuzzy sets, the statement ((D and H) or (D and not H)) is only equivalent to D in some algebras of fuzzy sets in which no law of duality holds.

After a concept is designed as a fuzzy set, accordingly with its technical use, it could be managed under the rules allowed in the corresponding algebra of fuzzy sets. In addition, when the representation of its negation is chosen, it can be approached by the crisp set whose elements are those in the universe that are more C than not C.

15.2 The Case of the Term 'small' in the Interval [0,10] of the Real Line

It seems reasonable to agree that a layperson does use the term 'small' in the real interval $[0,10]$ by following the four rules,

1. There are numbers in [0,10] that are small. For instance, at least 0 is small.
2. Not all the numbers in [0,10] are small. For instance, at least 10 is not small.
3. If x is small, and $y < x$, also y is small
4. There exists some number $e > 0$ such that if $|x - y| \leq e$, and one of the elements x or y is small, the other is also small.

Notice that from (4) follows immediatelly that if x is small, then it is also $x + e$ small, since $|x + e - x| = e$.

Can it exist a subset S of [0,10] containing all the small numbers and only them? In other words: Is the classical axiom of specification applicable to the predicate 'small'?

Obviously, and provided it exists the set $S = \{x \in [0,10]; x \text{ is small}\}$, it should be $S' = [0,10] - S = \{x \in [0,10]; x \text{ is not small}\}$, the complement of S in [0,10]. From (1) and (2), 0 is in S, and 10 is in S', that is, both sets are not-empty.

Since [0,10] is a compact set in the usual topology of the real line, and S is bounded by 10, it should exist $s = SupS \in [0,10]$, with elements of S arbitrarily close to s by the left. Thus, by (4) it should be s in S, and by (3) all numbers in S are small. But $s + e > s$ implies that also $s + e$ in S' is small, that by the set theoretic property $S \bigcap S' = \emptyset$, is a contradiction! Hence, there cannot exist any subset like S. The predicate 'small', as used by a layperson, is not representable by any subset of [0,10] since with it the axiom of specificity fails, and consequently Boolean algebra cannot be used to represent commonsense reasonings involving the linguistic term 'small'.

Remarks 1. *a) Notice that, once* $e > 0$ *is fixed, with the number* $(10 - s)/e = t$*, it is obtained* $10 = s + t \cdot e$*. It should be pointed out that if both s and e are with a finite number of decimal digits, then t is a positive integer. For instance, if* $e = 0.01$ *and* $s = 3.4$*, it results* $(10 - 3.4)/0.01 = 660$*, thus* $3.4 + 660.0.01 = 10$*. Keeping e as a negative power of 10, for instance if it were s = the number pi, it will suffice to take* $s* = 3.14 < s$ *to also have s∗ in S, and since* $(10 - 3.14)/0.01 = 686$ *it follows* $3.14 + 686e = 10$*, that implies the absurd* $10 \in S$*. Consequently, provided e is a negative power of 10, it always follows that 10 is small, and* $S = [0,10]$*: all numbers in [0,10] are actually small, that is the 'paradox'.*

This is exactly what is called the Sorites Paradox, that was classically posed with the number of hairs in a human head (In Greek, Sorites means 'bald man'). Nevertheless, and from a layperson point of view, what Sorites just shows is that there are some linguistic terms, like 'small', for which the axiom of specification fails. Thus, it is not possible to represent them by means of classical sets or elements in a Boolean algebra, in the corresponding universe of discourse. This conclusion is at the same origin of fuzzy sets.

b) To clarify the inference done to state that $s + te$ *is in S, let's notice that it is a deductive process reached by a t times reiteration of 'Modus Ponens':*

$$\begin{array}{ll} x \textit{ is small} & \to x+e \textit{ is small} \\ s \textit{ is small} & \\ \hline & s+e \textit{ is small} \\ x+e \textit{ is small} & \to x+2e \textit{ is small} \\ s+e \textit{ is small} & \\ \hline & s+2e \textit{ is small} \\ & \dots \\ \hline & s+te \textit{ is small} \end{array}$$

It should be pointed out that this successive application of 'Modus Ponens' is only formally correct provided the arrow $\to$*, representing the conditional statements is a 'conditional', that is, satisfies the Modus Ponens' inequality* $a \cdot (a \to b) \leq b$*, for all a and b. It happens for instance either with* $a \to b = a' + b$ *in the case all statements can be represented in a Boolean algebra, or* $a \to b = a \cdot b$*, if they are representable in just a lattice (at the end, the negation is not in the problem). In the current case. 'If x is small, then* $x+e$ *is small' either can be identified with 'Not(x is small) or (*$x+e$ *is small)', or with '(x is small) and (*$x+e$ *is small)'. Of course, in a Boolean algebra it is* $a \cdot (a' + b) = a \cdot a' + a \cdot b = 0 + a \cdot b = a \cdot b \leq b$*, and in any lattice it is* $a \cdot (a \cdot b) = (a \cdot a) \cdot b = a \cdot b \leq b$*.*

15.3 About the Black's Separation Point with 'small' in [0,10]

The philosopher Max Black asserted, in a more general setting, that a separation point B between the numbers that are small and those that are not, does exist, but is impossible to find. That is, that the before mentioned number p such that $h(p)$ is not a heap does exist but is not determinable. We will see in the following that this statement is not always correct, but that a different kind of separation points s for 'small' can always be found by employing something related with a partial contradiction of small with itself [8].

15.3.1

Accepting that 'small' is a gradable predicate in [0,10], and by using 'small' under the former four rules, it is possible to define which functions $\mu_S : [0,10] \to [0,1]$ can represent

$$\mu_S(x) = \text{degree up to which 'x is small'}.$$

Under those rules, those functions do verify:

a) $\mu_S(0) = 1$
b) $\mu_S(10) = 0$
c) If $x \leq y$, then $\mu_S(y) \leq \mu_S(y)$
d) If $\mu_S(x) > 0$, then there is no any $y \in (x-e, x+c)$ such that $\mu_S(y) = 0$.

(a) and (b) say that 0 is completely small, and that 10 is not small at all. (c) says that function μ_S shall be decreasing, and (d) says that no jumps to zero are allowed for μ_S. Some of those functions are depicted in figures 15.1a, 15.1b, 15.1c, 15.1d.

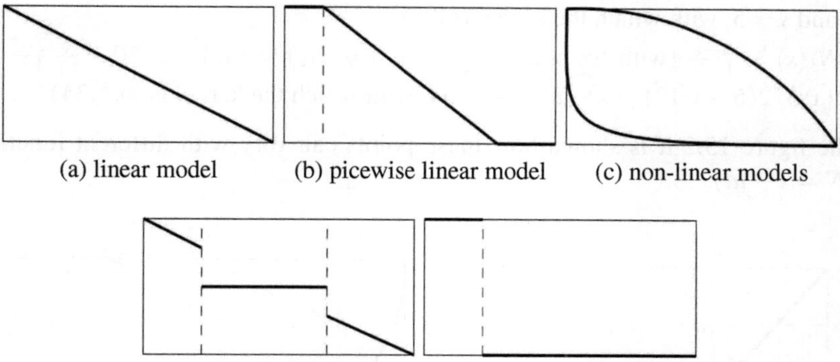

(a) linear model (b) picewise linear model (c) non-linear models

(d) picewise linear with jumps (e) not allowed jumps

Fig. 15.1

Obviously no function like that in figure 15.1e is allowed to represent 'small', that is, no *precisification* of the grade of 'small' by a classical predicate like 'less than s' is permitted by the use given by the former four rules.

15.3.2

Once one of those functions μ_S is taken as adequate to represent how 'small' is being used in a concrete case, it is supposed that also, the use of 'not small' should be known, that is, a strong negation function $N : [0,1] \to [0,1]$ is known to verify $\mu_{notS}(x) = N(\mu_S(x)) = \varphi^{-1}(1 - \varphi(\mu_S(x)))$, for all x in [0,10], with an order-antomorphism φ of the totally ordered unit interval [4]. Notice that it is $N(n) = n$, *if an only if* $n = \varphi^{-1}(1/2) \in (0,1)$, hence it is:

$$\mu_S(x) \geq \mu_{notS}(x) \Leftrightarrow \mu_S(x) \geq \varphi^{-1}(1/2),$$

and then the *Kernel* of μ_S is defined by:

$$K_N(\mu_S) = \{x \in [0,10]; \mu_S(x) \geq \mu_{notS}(x)\} = \{x \in [0,10]; \mu_S(x) \geq \varphi^{-1}(1/2)\},$$

that is, $K_N(\mu_P)$ is the subset of [0,10] containing those x that are 'more S than not S'. Of course, it exists $s = SupK_N(\mu_S) \in [0,10]$, a value that can be identified with a kind of separation point in a similar sense to that of Max Black since any $s + \varepsilon$ is 'more' not S than S.

For instance, if $\mu_S(x) = 1 - x/10$ and

1. $N_1(x) = \frac{1-x}{1+x}$ (with the fix point $2-\sqrt{2}$), it is $K_{N_1}(\mu_S) = \{x; 1-x/10 \geq 2-\sqrt{2}\} = \{x; \sqrt{2}-10 \geq x\}$, and $\sqrt{2}-10 \approx 4.14$, with which the Kernel is $[0, 4.14)$.
2. $N_2(x) = 1-x$ (fix point 1/2), is $K_{N_2}(\mu_S) = \{x; 1-x/10 \geq 1/2\} = \{x; 5 \geq x\}$, and $s = 5$, with which the kernel is $[0,5)$.
3. $N_3(s) = \frac{1-x}{1+2x}$ (with fix point $\frac{\sqrt{12}-2}{4}$), is $K_{N_3}(\mu_S) = \{x; 1-x/10 \geq \frac{\sqrt{12}-2}{4}\} = \{x; 5/2(6-\sqrt{12}) \geq x\}$, and $s \approx 6.34$, with which the kernel is $[0, 6.34)$.

In the figure 15.2 it is shown how these points can vary with different functions $\mu_S(N = 1 - id)$.

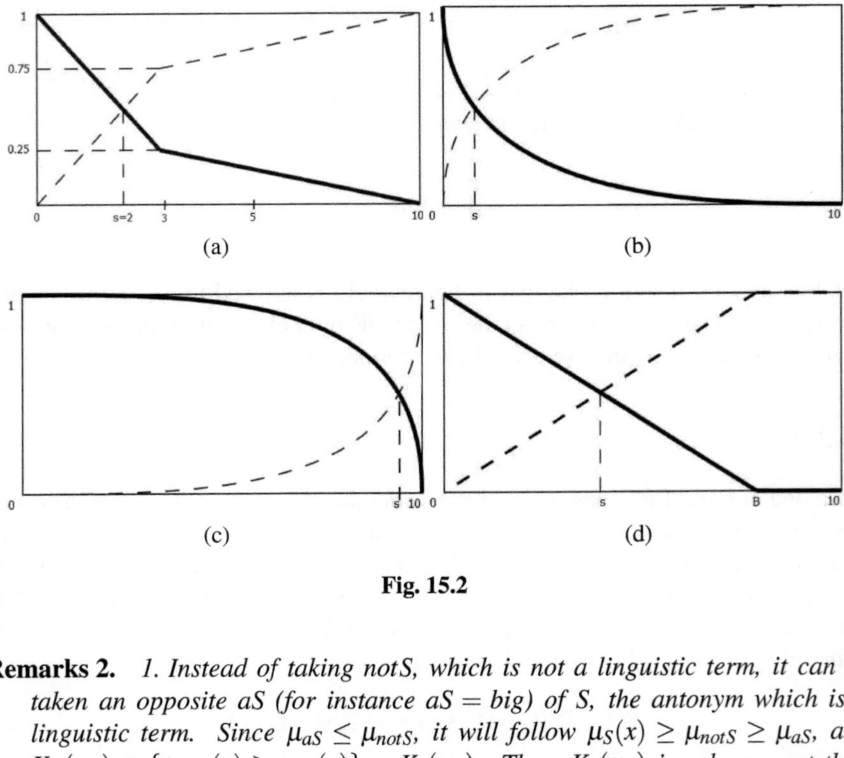

Fig. 15.2

Remarks 2. *1. Instead of taking notS, which is not a linguistic term, it can be taken an opposite aS (for instance aS = big) of S, the antonym which is a linguistic term. Since* $\mu_{aS} \leq \mu_{notS}$, *it will follow* $\mu_S(x) \geq \mu_{notS} \geq \mu_{aS}$, *and* $K_N(\mu_S) \subset \{x; \mu_S(x) \geq \mu_{aS}(x)\} = K_a(\mu_S)$. *Thus,* $K_a(\mu_S)$ *is a larger set than* $K_N(\mu_S)$, *therefore if* $s_a = supK_a(\mu_S)$, *it is* $s \leq s_a$.

For instance, with $\mu_{aS}(x) = \mu_S(\alpha(x))$ *and the symmetry* $\alpha(x) = 10 - x$, *it is* $\mu_{aS}(x) = 1 - \frac{10-x}{10} = \frac{x}{10} = \mu_{big}(x)$, *and*

$$\mu_S(x) \geq \mu_{aS}(x) \Leftrightarrow 1 - \frac{x}{10} \geq \frac{x}{10} \Leftrightarrow 5 \geq x,$$

that gives $K_a(\mu_S) = K_{N_2}(\mu_S) = [0,5)$, *so for* $\alpha(x) = 10 - x$ *and* N_2, $s = s_a = 5$.

2. *It should be pointed out that the separation point introduced in this paper is not the one advocated by Max Black [1]. Notice that in a, b, c, in the the figure 15.2 the Black's one is* $B = 10$*, and in figure (d) is the* $B < 10$ *marked there, and that in all the four cases it is* $s \leq B$ *(and* $s_A \leq B$*). Hence, contrarily to what he said, Black's point can be found in some cases, but is different from s (or* s_a*) that only classifies* $[0,10]$ *in the two subsets of points that are*
   - *more P than* not *P (*opposite of *P)*
   - *less P than* not *P (*opposite of *P)*
3. *There are cases in which point B does not exist. For instance, if the universe is the real semi-line* $[0,+\infty)$*, and* μ_S *tends asymptotically towards* 0 *(see the figure 15.3) it is clear that no point B can exist.*
   Nevertheless, as it appears in the figure, point s does exist.

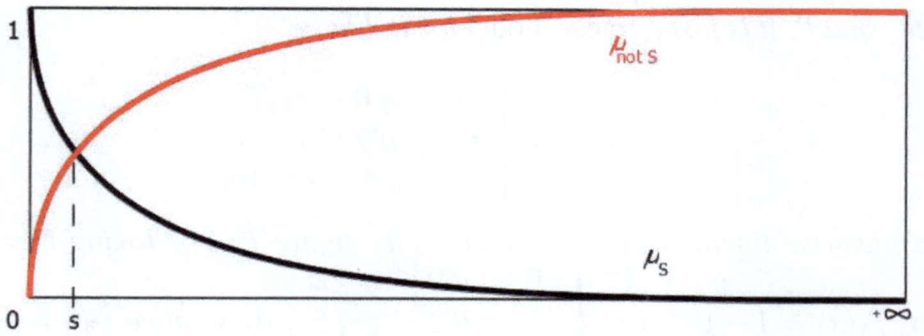

Fig. 15.3

For instance, if it is $\mu_S(x) = e^{-x} \in (0,1]$*, that verifies* $\lim_{x \to +\infty} e^{-x} = 0$*, it follows* $e^{-x} = 1 - e^{-x}$*, or* $e^{-x} = 0.5$*, but there is no a value B such that* $e^{-B} = 0$*. Provided 'not' is represented by the Sugeno's negation* $N(x) = \frac{1-x}{1+x}$*, from* $e^{-x} = N(e^{-x}) = \frac{1-e^{-x}}{1+e^{-x}}$*, it follows* $e^{-2x} + 2e^{-x} - 1 = 0$*, and* $e^{-x} = \sqrt{2} - 1$*. Hence,* $e^{-s_2} = \sqrt{2} - 1 < 0.5 = e^{-s_1}$*, and* $s_1 < s_2$*.*

4. *There are also cases in which points B and s are not unique and, hence, difficult to select. Of course, s is a supremum provided* μ_P *is decreasing, and a infimum if* μ_P *is non-decreasing. Hence, if* μ_P *is not monotonic, there can exist both an infimum and a supremum. This is, for instnace, the case with* $A4 =$*'around four' in* $X = [0,10]$ *whose membership function* μ_{A4} *is non monotonic. In the figure 15.4 it is clear the existence of the infimum* $i = 3.5$*, and the supremum* $s = 4.5$*, with which it is*

$$K_{1-id}(\mu_{A4}) = [3.5, 4.5].$$

It is analogously clear that there is not a point B after which the elements in $[0,1]$ *are not at all around 4.*

An analogous result is obtained dealing with s_a*.*

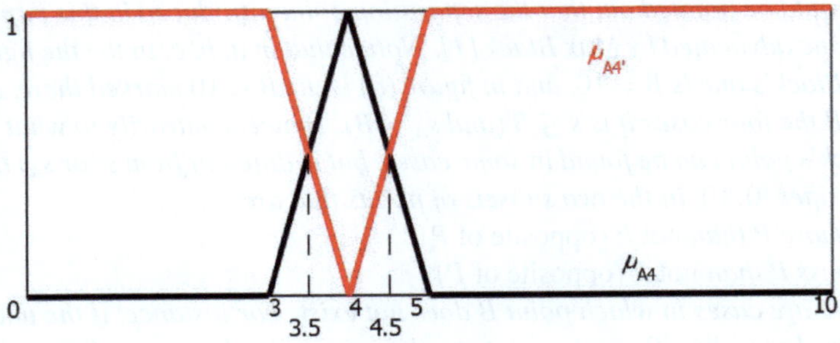

Fig. 15.4

5. *Function* $\mu_S(x) = 1 - \frac{x}{10}$ *is not, of course, the only that can represent the predicate 'small', it is just a* linear model *for it, like*

$$\mu_S(x) = \begin{cases} 1 & , \text{if } 0 \le x \le 2 \\ \frac{5-x}{3} & , \text{if } 2 \le x \le 5 \\ 0 & , \text{if } 5 \le x \le 10 \end{cases}$$

is a picewise linear model for 'small' (see figure 15.5). Taking $N = 1 - id$, *is* $\mu_{not\,S}(x) = 1 - \mu_S(x) = \begin{cases} 0 & , \text{if } 0 \le x \le 2 \\ \frac{x-2}{3} & , \text{if } 2 \le x \le 5 \\ 1 & , \text{if } 5 \le x \le 10 \end{cases}$, *thus, since* $\frac{5-x}{3} = \frac{x-2}{3}$, *it is* $s = 3.5$, *and the kernel is* $K_{1-id}(\mu_S) = [0, 3.5)$ *with* $s = 3.5$ *and* $B = 5$.
If instead of considering 'not small' it is considered the antonym 'big', and it is defined by $\alpha(x) = 10 - x$, *from*

$$\mu_{big}(x) = \mu_S(10 - x) = \begin{cases} 0 & , \text{if } 0 \le x \le 5 \\ \frac{x-5}{3} & , \text{if } 5 \le x \le 8 \\ 1 & , \text{if } 8 \le x \le 10 \end{cases}$$

in the figure 15.5 is obvious that it is $s_\alpha = B = 5$, *and hence* $K_\alpha(\mu_S) = [0, 5]$. *Thus,* $K_{1-id}(\mu_S) \subset K_\alpha(\mu_S)$.

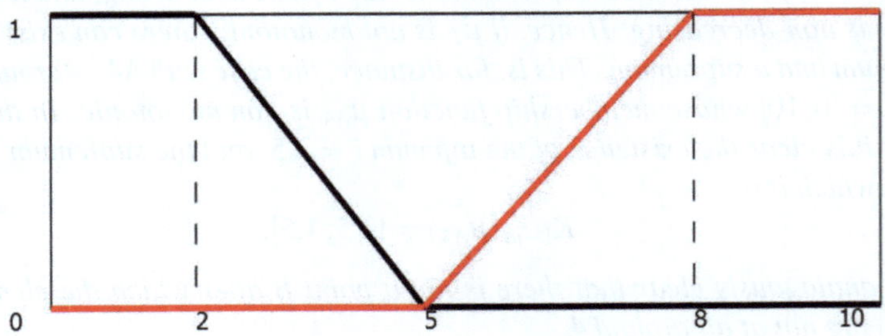

Fig. 15.5

That is, depending on the chosen particular model for representing 'small', and either on the negation N, or the symmetry α, *the points s and B can change. Of course, this variation is context-dependent on the concrete ways of using 'small', 'not small', and 'big'.*

6. *Provided the predicate P were crisp, then* $\mu_P \in \{0,1\}^X$ *and* $\mu_P(x) \geq \mu_{not\ P}(x) = 1 - \mu_P(x)$ *is equivalent to* $\mu_P(x) \geq 1/2$, *that is,* $\mu_P(x) = 1$. *Thus in these cases the kernel is* $K_{1-id}(\mu_P) = \{x \in X; \mu_P(x) = 1\}$, *that is, it is just the subset specified by P in X.*

15.4 Approaching the Use of the Term 'heap'

15.4.1

Like a correct linguistic use of the term 'small' in $[0,10]$ *requires to recognize, for instance, that '1 is small' and that '9 is big' or at least, that '9 is not small', also the use of the term 'heap' requires to recognize when something is not a heap, or that it is a 'flat'. Additionally, it should be known on which universe of discourse the term heap is applied to. Notice that, for instance, to correctly use the term 'odd' it is needed to know if it is being applied to the universe of the positive integers. In this way, the use of the word heap can be well learned, like it is learned the use of small, or that of odd.*

Under the typical philosophical hypothesis that a heap h only depends on the number of grains it contents, and by taking a sufficient big number N of grains, let us suppose that the universe is the interval $[0,N]$ *and that the degree up to which h is a heap can be described by the picewise linear function in the figure (15.6), in which it is clear that the threshold s is* $s = N/2$ *and* $K_{1-id}(\mu_H) = (N/2,N]$ *[8]. Of course, in this case it is* $B = 2N/3$. *For instance, if it were* $N = 2.500.000$, *it will be* $s = 834.000$, *and* $B = 1.666.667$, *grains of sand.*

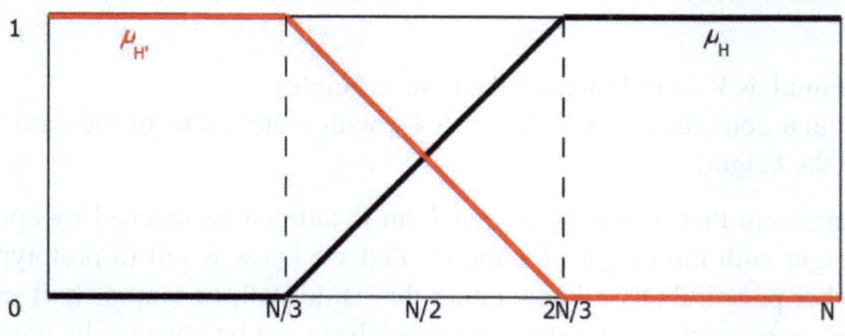

Fig. 15.6

That function is

$$\mu_{h'}(x) = \begin{cases} 0 & , \textit{if } x \leq N/3 \\ \frac{3x}{N} - 1 & , \textit{if } N/3 \leq x \leq 2N/3 \\ 1 & , \textit{if } 2N/3 \leq x \leq N \end{cases}$$

and then

$$\mu'_h(x) = 1 - \mu_h(x) = \begin{cases} 1 & , \textit{if } 0 \leq x \leq N/3 \\ 2 - \frac{3x}{N} & , \textit{if } N/3 \leq x \leq 2N/3 \\ 0 & , \textit{if } 2N/3 \leq x \end{cases}$$

and with them it can be recognized that an opposite, or antonym, of h is

$$\mu_{ah} = \mu_h(N-x) = \left\{ \begin{array}{ll} 1 & , \textit{if } 0 \leq x \leq N/3 \\ 2 - \frac{3x}{N} & , \textit{if } N/3 \leq x \leq 2N/3 \\ 0 & , \textit{if } 2N/3 \leq x \end{array} \right\} = \mu_{h'}(x).$$

Thus, under the representation of the antonym by the symmetry $\alpha(x) = N - x$, the antonym of heap coincides with the negation of heap given by the negation function $N(x) = 1 - x$, something that seems to be in agreement with the inexistence of antonyms of the term heap in the dictionaries of antonyms. Familiarity with the term heap requires, at least, familiarity with not-heap, once it is understood as an antonym (not regular, of course). On the contrary, how could a heap be recognized as such?

15.4.2

Undoubtedly, a heap is constitued by grains although it is not perceived through the number of grains it contents, but by its three-dimensional shape captured by a balance between the area of its basement, and its height. For instance, with a small basement and a large height, the heap will go down. A representation of this characteristic of heaps can be reached through its volume, that if, for instance, the heap is

- A pyramid, is $V = 1/3$ (area of the base $\times$ height)
- A circular cone, is $V = 1/3(\pi \times r^2 \times h)$, with r the radius of the circle's base, and h the height.

In the same vein that to recognize that John is tall can be reached by comparing John's height with the height of someone that we know is tall (a prototype), and with another person that we know either that is not tall, or that is short (an anty-prototype), to recognize that a set of grain is a heap can be obtained by comparison with something we know can be called a heap, and something that cannot be called a heap. To fix the universe, let us only consider heaps in the unit cube $[0,1]^3$.

1. *The prototype of heap is a pyramid, and its anti-prototype a flat collection of grains.*

The pyramid is that in the figure (a), with its vertex the point $(\frac{1}{2}, \frac{1}{2}, 1)$, height $h = 1$, and volumen $V = \frac{1}{3}$. The flat collection of grains can be supposed to be like in figure (b), with a small height ε, and volume=area of the base $\times \varepsilon = \varepsilon$. An instance of a heap is in figure (c).

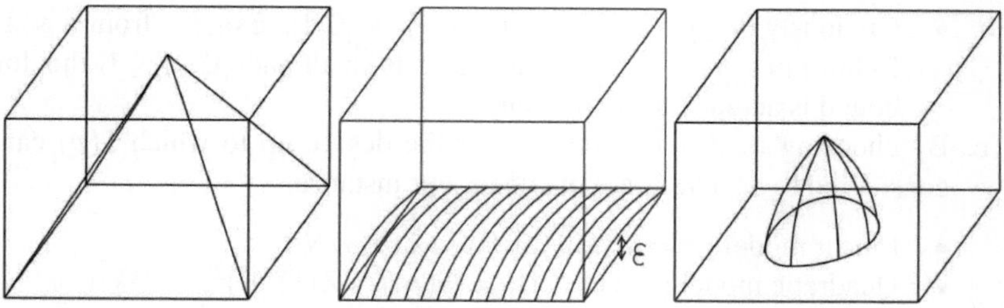

(a) (b) (c)

Let N a sufficiently big number and let us design by $S(p)$, $p \leq N$, a set of p grains, with which we will state 'S(p) is a heap'. That is, the universe of discourse in $X = \{S(p);\, p \leq N\}$, endowed with the partial order '$S(p) \leq^* S(q) \Leftrightarrow p \leq q$'.

The heap is undoubtedly constituted by the collection $S(p)$ of grains, but it is recognized that $S(p)$ is a heap by comparing it with a prototype like P. Such comparison is a matter of perceptive similarity. Thus, and provided the number of p can be estimated,

a. Let it be $\lambda(h)$, $0 < \lambda(h) \leq 1$, a coefficient perceptively established with which we compare the statement 'h is a heap' with the statements 'F is a heap' and 'P is a heap'. Clearly, $\lambda(h)$ comes from a perceptive comparison with the volumes of F and P. It will be supposed that if h_1 has p_1 grains, and h_2 has p_2 grains, $p_1 \leq p_2$, it is $\lambda(h_1) \leq \lambda(h_2)$. For instance, for h in figure (c) it could be taken $\lambda(h) = \frac{1}{3}$, that represents that the volume of P is around three times de volume of h in the figure (c).
b. Let it be $\varphi : [0,1] \to [0,1]$, continuous non-decreasing, and such that $\varphi(0) = 0$, $\varphi(1) = 1$ (an order-automorphism of the ordered unit interval). With φ, the degree up to which 'S(p) is a heap' could be defined by

$$\mu_h(S(p)) = \lambda(h)\varphi(\frac{p}{N}),$$

since $S(p) \leq^* S(q) \Leftrightarrow p \leq q \Leftrightarrow \frac{p}{N} \leq \frac{q}{N} \Rightarrow \varphi(\frac{p}{N}) \leq \varphi(\frac{q}{n})$, and provided λ also increases with the number of grains, is

$$S(p) \leq^* S(q) \Rightarrow \mu_h(S(p)) \leq \mu_h(S(q)).$$

Notice that:

- $\mu_P(S(p)) = \lambda(h)\varphi(\frac{p}{N}) = \varphi(\frac{p}{N})$, $\mu_F(S(p)) = \varepsilon\varphi(\frac{p}{N})$, and as it is supposed that it is $0 < \varepsilon < 1$, it follows $\mu_F(S(p)) \leq \mu_P(S(p))$, for all $p \leq N$.
- If p is fixed, and $\lambda(h_1) \leq \lambda(h_2)$, it follows $\mu_{h_1}(S(p)) \leq \mu_{h_2}(S(p))$.
- $\mu_h(S(0)) = \lambda(h)\varphi(\frac{0}{N}) = 0$, $\mu_h(S(N)) = \lambda(h)\varphi(\frac{N}{N}) = \lambda(h)$, and $\mu_P(S(N)) = 1$, $\mu_F(S(N)) = \varepsilon$.
- From $\lambda(h) \leq 1$ it follows $\lambda(h)\varphi(\frac{p}{N}) \leq \varphi(\frac{p}{N}) \leq 1$, by $p \leq N$. Hence, $\mu_h(S(p)) \leq 1$.
- Obviously $0 \leq \mu_h(S(p))$ and $\mu_h(S(p)) \in [0,1]$. Exactly, from $\varepsilon \leq \lambda(h)$ follows $\varepsilon\varphi(\frac{p}{N}) \leq \mu_h(S(p))$, and as ε is small and $\varphi(\frac{p}{N}) \leq 1$, this lower bound is actually a small number.

c. By choosing φ, different models for the degree up to which $S(p)$ can be considered to be a heap are obtained. For instance,

- Linear model ($\varphi = id$), $\mu_h(S(p)) = \lambda(h)p/N$
- Quadratic model ($\varphi(x) = x^2$), $\mu_h(S(p)) = \lambda(h)(\frac{p}{N})^2$,
- etc.

Finally, provided '$S(p)$ is not a heap' can be represented by a strong-negation N_{φ_1}, $\mu_{h'} = N_{\varphi_1} \circ \mu_h$, is

$$\mu_{h'}(S(p)) \geq \mu_h(S(p)) \Leftrightarrow \varphi_1^{-1}(1 - \varphi_1(\lambda(h)\varphi(\frac{p}{N}))) \geq \lambda(h)\varphi(\frac{p}{N})) \Leftrightarrow$$

$$\Leftrightarrow \frac{\varphi_1^{-1}(\frac{1}{2})}{\lambda(h)} \geq \varphi(\frac{P}{N}) \Leftrightarrow \varphi^{-1}(\frac{\varphi_1^{-1}(1/2)}{\lambda(h)}) \cdot N \geq p$$

with which the kernel is $[0, \varphi^{-1}(\frac{\varphi_1^{-1}(1/2)}{\lambda(h)}) \cdot N]$. For instance,

- If, $\varphi_1 = id$, $\varphi(x) = x^2$, the threshold between heap and not heap, is $N\sqrt{\frac{0.5}{\lambda(h)}} = N\sqrt{\frac{1}{2\lambda(h)}} = 0.71N\sqrt{\frac{1}{\lambda(h)}}$ that, for $h = P$ is $0.71N$.
- If $\varphi_1 = \varphi = id$, is $N\frac{0.5}{\lambda(h)} = \frac{N}{2\lambda(h)}$ that, for $h = P$ is $\frac{N}{2}$.

2. *Let us consider the case in which the prototype is a circular cone, C, of radius r and height h, whose volume is given by $V = \frac{1}{3}(\pi \times r^2 \times H)$, and suppose the heaps are in the unit cube of $\mathbb{R}^3$.*

If the cone C is in $[0,1]^3$ with its base in $[0,1]^2$, radius $r = 0.5$ and height $H = 1$, let us take the same F, as well as a perceptive similarity index $0 \leq \sigma(h) \leq 1$. For instance, the heap in figure (c) of 15.4.2 could have $\sigma(h) = \frac{1}{4}$, that represents that the volume of C is around four times de volume of figure (c). Since $Vol(C) = \pi/2$, $\sigma(h) = 1/4$ means an evaluation of the volume of h around $\pi/48$ cubic units.

Thus, we can take

$$\mu_h(S(p)) = \sigma(h)\varphi(\frac{p}{N}),$$

with which all has been said in the former paragraph can be repeated exactly by just changing $\lambda(h)$ by $\sigma(h)$.

Hence, no actual difference with the case of the pyramid appears.

15.5 Conclusion

This paper tries to turn-out the Sorites' Paradox from a different point of view than that of only considering heaps as sets of grains, the radical simplification on which base the paradox is classically reached by only using boolean deductive reasoning. Essentially, the only safe conclusion of those arguments is to show the existence of predicates to which the Specificity Axiom of Set Theory fails to be applicable, that is, that they cannot have set-extension. This is the most elemental reason among those for which Lotfi A. Zadeh introduced in 1965 the concept of a fuzzy set, or membership function of an imprecise predicate acting in a universe of discourse.

The new point of view this paper holds is based on the perceptive three-dimensional experience a layperson has on heaps, and that actually excludes to know the number of grains of sand in each one of them, a number nobody will never count in the real life.

After presenting the 'paradox' with the paradigm of 'small numbers in the real line', that enjoys the rich structure of real numbers, it is shown that a point of separation B between either small and not-small, or between small and big, exists in some (bounded) cases, but not always in the case of an unbounded interval of real numbers.Thus, and with an elemental use of mathematical concepts, the conclusion at which Max Black did arrive is shown to be erroneous in some important cases. Nevertheless, it is proven that with an imprecise concept named by a predicate P, describable by means of a monotonic real function (membership function), it always exists a point s separating those elements that are 'more P than not P' (the kernel of P), from those that are 'more not P than P'. The kernel offers a way of approaching the imprecise concept named by P, by a crisp or bivaluate one specifying the kernel. Usually, is $s < B$. If instead of not-P (that is not a linguistic term as it is P), is taken an antonym of P, something that is more in agreement with the commonsense way of reasoning [7], a second kernel, usually containing the first one, is also obtained and could also be used to obtain another and wider crisp 'approach of P'.

A way of obtaining a membership function for the three-dimensional perceptively imprecise concept named 'heap' (a term without antonyms), is introduced by means of a numerical index that could be attributed to a heap by perceptively comparing it with some specific prototypes, like either a well known pyramid or a well known circular cone, and the anti-prototype known as a 'flat-set' of grains. Once such membership function is given, both point s, and point B, are obtained and the corresponding kernels can facilitate some information on the number of grains a heap could be constitued of.

In the field of medicine, and particularly in its important part of the reasoning for diagnose (see [2]), there are many technical concepts that cannot be considered precise, and are subjected to degrees as i is, for instance, the concept 'diabetes'. These degrees allow to submit the corresponding concept to a Sorites' process, and to conclude that they are not representable by classical sets.

For instance, it is considered that a patient with 100mg/dl of glucose in blood does not suffer diabetes, and the same conclusion holds for 101 mg/dl, 102 mg/dl, ..., etc., up to 120 mg/dl, in which moment the patient is said to suffer diabetes.

Nevertheless, since the crisp mark 120 is not liable in all cases as it is a somehow arbitrary and changing threshold, it could be better to frame the diagnose in the setting of fuzzy logic by also taking into account the weight, the age, the kind of job, as well as the usual alimentation of the patient. The doctors cannot reason by only taking into account the amount of glucose in blood, and under the schemes of boolean reasoning. Once the current medical concepts are translated into fuzzy terms it is necessary to follow the reasoning under those schemes of fuzzy logic allowed in a suitably algebra of fuzzy sets designed accordingly with the context in which the concepts are inscribed.

In addition, since the processes conducting to diagnose try to find a good enough hypothesis, matching with the symptoms of the presumed illness, it is relevant for the researchers on medical reasoning to know what is concerned with abduction and speculation in both classical and fuzzy logic. It could be of some interest for those researchers to know something on the more general framework considering reasoning as the pair conjecturing + refuting) (see [5], [7], and [6]).

With all that, the authors are only trying to rescue the Sorites argument from the kingdom of classical logic, where only boolean tautological reasonings are allowed, and to place it into a total different kingdom where rational conjecturing based on either experience, or experiments, is pertinent for obtaining mathematical models with which knowledge can be controlled to progressively become deep and deep. This is in fact, in the line of Zadeh's Computing with Words [10] or, at least, the way the authors see it.

To some extent, to analyze Sorites' type problems with only strictly theoretic boolean reasoning, is close to analyze the universe without using the telescope and going back to times without the work of Kepler, Copernicus and Galileo.

Acknowledgement. The authors warmly thank Prof. Claudio Moraga (ECSC), for his help during the writing of this paper. This work has been supported by the Foundation for the Advancement of Soft Computing (ECSC) (Asturias, Spain), and by the Spanish Department of Science and Innovation (MICINN) under project TIN2008-06890-C02-01.

References

1. Black, M.: Reasoning with Loose Concepts. Dialogue 2, 1–12 (1963)
2. Masquelet, A.C.: Le Raisonnement Médical. PUF, Paris (2006) (in French)
3. Sorensen, R.A.: Vagueness and Contradiction. Clarendon Press, Oxford (2001)
4. Trillas, E.: On Negation Functions in Fuzzy Set Theory. In: Barro, S., Bugarin, A., Sobrino, A. (eds.) Advances of Fuzzy Logic, pp. 31–43. Universidad de Santiago de Compostela (1998)
5. Trillas, E.: Conjectures in De Morgan Algebras and with Fuzzy Sets. Submitted to NAFIPS 2012 (2012)
6. García-Honrado, I., Trillas, E.: On an Attempt to Formalize Guessing. In: Seising, R., Sanz González, V. (eds.) Soft Computing in Humanities and Social Sciences. STUDFUZZ, vol. 273, pp. 243–264. Springer, Heidelberg (2012)

7. Trillas, E., Guadarrama, S.: Fuzzy Representations Need a Careful Design. International Journal of General Systems 39(3), 329–346 (2010)
8. Trillas, E., Urtubey, L.A.: Towards the Dissolution of the Sorites Paradox. Applied Soft Computing 11(2), 1506–1510 (2011)
9. Williamson, T.: Vagueness. Routledge, London (1994)
10. Zadeh, L.A.: From Computing with Numbers to Computing with Words. IEEE Transactions on Circuits and Systems 46(1), 105–119 (1999)

16

Fuzziness in Medical Measurement and Approximate Reasoning

Ernesto Araujo

16.1 Introduction

Finding out autonomous mechanisms and structures that emulate the human reasoning is an important objective that has been pursuit in diverse areas [8, 10, 11, 18]. Making computers think like people is a challenging objective [39], especially in medicine and health care.

The field of artificial intelligence is, so far, an alternative for dealing with assessment, diagnosis, and therapeutic conduct. Probability is another approach largely employed in medicine and health care. A more recent alternative concerns the field of computational intelligence. Computational intelligence and artificial intelligence present differences and similarities. In the traditional perspective, the latter is understood as a top–down symbolic approach composed of case–based reasoning, deductive reasoning, expert systems, logic and symbolic machine learning systems. The former comprises neural networks, fuzzy systems, evolutionary computing, swarm intelligence, and immune systems mimicking nature for problem solving in a bottom–up approach [32]. The manner to select among these techniques relies on the sort of available information and the way to represent knowledge. Information that is (*a*) perfect, certain and precise; (*b*) imperfect, certain but imprecise; (*c*) imperfect, precise but uncertain, (*d*) imperfect, uncertain and imprecise – concerning vagueness, similarity, approximation, and truth – from the field of possibility theory; and (*e*) imperfect, uncertain and imprecise – related to occurrence, and confidence – from the field of probability theory are depicted in Figure 16.1.

Medicine and health care are a fertile environment for vague, conflicting, and not definitive decisions, and therefore diagnosis, assessment, and therapeutic conduct. When dealing with this kind of information, that is simultaneously uncertain and imprecise, then the decision is considered to be under approximation. In order to deal with this kind of problem, a general theory of approximate reasoning was proposed in [38]. This reasoning methodology addresses the interface between numbers and symbols by using the fuzzy set theory approach. In this case, the theory of fuzzy sets [35] is appropriate to express vague (approximate) information, since vagueness

R. Seising and M.E. Tabacchi (Eds.): *Fuzziness and Medicine*, STUDFUZZ 302, pp. 233–249.
DOI: 10.1007/978-3-642-36527-0_16

is related to the absence of crisp boundaries in the membership function. Humans have the ability to evaluate whether an information belongs gradually to a set, or not, and the definition of fuzzy membership functions describes this notion. While the fuzzy set theory is able to deal with information that is simultaneously imprecise and uncertain, the fuzzy logic allows aggregating different information entailing a conclusive condition. In the field of medicine, for instance, it is able to deal with signals and symptoms, laboratorial results, marks, environment etc. for achieving, only to mention few, risk analysis, assessment, diagnosis, therapeutic conduct.

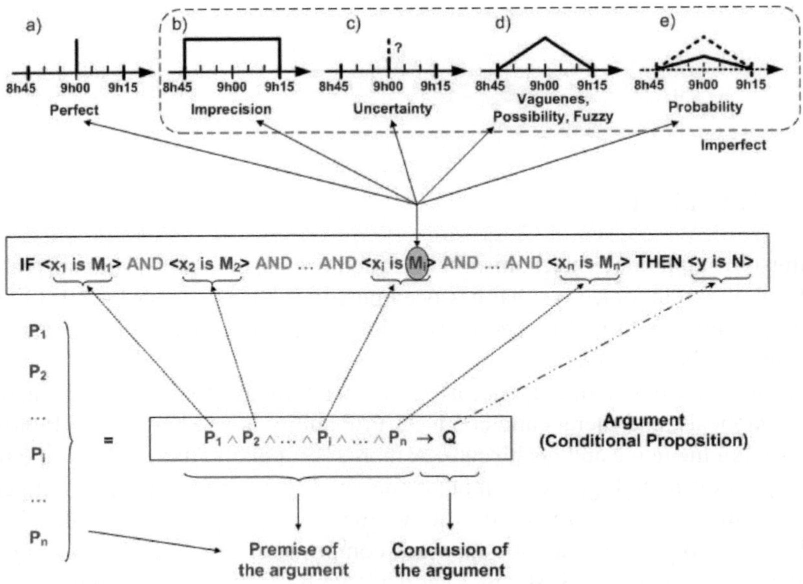

Fig. 16.1 Human reasoning when dealing with perfect and imperfect information [4]

A historical perspective on the use of the fuzzy set theory and fuzzy logic in medicine and bio–medical engineering is presented in [30]. Another historical analysis concerning vagueness as unsharp boundaries sewed with the haziness and fuzziness concepts in the field of medicine but philosophy, logic, mathematics, applied sciences, as well, is carried out in [26, 27]. A literature survey on fuzzy sets as a useful mechanism for medical artificial intelligence is given in [29]. A more specific survey on the current and future use of fuzziness in medical sciences, encompassing areas of (*i*) conservative, (*ii*) invasive, (*iii*) regionally (organ) defined, (*iv*) neural, medical disciplines as well as (*v*) image and signal processing, (*vi*) laboratorial analysis, and other (*vii*) basic science disciplines is described in [1]. In this sense, a review article in medicine and bioinformatics focusing on the geometrical interpretation of fuzziness in a fuzzy hypercube approach is presented in [31]. A philosophical background for applying the fuzzy logic to the medical theory and the understanding of fuzzy health, illness, and disease is discussed in [25]. Such a fuzziness approach concerning health, illness, and disease is somewhat contested meanwhile being in some part acquiesced in [17]. Another provocative philosophical and methodological approach on employing the fuzzy set theory, degrees of truth, and subjectivity in epidemiology, in particular, and medicine, in general, is available in [33]. The fuzzy epidemic approach in [13] endorses the importance of the fuzzy set theory and fuzzy logic in medicine and health care. The work on the fuzzy trace theory is also an instigating perception of fuzziness in the prevention behavior or in supporting medical decision making as given in [19]. A descriptive use of fuzziness to medical decision making in Intensive Care Units is reported in [7]. A cognitive presentation on fuzziness in pharmacy, in particular, and medicine, in general, can be found in the tutorial in [28]. Another source of elucidative papers on the use of the fuzzy set theory and fuzzy logic in etiology, nosology, and diagnosis in medicine is within the series [20–24]. Thus, the use of fuzzy sets and fuzzy logic seem to be appropriate to make computers carry out decision making, emulating paradigms and mechanisms assumed to be in action in medicine and health care.

The content herein exposed aims at presenting that fuzziness is inherent in measurement and reasoning through the approximate reasoning approach, in general, and proper for the field of medicine and health care, in particular. In so doing, the compositional rule of inference and conditional restrictions working as a fuzziness mechanism of measure are natural approaches for being employed in analysis, assessment, classification, therapeutic conduct.

16.2 Fuzziness in Reasoning and Measurement

When a computer carries out a decision, it relies on emulating paradigms and mechanisms assumed to be in action in the human mind. Equivalent in structure, the classical (Aristotelian) logic and the fuzzy logic differ according to the sort of information and the inference system. While the classic (Aristotelian) logic is based on bivalued propositions, describing perfect, crisp reasoning, the fuzzy logic uses multivalued propositions (infinite levels of truth), describing imperfect, uncertain–imprecise reasoning (vague, approximate reasoning).

The classic (Aristotelian) logic is based on the *third excluded principle* in which propositions are assumed to be either true or false. Nevertheless, requiring that propositions be only true or false is, in numerous situations, to evade the reality, since it requires information be perfect. Most of the information that humans, systems, or machines deal with are, actually, imperfect, being characterized as imprecise, uncertain, vague, or that corresponds to either partial truthiness or subjectiveness (Figure 16.1). An alternative to deal with imperfect information is to employ the fuzzy set theory and fuzzy logic, through the approximate reasoning approach.

The approximate reasoning is characterized by rules that (*i*) describe a functional input–output mapping by using linguistic terms, (*ii*) present as fundamental element the fuzzy graph, (*iii*) incorporate a fuzzy inference that involves a set of fuzzy rules (fuzzy model), such that the antecedents of the rule form the fuzzy partition of the input space, (*iv*) are designed and activated in groups and not individually, as explained onwards.

16.2.1 Approximate Reasoning

The approximate (fuzzy) reasoning is achieved when a feasible *uncertain* and *imprecise* conclusion, Q, is deduced from a collection of *imprecise* and *uncertain* premises, represented as vague (fuzzy) sets. A linguistic expression related to an argument can be represented as IF–THEN rules in the form:

$$\begin{aligned} \mathrm{R}: \mathrm{IF}\ \langle x_1 \text{ is } M_1(x_1)\rangle \text{ AND } \ldots \text{ AND } \langle x_j \text{ is } M_j(x_j)\rangle \text{ AND } \ldots \\ \text{AND } \langle x_n \text{ is } M_n(x_n)\rangle \text{ THEN } \langle y \text{ is } N\rangle\ . \end{aligned} \tag{16.1}$$

where $P_j = \langle x_j \text{ is } M_j\rangle$, for $j = 1,\ldots,n$, is the j–th input proposition and $Q = \langle y \text{ is } N\rangle$ is the inferred (deduced) proposition. The i–th rule, for $i = 1,2,\ldots,m$, compose a set of fuzzy rules:

$$\begin{aligned} &\mathrm{R}_1: \mathrm{IF}\ \langle x_1 \text{ is } M_{11}(x_1)\rangle \text{ AND}\ldots\text{AND } \langle x_j \text{ is } M_{1j}(x_j)\rangle \text{ AND}\ldots \\ &\qquad\qquad \text{AND } \langle x_n \text{ is } M_{1n}(x_n)\rangle \text{ THEN } \langle y \text{ is } N_1(y)\rangle \\ &\ldots \\ &\mathrm{R}_i: \mathrm{IF}\ \langle x_1 \text{ is } M_{i1}(x_1)\rangle \text{ AND}\ldots\text{AND } \langle x_j \text{ is } M_{ij}(x_j)\rangle \text{ AND}\ldots \\ &\qquad\qquad \text{AND } \langle x_n \text{ is } M_{in}(x_n)\rangle \text{ THEN } \langle y \text{ is } N_i(y)\rangle \\ &\ldots \\ &\mathrm{R}_m: \mathrm{IF}\ \langle x_1 \text{ is } M_{m1}(x_1)\rangle \text{ AND}\ldots\text{AND } \langle x_j \text{ is } M_{mj}(x_j)\rangle \text{ AND}\ldots \\ &\qquad\qquad \text{AND } \langle x_n \text{ is } M_{mn}(x_n)\rangle \text{ THEN } \langle y \text{ is } N_m(y)\rangle \end{aligned} \tag{16.2}$$

representing, for instance, a multi–input single–output (MISO) linguistic fuzzy logic system.

The elements x_j and y refer, respectively, to a j–th input and the output objects within distinct collections named *universe of discourse*, $x_j \in X_j$ and $y \in Y$, also assigned *linguistic variable*, as well. The amount of P_n propositions is related to the n–th dimensionality of the argument and so of the human thinking or reasoning. The input vector $x = [x_1,\ldots,x_n]^T$ is denominated as premise (antecedent of the rule) while the output, y, is associated to the conclusion (consequent of the rule). The linguistic expressions AND corresponds to the *set operation*, intersection, $\cap$, the *logic operation*, conjunction, $\wedge$, and the *Triangular norm* operation (*T-norm*), $t(x,y)$. The terms M_{ij} and N_j are assigned *linguistic terms* within the respective universes of discourse and built as fuzzy sets.

A fuzzy set represents the possibility, similarity, or conformity of an element, x, to belong to a set, M. Such a *fuzzy set*, M, within a universe of discourse, X, is defined by a *membership function*, $\mu_M(x) : X \mapsto [0,1]$. If the values of $\mu_M(x)$ are, in turn, associate to a degree of truthiness, this is equivalent to the multivalued logic in which the truth is assigned to continuous values in $[0,1]$ [35]. The null membership degree denotes that such an element is not in the set, being completely not compatible to M at all. Otherwise, the unitary membership degree states that an element is fully represented in the set, being completely compatible to M. When the element is mapped into this interval, $0 < \mu_{M_X}(x) < 1$, there is a partial degree of membership. The j–th approximate (fuzzy) proposition is, thus, associated to information (knowledge) that is simultaneously *uncertain* and *imprecise*, i.e., *vague*, being understood as the mechanism employed to build up the approximate (fuzzy) human reasoning. The antecedent in the expression (16.1) form a space within the premise space, $P_1 \times \ldots \times P_n$. A compound proposition connected by conjunctive logic operators, $\wedge$, form a fuzzy region, expressing flexibility (or in doubt) in making decisions, judgment or analysis. In so doing, it represents the fuzziness in reasoning.

An argument employed to make deductive inferences is known as an *inference rule* and can be built up by diverse manners, limited to be tautological. Arguments in the form of fuzzy IF–THEN rules may also be defined as *fuzzy relations*, R, with the membership grade:

$$R([x_1,\ldots,x_n],y) = f([M(x_1),\ldots,M(x_n)],N(y)) \,, \tag{16.3}$$

in $X_n \times Y$. Such a *nonlinear* mapping, $f : [0,1]^n \to [0,1]$ gives birth to a *relational fuzzy inference system.* A functional input–output mapping as given in (16.1) can be understood as the union of Cartesian products obtained by the association of fuzzy linguistic terms. The resulting fuzzy graph, f^*, concerning a set of fuzzy rules as presented in (16.2) is inherent to the fuzzy relation (16.3). A fuzzy graph, f^*, describes a functional mapping, $f : U \to V$, $X \in U$, $Y \in V$ from the linguistic variables, X_i for $i = 1,2,\ldots,m$, in the universes of discourse, U, to the linguistic variable, Y, in the output universe of discourse, V, given as:

$$\begin{aligned} f^* = [M_1(x_1),\ldots,M_1(x_n)] \times N(y)_1 + [M_2(x_1),\ldots,M_2(x_n)] \times N(y)_2 + \ldots \\ + [M_m(x_1),\ldots,M_m(x_n)] \times N(y)_m \end{aligned} \tag{16.4}$$

where the operations $+$ and $\times$ denote, respectively, the operations of disjunction and Cartesian product, $M_{1j}(x_1) \times \ldots \times M_{nj}(x_n)$. When understood as the combination of fuzzy relations or, particularly, the union of the Cartesian products concerning pairs of input, $[M(x_1),\ldots,M(x_n)]$, and output, $N(y)$, the fuzzy graph, f^*, from X^n to Y can be given as:

$$f^* = \bigcup_i [M(x_1),\ldots,M(x_n)]_i \times N(y)_i \tag{16.5}$$

and illustrated in Fig. 16.2.

16.2.2 Conditional Restriction as a Fuzziness Mechanism of Measure

Once the approximate (fuzzy) reasoning is available (16.1), it is required fact(s) to infer (induce) new facts, $(y = b, \mu([b1,b2]))$, from current facts, $(x = a, \mu(a))$, or previous decisions (Fig. 16.2). The primary fact represents, thus, a *conditional restriction* on the values of x imposed by the measure or observation. In the context of approximate reasoning such an input value is a subset in X and works as a singleton restriction on x or a fuzzy restriction *imposed* by $\tilde{M}$.

A linguistic term (value) can be interpreted as a label for a *fuzzy restriction* upon the linguistic variable being characterized by a *compatibility function*, as well. The calculus of the restriction is one of the most important concepts in the theory of fuzzy systems and approximate reasoning because it can be related to human cognition. In particular, it is related to situations that involve the construction of concepts, patter recognition, and decision– making processes in fuzzy environments or in the presence of uncertainties [37]. The area underneath a fuzzy set corresponds to an *elastic restriction* of the possible (also similar) values of elements $x \in X$, also denominated *possibility distribution function*. One of the most important roles assigned to the calculus of fuzzy constraints is to supply a kind of reasoning that is neither exact, nor inexact. Known as the main element to build up the approximate reasoning, the fuzzy restriction assumes a basic role not only in the process to form the approximate inference mechanism but the measurement, as well [36].

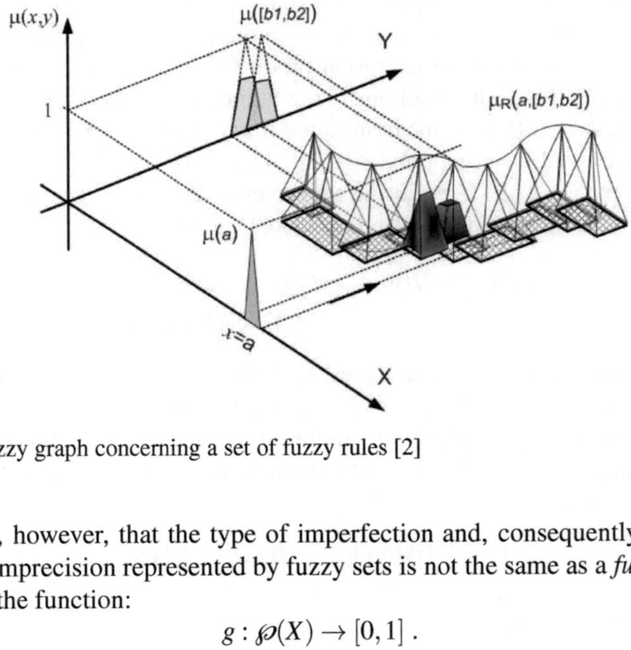

Fig. 16.2 Fuzzy graph concerning a set of fuzzy rules [2]

Observe, however, that the type of imperfection and, consequently, the uncertainty and imprecision represented by fuzzy sets is not the same as a *fuzzy measure* defined by the function:

$$g : \wp(X) \to [0,1] . \tag{16.6}$$

A fuzzy measure assigns to each *crisp set* of X a number in the unit interval $[0,1]$, where $\wp(X)$ is the power set of crisp set and not the power of fuzzy sets on X, i.e., $\tilde{\wp}(X)$. A fuzzy measure concerns the degree of evidence or belief associated to a fuzzy set that a particular element belongs to a crisp set, a set with sharp boundaries. It indicates the degree of evidence or subjective certainty that an element belongs to a subset is not known with certainty, even though the classes are disjoint intervals. In the presence of perfect evidence, a full membership is assigned to one and only one of the available crisp sets. The fuzzy measure is employed due to the fact that most of the time the evidence is not perfect, at all, even if the classes (subsets) are assumed to be perfect. The difference between the fuzzy measure and the measure of fuzziness relies on the fact that for the first the subsets (classes) are crisp not presenting fuzziness associated to their boundaries. In turn, a measure of fuzziness concerns the degree of evidence or belief associated to a fuzzy set (input) that a particular element belongs to a fuzzy set (class), one with unsharp boundaries. As before mentioned, a fuzzy set is related to each element of the universe of discourse be assigned a value representing the degree of membership in a fuzzy set and, due to that, related to fuzziness [12].

In the field of medicine and health care, the difference between fuzzy measure and the measure of fuzziness can be exemplified as follows. Given an ill patient and inconclusive evidence obtained by anamnesis or physical examination, how to classify or diagnosis this individual is not a simple task. If there are predetermined crisp subsets (classes) of diagnosis, where each individual must be allocated in, a fuzzy measure is, then, employed. Nevertheless, if the predetermined classes are not crisp at all and due to that present unsharp boundaries, then it is a matter of using fuzziness in measurement and approximate reasoning [12].

Table 16.1 Classification of Overweight and Obesity by %BF

Obesity	Women	Men
Adequate (AF)	< 25 %	< 15 %
Low (LF)	25–30 %	15–20 %
Moderate (MOD)	30–35 %	20–25 %
Elevate (ELEV)	35–40 %	25–30 %
Morbid (MOR)	> 40 %	> 30 %

(Source: WHO - World Health Organization)

Consider, for instance, the clinical guidelines on the identification, evaluation, and therapeutic conduct of overweight and obesity in adults in Table 16.1 referring to Percentage of Body Fat (%BF), as assigned by the World Health Organization (WHO). Observe that the classifications are crisp sets as depicted in Fig. 16.3 and these crisp classes were modified to fuzzy sets in order to accommodate the subjectivity in classification, as first presented in [14]. The fuzziness in the fuzzy %BF obesity classification is shown in Fig. 16.4. This novel approach not only presents fuzzy %BF classes (input) but fuzzy BMI (Body Mass Index) classes (input) that are aggregated by employing logical connectives for further being mapped into new fuzzy obesity classes (output), resulting in a new index named Miyahira–Araujo Fuzzy Obesity Index (MAFOI). Such a novel fuzzy obesity index introduces fuzziness in the manner to understand obesity and the relation between individuals to their obesity condition. MAFOI also establishes a criterion that provides a mechanism to deal with clinical analysis and syndrome assessment, classification, therapeutic conduct and surgical (bariatric) indication [16]. The MAFOI is, then, extended and validated by experimental data in [15]. In order to exemplify the difference between fuzziness in measure and fuzzy measure, consider the classic and fuzzy %BF obesity classifications. Take into account that according to the mechanism or methodology employed to measure the %BF, a fuzzy value (fuzzy set) or a singleton value is achieved, respectively, representing either a subjective (imperfect) or a certain and precise (perfect) evidence during diagnostic or analysis, as depicted in Fig. 16.3 and 16.4.

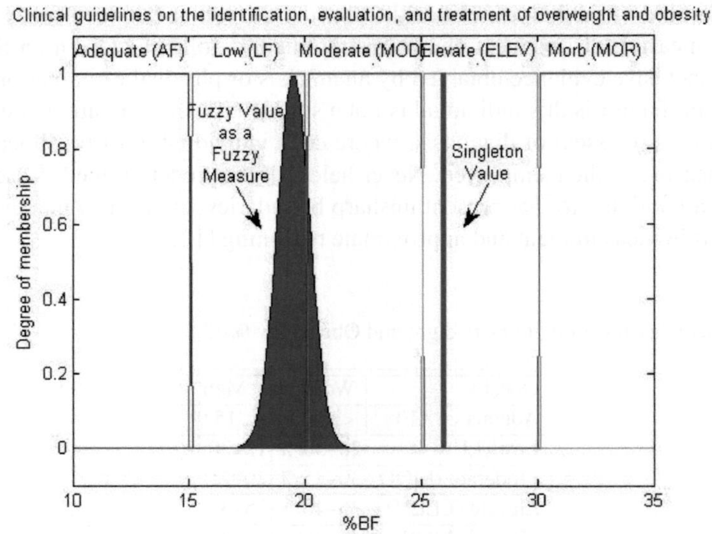

Fig. 16.3 Example of fuzzy measure to a *possible* crisp set

Observe that when dealing with crisp classes and there is a perfect evidence, a full membership value achieves only one class, M_{Elev}, such that $\mu^S_{M_{Elev}}(x) = 1$ (right measure in Fig. 16.3). In so doing, there is no fuzziness associated to their boundaries. The upper index, *S*, refers to the singleton measure. Otherwise, when dealing with subjective (or in doubt, inconclusive) classes, here associated to fuzzy sets, there may be either a full membership, when the singleton value coincides to the core of the membership function, or a partial membership, when such a measure achieves unsharp borders of the fuzzy set yielding distinct degrees of activation (right measure in Fig. 16.4). In this example, the measure of fuzziness is obtained when a measure, *x*, generates two degrees of activation, $\mu^S_{M_{Mod}}(x)$ and $\mu^S_{M_{Elev}}(x)$, respectively, by achieving the fuzzy moderate obesity set, M_{Mod}, and the fuzzy elevate obesity set, M_{Elev}, such that $0 < \mu^S_{M_{Mod}}(x) < \mu^S_{M_{Elev}}(x) < 1$. On the other hand, when the measure assumes fuzzy evidence, there is not a full membership value when dealing with crisp classes, yielding an inconclusive classification (left measure in Fig. 16.3). The example of fuzzy measure reflects the ambiguity, subjectivity associated to two disjoint, well–defined sets. The classic low obesity set, M_{LF}, and the classic moderate obesity set, M_{Mod}, are simultaneously activated by the fuzzy evidence indicating the degree of evidence or belief associated to two *possible* crisp sets. When dealing with fuzzy classes, there are partial membership values, as well. Such a measure achieves unsharp borders of fuzzy sets yielding distinct degrees of activation. In this example, the measure of fuzziness is obtained when a measure, $x = \tilde{M}$, generates two degrees of activation, $\mu^F_{M_{LF}}(\tilde{M})$ and $\mu^F_{M_{Mod}}(\tilde{M})$, respectively, by achieving the fuzzy low obesity set, M_{LF}, and the fuzzy moderate obesity set, M_{Mod}, such that $1 > \mu^F_{M_{LF}}(\tilde{M}) > \mu^F_{M_{Mod}}(\tilde{M}) > 0$ (left measure in Fig. 16.4). The upper index, F, refers to fuzzy set for representing the measure.

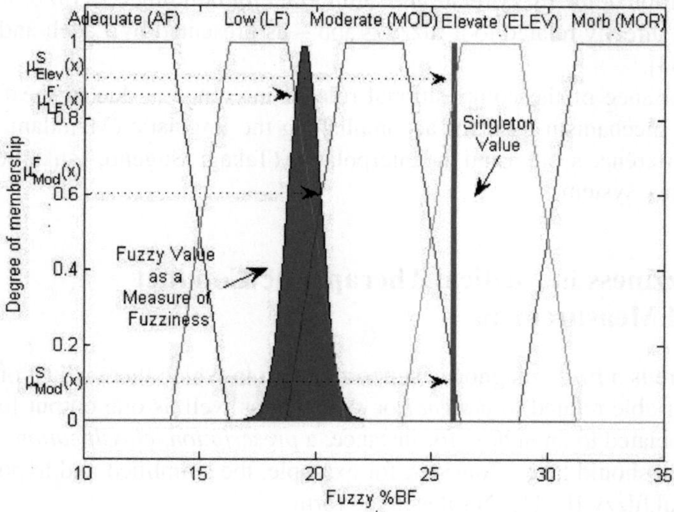

Fig. 16.4 Example of fuzziness in measure to a *fuzzy* set

16.2.3 *Fuzziness in the Compositional Rule of Inference*

An alternative to implement the fuzzy inference system is by using the *compositional rule of inference* (CRI), leading to a *generalized modus ponens*. The CRI embraces (*i*) the *projection principle*, (*ii*) the *conjunction principle*; and (*iii*) the *semantic global entailment*. This inference mechanism is a cornerstone in many applications of fuzzy systems, chiefly because it is regarded within a general category of fuzzy reasoning.

Two important operations in fuzzy relations are *projection* and *conjunction*. Moreover, the *extension principle* is used to transform fuzzy sets via functions into their fuzzy–set counterparts by using the *cylindrical extension*. Such an operation allows computing induced constraints into different universe of discourses. The outcome in Y is, thus, calculated as the *relational composition*:

$$N = \tilde{M} \circ R\,, \tag{16.7}$$

where R is a fuzzy relation (16.3) and $\tilde{M}$ is the input measure; fuzzy or singleton ones. The expression in (16.7) is decomposed into:

$$\begin{aligned} N(y) &= proj\left\{conj\left\{cyl\left[\tilde{M}(x)\right], R(x,y)\right\}\right\} \\ &= \sup_x \left[\tilde{M}(x) \wedge R(x,y)\right] \\ &= \sup_x \left[\tilde{M}(x) \wedge \vee_{i=1}^{N} R_i(x,u)\right] , \end{aligned} \tag{16.8}$$

since the operation $\circ$ is related to *proj*, *conj*, and *cyl* which refers, respectively, to the principle of projection, principle of conjunction, and cylindrical extension. The composition of the fuzzy relations is important for building up a fuzzy mapping by rules and directly related to a fuzzy graph – as presented by Zadeh and not by Rosenfeld [34].

The importance of the compositional rule of inference is due to the fact that it is the key mechanism used for accomplishing the linguistic (Mamdani, Larsen etc.) fuzzy inference system and the interpolative (Takagi–Sugeno, Tsukamoto etc.) fuzzy inference system.

16.3 Fuzziness in Medical Therapeutic Conduct and Measurement

Suppose there is a fuzzy diagnostic support system in which there is just one input linguistic variable related to a *signal* or *symptom* as well as one output linguistic variable associated to an *action*, for instance, a *prescription, classification etc.* that a professional should take. Consider, for example, the simplified and hypothetical set of medical fuzzy IF–THEN rules in the form:

$$\begin{aligned} &: \text{IF } x \text{ is Light THEN } y \text{ is Reduced} \\ f^* &: \text{IF } x \text{ is Mild THEN } y \text{ is Moderate} \\ &: \text{IF } x \text{ is Severe THEN } y \text{ is Strong .} \end{aligned} \tag{16.9}$$

The set of inference rules can be comprehended as the knowledge base to a certain domain of problem. Consider that the input linguistic variable, X, can be assigned, for instance, to *pain* meanwhile the output linguistic variable, Y, can be related to *opioid*, or the *dose of opioid* to be applied to the patient. In so doing, this set of rule works as a meta mental modeling representing the manner a professional would determine the dose of opioid to be administered according to the pain reported by the patient or measured by instruments. The input linguistic terms assigned *light*, *mild*, and *severe* have their respective membership functions shown in Fig. 16.5a. The output linguistic terms assigned *reduced*, *moderate*, and *strong* have their respective membership functions shown in Fig. 16.5b. These membership functions part, respectively, the universes of discourse associated to the input linguistic variable, $X = \text{pain}$, and the output linguistic variable, $Y = \text{opioid}$.

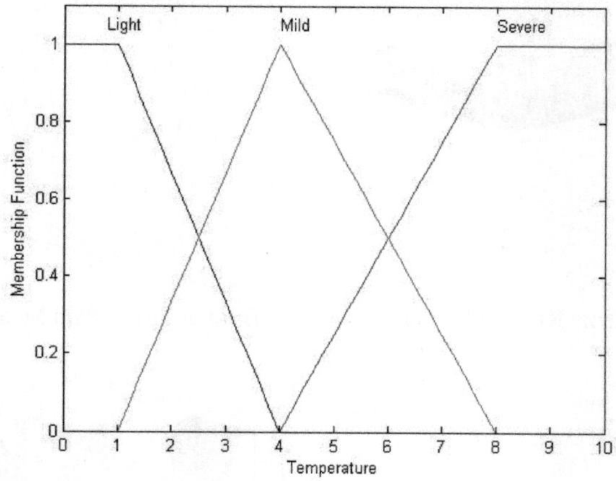

(a) Input Linguistic Terms, *Pain*.

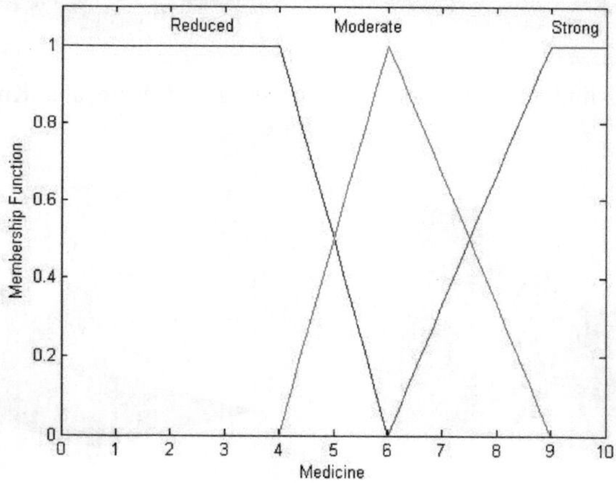

(b) Output Linguistic Terms, *Opioid*.

Fig. 16.5 Fuzzy sets that part the input and output universes of discourse

The fuzzy relation resulting from the fuzzy rules that stands for the diagnostic is depicted in Fig. 16.6a. Observe the level curves obtained with the projection of the set of rules that part the input–output space of the problem. There are three fuzzy regions corresponding each to a fuzzy rule that are aggregated by using the logical operator of disjunction, after the Cartesian product be obtained with the logical operator of conjunction. The choice of the logical operators (t–norm and t–conorm) directly affects the geometry of the fuzzy inference mechanism, determining the intersection of the fuzzy regions. In this example the conjunction operator is chosen to be the *min* while the disjunction operator is the *max*.

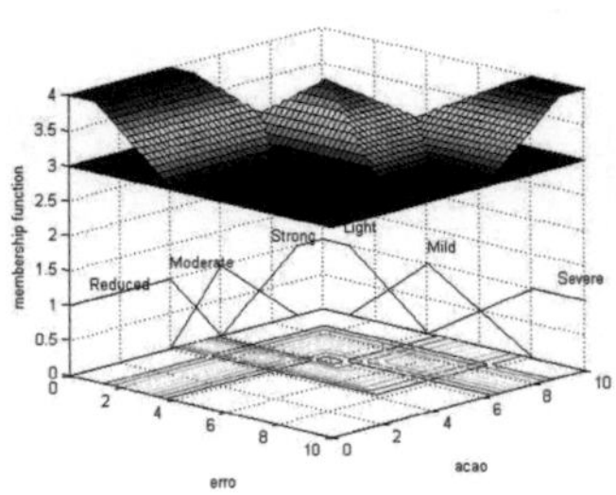

(a) Fuzzy Knowledge Base.

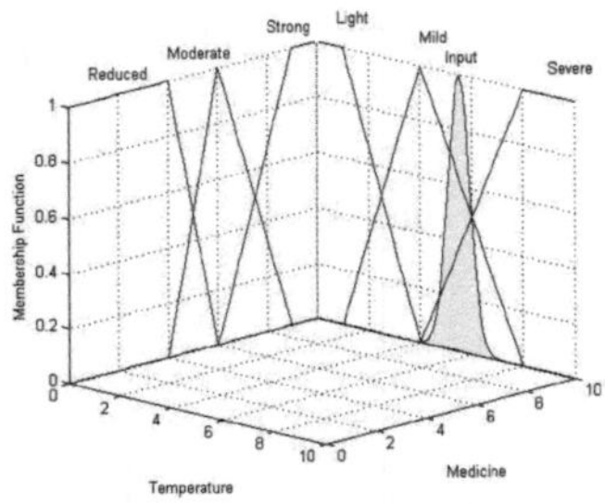

(b) Input Fuzzy Pain Measure.

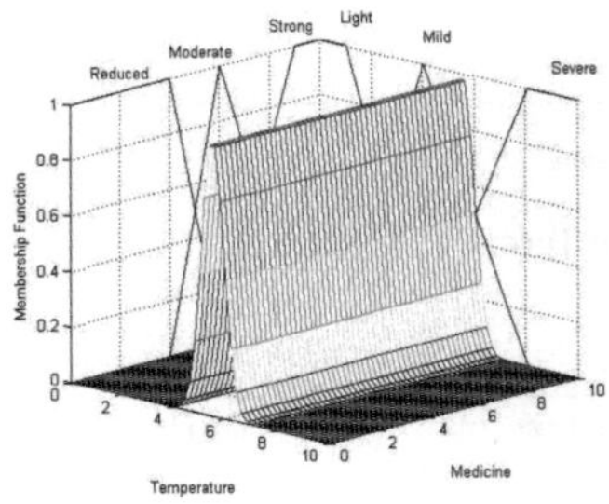

(c) Cylindrical Extension.

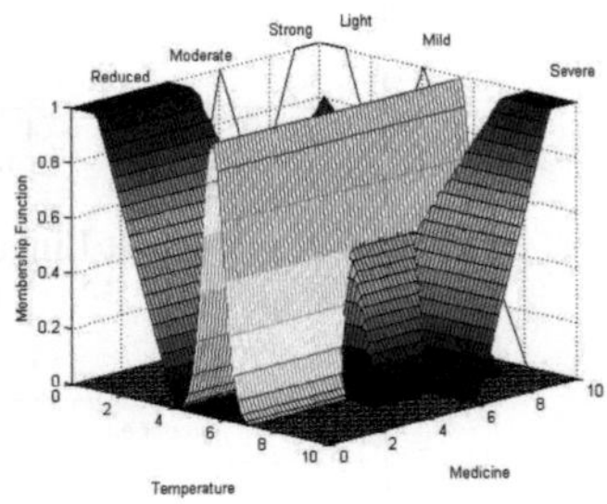

(d) Fuzzy Measure and Knowledge Base.

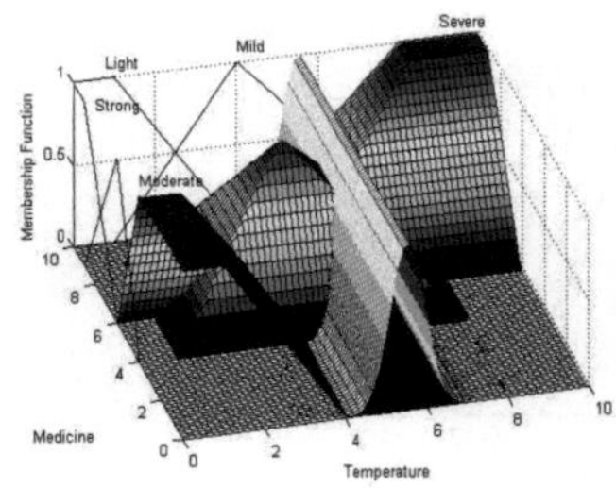

(e) Another Perspective of 16.6c.

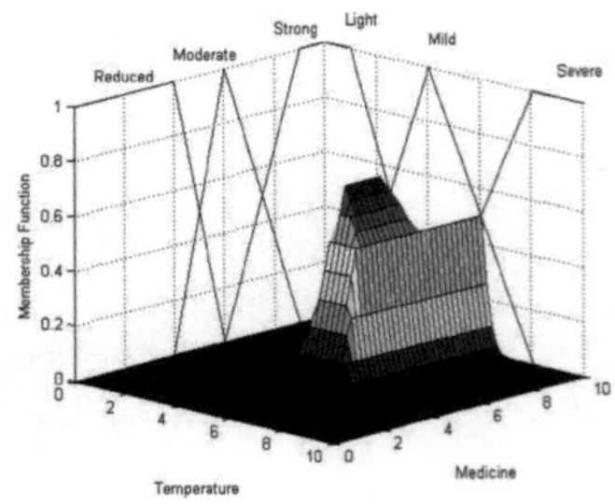

(f) Conjunction Principle.

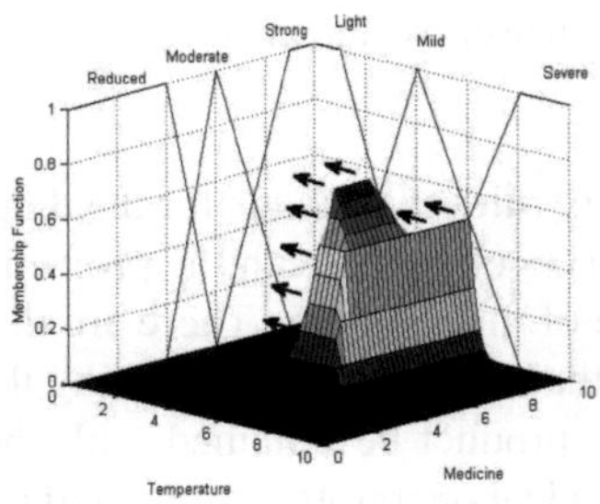

(g) Projection Principle.

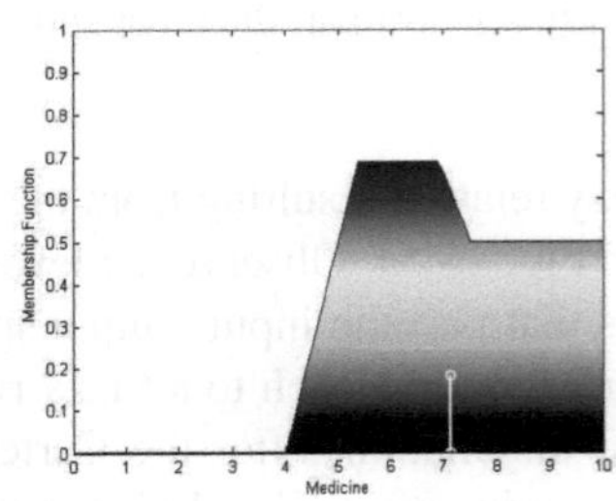

(h) Final Projection and Defuzzification.

Fig. 16.6 Fuzziness in the Pain Symptom Providing Evidence for Opioid Therapeutic Conduct

Take into account for such an example that the input linguistic variable, X, assumes values within the standardized domain $X = [0,10]$, whose associated linguistic terms are $T = \{Light,\ Mild,\ Severe\}$. Consider yet the membership functions of the term $M \in T$ be $\mu_M : X \to [0,1]$, such that $c(M) = \{x_0 \in X \mid \mu_M(x_0) = 1\}$ and $s(M) = \{x_0 \in X \mid \mu_M(x_0) > 0\}$ denote the core and the support, respectively. The support of M is the set of points in X in which $\mu_M(x)$ is positive while the core is the set of point in which $\mu_M(x)$ is unitary. The linguistic terms *Light* and *Severe* $\in T$ assumes the trapezoidal membership function being represented, respectively, by $\langle s_{1light}, c_{1light}, c_{2light}, s_{2light} \rangle$, such that $s(Light) = [s_{1light}, s_{2light}]$ and $c(Light) = [c_{1light}, c_{2light}]$ and by $\langle s_{1severe}, c_{1severe}, c_{2severe}, s_{2severe} \rangle$, such that $s(Severe) = [s_{1severe}, s_{2severe}]$ and $c(Severe) = [c_{1severe}, c_{2severe}]$. The term $Mild \in T$ is defined as a triangular membership function and represented by the triple $\langle s_{1mild}, c_{1mild}, s_{2mild} \rangle$, such that $s(Mild) = [s_{1mold}, s_{2mold}]$ and $c(Mild) = [c_{1mild}]$. Here, the fuzzy sets in T are defined by the following set of supports and cores: $Light = \langle 0,\ 0,\ 1,\ 4 \rangle$, $Mild = \langle 1,\ 4,\ 8 \rangle$ and $Severe = \langle 4,\ 8,\ 10,\ 10 \rangle$. Likewise the input linguistic variable, the output linguistic variable, Y, assumes values within the domain $Y = [0,10]$. The linguistic terms $T = \{Reduced, Moderate, Strong\}$ can also be defined by their supports and cores as given by $Reduced = \langle 0,\ 0,\ 4,\ 6 \rangle$, $Moderate = \langle 4,\ 6,\ 9 \rangle$ and $Strong = \langle 6,\ 9,\ 10,\ 10 \rangle$. The linguistic terms and their associated fuzzy sets are depicted in Fig. 16.5.

The mapping, f, of $X = \{x\}$ into $Y = \{y\}$, shown in (16.9) is obtained by employing the compositional operation, $\tilde{M} \circ R$, in such a way that $x = \tilde{M}$ represents the input measure or observation (cause), and y the output (consequence) that can be associated to decision, diagnosis, assessment, therapeutic conduct, and so on. Consider also a fuzzy restriction characterizing a signal measurement or a patient cognition concerning the symptom as depicted in Fig. 16.6b. A Gaussian function is employed to represent such a subjective measure:

$$g(e) = exp\left(-\frac{(e-\mu)^2}{2\sigma^2}\right), \tag{16.10}$$

where μ is the mean value and σ, the standard deviation. Assume, for instance, that $\mu = 5.5$ and $\sigma = 0.4$. Employing fuzzy sets to stand for the fifth vital sign of medical condition was first presented in [3] to represent the inherent imprecision, uncertainty and vagueness presented in the pain report and assessment. The unidimensional fuzzy pain intensity scales therein proposed extend the accepted classical unidimensional pain scales to fuzzy set theory obtaining the fuzzy visual analog scale (FVAS), fuzzy numerical rating scale (FNRS), fuzzy qualitative pain scale (FQPS), and fuzzy face pain scale (FFPS). The input measure as illustrated in Fig. 16.6b can immediately be associated to any of the FVAS, FNRS, FFPS by using traditional measurement systems or by a computer program [9]. When interested in representing physiological, behavioral, psychological, and cultural aspects of individual life experience encompassing pain–related disabilities, the tridimensional Fuzzy Professional–Social–Sexual Pain Assessment also furnishes both singleton or fuzzy pain measurement [6], as portrayed in Fig. 16.6b. Another source of fuzzy pain is the Fuzzy Musculoskeletal Pain Scale (FUMPS). Such a multi–criteria fuzzy pain assessment can be applied for pain measurement in patients with musculoskeletal disorder with reduction in the range of motion, as exemplified in [5].

This conditional restriction is the information that defines the actual reasoning process in the decision making and will affect the final and accurate decision as given in Fig. 16.6h. The compositional rule of inference states that the cylindrical extension, $cyl(\tilde{M}(x))$, is the first operation to extend this measure (Fig. 16.6c) upon the knowledge base (Fig. 16.6d and Fig. 16.6e). In sequence, the conjunction principle, $conj\left[cyl(\tilde{M}(x)), R(x,y)\right]$, is the operation that reduce the knowledge base according to the input fuzzy restriction, as illustrated in (Fig. 16.6f). The conjunction operation, $\{cyl(\tilde{M}(x)) \wedge R(x,y)\}$, is accomplished by using a t–norm that allows determining a partial fuzzy set in the relation R, restricted by the measure, $\tilde{M}$ through the cylindrical extension. The logical operator of conjunction is *min*. Finally, the projection principle, $proj\left\{conj\left[cyl(\tilde{M}(x)), R(x,y)\right]\right\}$, is the operation employed to obtain the final approximate decision (also classification, assessment, diagnosis, therapeutic conduct etc.), as show in Fig. 16.6h). The resulting projected surface upon the output fuzzy sets is accomplished by the logical operation of *max*. In the case a precise, exact output is required, the defuzzification method is employed. The most common defuzzification method is the *Center of Area* (COA):

$$opioid = \frac{\sum_{i \in M} a_i y_{opioid}(x_i)}{\sum_{i \in M} y_{opioid}(x_i)} . \tag{16.11}$$

The induced precise and exact output value concerning the opioid linguistic variable is 7.140950 for this example when computed by the COA for the input given in (16.10).

Determining a precise and certain therapeutic conduct from an imprecise and uncertain measure is a task not easily performed even by human beings. The resulting value obtained with this hypothetical Fuzzy Decision Support Systems (FDSS) for opioid administration – i.e., a Fuzzy Opioid Prescription System (FOPS) – means not prescribing an overdose that eliminates the pain but let the patient lethargic, or not administering a low dose that let the patient lucid but does not eliminate the pain. When designed according to experimental data and/or the heuristic, the FOPS can, thus, be a feasible alternative to reduce errors in prescribing the therapeutic conduct because it is a natural mechanism for dealing with vagueness, subjectivity, and fuzziness during the medical and healthcare process.

16.4 Conclusion

Fuzziness concerns all activity within the medical and healthcare context. The subjectivity, fuzziness, or vagueness is a constant in all aspects of sign and symptom measurements as a mechanism of providing evidence as well as during the decision, diagnosis, classification, analysis, therapeutic conduct, and so forth. In this sense, fuzzy systems and approximate reasoning are a natural mechanism for being employed by medical and healthcare professionals.

The difference and similarities among fuzzy measure and fuzziness in measure are presented, demonstrating how important these approaches assume in decision, diagnosis, analysis, assessment, classification, therapeutic conduct. Conditional restrictions represented as fuzzy sets are elastic restrictions associated to the possibility that an evidence can occur. It assumes, thus, a key role in the reasoning that is neither exact nor inexact. The role of approximate reasoning is then emphasized and the manner it is able to capture the subjectivity, vagueness, and inexact information is also described. The computational rule of inference is demonstrated to assume a fundamental mechanism not only to obtain both fuzzy and singleton inferred values but to understand the different stages that fuzziness is present.

Finally, the fuzzy inference system is advocated as a mechanism that allows mimicking the human reasoning to deal with environments (systems) that are complex, imperfect, and approximate. Such an approach is an alternative to substitute human beings in the task of modifying or helping in deciding how to modify systems to obtain safer, more effective, more efficient, higher quality, and lower costs. In particular, this technique has been investigated to help or to substitute professionals in diverse areas of medicine or health care, eliminating human mistakes due to human fails, tiring etc. In so doing, the fuzzy decision support system is an alternative for reducing the error in determining the therapeutic conduct.

References

1. Abbod, M.F., von Keyserling, D.G., Linken, D.A., Mahfouf, M.: Survey of Utilisation of Fuzzy Technology in Medicine and Healthcare. Fuzzy Sets and Systems 120, 331–349 (2001)
2. Araujo, E., dos Santos Coelho, L.: Piecewise Reference–driven Takagi-Sugeno Fuzzy Modelling Based on Particle Swarm Optimization (PSO). In: Nedjah, N., de Macedo Mourelle, L. (eds.) Systems Engineering using Particle Swarm Optimization, p. 133. Nova Science Publishers Inc., Hauppauge (2007)
3. Araujo, E., Miyahira, S.A.: Unidimensional Fuzzy Pain Scale. In: International Conference on Fuzzy Systems, pp. 185–190 (2009)
4. Araujo, E.: Introduction to Fuzzy Logic and Approximate Reasoning, Course Class Notes (Apostile), São José dos Campos (1994, 1995, 2005)
5. Araujo, E., Lazzareschi, L.: Fuzzy pain assessment in musculoskeletal disorder (2011) (Chapter in this volume)
6. Araujo, E., Miyahira, S.A.: Tridimensional fuzzy pain assessment. In: IEEE International Conference on Fuzzy Systems, pp. 1634–1639 (2011)
7. Bates, J.H.T., Young, M.P.: Applying Fuzzy Logic to Medical Decision Making in the Intensive Care Unit. American Journal of Respiratory and CriticalCare Medicine 167, 948–952 (2003)
8. Bellman, R., Zadeh, L.A.: Decision-making in a Fuzzy Environment. Management Science 17(4), 141–164 (1970)
9. Bocato, E.S., Araujo, E., Miyahira, S.: Fuzzy System for Pain Assessment by Using Api Swing and Java Computational Tools. In: Brazilian Congress of Health Informatics, CD (2010) (in Portuguese)

10. Edmonds, B.: The Constructibility of Artificial Intelligence (as Defined by the Turing Test). Journal of Logic, Language and Information 9(4), 419–424 (2000)
11. Harnard, S.: Minds, Machines and Turing. Journal of Logic, Language and Information 9(4), 425–445 (2000)
12. Klir, G.J., Folger, T.A.: Fuzzy Sets, Uncertainty, and Information. Prentice-Hall, Englewood Cliffs (1988)
13. Massada, E., Siqueira Ortega, N.R., Struchiner, C.J., Burattini, M.N.: Fuzzy Epidemics. Artificial Intelligence in Medicine 29, 241–259 (2003)
14. Miyahira, S.A., Araujo, E.: Fuzzy Obesity Index for Surgical Indication and Treatment. In: International Conference on Fuzzy Systems, pp. 2392–2397 (2008)
15. Miyahira, S.A., de Azevedo, J.L.M.C., Araujo, E.: Fuzzy Obesity Index (mafoi) for Obesity Evaluation and Bariatric Surgery Indication. Journal of Translational Medicine 9(134), 1–10 (2011)
16. Miyahira Susana, A., Araujo, E.: Miyahira–Araujo Fuzzy Obesity Index (mafoi) for Body Mass Index and Body Fat Clinical Analysis. In: Syndrome Assessment, Classification and Treatment, and Surgical Indication (2011) (submitted)
17. Nordenfelt, L.: On the Place of Fuzzy Health in Medical Theory. Journal of Medicine and Philosophy 25, 639–649 (2000)
18. Rapaport, W.J.: How to Pass a Turing Test. Journal of Logic, Language and Information 9(4), 467–490 (2000)
19. Reyna, V.F.: A Theory of Medical Decision Making and Health: Fuzzy Trace Theory. Medical Decision Making 28, 850–865 (2008)
20. Sadegh-Zadeh, K.: Fundamentals of linical ethodology: 1.differential indication. Artificial Intelligence in Medicine 6, 83–102 (1998)
21. Sadegh-Zadeh, K.: Fundamentals of clinical methodology: 2.etiology. Artificial Intelligence in Medicine 12, 227–270 (1998)
22. Sadegh-Zadeh, K.: Fundamentals of clinical methodology: 3.nosology. Artificial Intelligence in Medicine 17, 87–108 (1999)
23. Sadegh-Zadeh, K.: Erratum to "fundamentals of clinical methodology: 3. nosology. Artificial Intelligence in Medicine 17(1), 87 (1999); Artificial Intelligence in Medicine 18, p. 109 (2000)
24. Sadegh-Zadeh, K.: Fundamentals of clinical methodology: 4.diagnosis. Artificial Intelligence in Medicine 20, 227–241 (2000)
25. Sadegh-Zadeh, K.: Fuzzy Health, Illness, and Disease. Journal of Medicine and Philosophy, 605–638 (2000)
26. Seising, R.: From vagueness in medical thought to the foundations of fuzzy reasoning in medical diagnosis. Artificial Intelligence in Medicine 38, 237–256 (2006)
27. Seising, R.: On the Absence of Strict Boundaries —Vagueness, Haziness, and Fuzziness in Philosophy, Science, and Medicine. Applied Soft Computing Journal 8, 1232–1242 (2008)
28. Sproule, B.A., Naranjo, C.A., Türksen, I.B.: Fuzzy Pharmacology: Theory and Applications. Trends in Pharmacological Sciences 23, 412–417 (2002)
29. Steimann, F.: On the Use and Usefulness of Fuzzy sets in Medical AI. Artificial Intelligence in Medicine 21, 131–137 (2001)
30. Teodorrescu, H.-N., Kandel, A., Jain, L.C.: Fuzzy Logic and Neuro–fuzzy Systems in Medicine and Bio–medical Engineering: A Historical Perspective. In: Jain, L.C., Teodorrescu, H.-N., Kandel, A. (eds.) Fuzzy and Neuro-Fuzzy Systems in Medicine, CRC Press, Boca Raton (1988)

31. Torres, A., Nieto, J.J.: Fuzzy Logic in Medicine and Bioinformatics. Journal of Biomedicine and Biotechnology, 1–7 (2006)
32. Venayagamoorthy, G.K., Venayagamoorthy, G.K.K.: A Successful Interdisciplinary Course on Computational Intelligence. IEEE Computational Intelligence Magazine 4(1), 14–23 (2009)
33. Vineis, P.: Methodological Insights: Fuzzy Sets in Medicine. Journal of Epidemiology & Community Health 62(3), 273–278 (2008)
34. John, Y., Langari, R.: Fuzzy Logic: Intelligence, Control, and Information. Prentice Hall Ed., New Jersey (1998)
35. Zadeh, L.A.: Fuzzy Sets. Information and Control 8, 338–353 (1965)
36. Zadeh, L.A.: Fuzzy Logic and Approximate Reasoning. Synthese 30, 407–428 (1975)
37. Zadeh, L.A.: Fuzzy Sets and their Applications to Cognitive and Decision Process. In: Calculus of Fuzzy Restrictions, pp. 1–39. Academic Press Inc., London (1975)
38. Zadeh, L.A.: Machine Intelligence. In: Hayes, J.E., Michie, D., Mikulich, L.I. (eds.) A Theory of Approximate Reasoning, vol. 9, pp. 149–194. Ellis Horwood Limited, Chinchester (1979)
39. Zadeh, L.A.: Making Computers Think Like people. IEEE Spectrum 30, 6–32 (1984)

17

Approaching What-, How- and Why-Questions Using a Medical Example

Alejandro Sobrino and Cristina Puente

17.1 Introduction

Aristotle distinguished in [2] and [1] four types of causes:

- Material cause, involving the physical matter of which something is made; that is, the mass of which it consists.
- Formal cause, focusing on the way that a thing is intended and planned to be.
- Efficient cause, quoted as "the primary source of the change or rest"; the prior movement or the source energy that triggers the final effect.
- Final cause, i.e., the end, goal or aim that a process leads to. The final cause is the teleology (from the Greek *telos*) that something is supposed to serve.

The Aristotelian view of causality traditionally offered a frame to provide answers to causal What- or Why-questions.

In effect, Aristotle's typology serves to answer *What*- and *For-what* questions. For example, in the presence of a statue, we can ask the following questions, which would correspond to the types of cases aforementioned:

- '*What* is it made from?' It is made of metal (material cause);
- '*What* is its form?' A man in a praying attitude (formal cause);
- '*What* produced it?' The sculptor (efficient cause);
- '*For what* purpose?' To pay tribute to a virtuous person (final cause).

But Aristotle's typology enables to answer *why*-questions as well. Efficient causes seem to be appropriate for this task. In this paper we are inspired by this view.

Aristotle's efficient cause is intended as a way of performing explanations. Explanations are usually related to why-questions. A typical – although not academic – way to provide an explanation is to distinguish the components involved in a process identifying the first cause or impulse and the final effect or result. In the aforementioned example, the sculptor is who acted in the first place, but 'the sculptor' is not a reasonable answer to a why-q as *Why the statue was made?*

R. Seising and M.E. Tabacchi (Eds.): *Fuzziness and Medicine*, STUDFUZZ 302, pp. 251–265.
DOI: 10.1007/978-3-642-36527-0_17

Aristotle pointed out that efficient causes are "the primary source of change". The transmission of such changes in a causal network is a mechanism. In this paper we deal with the analysis of *what-*, *how-* and *why-*questions focusing not only on efficient or final causes, but also on the crisp or imperfect mechanisms grouping them; i. e., – in terminology of K. Sadegh-Zadeh –, focusing our attention in fuzzy causal spaces [9], causal systems that label the link between causes and effect not using crisp numbers, but vague percentages (about 80%) or vague intensifiers (*moderately*, *strongly* and so on) [10]. The following pyramid arranges interrogative particles depending on the potential complexity of their answers [13]:

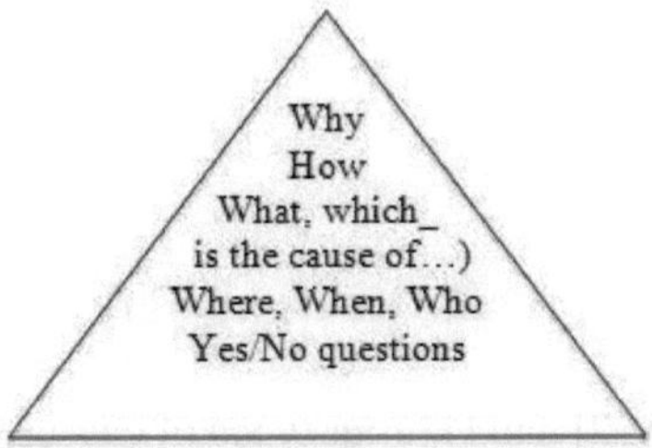

Fig. 17.1 Pyramid of questions' complexity

Ascending in the pyramid means demanding more and more complex answers instead of *yes*, *no* replies, stimulating reflective and deepest thinking. At the top, why-questions ask for some kind of explanation.

This paper will approach how to reach answers to causal questions: (1) what-questions as identifying the cause of a mechanism; (2) how-questions as selecting appropriate parts of a mechanism and (3) why-questions as extracting the prior cause, the final effect (contained in the posed question) and the information labeling relevant nodes.

Thus, this paper is organized as follows: in section 2 we analyze the mechanism to provide an answer to what-questions. In section 3 we will focus on the answer to how-questions. In section 4 why-questions will be approached. Finally, a section of conclusions and references close this work.

17.2 Answering What-Questions

In [8], Puente, Sobrino, Olivas & Merlo described a procedure to automatically display a causal graph from medical knowledge included in several medical texts.

Sentences from medical texts frequently show causality as imperfect or approximate in nature. This feature comes from the linguistic hedges or fuzzy quantifiers included in these sentences. A Flex and C program was designed to analyze causal phrases denoted by words like 'cause', 'effect' or their synonyms, highlighting vague words that qualify the causal nodes or the links between them. Another C program receives as input a set of tags from the previous parser and generates a template with a starting node (cause), a causal relation (denoted by lexical words), possibly qualified by fuzzy quantification, and a final node (effect), possibly modified by a linguistic hedge showing its intensity. Finally, a Java program automates this task. The next figure graphically shows the obtained mechanism:

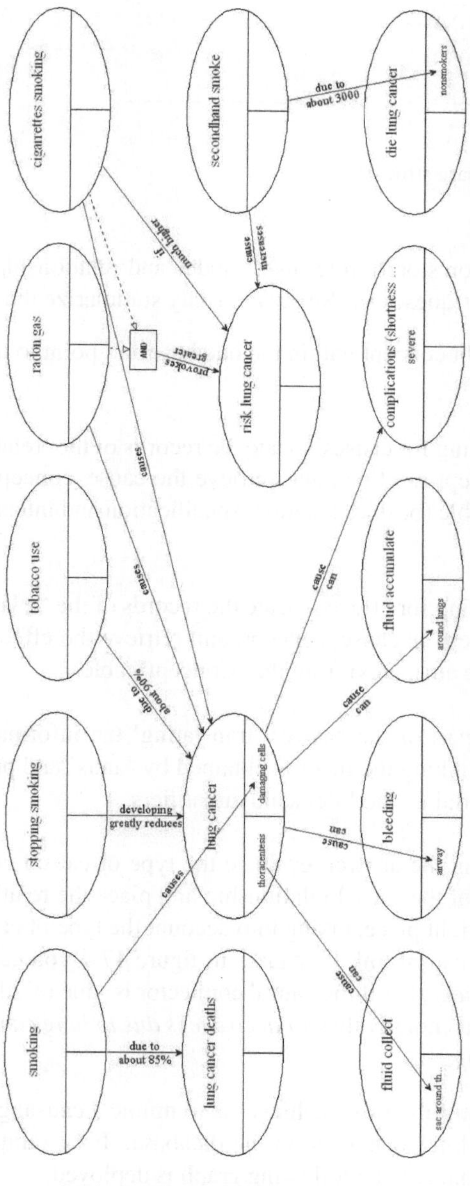

Fig. 17.2 Causal graph of a *lung cancer's mechanism*

Once the graph is performed, it is stored in a database attending to the following structure:

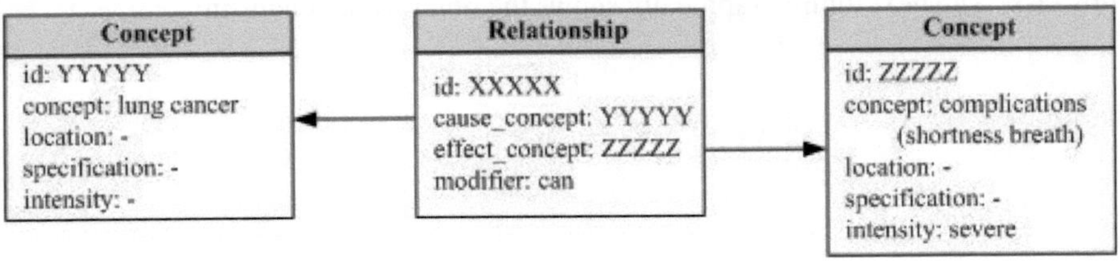

Fig. 17.3 Causal database structure

Causal information stored in terms of nodes and relationships will be useful to find answers to what-questions. Next, we briefly summarize the overall process:

- Locate the sought concept within the database and point to the records where it is contained.
- If the user is asking for causes, locate the records of the 'relationship' table with the sought concept as effect, and retrieve the cause_concept information from the 'Concept' table (besides location, specification and intensity attributes if exists).
- If the user is asking for effects, locate the records of the 'relationship' table with the sought concept as cause_concept, and retrieve the effect_concept information (with all the attributes) from the 'Concept' table.
- Compose each part of the answer 'translating' the information into these obtained records, linking the records obtained by 'ands' and processing the information contained; i.e., modifiers and quantifiers.
- When composing the answer, evaluate the type of causal connector to make a correct reading of the causal relationship and place the relationship modifier (if it exists) in the right place, taking into account the type of causal connector. For example, if the causal link is 'cause' in figure 17.4 you can say that *smoking* 'cause' *lung cancer*; but if the causal connector is 'due to', the reading is upside down: so, you can not say that *tobacco use is due to lung cancer but lung cancer is due to smoking*.

Graphically, what this algorithm achieves is to mimic a causal graph without drawing it, tracking the links contained in the database. For example, if the user asks What causes lung cancer?, the following graph is deployed:

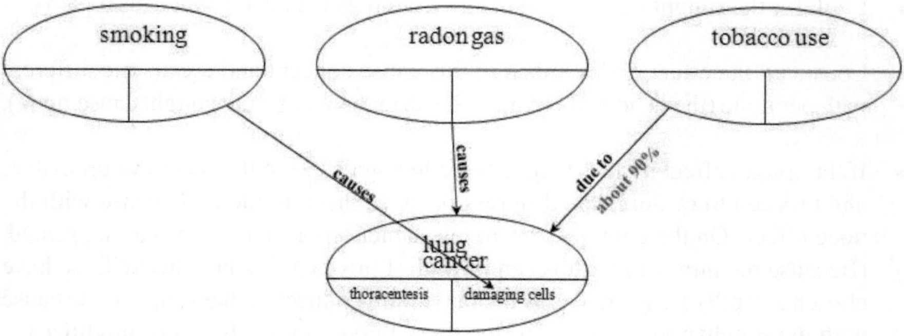

Fig. 17.4 Graph example to answer *What causes lung cancer?*

To compose an answer, we just have to gather the nodes and relationships pointing at the lung cancer node, e.g., in this case, *smoking*, *radon gas* and *tobacco* use. The algorithm with this information performs the answer displayed in figure 17.5. A simple interface, using Php and HTML languages, translates the graph into text:

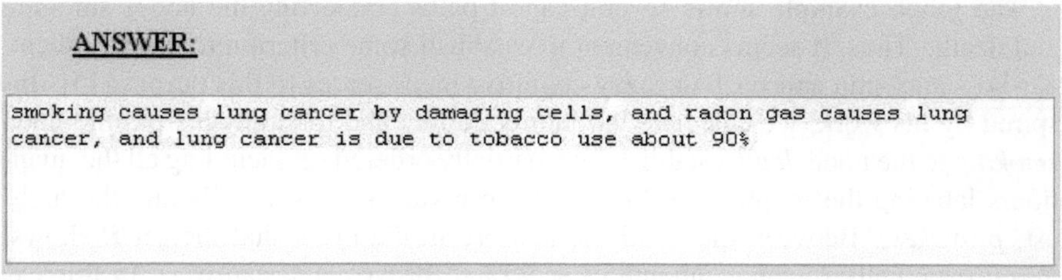

Fig. 17.5 Automated answer to the question *What causes lung cancer?*

17.3 Answering How-Questions

To address *how-questions*, the first step it to locate the causal paths connecting the concepts involved in the question. How-questions usually involve two concepts in the same question, the concept ‘cause’ and the concept ‘effect’. Thus, if we ask *How X causes Y?*, the objective is to find the causal path connecting X (as head of this path) to Y. Once the ‘cause’ concept has been located in the database (it will appear in the Relationship table as cause_concept), a recursive algorithm finds the possible paths connecting the concept cause with the concept effect. The main steps of it are the following:

- Look for the sought cause concept and store it as the head of all causal paths.

- Locate all the effect nodes linked to this cause concept and create one different path per node (the head node of all of these paths will be the sought cause node).

- If the sought effect node is among the effect nodes, stop the recursive procedure and proceed to evaluate the different paths connecting the node cause with the node effect. On the contrary, repeat this same step as many times as suggested. (Because the number of paths can be high if this factor is not checked, we have chosen a depth of eight nodes as the maximum connecting the sought node cause with the sought node effect. This number of nodes or levels can be modified).

- Once all the possible paths have been located, establish some criteria to order them on the basis of their relevance.

- Translate the information included in the three more relevant paths into a suitable answer (using the same procedure as in *What*-questions).

In the example presented in figure 17.6, the question *How smoking causes death?* has been made. That question displayed the following causal graph as a result.

The graph example shows several causal paths connecting the nodes smoking and death. Thus, it seems convenient to establish some criterion to classify them. Kosko's max-min approach to fuzzy cognitive maps serves to this purpose [5]. Inspired by his work, we calculate the indirect effect and total effect from the node *smoking* to the node *death* establishing a partially ordered set including all the quantifiers labeling the graph. The lowest of these values is eventually and the highest, *provokes*. Between them, all the rest are in the order that the set P shows: $P = \{$ eventually $<$ can $<$ about85% $<$ 90% $<$ provokes $\leq$ causes$\}$. In this example there are five possible paths linking *smoking* and *death*, so the indirect effect of each path is (the number indicates the node):

- $I\{n_1,n_2,n_3,n_4,n_6,n_7,n_9\} = min\{$causes, causes, eventually, can, can, provokes$\}$ $=$ eventually.

- $I\{n_1,n_2,n_3,n_4,n_5,n_8,n_9\} = min\{$causes, causes, eventually, can, can, can$\}$ $=$ eventually.

- $I\{n_1,n_4,n_6,n_7,n_9\} = min\{$about 90%, can, can, provokes$\} =$ can.

- $I\{n_1,n_4,n_5,n_8,n_9\} = min\{$about 90%, can, can, can$\} =$ can.

- $I\{n_1,n_9\} = min\{85\%\} = 85\%$.

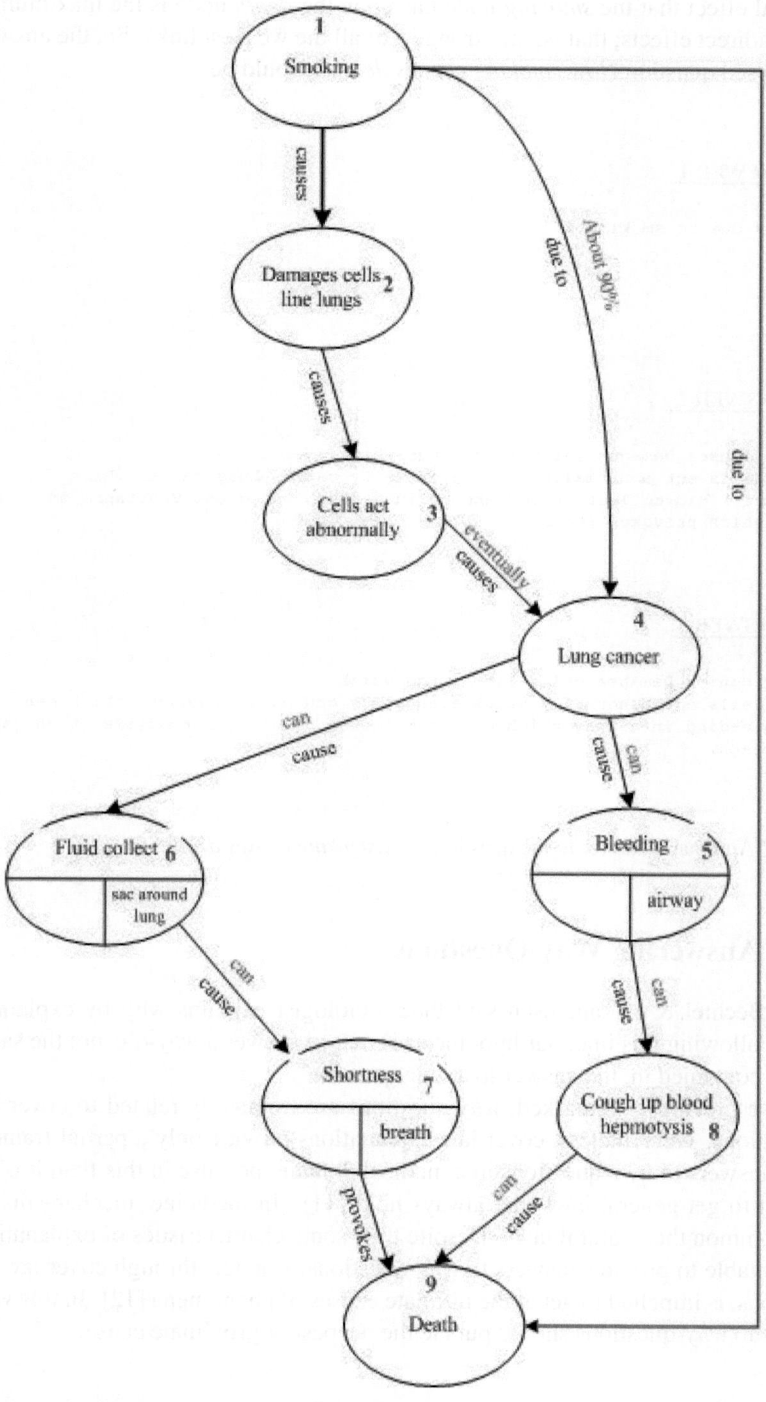

Fig. 17.6 Graph to answer the question *How smoking causes death?*

The total effect that the *smoking* node has upon the *death* node is the maximum of all the indirect effects; that is, the strongest of all the weakest links. So, the answers to the posed question *How smoking causes death?* would be:

ANSWER 1:

```
death is due to smoking 85%.
```

ANSWER 2:

```
Smoking causes Damages cells line lungs which
causes Cells act abnormally which eventually causes Lung cancer which
can cause Fluid collect in sac around lung which can cause Shortness in
breath which provokes Death.
```

ANSWER 3:

```
Smoking causes Damages cells line lungs which
causes Cells act abnormally which eventually causes Lung cancer which can
cause Bleeding in airway which can cause Cough up blood hepmotysis which can
cause Death.
```

Fig. 17.7 Automatic answer to the question *How smoking causes death?*

17.4 Answering Why-Questions

In [3], Bechtel & Abrahamsen said that: "biologist explains why by explaining how". Following this line, our hypothesis is that to answer a *why*-q is not the same, but it is contained in, the answer to a *how*-question.

As we previously remarked, *why*-questions are frequently related to cover law explanations. Nevertheless, cover law explanations provide only a partial frame to obtain answers to *why*-questions in a medical domain, because in this field it is not frequent to get general laws that always hold [11]. In medicine, mechanisms are more common than natural laws. Despite this, some characteristics of explanations are profitable to provide answers to *why*-questions: science, through cover law explanations, is impelled to get at the ultimate causes of phenomena [12]. In this vein, answers to *why*-questions should pursue the deepest or proximate cause.

An explanation is a kind of logical relation between the *explanans* and the *explanandum* [2]. In *why*-questions, the assertive part of the query can be chosen as the *explanadum* and, as a capital part of the *explanans*, we can select the prior cause, from which all the explicative process is triggered. In most cases, nevertheless, to invoke only to the primary cause is quite limited. Other information should join the prior cause in the explanation. A reasonable candidate will be the information included in the relevant nodes of the graph. Our hypothesis is that nodes with high centrality values would be relevant nodes. Depending on whether the answer is for a people with expertise in medicine (in the example at hand) or without it, we can select one or more central nodes to conduct the causal relation between the prior cause and the final effect (the assertive part of the question).

In order to advance in this task, we conceive a mechanism represented by a graph and we follow the widely shared conjecture that the higher the centrality of a node in the graph, the greater its relevance [4]. Next, here is some notation concerning centrality measures in a graph. A graph $G = (V,E)$ consists of a finite set V of vertices and a finite set $E \subseteq V \times V$ of edges. And edge connects two vertices u and v. The vertices u and v are said to be incident with the edge e and adjacent to each other. Centrality is a function C which maps every vertex v (of a given graph G) to a value $C(v) \in \Re$. A vertex u is more important than another vertex v iff $C(u) > C(v)$. Vertices have different relevance. Centrality measures provide a calculus to perform it. In the sequel, we will exemplify some centrality measures for the example depicted in figure 17.6:

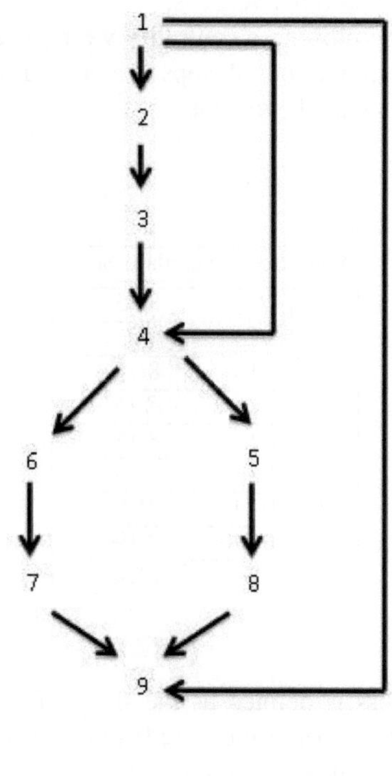

-Degree centrality: The degree $d(v)$ of a vertex is the number of its incident edges. For standardization, divide each score by $n-1$, n is the number of nodes. In directed graphs, edges have a direction associated. Accordingly, there are two different types of degree centrality: in-degree, which is the number of edges pointing into a node and out-degree centrality; i.e., the number of edges pointing out from a node.

Table 17.1 Out-Degree

Node	Score	Standard Score
1	*3*	*3/8*
2	2	1/8
3	2	1/8
4	2	2/8 = 1/4
5	2	1/8
6	2	1/8
7	2	1/8
8	2	1/8
9	2	1/8

-Closeness: In contrast with centrality, closeness uses not only the maximum distance between the vertex of reference and all other vertices, but the sum of the distances of this vertex and all other vertices.

In order to calculate the closeness centrality we need to calculate the inverted score after we count the total number of steps to a node. For standardization, divide a score by $(n-1)$ and then take the inverse.

Table 17.2 Closeness

Node	Score	Standard Score
1	1/30	8/23
2	1/23	8/23
3	1/18	8/18
4	*1/15*	*8/15*
5	1/18	8/18
6	1/18	8/18
7	1/19	8/19
8	1/19	8/19
9	1/24	8/24

-Betweenness: Betweenness is defined as the share of times that a node i needs a node k (whose centrality is being measured) in order to reach a node j via the shortest path. Putted bluntly, this measure basically counts the number of geodesic

paths (the shortest path between two nodes) that pass through a node k. To calculate the betweenness centrality, we take every pair of the network and count how many times a node can interrupt the geodesic distance between the two nodes of the pair. For standardization, the denominator is $(n-1)(n-2)/2$.

Table 17.3 Betweenness

	1	2	3	4	5	6	7	8	9
	1	2	3	4	5	6	7	8	9
1	—	1-2	1-2-3	1-4	1-4-5	1-4-6	1-4-7	1-4-5-8	1-9
2	— —	— —	2-3 —	2-3-4	2-3-4-5	2-3-4-6	2-3-4-6-7	2-3-4-5-8	2-3-4-6-7-9 2-3-4-5-8-9
3	—	—	—	3-4	3-4-5	3-4-6	3-4-6-7	3-4-5-8	3-4-6-7-9 3-4-5-8-9
4	—	—	—	—	4-5	4-6	4-6-7	4-5-8	4-6-7-9 4-5-8-9
5	—	—	—	—	—	—	—	5-8	5-8-9
6	—	—	—	—	—	—	—	6-8	6-7-9
7	—	—	—	—	—	—	—	—	7-9
8	—	—	—	—	—	—	—	—	8-9
9	—	—	—	—	—	—	—	—	—

For example, the betweenness centrality for the node 4 will be:

Betweenness centrality(4)= fraction_paths_broken
(1, 2)= 0 + (2, 3)= 0 + (3, 4)= 1 + (4, 5)= 1 +
+ (1, 3)= 0 + (2, 4)= 1 + (3, 5)= 1 + (4, 6)= 1 +
+ (1, 4)= 1 + (2, 5)= 1 + (3, 6)= 1 + (4, 7)= 1 +
+ (1, 5)= 1 + (2, 6)= 1 + (3, 7)= 1 + (4, 8)= 1 +
+ (1, 6)= 1 + (2, 7)= 1 + (3, 8)= 1 + (4, 9)= 2/2=1 +
+ (1, 7)= 1 + (2, 8)= 1 + (3, 9)= 2/2=1 +
+ (1, 8)= 1 + (2, 9)= 2/2=1 +
+ (1, 9)= 0 +

+ (5, 8)= 0 + (6, 7)= 0 + (7, 9)= 0 + (8, 9)= 0
+ (5, 9)= 0 + (6, 9)= 0 + N
= 0+0+1+1+1+1+1+0+0+1+1+1+1+1+1+1+1
+1+1+1+1+1+1+1+1+1+1+0+0+0+0+0+0
= 21/32
= 0,656

Operating a similar calculus for the node 5, the result is =
0+0+0+1+0+0+1+0+0+0+1+0+0+1+0,5+0+1
+0+0+1+0,5+1+0+0+1+0,5+1+1+0+0+0+0
= 11,5/32
= 0,334
significantly lower than the previous one as expected.

-*Out Eigenvector centrality*: It is based on the assumption that the value of a single vertex depends on the values of the neighboring vertices and not only on the position of a vertex within the graph. The moral is that the popularity of a node depends also on its proximity to other nodes highly connected. *Mathematica* shows the following out-eigenvector centrality measure for the graph of our example:

Table 17.4 Out-Eigenvector centrality

Node	Score
1	0.999991
2	0.004339
3	8.16933×10^{-8}
4	3.27441×10^{-15}
5	0.0000188273
6	1.77148×10^{-10}
7	$1{,}77326 \times 10^{-10}$
8	7.68872×10^{-13}
9	7.69543×10^{-13}

In the aforementioned example we can see that node 1 has a higher degree than node 4, but node four has a higher score in closeness and betweenness that node 1. As suggested by Obietat et al. in [7], we think that it is convenient to combine the degree, betweenness and closeness centrality measures in order to reach a consensus centrality measure. Combination is needed because the degree measure only takes into account the direct connections, ignoring the importance of indirect links. If we adopt as the consensus measure the arithmetical mean, we can see – attending our example – that node 1 has a consensus measure: $0,375$ (degree) $+0,348$ (closeness) $+0,25$ (betweenness)$/3 = 0,324$ and node 4: $0,25+0,533+0,656/3 = 0,480$. Thus, node 4 is the node with a highest centrality measure in the graph. Therefore, the content of node 4 complements the prior cause in the why-question explanation. This would be enough to answer to a lay audience. But if people involved in the inquiry are specialized, other than centrality nodes should provide technical information. Eigenvector centrality permits to select nodes not only because they are central, but because they are highly connected to central nodes. In our example, nodes with high eigenvalue score are: $1 > 2 > 5 > 3 > 6$. Perhaps we need to perform a selection in this set. Node 1 is out as it is the prior cause. Nodes 2 and 3 are before node 4, the central node par excellence. So nodes 2 and 3 are explanans of node 4, as node 4 is part of the explanans elicited by the why-q; thus, general information contained in nodes 2 and 3 is ruled out. Only nodes 5 and 6 remain.

In short, if we take the graph of the figure 17.6 and launch it against the query *Why John died?* some answers arise. The graph has a main node or prior cause that directly or indirectly connects with the effect. So, a tentative answer could be to locate the root node and say: *Because John was a smoker.* But, as previously said, why-questions are concerned – if accessible – with deepening in knowledge. Thus, other nodes should be explored. Our hypothesis is that central nodes in the mechanism include relevant content. In the quoted graph, the central node is node 4. But we can tune perhaps a little more. A why-question can be made by a skilled or a non-skilled, interrogator. If the questioner is not specialized, the causal link between the prior cause and the central node is perhaps enough to arrange the answer. As In the previous example, *Because John was a smoker, causing lung cancer*. But if the questioner is specialized, more specific knowledge is needed. Eingenvector centrality values detect nodes connected with a few neighbors of high importance. If the node with the highest centrality value is node 4, the nodes with more eingencentrality are 1, 2, 5, 3 and 6. Node 1 is ruled out by the root cause. Nodes 2 and 3 do not include specific content, as they are before node 4, the central node. Thus, nodes 5 and 6 are the candidates to express specific explanations about why lung cancer causes death. Thus, the answer for a specialized questioner will be the following causal chain: *Because John was a smoker, provoking lung cancer, that leads to fluid collect or bleeding* (*leads to a* synonym of causing, and included in the final answer in order to make it more linguistically expressible).

To provide an automatic answer, we have modified partially the algorithm used with how-questions. This procedure selected the possible paths linking the node cause with the node effect. Each one of these paths would be a cluster of nodes to summarize. So, the steps to answer (and summarize) a why question are the following:

- Locate the main cause node (head of the diagram), and the effect node.
- Calculate the centrality measure of each node (but the cause and effect nodes).
- Select the node with the highest centrality value.
- Select those nodes with the highest eingencentrality value related to the node with the highest centrality value.
- Reject those nodes selected in the previous step which number is lower than the node with the highest centrality value.
- Order the nodes to compose an appropriate answer.
- Compose an answer summarizing the retrieved nodes.

In the graph showed in figure 17.6, the algorithm would locate nodes 1 and 9 as cause and effect nodes. The node with the highest centrality value would be node 4, so the eingencentrality values will be calculated in base to this node. As a result four more nodes are obtained in this order, 2, 5, 3 and 6, but nodes 2 and 3 are rejected because they are lower than 4. On the other hand, nodes 5 and 6 will be included in the new answer, as well as the causal paths that link these nodes with the effect node.

The next step is to order the nodes to compose an answer. So, with all these nodes, the final answer would be the composition of nodes 1, 9, 4, 5, 6, and the causal paths derived from nodes 5 and 6 as seen in the following figure:

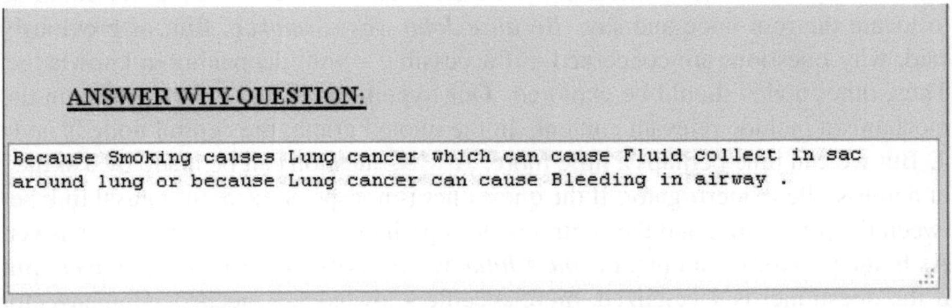

Fig. 17.8 Automatic answer to the question *Why smoking causes death?*

17.5 Conclusion

In this paper we have approached how to get answers to causal questions by mechanisms reflecting medical knowledge. In the pyramid of causal questions, what-q, how-q and - at the top - why-questions have been analyzed and preprocessed using templates. Solutions to automatically get answers for each of them are provided.

These solutions are dependent of the field selected – medical knowledge – and even of the furnished example. Clearly other domains or examples would request substantial improvements, although we think that the approach followed in this paper is a good start. A challenge for future work will be generalize this oncoming from a medical example to a medical domain.

Note

Points 1, 2 and 3 of this paper are largely based in the author's contribution (with J. A. Olivas) to the ISDA 2011 Congress, November 22-24, Córdoba, Spain.

Acknowledgement. This work was supported by the Spanish Ministry for Economy and Innovation and by the European Regional Development Fund (ERDF/FEDER) under grant TIN2011-29827-C02-02

References

1. Aristotle: The metaphysics. Penguin Books, London (1998); (translated by Hugh Lawson-Tancred)
2. Aristotle (ed.): Aristotle: Physics. Oxford University Press, Oxford (1996); (translated by Robin Waterfield)

3. Bechtel, W., Abrahamsen, A.: Explanation: A Mechanist Alternative. Studies in History and Philosophy of Biology and Biomedical Sciences 36, 421–441 (2005)
4. Koschützki, D., Schreiber, F.: Comparison of Centralities for Biological Networks. In: Proceedings of German Conference of Bioinformatics (GCB 2004), vol. P-53, pp. 199–206 (2004)
5. Kosko, B.: Fuzzy Cognitive Maps. International Journal of Man-Machine Studies 24, 65–75 (1986)
6. Mackie, J.L.: The Cement of the Universe: A Study in Causation. Clarendon Press, Oxford (1988)
7. Obiedat, M., Samarasinghe, S., Strickert, G.: A New Method for Indentifying the Central Nodes in Fuzzy Cognitive Maps Using Consensus Centrality Measure. In: 19th. International Congress on Modelling and Simulation, Perth, Australia, December 12-16 (2011)
8. Puente, C., Sobrino, A., Olivas, J.A., Merlo, R.: Extraction, Analysis and Representation of Imperfect Conditional and Causal Sentences by Means of a Semi-Automatic Process. In: Proceedings IEEE International Conference on Fuzzy Systems (FUZZ-IEEE 2010), Barcelona, Spain, pp. 1423–1430 (2010)
9. Sadegh-Zadeh, K.: Fundamentals of clinical methodology: 2. Etiology. Artificial Intelligence in Medicine 12, 227–270 (1998)
10. Sadegh-Zadeh, K.: Handbook of Analytical Philosophy of Mecedine. Springer, Amsterdam (2011)
11. Thagard, P.: Explaining Disease: Correlations, Causes and Mechanisms. Mind and Machines 8, 61–78 (1998)
12. Thagard, P.: Coherence, Truth and the Development of Scientific Knowledge. Philosophy of Science 74, 28–47 (2007)
13. Vogt, E.E., Brown, J., Isaacs, D.: The Art of Powerful Questions. Whole Systems Associates, Mill Valley (2003)

Part V

Statistical Approaches

18

On Examination of Medical Data with Approximate Reasoning

Vesa A. Niskanen

18.1 Introduction

Modern medicine applies both quantitative and qualitative methods because its scope covers both natural and human sciences. In the former case numerical data, computer modeling and mathematical and statistical methods are essential, whereas the latter mainly operates with non-numerical materials, manual work and with such reasoning as interpretation.

We will consider how computational intelligence (which is sometimes also referred to as soft computing) may be applied to quantitative medical research, and this study is inspired by Lotfi Zadeh's recent work and the book of Kazem Sadegh-Zadeh [17]. Computational intelligence comprises such methods as fuzzy systems, neural nets, probabilistic reasoning and evolutionary computing, and it provides us with usable tools for examining empirical data and medical phenomena in a more thorough and convenient manner. Today we have mainly applied computational intelligence to quantitative studies, but it also seems usable in qualitative research.

In particular, we consider below the role of computational intelligence in statistical research in the light of medical data. Hence, we examine how we may replace or enhance certain statistical analyses with our novel methods in order to achieve better results. Our methods stem from Lotfi Zadeh's novel fuzzy extended logic, fuzzy cluster analysis and fuzzy modeling in general, and then we apply them to regression analysis. We also provide some ideas for applying our models to analysis of covariance and novel clustering techniques.

Chapter 18.2 presents some basic principles of linguistic reasoning and fuzzy extended logic. Chapter 18.3 considers regression modeling from both the traditional and computational intelligence standpoint. Chapter 18.4 deals with discriminant analysis. Chapter 18.5 provides some ideas on applying computational intelligence to analysis of covariance and cluster analysis. Chapter 18.6 concludes our examination.

R. Seising and M.E. Tabacchi (Eds.): *Fuzziness and Medicine*, STUDFUZZ 302, pp. 269–290.
DOI: 10.1007/978-3-642-36527-0_18

18.2 Measuring and Reasoning with Imprecise Concepts in Statistics

18.2.1 Linguistic Variables and Approximate Reasoning

In traditional measuring we may draw a distinction between qualitative, comparative and quantitative concepts or variables, but in statistical analysis we usually regard them as being precise entities. For example, when Likert or Osgood scales are used, their values are assumed to be precise values although they are actually imprecise by nature. Thanks for the fuzzy systems, we can also operate with both precise and imprecise values, as well as with the linguistic values. Hence, in addition to the precise (or crisp) numerical values or intervals, we may also use such values as *approximately 5, approximately from 4 to 6 or very young*. In statistics this means that we may also use fuzzy linguistic variables. One usable method for generating linguistic values for linguistic variables within Likert or Osgood scales is as follows [15]:

1. Specify such two primitive terms for each variable which are antonyms (if possible). *Young* and *old* seem appropriate to age on Osgood scale. *Fully agree* and *fully disagree* on Likert scale.
2. Specify such linguistic modifiers (adverbs) as *very*, *fairly* or *more or less*, and construct usable symmetrical scales with the modifiers and primitive terms. Five or seven values are widely used in this context. For example, *young – fairly young – middle-aged (neither young nor old) – fairly old – old.*
3. We can also use negation not. For example, *not fairly young*.
4. Use such connectives for compound expressions as *and*, or *and if – then*.
5. If necessary, specify such quantifiers as *all*, *most*, *some* or *none*.
6. We may also use crisp numerical values or such fuzzy numbers as *approximately 5* or *approximately between 4 and 6*.

Given a linguistic variable and its reference set (universe of discourse), each linguistic value refers to a certain fuzzy set, and in practice we operate with the corresponding membership functions of these sets in a computer environment (Fig. 18.1). Various shapes for these functions, such as triangular, bell-shaped and trapezoidal, are available, and we may specify them according to our expertise or empirical data [1],[5], [21].

The fuzzy systems have already proved their applicability in various disciplines even though several models still use only more or less numerical methods. In a sense, they have mainly applied fuzzy sets and not fuzzy linguistic logic. However, recently Zadeh has established the principles of his novel fuzzy extended logic, *FLe*, which is a combination of "traditional" provable and "precisiated" fuzzy logic as well as a novel meta-level "unprecisiated" fuzzy logic [25]. He states that in the precisiated case the objects of discourse and analysis can be imprecise, uncertain, unreliable, incomplete or partially true, whereas the results of reasoning, deduction and computation are expected to be provably valid in the traditional sense. In his meta-level unprecisiated logic, in turn, membership functions and generalized

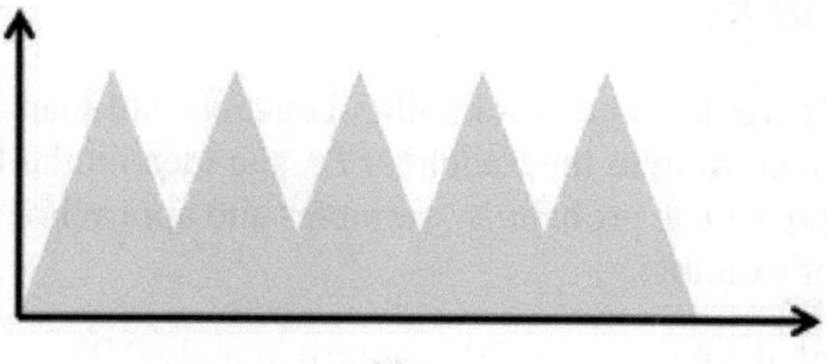

Fig. 18.1 Tentative membership functions for denoting the linguistic values young, fairly young, middle-aged, fairly old and old in the context of age (horizontal axis)

constraints are not specified, and they are a matter of perception rather than measurement. In addition, we apply informal and approximate reasoning in this context.

The *FLe* stems from Zadeh's previous theories on information granulation, precisiated language and computing with words, as well as on the theory of perceptions [21],[22–27]. His ideas mean that we can apply both traditional bivalent-based and novel approximate validity, definitions, axioms, theories and explanations, inter alia. The well-known syllogism, the fuzzified Modus Ponens, is an example of his approximate reasoning. Hence, instead of the traditional Modus Ponens,

A
If A, then B
Thus, B

in the fuzzified version the first premise need not to be identical with the antecedent of the second premise, and thus we use the fuzzified Modus Ponens in a form

A_1
If A, then B
Thus, B_1

For example,

John is 22 years old.
If John is 20 years old, then he is young.
Thus, John is approximately young

The *FLe* opens several prospects for conduct of inquiry [11–14],[16]. Below we apply its ideas to statistical reasoning and modeling.

18.2.2 Statistical Reasoning

In statistical analysis we use much probability concepts and many of these are imprecise by nature. According to the Zadeh's *FLe*, the idea on the fuzzy probability generally means approximate probability variables and approximate values of these variables [3, 25]. For example,

- The probability that John's age is 20 is approximately 0.95.
- The probability that John's age is 20 is very high.
- The probability that John's age is approximately 20 is very high.
- The probability that John is young is very high.

In particular, statistical tests apply much probability and random distributions when we consider the acceptance of the null and alternative hypotheses according to the tests of significance [6],[11],[12],[28]. We accept the null hypothesis if the value of our test variable does not deviate too much from the "usual" case, otherwise we reject it and accept the alternative hypothesis. In practice we operate with the p-values (level of significance, ($0 \leq p \leq 1$) in a computer environment in which case we consider the rejection of the null hypotheses if the obtained p-value is sufficiently small. In other words, the p-value is our risk to draw an erroneous conclusion if we reject the null hypothesis.

Traditionally the statistical hypothesis verification is based on bivalent reasoning, and thus the rejection of one hypothesis automatically means the acceptance of the other. Hence, formally we reason that if the p-value is greater than a given limit point, we accept the null hypothesis, otherwise we reject it. The usual threshold values for p are .05 or .01 (5 % and 1 % levels of significance, respectively). For example, when the t-test is applied to two independent samples of data (the two-tailed case), we have the null hypothesis that there is no difference in the means between the groups, whereas the alternative hypothesis asserts that this difference prevails.

In practice we nevertheless take into account the borderline cases when the acceptance of the null hypothesis is considered. For example, we may pay special attention to the p-values which are in the close neighborhood of $p = .05$ in order to avoid erroneous conclusions. Hence, we actually apply approximate reasoning and probability.

In approximate reasoning we may operate with the degrees of acceptance and rejection in this context and thus acquire more informative outcomes. For example, we can establish the meta-rule that the smaller the p-value, the lower the risk of error for rejecting the null hypothesis, in other words, the higher the degree of rejection for the null hypothesis. Simultaneously, then it also holds that the higher the degree of accepting the alternative hypothesis. On Osgood scale it would mean such values as *high degree of acceptance*, *fairly high degree of acceptance*, *borderline case*, *fairly high degree of rejection* and *high degree of rejection*. We may even construct a fuzzy inference engine including this type of fuzzy rule base for this task.

In general, possible approximate statistical hypotheses are

- In Germany the heights of the males are approximately normally distributed.
- The Swedish males are slightly taller than the Italian males.
- Most Swedish males are very likely fairly tall.
- The people in the Nordic countries usually drink coffee quite much.
- There is often fairly high positive correlation between the grades in mathematics and physics among pupils at school.
- One-dollar bills fairly likely contain a few particles of cocaine.

Within statistical explanations we may also use probabilistic or statistical statements. For example, consider first the fact that the tossing of the coin in the real world yields approximately 50 % of heads. If we now ask why approximately 50 % of these outcomes are heads, we can provide an approximate explanation that it is due to this approximate frequency probability. Second, we may explain that most Swedish men are tall because, according to the statistics, their average height is approximately 180 cm.

In addition to statistical decision making, computational intelligence may provide us with enhanced methods in model construction. We consider this aspect next.

18.3 Model Construction for Regression Analysis

Regression models are used when we aim at explaining or predicting the behavior of a given variable, the dependent variable, according to the other variables known as the independent variables. In the traditional case we presuppose that the independent variables have linear correlations with the dependent variable, and thus linear models are widely used. In practice we apply then the linear regression equation

$$Y = \sum_i a_i X_i + b, \quad i = 1, 2, \ldots, n. \tag{18.1}$$

in which Y is the dependent variable and X_i are the independent variables. When the regression coefficients, a_i and b, are specified correctly, this equation yields a plane in a space with $n+1$ dimensions according to the given data points [9],[28] .

Unfortunately, the linear models often seem to be too coarse for our purposes because the real world is usually non-linear by nature. Thus, we may also attempt to apply non-linear models, but then we do not necessarily know which regression function would be appropriate to us, and we may have thousands of alternatives. Even if we can find such function, it may be complicated and laborious with respect to calculations, and naturally deep mathematical knowledge is also required.

Computational intelligence may resolve several of these problems, and we will apply it with a synthetic data set of 98 persons which for the sake of simplicity only comprises three variables, age in years, body mass index (*Bmi*) and systolic blood pressure in mmHg (*Syst*). This data set is a modified version that is presented in [10]. We apply SPSS™ and MATLAB™ software to our analyses below.

Figure 18.2 depicts the histograms and scatter plots of this set. We notice that there seems to be a positive correlation between *Bmi* and *Syst*, whereas the rest of the correlations are less obvious.

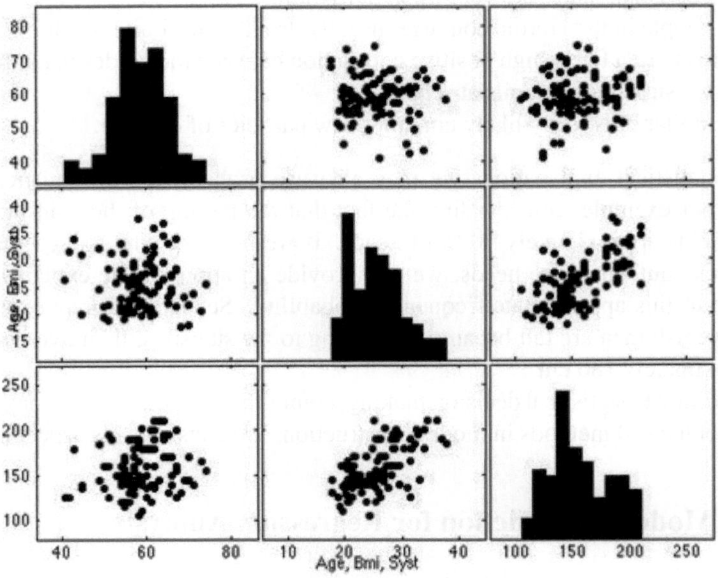

Fig. 18.2 Histograms and scatter plots of 98 persons in the case of variables age, body mass index and systolic blood pressure

18.3.1 Prelude – Fuzzy Cluster Analysis

In computational intelligence modeling we mainly apply fuzzy systems and their fine-tuned versions below, viz. neuro-fuzzy and genetic-fuzzy systems. Hence, if a data set is available, we first examine the data clusters in a multi-dimensional space and then we construct our models according to these clusters.

If the traditional *k*-means clustering is used, we obtain the cluster centers in Table 18.1 Seven clusters were selected because then the *F* ratio, the ratio of the variance between the clusters to the variance within the clusters, was high. However, now we operate with crisp clusters, and thus each person is forced to have a full membership to a certain cluster and a full non-membership to the other clusters [18].

The fuzzy clustering methods, such as the fuzzy *c*-means (FCM) and mountain clustering methods (MC), will also take into account the borderline cases, and thus the persons or objects may also have partial memberships to clusters [2–4], [8],[20]. In this manner we may acquire more thorough information on our data set and even avoid misclassifications. Table 18.2 shows the corresponding cluster centers when the FCM, which is the fuzzified version of the *k*-means clustering, is used in our data.

Table 18.1 Final cluster centers when traditional k-means clustering is used

	Cluster						
	1	2	3	4	5	6	7
Age	57	56	57	47	64	62	63
Bmi	21	24	30	26	26	23	31
Syst	119	151	185	132	164	139	202

Table 18.2 Cluster centers when FCM is used

	Cluster						
	1	2	3	4	5	6	7
Age	58	62	56	56	64	62	56
Bmi	30	26	24	24	23	31	22
Syst	184	165	139	151	140	201	120

In practice the FCM calculates the weighted distances between the data points and the tentative cluster centers, and these weights base on the degrees of memberships of the points to the cluster centers. We obtain the optimal outcomes when the centers in the densest clusters are selected.

Figure 18.3 depicts the degrees of membership of the persons to the first cluster the center of which is $Age = 58$, $Bmi = 30$ and $Syst = 184$. This means that one typical group of persons in our data is having this approximate age, body mass index

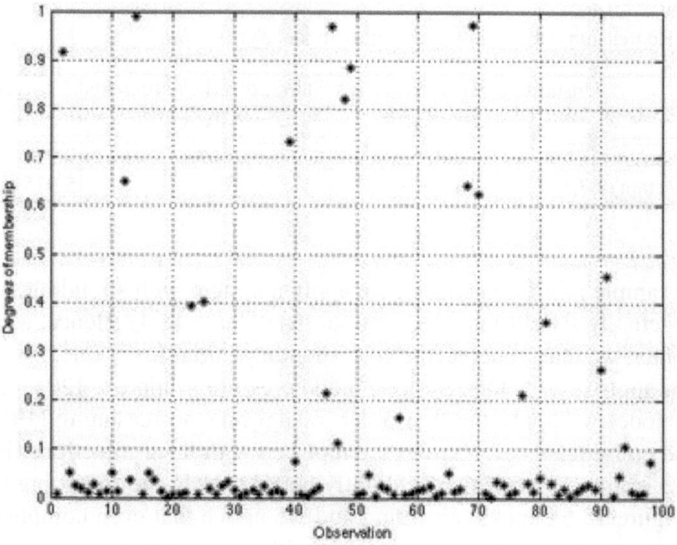

Fig. 18.3 Degrees of membership of persons to the first cluster in Table 3.2 in our data set when FCM is applied

and systolic blood pressure. We notice that, in addition to the clear cases, we also have such borderline cases which only have a partial membership to this cluster.

Fuzzy cluster methods are often the corner stones when fuzzy model construction with empirical data is carried out. Fuzzy clusters reveal us the typical cases in the data set, and the rest of the predicted values of the models are specified according to these objects. This approach is widely used in the regression models, and we will consider them next with our data set.

18.3.2 Regression Models

Consider first a simple regression model in which we have *Bmi* as the independent and *Syst* as the dependent variable. Figure 18.4 shows us that a more or less linear correlation seems to prevail between these variables and thus a linear model is first constructed with SPSS (Table 18.3). This model yields us the regression equation

$$Syst = 3.454Bmi + 67.563$$

with the root mean square of error (RMSE) = 19.66 when

$$RMSE = (\sum_i \frac{e_i}{n})^{1/2}, \quad i = 1,2,\ldots,n$$

in which e_1, e_2, ..., e_n are the error terms (residuals) and n is the number of cases. A cubic curve, i.e., a third degree polynomial, would now yield an almost similar RMSE.

Table 18.3 Regression coefficients for a linear model *Syst* vs. *Bmi*

	Unstardardized Coefficients		Stardardized Coefficients	t	Sig.
	B	Std. Error	Beta		
Bmi	3.454	.435	.630	7.940	.000
(Constant)	67.563	11.308		5.975	.000

As an example of a fuzzy model, we apply a system with six initial fuzzy rules which are actually six cluster centers of our data (Table 18.4). Hence, according to the first center, we may generate the corresponding initial fuzzy rule.

If *Bmi* is approx. 20.5, then Systolic blood pressure is approx. 120.

In our model we apply the first-order Takagi-Sugeno reasoning [19] and thus the original consequents of the rules are replaced with linear functions (Fig. 18.5). Our RMSE is now 18.86 which is slightly better than in the foregoing traditional models. Figure 18.6 depicts our fitting and we notice that even complicated non-linear fittings may be obtained conveniently with fuzzy systems.

Next, we add another independent variable to our model, viz. the age of persons. Figure 18.7 depicts our data set in a 3-D space, and our task is now to specify such

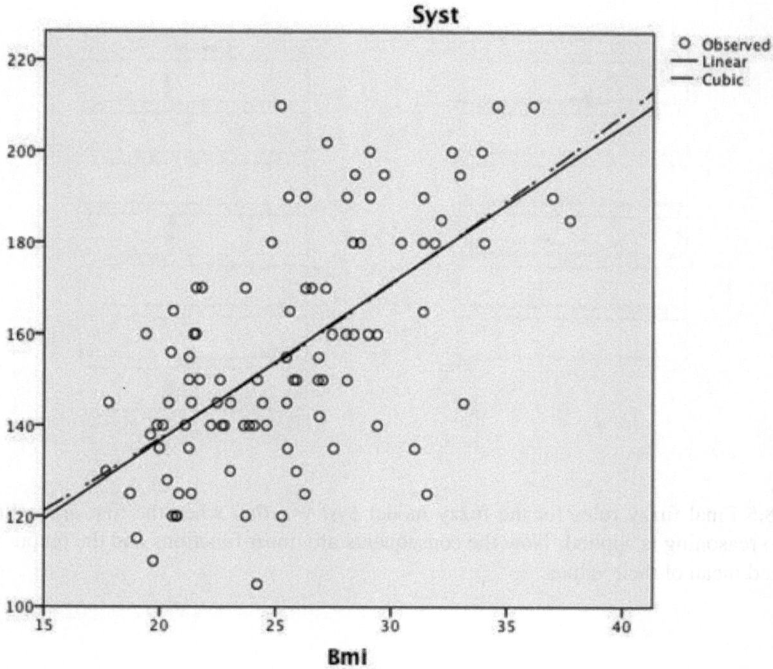

Fig. 18.4 Linear and cubic fittings to the regression model *Syst* vs. *Bmi*

Table 18.4 Cluster centers (fuzzy rules) for the regression model *Syst* vs. *Bmi*

Rule	If *Bmi*	then *Syst*
1	20.5	120
2	22.5	145
3	27.4	160
4	27.5	135
5	29.1	190
6	33.9	2

fitting plane or surface which is optimally close to our data points. Table 18.5 shows the linear resolution and thus we obtain the regression equation

$$\text{Syst} = 0.856\,Age + 3.524\,Bmi + 15.421.$$

According to t-tests in Table 18.5 , both independent variables seem to be relevant in our model. The RMSE is 18.87 (adjusted Rsquare = .432) which smaller than in the foregoing linear model Syst vs. Bmi and almost similar to our fuzzy model with one independent variable. Figure 18.8 depicts this linear fitting.

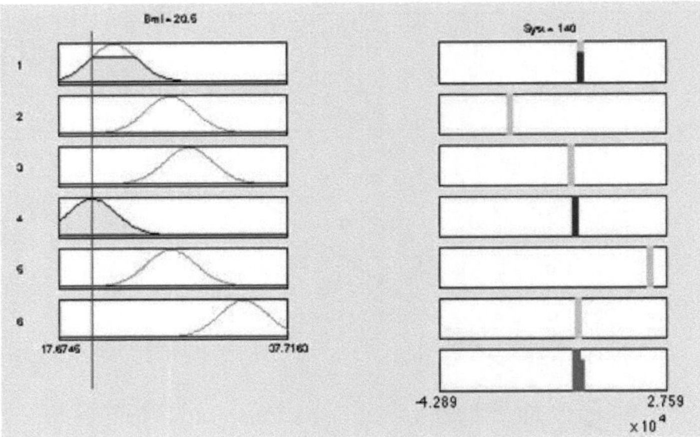

Fig. 18.5 Final fuzzy rules for the fuzzy model *Syst* vs. *Bmi* when the first-order Takagi-Sugeno reasoning is applied. Now the consequents are linear functions and the output is the weighted mean of their values.

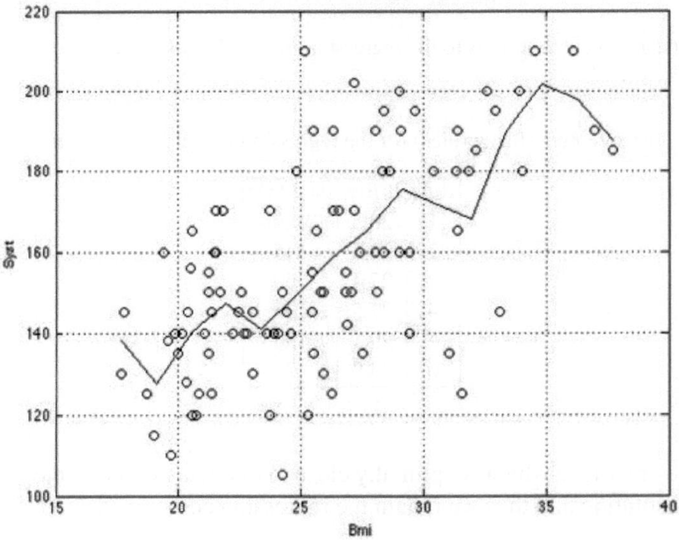

Fig. 18.6 Fitting curve of the fuzzy model *Syst* vs. *Bmi*

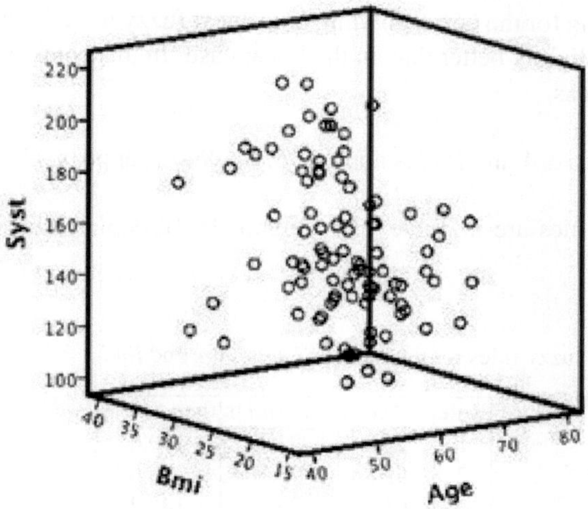

Fig. 18.7 Our data points for the regression model *Syst* vs. *Age* and *Bmi*

Table 18.5 Regression coefficients for the linear model *Syst* vs. *Age* and *Bmi*

	Unstardardized Coefficients		Stardardized Coefficients	t	Sig.
	B	Std. Error	Beta		
(Constant)	15.421	21.258		.725	.470
Age	.856	.3	.219	2.858	.005
Bmi	3.524	.420	.642	8.384	.000

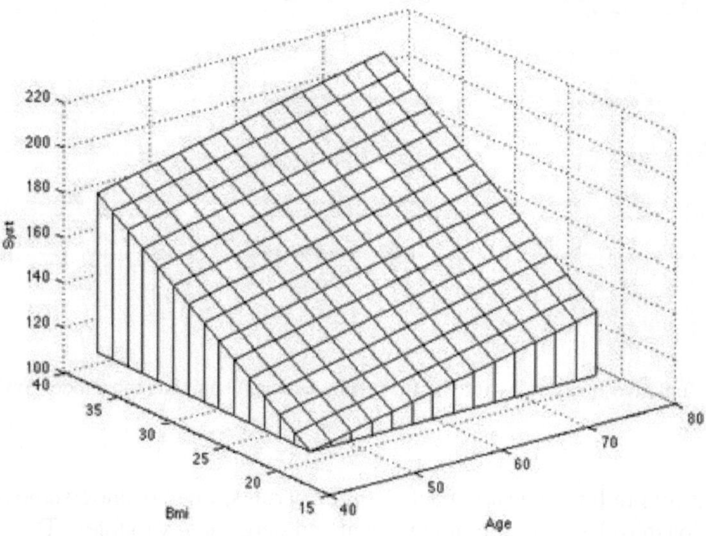

Fig. 18.8 Fitting plane for the linear model *Syst* vs. *Age* and *Bmi*

Figure 18.9 depicts an example of a fuzzy rule set (seven rules) with Takagi-Sugeno reasoning for the corresponding non-linear fuzzy model. Our RMSE is now 16.48 and thus slightly better than in the linear case. In this context we operate with such fuzzy rules as

If *Age* is approx. *A* and *Bmi* is approx. *B*, the *Syst* is approx. *C*

and our initial rules are in Table 18.6. Figure 18.10 depicts our non-linear fuzzy fitting surface.

Table 18.6 Initial fuzzy rules for the model *Syst* vs. *Age* and *Bmi*

Rule	If *Age* is	and *Bmi* is	then *Syst* is
1	55.8	21.7	119.6
2	55.8	23.5	138.6
3	63.7	23.2	140.2
4	56.5	24.4	151.0
5	61.9	25.9	165.5
6	57.9	29.9	184.4
7	62.3	31.2	201.4

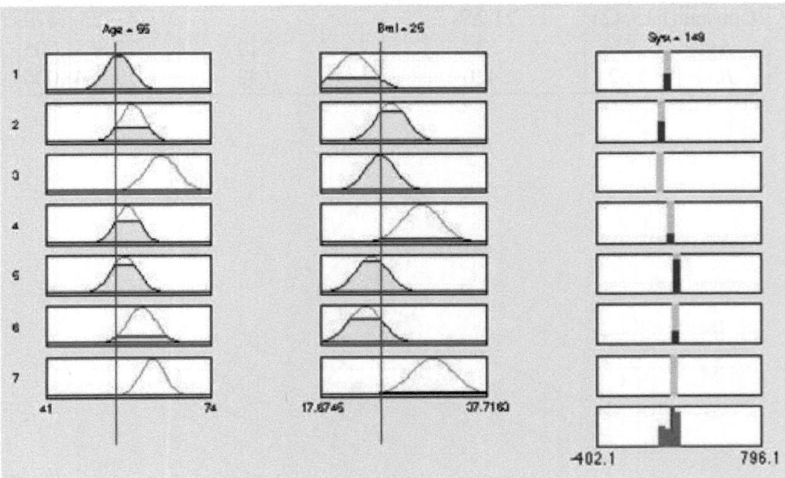

Fig. 18.9 Tentative fuzzy rules for the fuzzy first-order Takagi-Sugeno model *Syst* vs. *Age* and *Bmi*

Thanks for our linguistic approach with fuzzy rules, we may understand better the interrelationships between the independent and dependent variables. This is essential particularly in the non-linear models because then corresponding mathematical resolutions may be much more complicated and inconceivable.

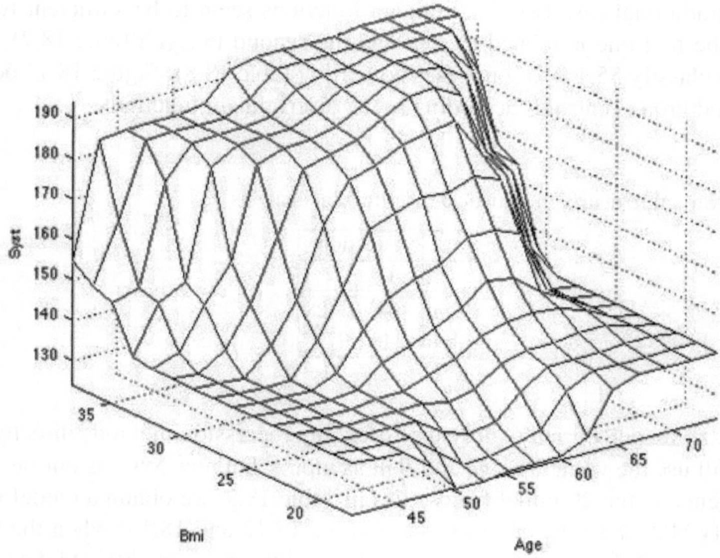

Fig. 18.10 Non-linear fitting surface for the fuzzy model *Syst* vs. *Age* and *Bmi*

The foregoing fuzzy modeling provides us with a basis for various such analyses in which we consider the interrelationships between the variables. Below we sketch some typical modelings.

18.4 Discriminant Analysis

In discriminant analysis we aim to classify the objects of our data set into groups according to such previously performed methods as cluster analysis. Hence, for example, if we have previously specified three groups for our objects in a space of n variables, in discriminant analysis we aim to provide a method for classifying our objects into these groups correctly. From the neural nets standpoint, clustering of objects and their classification according to the clustering are examples of unsupervised and supervised learning, respectively [2]. We thus "supervise" our model to carry out correct classification by using representative training data in this task.

Consider our data set above. If we have created such a discrete variable, *Syst3*, for the systolic blood pressure which has three values, low pressure (= 1), average pressure (= 2) and high pressure (= 3), we could next construct a model for classifying our persons into these groups correctly according to the variables *Age* and *Bmi* (Fig. 18.11). If our model is sufficiently good, we can also apply it to the other data sets collected from the same population. Corresponding methods in statistics for this task are logistic and multinomial regression analyses and Cox's regression analysis, for example. In computational intelligence we may apply neural nets or the foregoing fuzzy approach. We sketch first the traditional discriminant analysis.

In the traditional case two discriminant functions seem to be sufficient for our data and the first one is related to *Bmi* and the second to *Age* (Table 18.7). This model can classify 55.1 % of our cases correctly (Table 18.8). Figure 18.11 depicts the obtained group centroids according to the discriminant functions.

Table 18.7 Structure matrix in statistical discriminant analysis

	Function	
	1	2
Bmi	.904*	-.428
Age	.243	.970*

In a fuzzy model we may apply the foregoing regression methods directly, and thus we still use the variables *Age* and *Bmi* as inputs, but now *Syst3* is our output.

If we generate the 20 initial fuzzy rules in Table 18.9, we obtain a model which can classify 80.6 % of the cases correctly (Fig. 18.12 and 18.13) when the initial outputs are rounded into integers, and thus better outcomes are obtained than in the traditional case. The fuzzy model is also simpler and more conceivable. Naturally

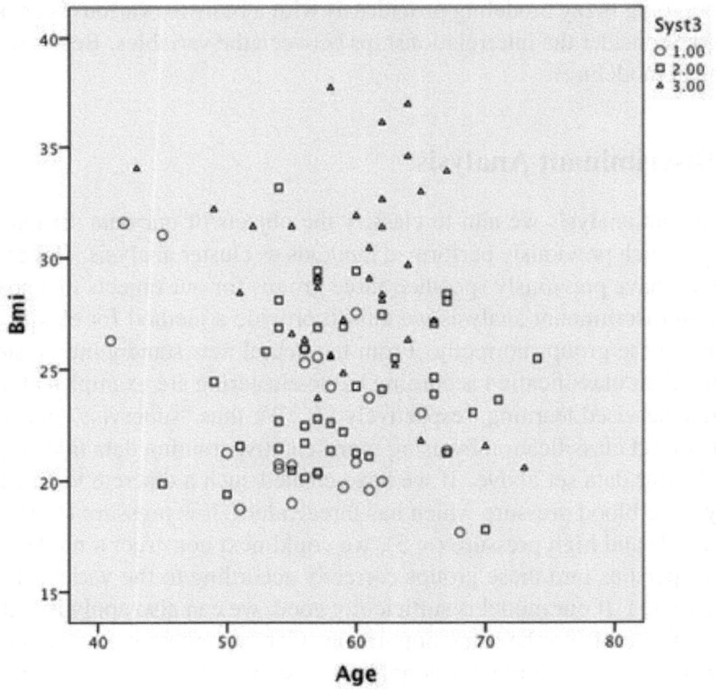

Fig. 18.11 Three systolic blood pressure groups

Table 18.8 Classification results in discriminant analysis; 55.1% of original grouped cases correctly classified

		Syst3	Predicted Group Membership			Total
			1.	2.	3.	
Original	Count	1.	6	14	3	23
		2.	5	27	9	41
		3.	0	13	21	34
	%	1.	26.1	60.9	13.0	1.0
		2	12.2	65.9	22.0	1.0
		3.	0	38.2	61.8	1.0

Table 18.9 Fuzzy rules for discriminant analysis model

Rule	If *Age* is	and *Bmi* is	then *Syst3* is	Rule	If *Age* is	and *Bmi* is	then *Syst3* is
1	54.4	20.8	1.3	11	59.1	26.9	2.1
2	56.2	25.6	1.3	12	63.0	25.1	2.4
3	42.9	31.7	1.5	13	65.9	26.7	2.4
4	50.1	20.5	1.5	14	70.8	21.9	2.6
5	60.5	20.8	1.5	15	49.4	31.9	2.9
6	67.1	21.3	1.6	16	56.9	28.9	2.9
7	56.9	20.9	1.8	17	58.1	25.3	2.9
8	67.0	28.1	2.0	18	61.9	28.3	2.9
9	53.8	26.9	2.1	19	61.8	31.8	3.0
10	56.9	29.3	2.1	20	63.4	35.8	3.0

we may also apply the initial outputs directly in which case their values represent both full and partial memberships to the systolic blood pressure groups.

Discriminant analysis a good example of such modeling in which the traditional approach is quite complicated and thus, despite its important role in medicine, it is not widely used in the research work.

Finally, we sketch some ideas how to apply the foregoing methods to other areas of statistics.

18.5 Prospects for Enhanced Models

One enhanced version of the traditional regression model is the switching regression model (e.g. [7]) which is appropriate to data sets containing clusters (Fig. 18.15). Then we may specify several fittings, one for each cluster. The specifications of these fittings correspond to the idea already used in the analysis of variance, viz. the point-wise distances to the fittings within the clusters should be minimized, whereas the distances between the fittings should be maximized. In the latter case we thus calculate the distances between the functions. As above, linear or nonlinear mathematical functions can be used in the traditional case, whereas the fuzzy models can

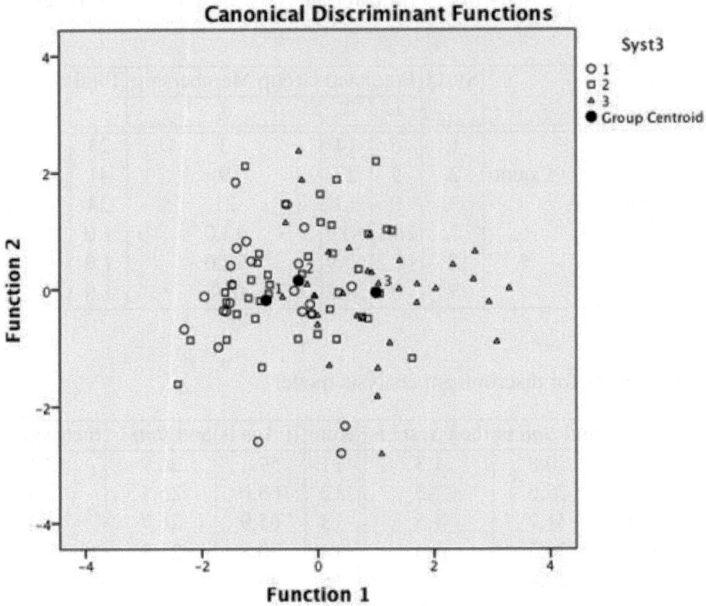

Fig. 18.12 Group centroids for three systolic blood pressure groups in discriminant analysis with two discriminant functions

operate with fuzzy rule bases and inference engines. Instead of functions, in the fuzzy case we now construct one fuzzy model for each cluster.

The switching regression approach has an interesting analogy to analysis of covariance (ANCOVA) when we examine the data groups of a test variable with its covariates. Since we now consider whether these groups have similar means when the effects of the covariates are excluded, we do not use the original group means directly, but rather their "corrected" values. In statistics we thus specify (usually linear) fitting functions for these groups and then we evaluate the distances, the corrected groups distinctions, between these fittings (Fig. 18.16).

We notice that ANCOVA modeling is in a sense a special case of switching regression modeling. In both cases we first specify the sufficiently good fittings to our data clusters, but in the former case we usually evaluate the distances between these fittings, whereas the latter aims at finding for good fittings. Hence, we could also apply fuzzy modeling and switching regression technique to ANCOVA, even when nonlinear correlations prevail between the covariates and the test variable. Given the fittings based on fuzzy models, we may evaluate the distances between these fittings, and these distances would be the correct distinctions between the groups. As above, we may aim at minimizing the errors within the clusters and maximizing the distances between the cluster fittings. However, we still expect more extensive studies on this topic (Fig. 18.17).

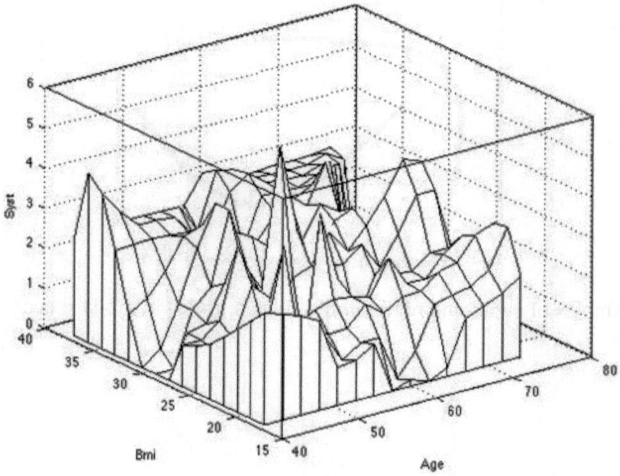

Fig. 18.13 Original fitting of the fuzzy model for discriminant analysis, *Syst3* vs. *Age* and *Bmi* (the first-order Takagi-Sugeno model)

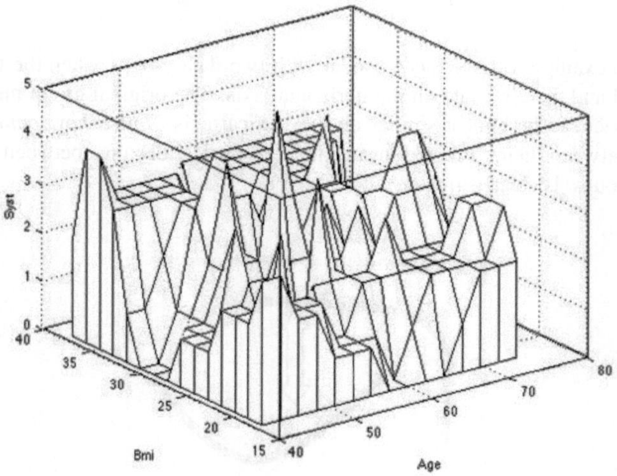

Fig. 18.14 Fitting of the fuzzy model for discriminant analysis when the outputs are rounded into integers. *Syst3* vs. *Age* and *Bmi*.

In fact, the ideas on switching regression modeling and fuzzy clusters are also applied to the first-order Takagi-Sugeno reasoning algorithm because it generates fuzzy rules the consequents of which are linear functions based on the data clusters [19]. In this case the output fitting is nevertheless the weighted sum of these functions (Fig. 18.18).

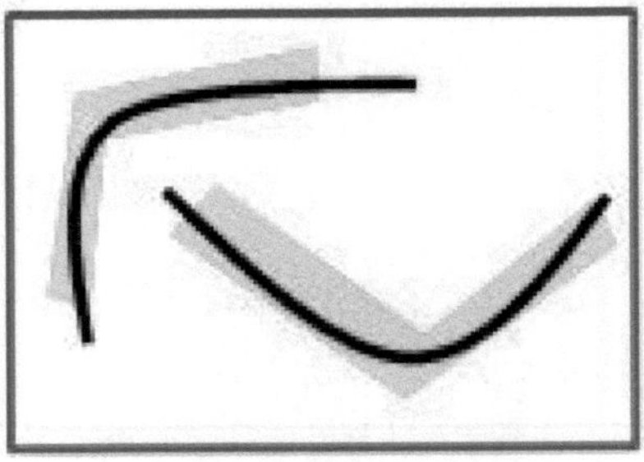

Fig. 18.15 Examples of switching regression fittings (curves) in a 2-D space

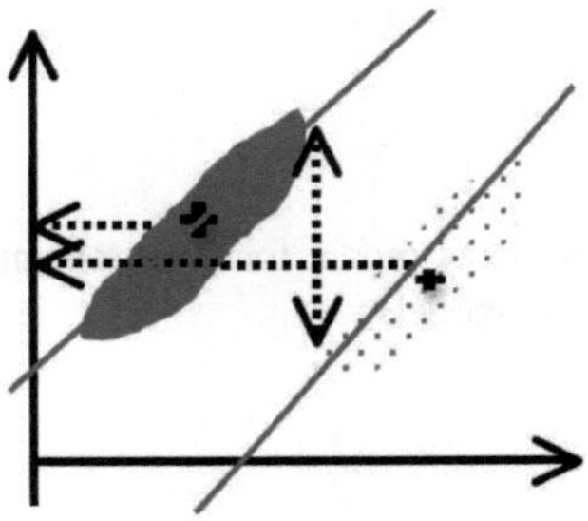

Fig. 18.16 An example of ANCOVA model with two data groups when the test variable is on the vertical and the covariate on the horizontal axis. The original group means (+) of the test variable seem to be almost similar on the vertical axis (*dotted horizontal arrows*), but the distance between their corrected means, i.e., the vertical distance between the regression lines of the groups, is clearly greater.

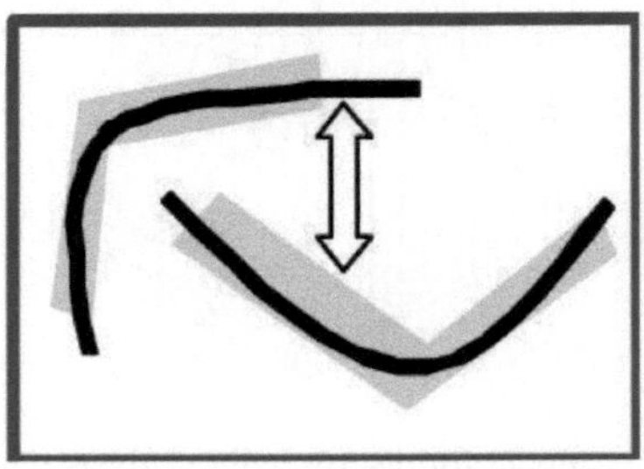

Fig. 18.17 In ANCOVA we can also apply switching regression and fuzzy models for evaluating the distances between the fitting curves

We may also apply the foregoing fuzzy switching regression method to such cluster analyses in which the prevailing methods are insufficient. Most cluster analysis methods can only cope with spherical data clusters in a satisfactory manner. In this context the obtained cluster centers, which are points, usually represent well the corresponding clusters.

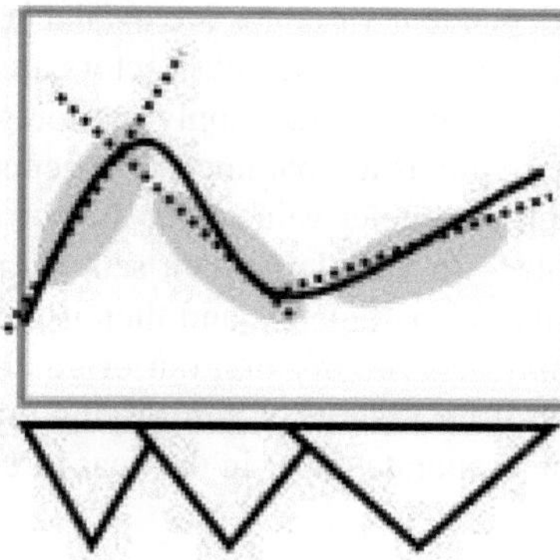

Fig. 18.18 The first-order Takagi-Sugeno algorithm generates linear fitting functions for data clusters (dotted lines). The output fitting (solid curve) is the weighted sum of these fittings.

If, in turn, non-spherical clusters are involved, we may specify such fittings for these clusters which represent the cluster centers [8]. However, now we do not have any dependent variables in our model. If we use such mathematical functions as linear functions for the cluster centers, we optimize a set of parameters for determining these functions in practice. Our task may nevertheless be more challenging if the appropriate cluster centers should be non-linear fittings, and then fuzzy systems may provide us with a better resolution (Fig. 18.19).

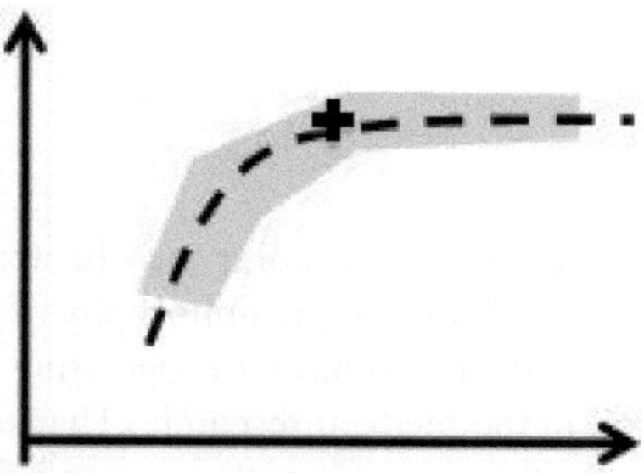

Fig. 18.19 Two possible cluster centers for a non-spherical cluster in a 2-D space, a point (+) and a curve (- -)

Within fuzzy systems we specify a fuzzy relation for each non-spherical cluster and the maximal intensities of these relations are obtained in the cluster centers. In other words, we may specify fittings for the clusters and the closer the data points are to these fittings, the higher intensities are obtained. On the other hand, these fittings should locate in the densest areas of the clusters. For example, in Fig. 18.20 the highest intensities are obtained close to the dotted curve.

However, since only independent variables are available, we first generate tentative data points for the fittings, and these data vectors are regarded as being our dependent variables. Hence, we may in fact apply the foregoing switching regression models. In practice these points are parameters in genetic algorithm optimization and we aim to find such parameter values that the corresponding data vectors are good dependent variables. In very large data sets we may first specify these fittings with a smaller number of parameters and then use the obtained fittings for the original data set. We may also modify first our original data set by using their standardized values instead, if necessary for simplifying our task. This clustering approach is studied more in a separate paper in the near future.

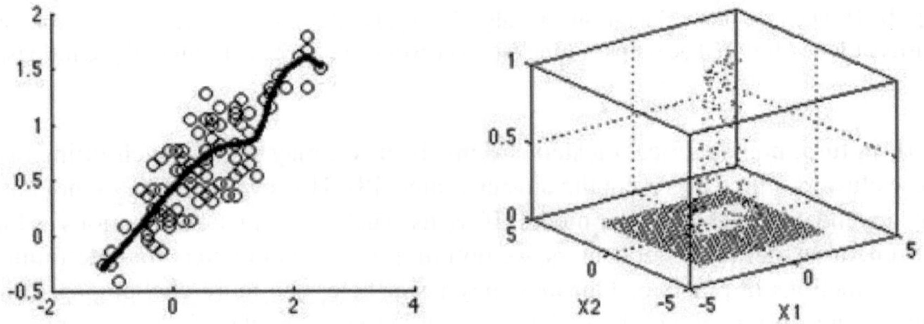

Fig. 18.20 The fitting curve which represents a cluster center in a 2-D space (left), and the corresponding fuzzy relation with its degrees of cluster membership (intensities, right)

18.6 Conclusions

We have considered above how fuzzy reasoning may be applied to statistical analysis in medicine. From the standpoint of the philosophy of science, Zadeh's fuzzy extended logic seems to provide a firm basis for operating with imprecise entities and approximate reasoning in the medical research. Thanks for this approach, we may apply approximate scientific reasoning, theories and explanations, as well as approximate hypothesis verification to our studies. We may also utilize imprecise and linguistic variables, scales, values and relations in data analysis.

At a general level, in medical statistical analysis fuzzy systems, as well as neuro-fuzzy and genetic-fuzzy systems, may replace or enhance many traditional methods. In particular, the traditional methods are often too coarse due to their linear or parametric nature, and these cause various limitations for their usage because the real world is usually non-linear by nature. Typical analyses for fuzzy modeling are analysis of variance, analysis of covariance, various regression models, cluster analysis, discriminant analysis and time series analysis. Additional examples would be principal component and factor analysis. Fuzzy cognitive maps, in turn, could often replace canonical correlation methods.

We considered cluster and discriminant analysis as well as regression modeling with a medical data. We also sketched how fuzzy switching regression analysis, analysis of covariance and sophisticated cluster analysis could be carried out. We aimed to justify that fuzzy models are often more usable and conceivable as well as simpler than the corresponding traditional models. Our results were in accordance with these aims. At a more general level, we aimed to show that we may acquire more thorough information on our data and thus enhance the quality of the quantitative medical research. Good medical research, in turn, plays an essential role when we work for the benefit of humanity.

References

1. Bandemer, H., Näther, W.: Fuzzy Data Analysis. Kluwer, Dordrecht (1992)
2. Bezdek, J.C., Pal, S.K.: Fuzzy Models for Pattern Recognition. IEEE Press, New York (1992)
3. Celikyilmaz, A., Burhan Türksen, I.: Enhanced Fuzzy System Models with Improved Fuzzy Clustering Algorithm. IEEE Transactions on Fuzzy Systems 16(3), 779–794 (2008)
4. Chiu, S.L.: Fuzzy Model Identification Based on Cluster Estimation. Journal of Intelligent and Fuzzy Systems 2, 267–278 (1994)
5. Grzegorzewski, P., Hryniewicz, O., Gil, M.-Á.: Soft Methods in Probability, Statistics and Data Analysis. Physica Verlag, Heidelberg (2002)
6. Guilford, J.P., Fruchter, B.: Fundamental Statistics in Psychology and Education. McGraw-Hill, London (1978)
7. Hathaway, R.J., Bezdek, J.C.: Switching Regression Models and Fuzzy Clustering. IEEE Transactions on Fuzzy Systems 1(3), 195–204 (1993)
8. Hruschka, E.R., Cambello, R.J.G.B., Freitas, A.A., de Carvalho, A.C.P.L.F.: A Survey of Evolutionary Algorithms for Clustering. IEEE Transactions on Systems, Man and Cybernetics, Part C 39(2), 133–155 (2009)
9. Kacprzyk, J., Fedrizzi, M.: Fuzzy Regression Analysis. Physica Verlag, Heidelberg (1992)
10. Karhunen, V., Rasi, I., Kanniainen, A.: IBM SPSS Statistics, Menetelmiä (methods). University of Oulu, Oulu (2010)
11. Niskanen, V.A.: A Meta-level Approach to Approximate Probability. In: Setchi, R., Jordanov, I., Howlett, R.J., Jain, L.C. (eds.) KES 2010, Part IV. LNCS, vol. 6279, pp. 116–123. Springer, Heidelberg (2010)
12. Niskanen, V.A.: Application of Approximate Reasoning to Hypothesis Verification. Journal of Intelligent & Fuzzy Systems 21(5), 331–339 (2010)
13. Niskanen, V.A.: Application of Zadeh's Impossibility Principle to Approximate Explanation. In: Proceedings of the IFSA 2009 Conference, Lisbon, pp. 352–360 (2009)
14. Niskanen, V.A.: Fuzzy Systems and Scientific Method – Meta-level Reflections and Prospects. In: Seising, R. (ed.) Views on Fuzzy Sets and Systems from Different Perspectives. STUDFUZZ, vol. 243, pp. 37–65. Springer, Heidelberg (2009)
15. Niskanen, V.A.: Soft Computing Methods in Human Sciences. STUDFUZZ, vol. 134. Springer, Berlin (2004)

16. Niskanen, V.A.: Meta-Level Prospects for Scientific Theory Formation by Adopting the Information Granulation Approach. In: Proceedings of the IMS 2008 Conference, pp. 33–41. Sakarya University (2008)
17. Sadegh-Zadeh, K.: Handbook of Analytic Philosophy of Medicine. Springer, Heidelberg (2012)
18. Sneath, P., Sokal, R.R.: Numerical Taxonomy. Freeman, San Francisco (1973)
19. Takagi, T., Sugeno, M.: Fuzzy Identification of Systems and Its Applications to Modeling and Control. IEEE Transactions on Systems, Man and Cybernetics 15(1), 116–132 (1986)
20. Yager, R.R., Filev, D.: Generation of Fuzzy Rules by Mountain Clustering. Journal of Intelligent and Fuzzy Systems 2, 209–219 (1994)
21. Zadeh, L.A.: From Computing with Numbers to Computing with Words – From Manipulation of Measurements to Manipulation of Perceptions. IEEE Transactions on Circuits and Systems 45, 105–119 (1999)
22. Zadeh, L.A.: From Search Engines to Question Answering Systems? The Problems of World Knowledge, Relevance, Deduction and Precisiation. In: Sanchez, E. (ed.) Fuzzy Logic and the Semantic Web, pp. 163–210. Elsevier, Amsterdam (2006)
23. Zadeh, L.A.: Fuzzy Logic and Approximate Reasoning. Synthese 30, 407–428 (1975)
24. Zadeh, L.A.: Fuzzy Logic = Computing with Words. IEEE Transactions on Fuzzy Systems 2, 103–111 (1996)
25. Zadeh, L.A.: Toward Extended Fuzzy Logic – A First Step. Fuzzy Sets and Systems 160, 3175–3181 (2009)
26. Zadeh, L.A.: Toward a Theory of Fuzzy Information Granulation and Its Centrality in Human Reasoning and Fuzzy Logic. Fuzzy Sets and Systems 90(2), 111–127 (1997)
27. Zadeh, L.A.: Toward a Perception-Based Theory of Probabilistic Reasoning with Imprecise Probabilities. Journal of Statistical Planning and Inference 105(2), 233–264 (2002)
28. Zar, J.H.: Biostatistical Analysis. Prentice-Hall, Englewood Cliffs (1984)

19

Statistical Procedures for Fuzzy Data in Medical Research

Takehiko Nakama

19.1 Introduction and Summary

Observations or measurements in many real-world problems tend to be inherently imprecise, uncertain, or linguistic. In medical research, there has been an increasing interest in statistical analysis of such observations—perceived breathlessness, general fatigue, and self images, for example (e.g., Grant et al. [9], Laerhoven et al. [19]). Fuzzy sets can effectively encode those observations. Nominal or ordinal measurements can also be used to represent them, but statistical analyses are quite limited for those measures (see Section 19.2).

In this paper, we examine advantages of using fuzzy sets to represent observations in medical research and review some of the statistical procedures that have been developed for quantitatively analyzing fuzzy data. Various statistical tests are available for analyzing fuzzy data. For instance, Körner [10], Montenegro et al. [13], and González-Rodríguez et al. [8] developed one-sample methods for hypothesis testing about the fuzzy population mean. Montenegro et al. [12] and González-Rodríguez et al. [7] established a two-independent-sample test of equality of fuzzy means, and González-Rodríguez et al. [7] developed a paired-sample test of the same type. These are considered extensions of classical t tests to fuzzy data. Gil et al. [5] and González-Rodríguez et al. [6] developed a multiple-sample test of equality of fuzzy means; this is one-way analysis of variance (ANOVA) for fuzzy data. Recently, Nakama et al. [14, 15] have established factorial analysis of variance for fuzzy data. Using examples, we will explain how they can be applied to medical research.

Instead of describing mathematical details of the statistical procedures for fuzzy data, we provide a tutorial exposition of the methods in this paper. We will direct the reader interested in the technical details to relevant papers.

19.2 Scales of Measurement

Suppose that we are concerned with a patient's mental health and that we wish to measure the degree of happiness that the patient feels. First we consider the

R. Seising and M.E. Tabacchi (Eds.): *Fuzziness and Medicine*, STUDFUZZ 302, pp. 291–299.
DOI: 10.1007/978-3-642-36527-0_19

following two procedures, which have been typically used for this type of measurement in medical research (see, for instance, Wewers and Lowe [20], Grant et al. [9], Laerhoven et al. [19]):

(i) The patient is given a list of five categories: (1) very unhappy, (2) unhappy, (3) neither unhappy nor happy, (4) happy, and (5) very happy. The patient is asked to choose one of them.
(ii) The patient is asked to mark a point on the interval $[-100, 100]$. Here -100 indicates the greatest degree of unhappiness, and 100 indicates the greatest degree of happiness.

The scale of measurement used in (i) is categorical. In this example, the five categories can be ordered according to the degree of happiness, so it can also be considered an ordinal scale. To process the five categories numerically, integers 1–5 can be assigned to the five categories (1 and 5 represent the lowest and the greatest degrees of happiness); the resulting scale is a Likert-type scale. The scale used in (ii) is an example of visual analogue scale, which can be considered an interval scale or a ratio scale for subjective measurements. Figure 19.1 shows a sample response using the visual analogue scale in (ii).

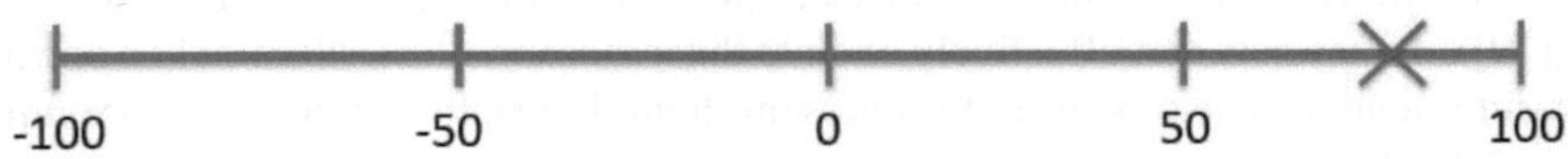

Fig. 19.1 A perceived degree of happiness on the visual analogue scale described in (ii)

Grant et al. [9] and Laerhoven et al. [19] compared these scales in medical research.

There are several disadvantages to using the scale in (i). The scale provides the patient with only five possible responses, so it is not suitable for fully capturing the details of the patient's response. Another disadvantage is that the scale fails to fully record the variability of responses. For example, suppose that two patients, call them A and B, choose (4). In this case, it is highly unlikely that their degrees of happiness are exactly the same—A's "true" degree of happiness may be between (4) and (5), whereas B's may be between (3) and (4). As illustrated here, the scale disregards the variability within each category. Also, it is important to note that Likert-type scales are not interval scales; although integers are often assigned to represent possible responses, it may be unreasonable to assume that the intervals between two adjacent responses have the same length (e.g., Wu [21]). Abrupt transitions between these measures are often undesirable for encoding imprecise observations. These characteristics severely limit the type of statistical analysis that we can apply to the measurements with this scale.

The scale in (ii) provides the patient with infinitely many (in fact, uncountably many) possible responses. It can be considered an interval scale, so it permits a variety of statistical analyses (e.g., Stevens [17], Chimka and Wolfe [1]). However,

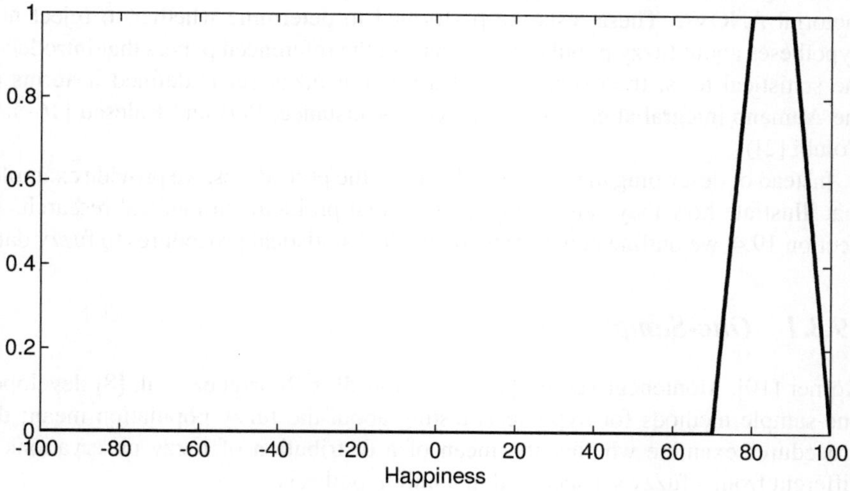

Fig. 19.2 A fuzzy set representing a perceived degree of happiness

the patient is required to provide a single number (which can be computed from the single point that she marks) for the inherently imprecise measurement, and it is unrealistic to assume that the number accurately reflects the perceived degree of happiness.

Fuzzy sets are effective in encoding the type of measurement described in the example. Figure 19.2 shows a sample response that represents a perceived degree of happiness. The horizontal axis represents the degree of happiness; as in the case of the visual analogue scale described above, -100 represents the greatest degree of unhappiness, whereas 100 represents the greatest degree of happiness. Clearly, the patient must be given proper instructions for using a fuzzy set to report her degree of happiness. For example, the patient must be told to assign 1 to those values in the interval $[-100, 100]$ that are most compatible with his/her degree of happiness. This fuzzy set reveals the imprecise or uncertain nature of the measurement. Also, the patient is provided with infinitely many possible responses, and the scale can capture subtle differences or variability.

Even though fuzzy sets can effectively represent imprecise, uncertain, or linguistic measurements, they would not be useful for statistical studies if they could not be analyzed statistically. Fortunately, various quantitative procedures are available for statistically analyzing fuzzy data. We will review some of them in the next section.

19.3 Statistical Procedures for Fuzzy Data: A Tutorial Exposition

Some of the most frequently used classical statistical tests have been successfully extended to fuzzy data. In this section, we review the following procedures for analyzing fuzzy data: one-sample and two-sample t tests, one-way ANOVA, and factorial ANOVA. These tests are performed to determine whether to reject null hypotheses about fuzzy population means. (In the referenced papers that introduced the statistical tests, the expectation of a random fuzzy set is defined in terms of the Aumann integral at each α level; see, for instance, Puri and Ralescu [16] and Colubi [2]).

Instead of describing the technical details of the procedures, we provide examples that illustrate how they can be applied to actual problems in medical research. In Section 19.4, we outline how to extend classical statistical procedures to fuzzy data.

19.3.1 One-Sample t Test

Körner [10], Montenegro et al. [13], and González-Rodríguez et al. [8] developed one-sample methods for hypothesis testing about the fuzzy population mean; the procedures examine whether the mean of a distribution of fuzzy observations is different from a fuzzy set specified in a null hypothesis.

Consider the fuzzy set graphed with a black line in Figure 19.3. We can describe it as a fuzzy set representing a neutral degree of happiness, "neither happy nor unhappy". Suppose that we want to know whether the mean degree of happiness of patients at a hospital is different from this fuzzy set, call it μ_0. Let μ denote the mean degree of happiness at the hospital. The null hypothesis H_0 is that $\mu_0 = \mu$, and the alternative hypothesis H_A is that $\mu_0 \neq \mu$.

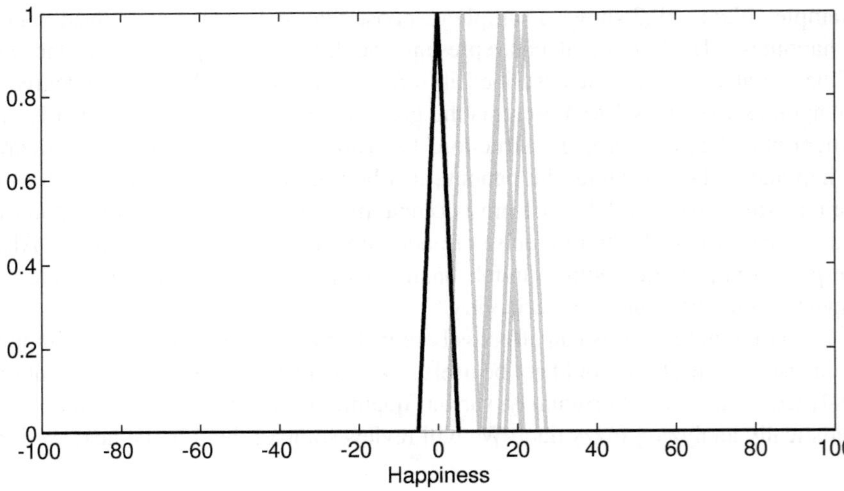

Fig. 19.3 A fuzzy set μ_0 representing a neutral degree of happiness, "neither happy nor unhappy" (shown in black), and hypothetical responses obtained from a hospital (shown in gray)

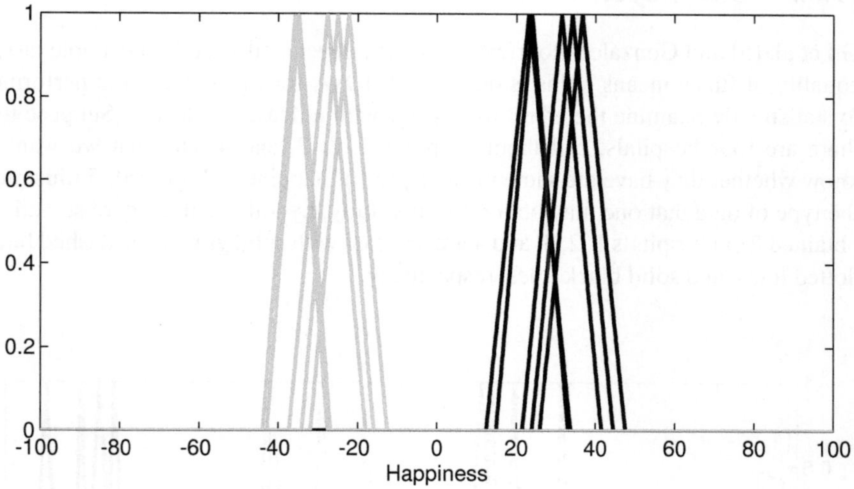

Fig. 19.4 Hypothetical fuzzy responses obtained from hospital 1 (show in gray) and from hospital 2 (shown in black)

We ask a group of patients at the hospital to report their degrees of happiness using fuzzy sets. We may obtain fuzzy responses similar to the ones plotted with gray lines in Figure 19.3. By applying a one-sample *t* test to the data, we can determine whether to reject H_0 with a predetermined significance level. For mathematical details, see Körner [10], Montenegro et al. [13], and González-Rodríguez et al. [8].

19.3.2 Two-Sample t Tests

Montenegro et al. [12] and González-Rodríguez et al. [7] established a two-independent-sample test of equality of fuzzy means, and González-Rodríguez et al. [7] developed a paired-sample test of the same type. These are considered extensions of classical two-sample *t* tests to fuzzy data, and they assess whether the means of two populations of fuzzy sets are different.

We will explain how to perform an independent-sample *t* test. Suppose that there are two hospitals, call them hospital 1 and hospital 2, and that we want to know whether the mean degree of happiness at hospital 1 is the same as that at hospital 2. Let μ_1 and μ_2 denote the mean degrees of happiness at hospitals 1 and 2, respectively. The null hypothesis H_0 is that $\mu_1 = \mu_2$. The alternative hypothesis H_A is that $\mu_1 \neq \mu_2$. We collect fuzzy data from the two hospitals. Suppose that we obtain fuzzy responses plotted in Figure 19.4. Assume that responses obtained from hospital 1 are shown in gray and that those obtained from hospital 2 are shown in black. By applying an independent-sample *t* test to the data, we can determine whether to reject H_0 with a predetermined significance level. See Montenegro et al. [12] and González-Rodríguez et al. [7] for mathematical details.

19.3.3 One-Way ANOVA

Gil et al. [5] and González-Rodríguez et al. [6] developed a multiple-sample test of equality of fuzzy means. This is one-way ANOVA for fuzzy data; it is performed to statistically examine the effect of a factor with at least two levels. Suppose that there are four hospitals, call them hospitals 1, 2, 3, and 4, and that we want to know whether they have the same mean degree of happiness. Figure 19.5 illustrates the type of data that one may obtain for this study; hypothetical fuzzy observations obtained from hospitals 1, 2, 3, and 4 are graphed with solid gray lines, dashed lines, dotted lines, and solid black lines, respectively.

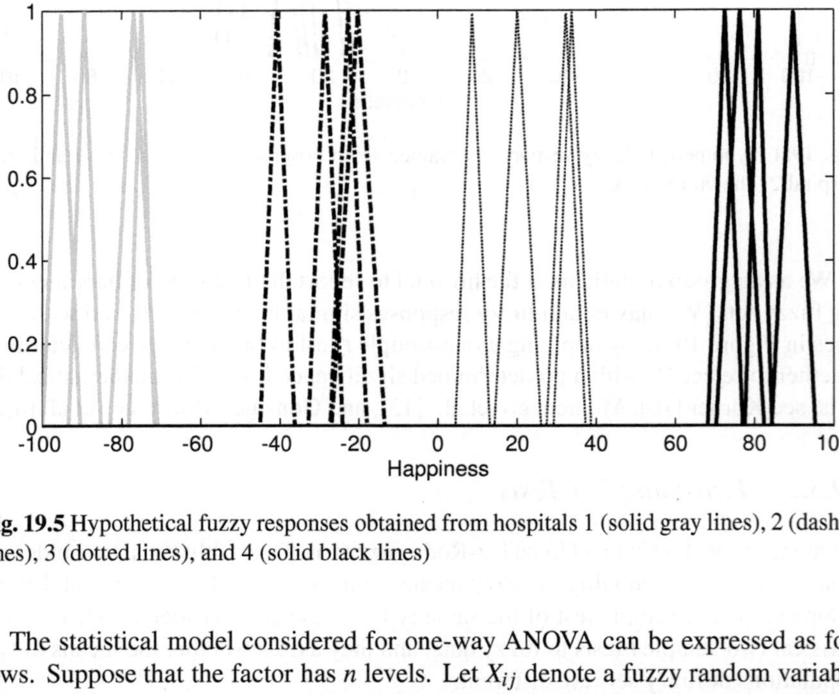

Fig. 19.5 Hypothetical fuzzy responses obtained from hospitals 1 (solid gray lines), 2 (dashed lines), 3 (dotted lines), and 4 (solid black lines)

The statistical model considered for one-way ANOVA can be expressed as follows. Suppose that the factor has n levels. Let X_{ij} denote a fuzzy random variable (also described as a random fuzzy set) that represents the jth observation under the ith level of the factor. Denote the overall mean and the mean of the ith level by μ and α_i, respectively. Then for each i and j, the model is expressed as

$$X_{ij} = \mu + \alpha_i + \varepsilon_{ij}.$$

where ε_{ij} represents the random component of the measurement. The null hypothesis is that $\alpha_1 = \alpha_2 = \cdots = \alpha_n$. The alternative hypothesis is that there exist α_{i_1} and α_{i_2} such that $\alpha_{i_1} \neq \alpha_{i_2}$.

We can perform one-way ANOVA to determine whether to reject the null hypothesis with a predetermined significance level. For mathematical details, see Gil et al. [5] and González-Rodríguez et al. [6].

19.3.4 Two-Way ANOVA

Recently, Nakama et al. [14, 15] have established factorial (m-way with $m \geq 2$) ANOVA for fuzzy data. A factorial layout is designed to statistically examine the effects of two or more factors that each involve at least two levels. For concreteness, we will describe two-way ANOVA.

Two-way ANOVA statistically determines wether two factors affect a response significantly. For example, suppose that we measure a response to two different drugs, drugs 1 and 2, in both men and women. Here the two factors are drug treatment and gender. In statistics, the two factors are described as independent variables, and the response is described as the dependent variable of this experiment. Two-way ANOVA tests the following null hypotheses:

(a) Drug treatment has no effect on the response.
(b) Gender has no effect on the response.
(c) There is no interaction between drug treatment and gender in affecting the response.

By (c), we mean that the effect of drug treatment does not depend on gender. The following is an example of interaction between the two factors: For men, the response is increased by drug 1 but decreased by drug 2, whereas for women, the response is decreased by drug 1 but increased by drug 2.

Suppose that we examine the effects of factors 1 and 2 that have I and J levels, respectively. In the example described above, drug treatment has two levels (drugs 1 and 2), and gender also has two levels (male and female). Let X_{ijk} denote a fuzzy random variable that represents the kth observed value of the dependent variable measured under level i of factor 1 and under level j of factor 2. In two-way ANOVA (and more generally factorial ANOVA), an unbalanced design may introduce artificial differential effects of one factor (or of interactions) on the marginal means of the other factor. Thus we assume that for each level of factor 1 and for each level of factor 2, there are K observations (thus $1 \leq k \leq K$). In two-way ANOVA, we consider the following additive statistical model:

$$X_{ijk} = \mu + \alpha_i + \beta_j + \gamma_{ij} + \varepsilon_{ijk}, \tag{19.1}$$

where ε_{ijk} represents the random component of the model. In (19.1), α_i denotes the main effect of level i of factor 1 on the dependent variable, and β_j denotes the main effect of level j of factor 2. The interaction between the two factors is quantified by γ_{ij}, which denotes the effect of concurrently having both level i of factor 1 and level j of factor 2.

Using this notation, the null hypotheses corresponding to (a)–(c) can be expressed as follows:

$H_0^{(1)}$: Factor 1 has no effect: $\alpha_1 = \alpha_2 = \cdots = \alpha_I$.
$H_0^{(2)}$: Factor 2 has no effect: $\beta_1 = \beta_2 = \cdots = \beta_J$.
$H_0^{(1,2)}$: There is no interaction between factors 1 and 2: $\gamma_{1,1} = \gamma_{1,2} = \cdots = \gamma_{IJ}$.

We can perform two-way ANOVA to determine whether to reject the null hypotheses with a predetermined significance level. See Nakama et al. [14, 15] for mathematical details.

19.4 Extending Classical Statistical Procedures to Fuzzy Data

In this section, we outline a methodology for extending classical statistical procedures to fuzzy data. Mathematical details are omitted.

We assume that for each α greater than 0 and less than or equal to 1, the α level of each fuzzy set is a nonempty compact convex set. We define two basic arithmetic operations on fuzzy sets: addition and scalar multiplication. There are several ways to define them. Typically addition is defined as the Minkovski addition at each alpha level, and scalar multiplication is also defined in a level-wise manner.

The Minkowski support function can be used to define a metric for fuzzy sets and to transform them to Hilbert-space-valued functions. The transformation isometrically embeds the class of fuzzy sets in a closed convex cone of a Hilbert space. As a result, various convergence results for random fuzzy sets can be derived from essential theoretical results for Hilbert-space-valued random variables. For mathematical details, see, for instance, Colubi [2].

19.5 Discussions

In many research areas, including medical research, we must often deal with observations that can be effectively represented by fuzzy sets. In addition to the hypothesis-testing procedures that we have reviewed, many other types of statistical analysis have also been developed for fuzzy data (for a review, see, for example, Taheri [18]). These procedures are not only theoretically rigorous but also practical. For instance, Colubi and González-Rodríguez [4] and Colubi [2] conducted statistical analyses of fuzzy data regarding forestry expert evaluations. Colubi et al. [3] analyzed bank managers' investment aversion assessments represented by fuzzy sets. Lubiano and Trutschnig [11] developed an R-package called SAFD, with which one can easily perform one-way ANOVA for fuzzy data. We hope that this paper will motivate the reader to use fuzzy measurements for statistical studies.

References

1. Chimka, J.R., Wolfe, H.: History of Ordinal Variables Before 1980. Scientific Research and Essays 4, 853–860 (2009)
2. Colubi, A.: Statistical Inference about the Means of Fuzzy Random Variables: Applications to the Analysis of Fuzzy- and Real-valued Data. Fuzzy Sets and Systems 160, 344–356 (2009)
3. Colubi, A., Coppi, R., D'Urso, P., Gil, M.A.: Statisitcs with Fuzzy Random Variables. Metron–International Journal of Statistics 65, 277–303 (2007)

4. Colubi, A., González-Rodríguez, G.: Triangular Fuzzification of Random Variables and Power of Distribution Tests: Empirical Discussion. Computational Statistics and Data Analysis 51, 4742–4750 (2007)
5. Gil, M.A., Montenegro, M., González-Rodríguez, G., Colubi, A., Casals, M.R.: Bootstrap Approach to the Multi-sample Test of Means with Imprecise Data. Computational Statistics and Data Analysis 51, 148–162 (2006)
6. González-Rodríguez, G., Colubi, A., Gil, M.A.: Fuzzy Data Treated as Functional Data: A One-way ANOVA Test Approach. Computational Statistics and Data Analysis 56(4), 943–955 (2012)
7. González-Rodríguez, G., Colubi, A., Angeles, M., D'Urso, P.: An Asymptotic Two Dependent Samples Test of Equality of Means of Fuzzy Random Fuzzy Random Variables. In: Proceedings of the 17th IASC-ERS, pp. 689–695 (2006)
8. González-Rodríguez, G., Montenegro, M., Colubi, A., Gil, M.A.: Bootstrap Techniques and Fuzzy Random Variables: Synergy in Hypothesis Testing with Fuzzy Data. Fuzzy Sets and Systems 157, 2608–2613 (2006)
9. Grant, S., Aitchison, T., Henderson, E., Christie, J., Zare, S., McMurray, J., Dargie, H.: A Comparison of the Reproducibility and the Sensitivity to Change of Visual Analogue Scales, Borg Scales, and Likert Scales in Normal Subjects During Submaximal Exercise. Chest 116, 1208–1217 (1999)
10. Körner, R.: An Asymptotic α-test for the Expectation of Random Fuzzy Variables. Journal of Statistical Planning and Inference 83, 331–346 (2000)
11. Lubiano, M.A., Trutschnig, W.: ANOVA for Fuzzy Random Variables Using the R-package SAFD. In: Borgelt, C., González-Rodríguez, G., Trutschnig, W., Lubiano, M.A., Gil, M.Á., Grzegorzewski, P., Hryniewicz, O. (eds.) Combining Soft Computing and Statistical Methods in Data Analysis. AISC, vol. 77, pp. 449–456. Springer, Heidelberg (2010)
12. Montenegro, M., Casal, M.R., Lubiano, M.A., Gil, M.A.: Two-sample Hypothesis Tests of Means of a Fuzzy Random Variable. Information Sciences 133(1-2), 89–100 (2001)
13. Montenegro, M., Colubi, A., Casal, M.R., Gil, M.A.: Asymptotic and Bootstrap Techniques for Testing the Expected Value of a Fuzzy Random Variable. Metrika 59, 31–49 (2004)
14. Nakama, T., Colubi, A., Lubiano, M.A.: Two-Way Analysis of Variance for Interval-Valued Data. In: Borgelt, C., González-Rodríguez, G., Trutschnig, W., Lubiano, M.A., Gil, M.Á., Grzegorzewski, P., Hryniewicz, O. (eds.) Combining Soft Computing and Statistical Methods in Data Analysis. AISC, vol. 77, pp. 475–482. Springer, Heidelberg (2010)
15. Nakama, T., Colubi, A., Lubiano, M.A.: Factorial Analysis of Variance for Fuzzy Data. Manuscript in Preparation (2011)
16. Puri, M.L., Ralescu, D.A.: Fuzzy Random Variables. Journal of Mathematical Analysis and Applications 114, 409–422 (1986)
17. Stevens, S.S.: On the Scales of Measurement. Science 103, 677–680 (1946)
18. Taheri, S.M.: Trends in Fuzzy Statistics. Austrian Journal of Statistics 32, 239–257 (2003)
19. van Laerhoven, H., van der Zaag-Loonen, H.J., Derkx, B.H.F.: A Comparison of Likert Scale and Visual Analogue Scales as Response Options in Children's Questionnaires. Acta Pædiatr 93, 830–835 (2004)
20. Wewers, M.E., Lowe, N.K.: A Critical Review of Visual Analogue Scales in the Measurement of Clinical Phenomena. Research in Nursing and Health 13, 227–236 (1990)
21. Wu, C.-H.: An Empirical Study on the Transformation of Likert-scale Data to Numerical Scores. Applied Mathematical Sciences 1, 2851–2862 (2007)

20

Probability, Fuzziness and Information: Defining Missions in Medicine

Luis Argüelles Méndez

20.1 Probability and Perception in Medicine

Like a representation of probabilistic concepts in formal terms, probability theory is a well developed area of mathematics, and an extensive number of physiological, biochemical and biophysical magnitudes closely adhere to probability distributions, specially to the Gaussian or Normal distribution, $N(\mu, \sigma^2)$, defined by its intrinsic parameters mean, μ, and variance, σ^2). When both parameters are known, that is, if the Gaussian distribution representing a subject of interest in medicine is well defined, the probability of appearance of a given observed value can be easily calculated. In particular, every health sciences practitioner knows that an observed feature with value x in a patient obeys the following probabilistic expressions:

$$P(\mu - \sigma \leq x \leq \mu + \sigma) \approx 0.6827$$

$$P(\mu - 2\sigma \leq x \leq \mu + 2\sigma) \approx 0.9545$$

$$P(\mu - 3\sigma \leq x \leq \mu + 3\sigma) \approx 0.9973$$

That is, a direct interpretation can be made in order to know how far is the observed value x from the mean in the population following a Gaussian distribution [3].

Very interestingly, probability laws produce numerical results that, as real numbers, generate a conscience of precision and accuracy that usually affects the perception and confidence of a physician, generating absolute and ultimate reference values. However, and as a philosophical reflection, we should ask ourselves about absolute probability and more precisely, about its own existence, or in other words: does absolute probability in medicine really exist? An example on autosomal recessive diseases will help us to clarify this point.

As it is well known, an autosomal recessive mechanism is one of several ways that a trait, disorder, or disease can be passed down through families. In these instances, two copies of an abnormal gene must be present in order for the disease or trait to develop [9]. If we name the following elements, $A =$ "to be an affected

R. Seising and M.E. Tabacchi (Eds.): *Fuzziness and Medicine*, STUDFUZZ 302, pp. 301–312.
DOI: 10.1007/978-3-642-36527-0_20

patient", $C =$ "to be a carrier patient" and $U =$ "to be an unaffected patient", descendants from a couple, both being carriers of an autosomal recessive disease Z have the following associated probabilities: $P(A) = 0.25$; $P(C) = 0.25 + 0.25 = 0.5$; $P(U) = 0.25$. Thus, the probability of having a descendant that will enjoy a good quality of life is $P(U) + P(C) = 0.75$. If we think for a while in this situation, and from a purely mathematical viewpoint, the decision of having a child under normal circumstances is no more and no less than a common accorded bet between two adults for "producing" a healthy child with an associated perceived probability of such an occurrence that can at least be described as "very high". In this point, we must remark the fact that the perceived probability from wealthy parents of having a healthy child is usually just 100%. Needless to say, such a perception is never completely true, among other reasons, because a Gaussian distribution has asymptotic tails.

To speak about bets implies to speak about games. In order to better express the idea behind this section, we can modify the autosomal recessive transmission example, transform it with other words, and enunciate the following game, where we bet one Euro (i.e. through a random device or system, like extracting some coloured balls from a bag) with the associated probabilities shown in table 20.1:

Table 20.1 The case of 1 Euro bet and associated probabilities (read text)

Event	Probability value	Result
To win	0.25	We win 1 Euro.
To tie	0.50	Neither lose nor win.
To lose	0.25	We lose 1 Euro.

It seems a good, equitable game at first. Now, we can develop another transformation for the same game, this time changing the bet value. Let us imagine we bet $50,000$ Euros from our own savings. The probabilities and derived results are shown in table 20.2:

Table 20.2 The case of 50,000 Euros bet and associated probabilities (read text)

Event	Probability value	Result
To win	0.25	We win 50,000 Euros.
To tie	0.50	Neither lose nor win.
To lose	0.25	We lose 50,000 Euros.

Now, our perception of probability has changed and the risk of losing our bet seems to have dramatically grown. This is known as "subjective probability", that is, a probability derived from an individual's personal judgement about whether a specific outcome is likely to occur. In broad terms, subjective probabilities contain no formal calculations and only reflect the subject's opinions and past experiences.

In this domain of human perception it helps to think of subjective probabilities as expectations of particularly simple random variables called "indicators" [5]. Then, the indicator of a hypothesis H is a constant, I_H, which is 1 if H is true and 0 if H is false. Now we can write:

$$P_S(H) = Ex(I_H)$$

In our case, and as said previously, the indicator I_H = "wealthy parents having a healthy child" usually has an expectation $Ex(I_H) = 1$, so the subjective probability will be $P_S(H) = 1$. On the other hand, when dealing with an autosomal recessive disease, the indicator I_H = "carrier parents having a child that will enjoy a good quality of life", the expectation becomes $Ex(I_H) = P_S(H) \leq 1$, although the real probability P of this hypothesis equals exactly 0.75, as stated previously.

Subjective probabilities deserve another important remark: they differ from person to person and some carrier parents will experience a $P_S(H) = 0.9$, while for others it will be, for example, $P_S(H) = 0.2$ or maybe less. Because now the probability is subjective, it contains a high degree of personal bias, so the expectation of a physician about a given condition or disease can be, and usually it is, different from the patient, patient's relatives or even the society, so we can see that subjective probability is a personal perception, but plays and important role in medicine since many human decisions rest on such type of information. We shall tackle again this concept from another point of view in section 20.3 of this work.

20.2 From Aristotle to Plato and Then Zadeh

There is no doubt about the influence that Aristotle has had not only in philosophy but also in science, including health sciences and medicine along the history of the western culture. Such an authority in the established way of thinking has brought as a result the use of sharp classifications in every branch of science, that is, classifications where the law of excluded middle holds. We can read an example of sharp classification for the concept of "being a man" by Aristotle himself:

> "It is impossible, then, that "being a man" should mean precisely "not being a man", if "man" not only signifies something about one subject but also has one significance. ... And it will not be possible to be and not to be the same thing, except in virtue of an ambiguity, just as if one whom we call "man", and others were to call "not-man"; but the point in question is not this, whether the same thing can at the same time be and not be a man in name, but whether it can be in fact." [1]

In medicine, every type of symptom, state of the organism, disease, or therapy, for naming just a few families of concepts used everyday by physicians, is categorized into a sharp, clearly defined and bounded group, partition or classification. In essence, an observable magnitude x belongs to a traditional set S of symptoms and diseases, while a knowledge-based element y belongs to a traditional set T of treatments. In this simple but conceptually significant model, medicine can be seen as a function f that relates x_i symptoms and diseases to y_j treatments:

$$x_i \in S, y_j \in T / y_j = f(x_i)$$

From this expression, we can derive the traditional mission of a physician: To precisely identify symptoms and diseases and then find a suitable treatment for it. Let's see an example expressed by a composed expert rule: "if blood glucose levels are high at fasting in patient A, and he is usually tired, and he is usually very thirsty (polydipsia), and he urinates frequently (polyuria), and he is usually hungry (polyphagia), and he has lost weight, then patient A suffers from Diabetes, so treatment is diet, exercise and insulin."

Nevertheless, sharp classifications suffer from an important drawback: real life is extremely complex and usually sharp partitions don't fit well with the real physical models (human beings, in this case). As an example, hypoglycemia is defined as sugar concentrations in blood of less or equal to $70mg/dl$, while severe hypoglycemia is given for glucose levels of less to $45mg/dl$. Now, we can reflect on the following questions: a) Is $71mg/dl$ a case of normal glycaemia levels? b) Is $69mg/dl$ an absolutely clear example of hypoglycemia? And even more interestingly, c) can be $69mg/dl$ considered in the same category of sugar concentrations as $46mg/dl$?

These are questions that strongly put stress on Aristotle-type classification systems. Plato had been also interested on these ideas in his *Theory of forms* and as we can read from his *Dialogues*, he thought that all the forms in the real world are imperfect, being perceived as such by our senses. In his line of reasoning only ideal forms are perfect and only through the human reason we can perceive them. While less precise than the ideas of his disciple on this matter, from our point of view we suspect that if only Plato had had a strong knowledge in algebra and functions, maybe he had anticipated fuzzy sets by more than 2,000 years because the inherent foundations of fuzziness were already present in his mind. Sadly it was not the case, so classic logic appeared with Aristotle, reigning supreme until the 20th century.

The shift of paradigm about the very concept of classifications and classical sets and then logic had a sharp launch in a seminal paper from Lofty A. Zadeh in 1965 [10], unambiguously titled "Fuzzy sets". As it is well known at present, boundaries of a fuzzy set are not precise, so the membership of a given element to a given fuzzy set is not a binary, yes or no question, but it converts to a question of degree [7].

If we say an element x is a member of A, we are not speaking about something completely true or completely false, but it may be true only to some degree, usually expressed in the closed interval $[0,1]$, the degree to which x is actually a member of A. For defining fuzzy-sets, a membership function maps elements from a given universe of discourse into real numbers inside the unit interval $[0,1]$ [6]

$$\mu_A : X \longrightarrow [0,1]$$

In this expression, the function μ_A completely defines the fuzzy set A. Now let us design some trapezoidal membership functions for the fuzzy sets "hypoglycemia" and "normal" for sugar concentrations in blood. For hypoglycemia we shall have the membership function $\mu_h(x) = 1$ when x belongs to the interval $[0,60)$ and $\mu_h(x) = (60-x)/20+1$ when x belongs to the interval $[60,80]$. On the other hand, for defining normal glycaemia, we shall use $\mu_n(x) = (x-80)/20+1$ when x belongs to the interval $[60,80]$, $\mu_n(x) = 1$ when x is inside the interval $(80,120)$, and $\mu_n(x) = (120-x)/20+1$ when x belongs to the interval $[120,140]$. The resulting fuzzy-sets can be observed in figure 20.1:

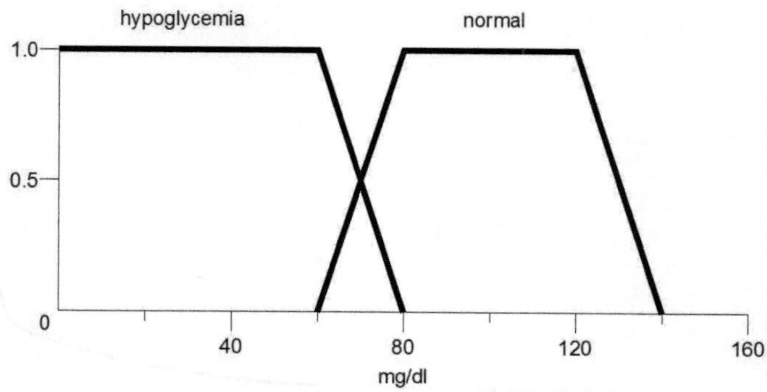

Fig. 20.1 Fuzzy-sets for representing hypoglycemia and normal glycaemia levels

In this moment we can obtain the following membership degrees for the aforementioned values $x = 71,69,46$: $\mu_h(71) = 0.45$, $\mu_h(69) = 0,55$, $\mu_h(46) = 1,0$ and $\mu_n(71) = 0.55$, $\mu_n(69) = 0.45$, $\mu_n(71) = 0.0$. Now we can see that the "hypoglycemia paradox" is solved and only exists under the strict aristotelian logic. For a concentration of $69mg/dl$ of sugar in blood, this value has a membership degree of 0.55 to the fuzzy set of hypoglycemia and 0.45 membership degree to the fuzzy set of normal glucose levels. Needles to say, a value of $46mg/dl$ is now correctly represented, with a 0.0 membership degree to the set of normal glucose levels and 1.0 membership degree to the fuzzy set of hypoglycemia.

Kazem Sadegh-Zadeh in his *Handbook of Analytic Philosophy of Medicine* makes the point that "almost everything in medicine is inevitably vague" [8], including the following families of health-related concepts: Patient complaints, Symptoms, States of the organism, Diseases, Therapies and Recoveries. We not only agree, but would like to add also Life Illness Curves and Life Quality Curves, as discussed on the following section.

20.3 Life Illness Curves (LIC) and Life Quality Curves (LQC)

We define a Life Illness Curve as a graphical representation of the membership degree that a person has to the fuzzy set I of Illness over time, that is $y = \mu_I(x), t$. In these graphics, the vertical axis represents the membership $\mu_I(x)$, defined as usually in the interval $[0,1]$. The value $\mu_I(x) = 0$ means an absolutely absence of illness that is experienced by the human being only at birth, when no congenital disorder is present. We emphasize the condition "only at birth" because cellular deterioration begins just with life, albeit usually extremely slowly. The value $\mu_I(x) = 1$ means an integral and definitive presence of illness that happens only at the individual's exitus. On the other hand, the value t is expressed in years. We have taken an interval from 0 to 80, because 80 years old is an approximation to the average duration of the life of a human being in modern countries of the occidental culture. In the next paragraphs we present some examples of Life Illness Curves.

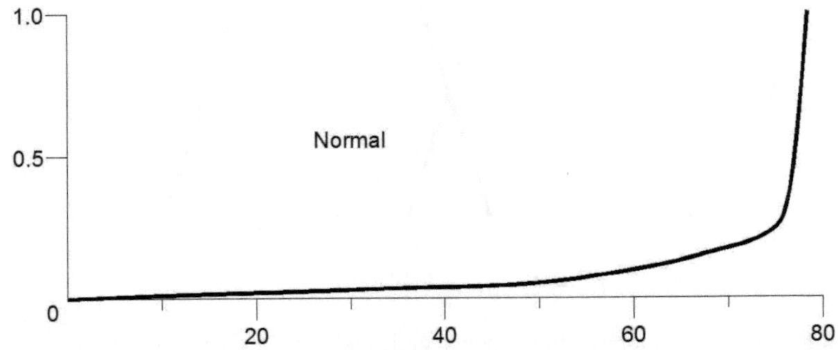

Fig. 20.2 LIC of a healthy person

Figure 20.2 shows a LIC of a normal, healthy individual. The value $\mu_I(x)$ remains low for almost the entire life of the person and only in the last months of his/her life the organism looses its healthy state.

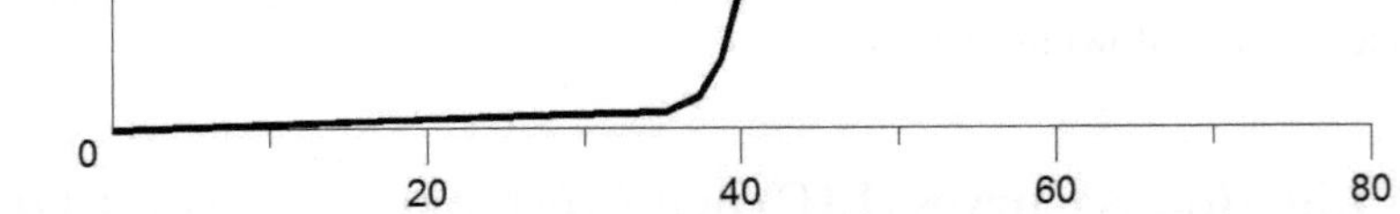

Fig. 20.3 LIC of a patient suffering Amyotrophic Lateral Sclerosis. Lou Gehrig's case.

Figure 20.3 represents the evolution in time of a patient affected by amyotrophic lateral sclerosis (ALS), where the value $\mu_I(x)$ remains low and normal until the disease's debut that leads into a relatively quick outcome [2]. This figure represents exactly the case of the famous baseball player Lou Gehrig, that suffered this condition from 1938 to 1941. Interestingly, figure 20.4 shows the LIC of the same illness, this time representing the case of the known cosmologist Stephen Hawking. The curve shows the debut of the condition in his twenties, a tracheotomy that resulted into a permanent aphonia in his forties and some severe infectious disorders at his sixties.

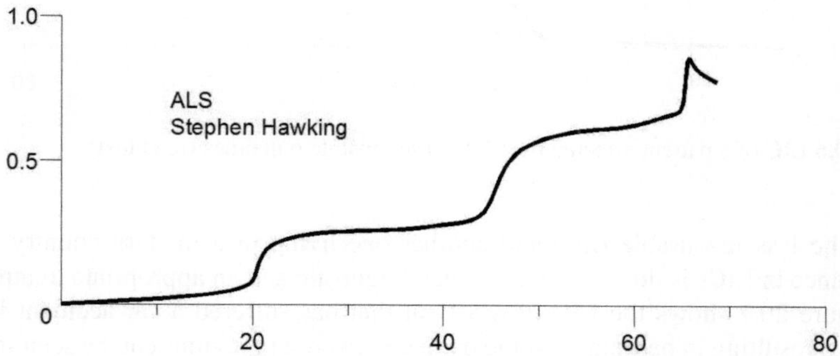

Fig. 20.4 LIC of a patient suffering Amyotrophic Lateral Sclerosis. Stephen Hawking case.

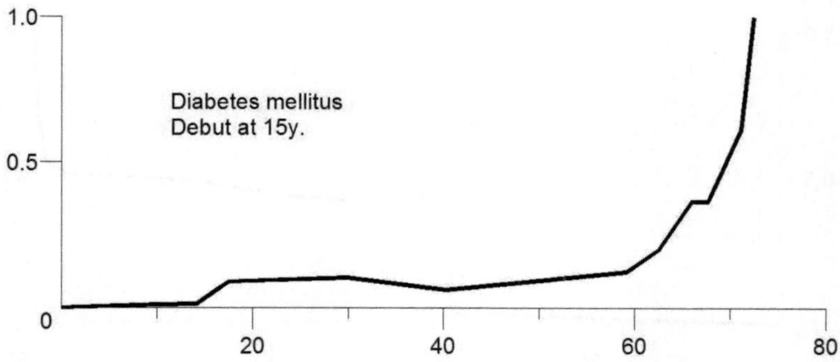

Fig. 20.5 LIC of a patient affected by diabetes with good diagnostic and treatment

Figure 20.5 shows the LIC of a patient affected by type-1 diabetes mellitus that debuts at 15 years old, is correctly diagnosed and is treated adequately by means of insulin therapy, diet and exercise. As can be seen, under such circumstances the values $\mu_I(x),t$ remain relatively low through his life and only from his sixties he can start to suffer diabetes-related complications that spark the apparition of other conditions such as blindness, kidney failure and so on [4].

Figure 20.6 shows two possible evolutions of patients suffering acquired immune deficiency syndrome (AIDS), one of them living in a third world country (the one

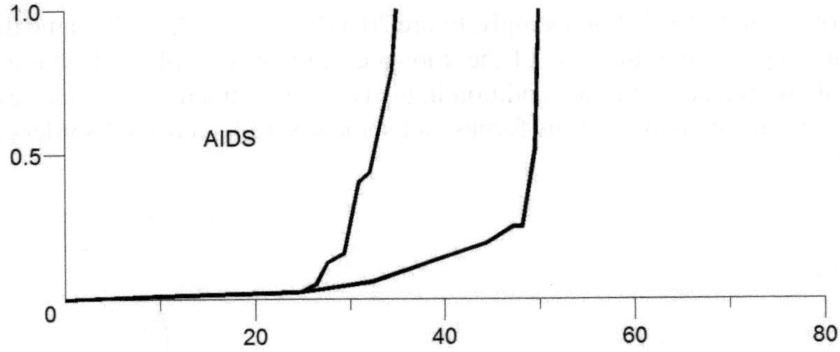

Fig. 20.6 LIC of a patient affected by AIDS. Two posible outcomes (read text).

with the less favourable LIC) and another one living in a modern country. The difference in LICs is due to both a correct diagnostic and an appropriate treatment.

Figure 20.7 shows the LIC of a patient that has suffered a car accident in his thirties, resulting in permanent spine damage. Two main regions can be seen for the LIC: the one before the accident and the one after. Despite the sharp increase in the $\mu_I(x)$ value resulting from the accident, the shape of each region resembles that of a normal life, like in figure 2.

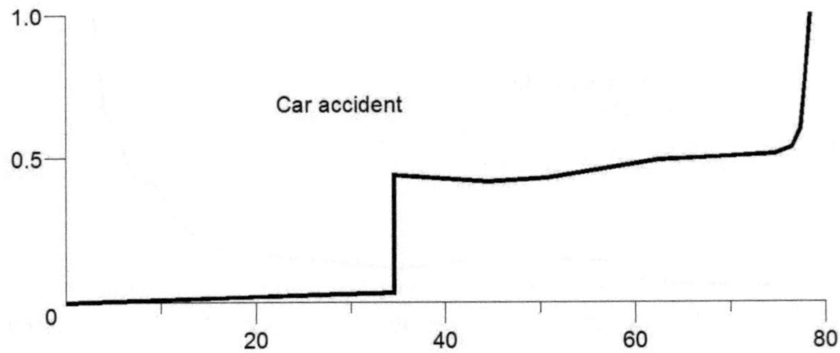

Fig. 20.7 LIC of a patient with permanent spine damage caused by an accident

We define a Life Quality Curve (LQC) as a graphical representation of the membership degree that a person has to the fuzzy set L of good quality of life over time. This curve is defined by the expression:

$$y = \mu_L(x) = (1 - \mu_I(x)), t$$

As can be easily seen, such an expression generates a symmetrical curve from LICs whose axis of symmetry is $y = 0.5$. Since the meaning of such type of curves is

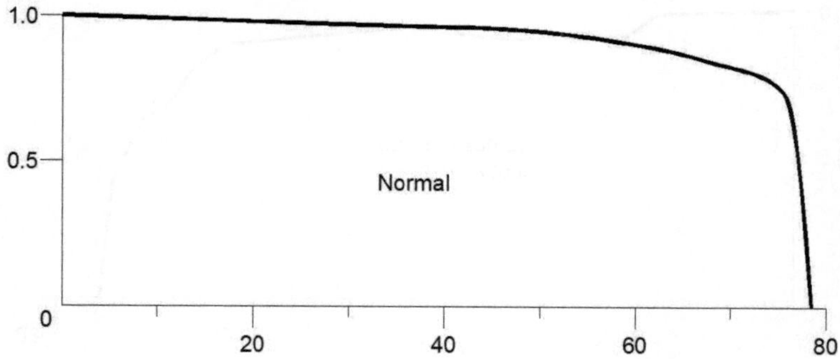

Fig. 20.8 LQC of a normal individual

immediate after having exposed LICs, we shall offer only two examples of LQCs, shown in figures 20.9 and 20.10 :

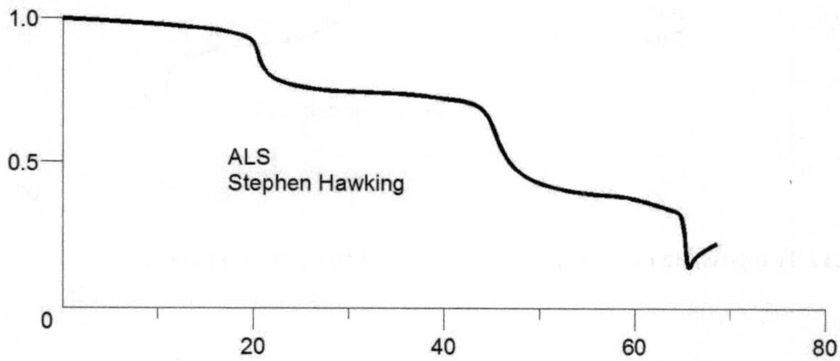

Fig. 20.9 LQC of a patient suffering Amyotrophic Lateral Sclerosis. Stephen Hawking case.

At this point we must note an important remark: both LIC and LQC curves are fuzzy and are not carved in stone, as we can immediately realize from figures 20.3 and 20.4 where the same illness, ALS, show two dramatically different behaviours in two different patients, although we must concede that Hawking's case is certainly rare. In any case, it's really interesting to note that the shape of LIC and LQC curves are affected by the perception of the person who observes the condition. Let us take again as an example the LQC of Stephen Hawking as shown in figure 20.11: While we can interpret the bold curve as the perception of a neurologist, it is more than likely that the own patient's perception is different, expressed as an example by the thin curve in the graphic.

The difference in perception between patient and physician is not the only one at play. Society also usually perceives a given condition from a different point of view that the one from the affected person, as we can observe in figure 12 for diabetes,

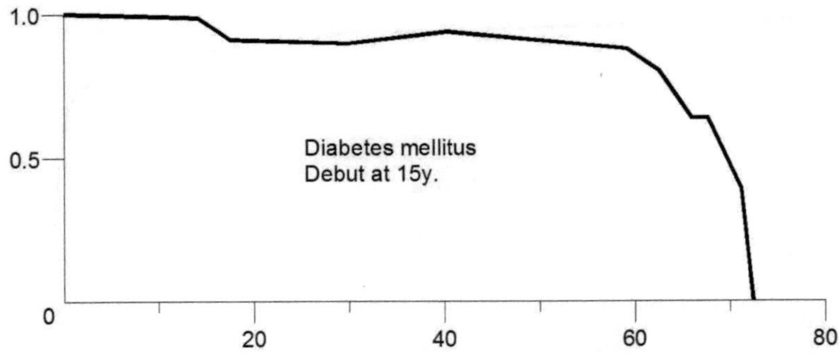

Fig. 20.10 LIC of a patient affected by diabetes with good diagnostic and treatment

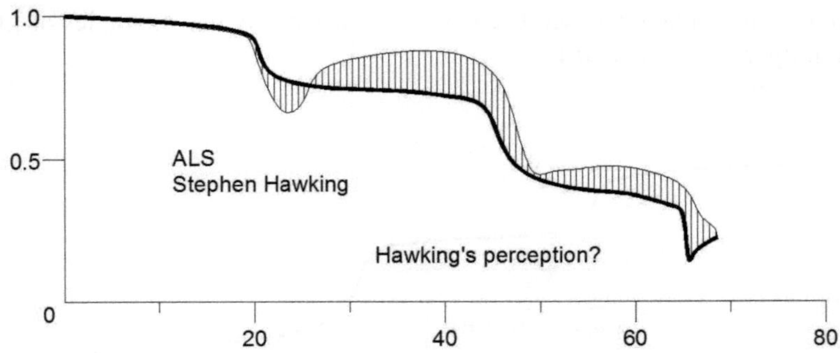

Fig. 20.11 Two possible LQC perceptions for ALS: Physician and patient

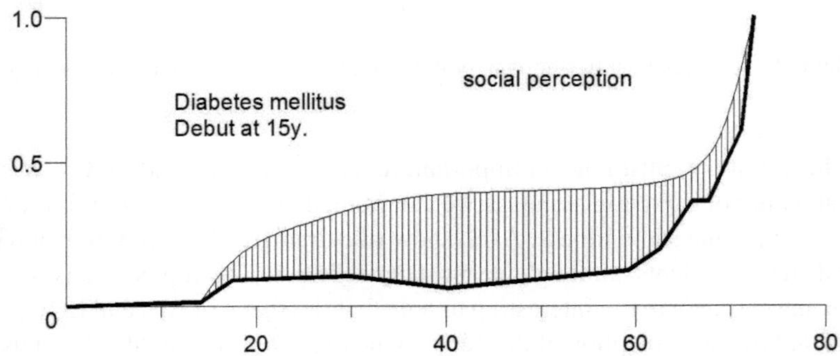

Fig. 20.12 Two possible LIC perceptions for diabetes: Patient and society

where the bold line shows a patient's possible own perception of the condition, used to daily subcutaneous insulin injections, while the fine line expresses a possible generalized perception as a result of social lack of information about diabetes.

Needless to say, the shape of Life Illness Curves and Life Quality Curves are not only dependent on the perception of the patient, physician or society, but also from the family environment, social class, economic scenario, politics, etc.

20.4 Conclusions

Through this work, we have explored the concepts of probability and fuzziness in medicine and how they are based on the information available at hand. Perceptions play a pivotal role in understanding and interpreting the world and every individual has his or her own particular and subjective vision on patient complaints, symptoms, states of the organism, diseases, therapies and recoveries. In order to battle this subjectivity, physicians use numerical indicators such as biochemical laboratory values and endless raw data from many types of clinical tests. However, and as we have seen, many of the data obtained from a patient are fuzzy in nature. Since the classical mission of a physician is to interpret the available information and to relate a set of symptoms with a precise disease or condition and then to find a suitable treatment, we can realize that physicians live in a world composed by rules, knowledge, information and experience where no sharp partitions do exist.

In this context, Life Illness Curves and Life Quality Curves are graphic representations of a perception of something that already exist (i.e., the health evolution of a patient through his or her life), an interpretation of reality in strong contrast to subjective probability, a perception or personal judgement of something unknown with respect to its future outcome. From this perspective it doesn't matter that LIC and LQC curves are heuristic and fuzzy in nature. Every LIC/LQC curve is unique and shows that the concept of "patient" entails a larger set of information that the concept of "illness". Under this perspective, we can even suggest that instead of speaking about diseases, it's usually better to speak about patients. With this vision in mind, we ultimately can realize that the mission of a physician is to diminish the $\mu_I(x),t$ values in LIC and to raise the $\mu_L(x)$ values in the family of LQC.

Acknowledgement. I would like to thank my wife, Dr. (MD) Ana Fernandez-Andrés, for her comments and suggestions in the development of this work.

References

1. Aristotle, R., William, D. (trans.): Metaphysics. NuVision Publications (2009)
2. Brown, R.H.: Amyotrophic Lateral Sclerosis and Other Motor Neurone Diseases. In: Hauser, S., Josephson, S. (eds.) Harrison's Neurology in Clinical Medicine. McGraw-Hill, Asia (2010)
3. Canavos, G.C.: Applied Probability and Statistical Methods. Brown and Company, Little (1984)
4. Guyton, A.C., Hall, J.E.: Textbook of Medical Physiology. W. B Saunders Company, Toronto (1996)

5. Jeffrey, R.: Subjective Probability. The Real Thing, Princeton University (2002) http://www.princeton.edu/~bayesway/Book*.pdf, (acceded January 2012)
6. Klir, G., Yuan, B.: Fuzzy Sets and Fuzzy Logic: Theory and Applications. Prentice Hall (1995)
7. Nguyen, H.T., Walker, E.A.: A First Course in Fuzzy Logic. Chapman and Hall/CRC (2006)
8. Sadegh-Zadeh, K.: Handbook of Analytic Philosophy of Medicine. Springer, Dordrecht (2011)
9. Thompson, J.S., Thompson, M.W.: (Authors: Nussbaum, R.L., McInnes, R.R., Willard, H.F., Thompson, M.W.) Genetics in Medicine. W. B Saunders Company, Elsevier Health Sciences, Toronto (2004)
10. Zadeh, L.A.: Fuzzy Sets. Information and Control 8, 338–353 (1965)

21

Medical Decision Making as a Group Choice Process: Consensual Dynamics in Fuzzy Diagnosis

Silvia Bortot and Mario Fedrizzi

21.1 Introduction

When addressing a medical decision making process, experts from different medical fields share information and knowledge to find a consensus, i.e. a common diagnosis and a common therapeutic decision. Diagnosis by a group consensus needs a wide range of organizational and technological support and therefore is very challenging to be developed. It's well known that the improvement of computer technology in the last twenty years made possible the implementation of the so called Group Decision Support Systems (GDSS). As pointed out in DeSanctis and Gallupe [8], a GDSS combines communication, computing and decision support technologies to facilitate formulation and solution of unstructured problems by a group of people. Accordingly, GDSS are very useful when teams of medical experts are involved in decision processes aiming at transforming medical evidence collected from a patient into a diagnosis. The development of a GDSS architecture to support collaborative medical decision making should cover several issues related to medical reasoning like data representation features, clinical algorithms, hypermedia techniques, cognitive models, communication tools, and so on. The reader interested in the development of a GDSS supporting the collaborative work conducted by a multidisciplinary medical team, based on cognitive processes incorporating clinical reasoning and problem solving features can refer to [24]. The authors introduce an hypermedia-based GDSS architecture to support collaborative medical decision making, showing the applicability of various models, techniques and reasoning methods at different levels of medical support to assist group members adaptation to a wide spectrum of problem solving patterns.

Since the diagnostic work is carried on through collaboration and information sharing among specialists, i.e. data presentation, analysis and interpretation are negotiated interactively and awareness of the outcome is shared by all of the team [20], one of the key issues to address is how to model consensual dynamics. Since the notion of consensus combines many significant aspects of preference modeling in group decisions, it plays a an important role when the social choice scheme is

R. Seising and M.E. Tabacchi (Eds.): *Fuzziness and Medicine*, STUDFUZZ 302, pp. 313–322.
DOI: 10.1007/978-3-642-36527-0_21

based on a dynamical model of preference aggregation. The fundamental problem becomes the construction of an appropriate consensus measure. In this paper, assuming that the opinions of medical specialists are represented by numerical fuzzy preferences, we develop a soft consensus model combining a measure of collective dissensus with an inertial mechanism of opinion changing aversion.

The structure of the paper is as follows. In section 2 a background explanation of the diagnostic framework in which our consensus module is embedded will be given. Section 3 focuses on a short historical overview of the main contributions in the area of group decision making and consensus modeling under fuzziness. In section 4 the model describing the consensual dynamics is presented.

21.2 A Diagnostic Frame

Sadegh-Zadeh in [25] wrote: "Medical diagnostics is a spatio-temporal network of collective action, a node of which accommodates an individual patient or a group of patients ... medical diagnosis is a social construct because the process of diagnostics that produces the diagnosis is itself socially shaped"

And then introduced the following 10-tuple diagnostic frame

- P, set of patients
- PO, a population that P is a subset of
- E, set of diagnosticians (experts)
- D and Δ, sets of categorical and conjectural abnormality statements on P
- G, set of goals the diagnosticians pursue
- A, set of actions available in pursuing goals
- KB, knowledge-base used by diagnosticians
- M, set of models (KBMS, optimization algorithms, reasoning processes, etc) that guides the diagnosticians from (D, KB) to Δ.
- T, the time period

In this frame, a central role is played by the collective medical decision process where experts from different medical fields, mostly in a "same place same time" meeting, sharing text and images, have to discuss and to agree about a common diagnosis and treatment.

Therefore, since evidence suggests that diagnoses made through collaboration achieve a higher performance then ones made by an individual clinician, addressing the problem involving several different specialists aiming at finding a consensual diagnosis is an approach becoming in more widespread use day by day. Accordingly, the architecture of the GDSS supporting the collaborative work of the group of clinical experts can be summarized as in Fig.21.1.

From the point of view of group decision theory, reaching a consensual diagnosis means updating opinions with respect to a given set of alternative diagnoses where these opinions are usually represented by preference relations. The uncertainty generated by imperfect, imprecise, information is a vital part of the diagnosis problem itself which should be combined with the vagueness in the clinicians' way of thinking (fuzzy mode of thinking). Consequently, the use of fuzzy relations in medical

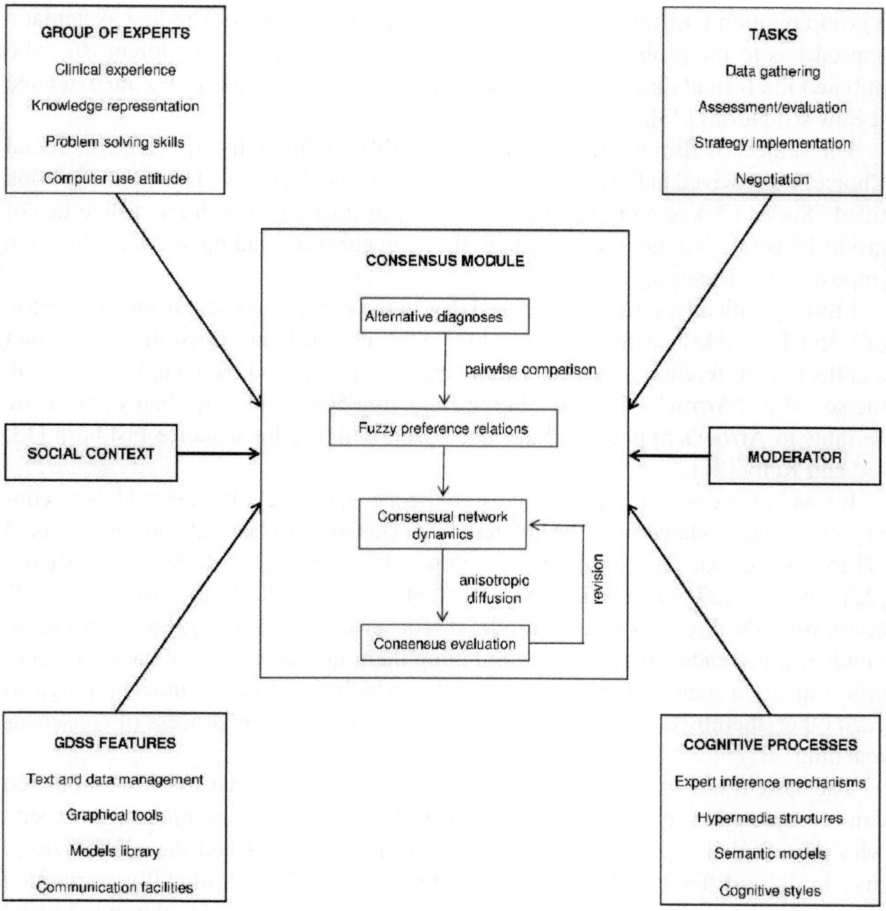

Fig. 21.1 GDSS architecture

diagnosis and their application in computer-assisted consensus reaching is useful to deal with the lack of sharp boundaries in the set of symptoms, diagnoses, and phenomena of diseases (see [26]).

Since our basic assumption in this paper is that for effectively representing medical collective decision processes we have to make reference to the theoretical framework of social choice theory and the related consensus models, the next session will be devoted to a short overview of the issue.

21.3 Group Decision Making and Consensus

The construction of models for making decisions when a group of two or more decision makers must aggregate their opinions (individual preferences) in order to get a group opinion (collective preference) is a very old problem. The first systematic approaches to the problem were pioneered by Borda [3] and Condorcet [6], who initiated the formal discipline of Social Choice in terms of voting. For an extended review see Nurmi [23].

The subject of Group Decision Making (GDM), traditionally equated with Social Choice, was revived in the twentieth century by Kenneth Arrow [1], who in his book titled "Social Choice and Individual Values" was concerned with the difficulties of group decisions and the inconsistencies they can generate leading to the well-known Impossibility Theorem.

More specifically, Arrow has proved that in the context of ordinal and symmetric (all decision makers with equal weight) preferences it is not possible to construct a collective preference structure without this being imposed by a single individual, the so-called "Arrow's dictator". In the following 50ies and 60ies many axiomatic variants to Arrow's hypothesis have been proposed, see for instance Fishburn [13, 14] and Kelly [21].

It was in the context of group decision theory that the traditional models of consensual dynamics have been formulated, from De Groot's classical consensus model [7] to various extended or alternative proposals: French [15], Lehrer and Wagner [22], and Sen [27], mostly in the probabilistic framework. In the spirit of "hard" consensus, De Groot's classical model of consensual dynamics [7] acts on the individual preference structures by combining them iteratively on the basis of a specific transition matrix of reciprocal weights which the decision makers assign to each other, thereby quantifying the reciprocal influence in the process of consensus reaching.

The basic framework within which most of the consensus processes are modelled can be depicted in the following way. There is a set of decision makers or experts who present their opinions concerning a set of alternatives and these alternatives may initially differ to a large extent. If the individuals are rationally committed to consensus, via some exchange of information, bargaining, etc. the individuals' opinions can be modified and the group may get closer to consensus.

Almost all of these approaches treat consensus as a strict and unanimous agreement, however, since various decision makers have different more or less conflicting opinions the traditional strict meaning of consensus is unrealistic. The human perception of consensus is much "softer", and people are willing to accept that a consensus has been reached when most or the more predominant decision makers agree on the preferences associated to the most relevant alternatives.

This degree of consensus takes on it values in the unit interval, and it's more realistic and human consistent than conventional degrees, mostly developed in the probabilistic framework.

The "soft" consensus paradigm developed in Kacprzyk and Fedrizzi [18], Fedrizzi et al. [9], Carlsson et al. [5], Kacprzyk et al. [19] in the standard framework of numerical fuzzy preferences was extended to a more dynamical context in Fedrizzi, Fedrizzi, Marques Pereira [10, 11]. The new model combines a soft measure of collective disagreement with an inertial mechanism of opinion changing aversion. It acts on the network of single preference structures by a combination of a collective process of (nonlinear) diffusion and an individual mechanism of (nonlinear) inertia. The overall effect of the dynamics is to outline and enhance the natural segmentation of the decision makers group into homogeneous preference subgroups. For extended review see [12].

In the meantime a number of different fuzzy approaches have been proposed. The linguistic approach of Zadeh [28–30] is applicable when the information involved either at individual level or at group level present qualitative aspects that cannot be effectively represented by means of precise numerical values. Innovative approaches to the modelling of consensus in fuzzy environments were developed under linguistic assessments and the interested reader is referred, among others, to Ben Arieh et al. [2], Cabrerizo et al. [4], and Herrera-Viedma et al. [16, 17]. The typical problem addressed is that in which decision makers have different levels of knowledge about the alternatives and use linguistic term sets with different cardinality to assess their preferences. This is the so-called group decision making problem in a multigranular fuzzy linguistic context.

21.4 Fuzzy Preference-Based Consensus in Diagnosis

By following the approach adopted in [10] now we introduce the dynamical consensus model aiming at finding the consensual diagnosis alternative.

If $A = \{a_1, \ldots, a_m\}$ is a set of alternative diagnoses considered and $E = \{e_1, \ldots, e_n\}$ is a set of experts, then the fuzzy preference relation R_i of expert e_i is given by its membership function $R_i : A \times A \longrightarrow [0,1]$, such that

$$R_i(a_k, a_l) = \begin{cases} 1 & \text{if } a_k \text{ is definitely preferred over } a_l \\ \xi_1 \in (0.5, 1) & \text{if } a_k \text{ is preferred over } a_l \\ 0.5 & \text{if there is indifference between} a_k \text{ and } a_l \\ \xi_2 \in (0, 0.5) & \text{if } a_l \text{ is preferred over } a_k \\ 0 & \text{if } a_l \text{ is definitely preferred over } a_k \end{cases}$$

where $i = 1, \ldots, n$ and $k, l = 1, \ldots, m$. Moreover, with $r^i_{kl} := R_i(a_k, a_l)$, we impose $r^i_{kl} + r^i_{lk} = 1$. This implies that $r^i_{kk} = 0.5$ for all $i = 1, \ldots, n$ and $k = 1, \ldots, m$. Here, for the sake of simplicity, we assume that the alternative diagnoses available are only two ($m = 2$), which means that each individual preference relation R_i has only one degree of freedom, denoted by $x_i = r^i_{12}$.

In the dynamical consensus model each expert e_i for $i = 1, \ldots, n$, is represented by a pair of connected nodes, a primary node (dynamic) and a secondary node (static). The n primary nodes, denoted $r_i \in [0,1]$, form a fully connected subnetwork and each of them encodes the individual opinion of a single expert. The n secondary nodes, denoted $s_i \in [0,1]$, on the other hand, encode the individual opinions originally declared by the experts, and each of them is connected only with the associated primary node.

The iterative process of opinion transformation corresponds to the gradient dynamics of a cost function W, depending on both the present and the original network configurations. W combines a measure V of the overall agreement in the present network configuration and a measure U of the overall change from the original network configuration.

The various interactions involving node i are mediated by interaction coefficients whose role is to quantify the strength of the interaction. The diffusive interaction between primary nodes i and j is mediated by the interaction coefficient $v_{ij} \in [0,1]$

$$v_{ij} = f'((x_i - x_j)^2). \tag{21.1}$$

The interaction coefficient $v_i \in [0,1]$ of this aggregated consensual interaction controls the extent to which expert e_i is influenced by the remaining experts in the group.

$$v_i = \sum_{j \neq i} v_{ij}/(n-1). \tag{21.2}$$

The inertial interaction between primary node i and the associated secondary node is mediated by the interaction coefficient $u_i \in [0,1]$ which controls the extent to which the expert e_i resists to opinion changes due to the collective consensual trend

$$u_i = f'((x_i - s_i)^2). \tag{21.3}$$

The values of these interaction coefficients are given by the first derivative of the scaling function

$$f(x) = -\frac{1}{\beta}\ln(1 + e^{-\beta(x-\alpha)}) \tag{21.4}$$

where $\alpha \in (0,1)$ is a threshold parameter and $\beta \in (0,\infty)$ is a free parameter. The graph of the scaling function f is shown in Fig. 2.

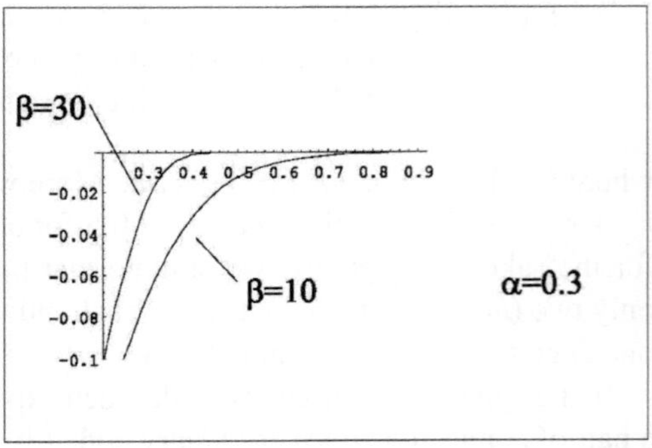

Fig. 21.2 The graph of the scaling function f

The sigmoid function $f'(x)$, plays a crucial role in the network dynamics and is obtained as the derivative of the scaling function $f(x)$ which, in turn, enters the construction of the soft consensus cost function from which the network dynamics derives

$$f'(x) = \frac{1}{1 + e^{\beta(x-\alpha)}}. \tag{21.5}$$

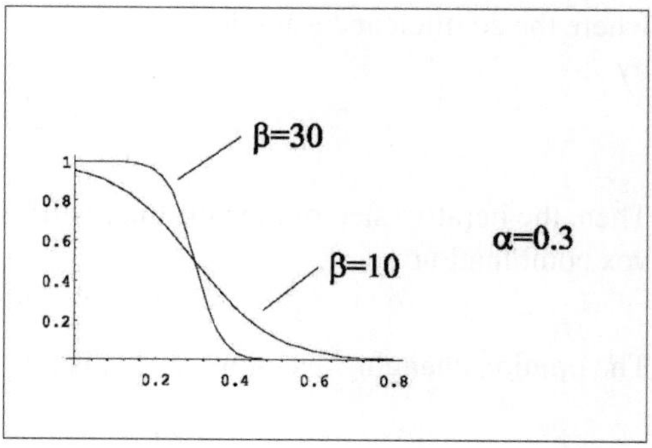

Fig. 21.3 The graph of the sigmoid function f'

The graph of the sigmoid function f' is shown in Fig. 3.

The diffusive component of the network dynamics results from the consensual interaction between each node x_i and the remaining $n-1$ nodes $x_{j\neq i}$ in the network. The aggregated effect of these $n-1$ interactions is represented as a single consensual interaction between node x_i and a virtual node containing a particular weighted average of the remaining opinion values.

The individual dissensus cost is given by

$$V(i) = \sum_{j\neq i} V(i,j)/(n-1) \tag{21.6}$$

where

$$V(i,j) = f((x_i - x_j)^2) \tag{21.7}$$

and the individual opinion changing cost is

$$U(i) = f((x_i - s_j)^2)\,. \tag{21.8}$$

Summing over the various experts we obtain the collective dissensus cost V and inertial cost U

$$V = \frac{1}{4}\sum_i V(i) \qquad\qquad U = \frac{1}{2}\sum_i U(i) \tag{21.9}$$

where $1/4$ and $1/2$ are conventional multiplicative factors. The full cost function W is then

$$W = (1-\lambda)V + \lambda U \qquad\qquad 0 \leq \lambda \leq 1\,. \tag{21.10}$$

The consensual network dynamics, which can be regarded as an unsupervised learning algorithm, acts on the individual opinion variables through the iterative process

$$x_i \longrightarrow x_i' = x_i - \varepsilon \frac{\partial W}{\partial x_i}\,. \tag{21.11}$$

The dissensus cost V induces a non-linear process of diffusion based on the gradient term

$$\frac{\partial V}{\partial x_i} = v_i(x_i - \bar{x}_i) \tag{21.12}$$

where the coefficients v_i are defined in (21.2) and the average preference $\bar{x}_i$ is given by

$$\bar{x}_i = \frac{\sum_{i \neq j} v_{ij} x_j}{\sum_{i \neq j} v_{ij}}. \tag{21.13}$$

Then, the iterative step of the non-linear diffusion mechanism corresponds to a convex combination

$$x_i' = (1 - \varepsilon v_i) x_i + \varepsilon v_i \bar{x}_i. \tag{21.14}$$

The opinion changing aversion mechanism is based on the gradient term

$$\frac{\partial U}{\partial x_i} = u_i (x_i - s_i). \tag{21.15}$$

The non-linearity of the opinion changing aversion mechanism is encoded in the inertial coefficient u_i which modulates the convex combination between the opinion value x_i and the original opinion value s_i

$$x_i' = (1 - \varepsilon u_i) x_i + \varepsilon u_i s_i. \tag{21.16}$$

The full dynamics associated with the cost function W acts iteratively on each expert e_i through convex combinations of the opinion value x_i, the average opinion value $\bar{x}_i$, and the original opinion value s_i

$$x_i' = (1 - \varepsilon(v_i + u_i)) x_i + \varepsilon v_i \bar{x}_i + \varepsilon u_i s_i. \tag{21.17}$$

The expert e_i is in dynamical equilibrium, in the sense that $x_i' = x_i'$, if the following stability equation holds

$$x_i = (v_i \bar{x}_i + u_i s_i)/(v_i + u_i) \tag{21.18}$$

that is, if the present opinion x_i coincides with an appropriate weighted average of the original opinion s_i and the average opinion $\bar{x}_i$.

21.5 Conclusions

In the first part of this paper we introduced a GDSS architecture based on the Sadegh-Zadeh's diagnostic framework as a spatio-temporal network of collective actions. Then we discussed some basic issues related to the representation of group decision making processes, summarizing key concepts stemming from the seminal work of Kenneth Arrow and mostly focused on the modeling of consensual dynamics. By referring to the fuzzy representation of individual binary fuzzy relations, an approach to consensus modeling in group based-diagnosis was introduced combining a soft measure of collective disagreement with an inertial mechanism of opinion changing aversion. For the future, we would like to extend the analysis of consensual dynamics considering linguistic preference relations defined on sets of linguistic summaries coming out from different knowledge sources.

References

1. Arrow, K.J.: Social Choice and Individual Values. Cowles Foundation and Wiley, New York (1951)
2. Ben-Arieh, D., Chen, Z.: Linguistic Labels Aggregation and Consensus Measures for utocratic Decision Making Using Group Recommendations. IEEE Transactions on Systems, Man, and Cybernetics, Part A 36(3), 258–268 (2006)
3. de Borda, J.C.: Mémoire sur les élections au scrutin. Histoire de l'Académie Royale des Sciences (1781)
4. Cabrerizo, F.J., Alonso, S., Herrera-Viedma, E.: A Consensus Model for Group Decision Making Problems with Unbalanced Fuzzy Linguistic Information. International Journal of Information Technology and Decision Making 8(1), 109–131 (2009)
5. Carlsson, C., Ehrenberg, D., Eklund, P., Fedrizzi, M., Gustafsson, P., Lindholm, P., Merkuryeva, G., Riissanen, T., Ventre, A.: Consensus in Distributed Soft Environments. European Journal of Operational Research 61, 165–185 (1992)
6. Condorcet, M., de Caritat, J.A.N., Marquis de: Essai sur l'Application de l'Analyse à la Probabilitié des Décisions rendues à la pluralité des voix. L'Imprimerie Royale, Parigi (1785)
7. DeGroot, M.H.: Reaching a Consensus. Journal of the American Statistical Association 69, 118–121 (1974)
8. DeSanctis, G., Brent Gallupe, R.: A Foundation for the Study of Group Decision Support Systems. Management Science 33(5), 589–609 (1987)
9. Fedrizzi, M., Kacprzyk, J., Zadrozny, S.: An Interactive Multi-user Decision Support System for Consensus Reaching Processes Using Fuzzy Logic with Linguistic Quantifiers. Decision Support Systems 4, 313–327 (1988)
10. Fedrizzi, M., Fedrizzi, M., Marques Pereira, R.A.: Soft Consensus and Network Dynamics in Group Decision Making. International Journal of intelligent Systems 14, 63–77 (1999)
11. Fedrizzi, M., Fedrizzi, M., Marques Pereira, R.A.: Consensus Modelling in Group Decision Making: a Dynamical Approach Based on Fuzzy Preferences. New Mathematics and Natural Computation 3(2), 219–237 (2007)
12. Fedrizzi, M., Fedrizzi, M., Marques Pereira, R.A., Brunelli, M.: The Dynamics of Consensus in Group Decision Making: Investigating the Pairwise Interactions Between Fuzzy Preferences. In: Greco, S., Pereira, M., Ricardo, A., Squillante, M., Yager, R.R., Kacprzyk, J. (eds.) Preferences and Decisions: Models and Applications, pp. 159–182. Springer, Heidelberg (2010)
13. Fishburn, P.C.: The Theory of Social Choice. Princeton University Press, Princeton (1973)
14. Fishburn, P.C.: Interprofile Conditions and Impossibility. Fundamentals of Pure and Applied Economics, vol. 18. Harwood Academic Publishers, London (1987)
15. French, S.: Consensus of Opinion. European Journal of Operational Research 7(4), 332–346 (1981)
16. Herrera, F., Herrera-Viedma, E., Verdegay, J.L.: A Model of Consensus in Group Decision Making under Linguistic Assessments. Fuzzy Sets and Systems 78, 73–88 (1996)
17. Herrera-Viedma, E., Martinez, L., Mata, F., Chiclana, F.: A Consensus Support System Model for Group Decision Making Problems with Multigranular Linguistic Preference Relations. IEEE Transactions on Fuzzy Systems 13(5), 644–658 (2005)
18. Kacprzyk, J., Fedrizzi, M.: A "Soft" Measure of Consensus in the Setting of Partial (Fuzzy) Preferences. European Journal of Operational Research 34, 316–325 (1988)

19. Kacprzyk, J., Nurmi, H., Fedrizzi, M. (eds.): Consensus Under Fuzziness. International Series in Intelligent Technologies. Kluwer Academic Press, Dordrecht (1997)
20. Kane, B., Luz, S.: Achieving Diagnosis by Consensus. Computer Supported Cooperative Work 18(4), 357–392 (2009)
21. Kelly, J.S.: Arrow Impossibility Theorems. Academic Press, New York (1978)
22. Lehrer, K., Wagner, C.: Rational Consensus in Science and Society. Reidel Publishing Company, Dordrecht (1981)
23. Nurmi, H.: Voting Procedures under Uncertainty. Springer, Heidelberg (2002)
24. Rao, G.R., Turoff, M.: A Hypermedia-based Group Decision Support System to Support Collaborative Medical Decision-making. Decision Support Systems 30(2), 187–216 (2000)
25. Sadegh-Zadeh, K.: Fundamentals of Clinical Methodology: 4. Diagnosis. Artificial Intelligence in Medicine 20(3), 227–241 (2000)
26. Seising, R.: From Vagueness in Medical Thought to the Foundations of Fuzzy Reasoning in Medical Diagnosis. Artificial Intelligence in Medicine 38(3), 237–256 (2006)
27. Sen, A.: Choice, Welfare and Measurement. Basil Blackwell, Oxford (1982)
28. Zadeh, L.A.: The concept of a linguistic variable and its application to approximate reasoning I. Information Sciences 8(3), 199–249 (1975)
29. Zadeh, L.A.: The concept of a linguistic variable and its application to approximate reasoning II. Information Sciences 8(4), 301–357 (1975)
30. Zadeh, L.A.: The concept of a linguistic variable and its application to approximate reasoning III. Information Sciences 9(1), 43–80 (1975)

22

Towards an Interpretation of the Medical Expert System CADIAG 2

David Picado Muiño, Agata Ciabattoni, and Thomas Vetterlein

22.1 Introduction

CADIAG2 (Computer Assisted DIAGnosis) is a well known rule-based expert system that aims at providing support in diagnostic decision making in the field of internal medicine. Its design and construction was initiated in the early 80's at the University of Vienna Medical School (now Medical University of Vienna) by Klaus-Peter Adlassnig –see [20] for a historical perspective on the origins and motivations of the system–.

CADIAG2 consists basically of two pieces: a knowledge base and an inference engine. CADIAG2's knowledge base is given by a set of *IF-THEN* rules, also known as production rules in the literature, intended to represent relationships between distinct medical entities: symptoms, findings, signs and test results on the one hand (to which we will commonly refer as *symptoms*) and diseases and therapies on the other one (to which we will commonly refer as *diagnoses*). The rules in CADIAG2 are defined along with a certain *degree of confirmation* which is intended to express the degree to which the antecedent confirms the consequent. For example,

IF suspicion of liver metastases by palpation
THEN pancreatic cancer
with degree of confirmation 0.3

The inference engine in CADIAG2 takes as its input (possibly) imprecise medical information about the patient, normally in the form of a set of symptoms present to some degree in the patient, and yields as its output a set of possible diagnoses, each along with a value intended to represent some degree of certainty about its presence in the patient. The inference rules in the knowledge base of the system are brought into play along the inference process, which is mostly based on methodology and techniques derived from fuzzy set theory, in the sense of [23] and [24].

The main aim of the present paper responds to an attempt to interpret the inference process in CADIAG2, and ultimately the output of the system, on the grounds

R. Seising and M.E. Tabacchi (Eds.): *Fuzziness and Medicine*, STUDFUZZ 302, pp. 323–338.
DOI: 10.1007/978-3-642-36527-0_22

of a *sound* semantics. Two semantics will be taken as reference in our attempt: probabilistic semantics and fuzzy (*t-norm*-based) semantics –see for example [10] or [12] for more on *t-norms* and some other concepts mentioned below that are related to them–. The use of probabilistic semantics is motivated by the natural identification of the degrees of confirmation in the rules of the system with probabilities (in principle with frequencies, as suggested in [3], estimated from medical databases and patient records, although not all degrees of confirmation were obtained in this way) and the rules themselves with probabilistic conditional statements. The use of a fuzzy semantics is mostly motivated by the natural identification of the degrees of presence of symptoms in the patient with *membership degrees* in fuzzy set theory (also called *truth degrees*) and by some inferential methodology derived from fuzzy set theory. It is common practice in the field to choose a *t-norm* as the interpretation of the conjunction and its *residuum* as the interpretation of the implication with which we will characterize the rules of the system: rules in this context will be formalized as graded implications in the context of many-valued logics, in a sense that will be made clear later.

The outcome of such an attempt can be at least partially anticipated. The inference mechanism in CADIAG2 is partially based on methodology from fuzzy set theory and thus it is bound to be unsound with respect to probabilistic semantics. Some aspects of the probabilistic unsoundness of the inference mechanism in CADIAG2 were soon observed in earlier studies concerning the celebrated rule-based expert system MYCIN (that shares some background methodology with CADIAG2) –see [4] or [21] for a description of MYCIN, [8] for a comparison of CADIAG2 and MYCIN-like systems and [11], [13], [14], [22] for some probabilistic approaches to it–. However, it remains to be seen how far the system CADIAG2 is from probabilistic soundness and thus how much of its inference process could be interpreted probabilistically. A better match of the inference process may be expected with respect to some *t-norm*-based fuzzy semantics (in particular, as will be clear later, with the semantics based on the indentification of the *t-norm* with the *minimum* operator) yet, as with probabilistic semantics, it needs to be seen how much of the inference process can be interpreted on the grounds of this semantics.

It is worth mentioning here that, although the interest among theoretical AI researchers in rule-based expert systems seems to be lesser today than some years ago, rule-based expert systems are very popular among AI engineers. Many CADIAG2-like systems are in use and more are being built for future implementation. It is mainly for this reason that we believe that further analysis and understanding of CADIAG2-like systems is of relevance (CADIAG2 is presented in some monographs as an example of a fuzzy expert system –for example in [15] or [25]– and thus is used as a reference for some newly developed knowledge-based systems).

The paper is structured as follows: in Section 22.2 we introduce some notation and give some preliminary definitions necessary for the description of the inference mechanism of the medical system CADIAG2, which is done in Section 22.3, where we also describe the knowledge base of the system. In Section 22.4 we introduce the logical system **CadL** that consists of a collection of rules that formalize the steps made along the inference process. Such a formalization will facilitate the semantic analysis of the system carried out in Section 22.5. Section 22.6 summarizes results.

22.2 Preliminary Definitions

In this section we define a pair of concepts that we will need to describe the inference process in CADIAG2.

First we define a partial ordering relation.

Definition 27. *Let* $\preceq$ *be the partial ordering relation on* $[0,1]$ *defined as follows: for* $a,b \in [0,1]$, $a \preceq b$ *if and only if* $0 < a \leq b$ *or* $0 \leq a < 1$ *and* $b = 0$.

We define the strict partial ordering $\prec$ from $\preceq$ in the conventional way.

As we will see later, the definition of the ordering $\preceq$ responds to the use of both 0 and 1 as maximal values in CADIAG2 for the interval $[0,1]$. The value 0 denotes certainty in the non-occurrence of an event or falsity of a statement and the value 1 denotes certainty in its occurrence or its truth.

For the next definition let

$$\mathbb{D} = [0,1] \times [0,1] - \{(0,1),(1,0)\}.$$

Definition 28. *The function* $\max^* : \mathbb{D} \longrightarrow \mathbb{R}$ *is defined as follows, for all* $(a,b) \in \mathbb{D}$*:*

$$\max^*(a,b) = \begin{cases} a & \textit{if } b \prec a \\ b & \textit{otherwise} \end{cases}$$

In words, $\max^*(a,b)$ returns the biggest value among a and b with respect to the ordering $\preceq$ just defined.

22.3 The Medical Expert System CADIAG2

In this section we briefly introduce the medical expert system CADIAG2 –for more details on its design one can look at [1], [2] or [3]–.

As already mentioned in the introduction, CADIAG2 consists of two fundamental pieces: the knowledge base and the inference engine. We first describe the different types of rules in the system, mostly in relation to the role they play along the inference process, and later describe the essentials of the inference mechanism. Before getting started some notation is needed.

Let $p_1,\ldots,p_l$ denote the *basic* medical entities that occur in CADIAG2 (i.e., the symptoms and diagnoses in the system), for some $l \in \mathbb{N}$. CADIAG2 deals also with *compound* entities, build from basic ones by means of conjunction ($\wedge$), disjunction ($\vee$) and negation ($\sim$) (i.e., built as Boolean combinations of basic ones).

Strictly speaking, the system regards two additional types of connectives called *at least n out of m* and *at most n out of m*, with $n,m \in \mathbb{N}$ and $n \leq m$. However, these can be expressed in terms of conjunction and disjunction and thus are not taken into account in this paper. As an example,

$$\textit{at least } 2 \textit{ of } (\phi_1, \phi_2, \phi_3)$$

can be rewritten as

$$(\phi_1 \wedge \phi_2) \vee (\phi_1 \wedge \phi_3) \vee (\phi_2 \wedge \phi_3),$$

for ϕ_1, ϕ_2, ϕ_3 some arbitrary medical entities in CADIAG2.

The Knowledge Base. The knowledge base of CADIAG2, to which we will commonly refer as *KR*, consists of a collection of approximately 40.000 *IF-THEN* rules that express possibly uncertain relationships among distinct medical entities.

Rules in CADIAG2 can be characterized by triples of the form $\langle \theta, \phi, \eta \rangle$, where θ is the *antecedent*, ϕ the *consequent* and η is the degree to which θ confirms ϕ (i.e., the degree of confirmation), for θ, ϕ medical entities and $\eta \in [0,1]$.

In some literature about CADIAG2 –see for example [1] or [7]– rules are defined as 4-tuples of the form $\langle \theta, \phi, \eta, \zeta \rangle$, for θ, ϕ medical entities and $\eta, \zeta \in [0,1]$, where η stands for the degree to which θ (the antecedent) confirms ϕ (the consequent) and ζ for the degree to which ϕ confirms θ, sometimes referred to in the corresponding literature as the *strength of confirmation* and the *frequency of occurrence* of the rule respectively. The 4-tuple $\langle \theta, \phi, \eta, \zeta \rangle$ corresponds in our notation to the pair of triples $\langle \theta, \phi, \eta \rangle$ and $\langle \phi, \theta, \zeta \rangle$.

We can distinguish among three different types of rules by considering their form and how they are used along the inference process in relation to the values assigned to their antecedent or consequent.

- Type ***confirming to the degree*** η (c_η). A rule of this type is of the general form $\langle \theta, \phi, \eta \rangle$, for θ, ϕ medical entities (ϕ a basic medical entity) and $\eta \in (0,1]$. It is triggered in a run of the inference mechanism in CADIAG2 for strictly positive values or grades of its antecedent (in a way that will be made clear below, where we describe the inference engine of CADIAG2). We will generally refer to rules of this kind as rules of type **c**.

A rule of type **c** formalizes (possibly) uncertain interrelations among medical entities, the bigger the degree of confirmation η the more certain the presence of the consequent given the antecedent of the rule.

What follows is an example of a rule of type **c**, taken from [1]:[1]

IF *suspicion of liver metastases by liver palpation*
THEN *pancreatic cancer*
with degree of confirmation 0.3.

- Type ***mutually exclusive*** (**me**). A rule of type **me** is of the form $\langle \theta, \phi, 0 \rangle$, for θ, ϕ medical entities (ϕ a basic medical entity). It is only triggered in a run of the inference engine of the system when there is certainty about the truth or occurrence of θ.

A rule of type **me** expresses mutual exclusiveness between antecedent and consequent (i.e., the presence of one of them excludes the other).

[1] The subsequent examples in this subsection are also taken from [1].

The one that follows is an example of a rule of this type:

IF *positive rheumatoid factor*
THEN NOT *seronegative rheumatoid arthritis*

- Type ***always occurring*** (**ao**). A rule of type **ao** is of the form $\langle \theta, \phi, 1 \rangle$, for θ, ϕ medical entities. It can be triggered by the system only when there is certainty about the falsity or non-occurrence of ϕ.

A rule of type **ao** expresses the fact that the antecedent implies the consequent. It follows that, if the consequent is excluded, the presence of the antecedent is also excluded.

Notice that a rule $\langle \theta, \phi, 1 \rangle$ of type **ao** can be alternatively formalized by the triple $\langle \sim \phi, \sim \theta, 1 \rangle$ and that it is not a special case of a rule of type **c** due to the fact that $\sim \theta$ is not a basic medical entity.

Next we give an example of a rule of this type:

IF NOT (*rheumatoid arthritis* AND *splenomegaly* AND *leukopenia* $\leq$ $4000/\mu l$)
THEN NOT *Felty's syndrome*

There are other typologies for the rules in *KR* that will prove useful in further sections in this paper. A very general typology is the one that follows:

- ***Binary* rules.** Rules of the form $\langle \theta, \phi, \eta \rangle$ where θ, ϕ are basic entities.
- ***Compound* rules.** Rules of the form $\langle \theta, \phi, \eta \rangle$ where θ is a compound medical entity and ϕ is a basic entity.

The vast majority of rules in *KR* are binary. There are less than one hundred compound rules in *KR* yet, despite the number, they are important for the functioning of the system.

We have a further distinction among binary rules of use in further sections:

- ***Symptom-symptom* rules.** Rules of the form $\langle \theta, \phi, \eta \rangle$ where both θ, ϕ are symptoms and $\eta \in \{0, 1\}$.
- ***Diagnose-diagnose* rules.** Rules of the form $\langle \theta, \phi, \eta \rangle$ where both θ, ϕ are diagnoses and $\eta \in \{0, 1\}$.
- ***Symptom-diagnose* rules.** Rules of the form $\langle \theta, \phi, \eta \rangle$ where θ is a symptom, ϕ a diagnose and $\eta \in [0, 1]$.
- ***Diagnose-symptom* rules.** Rules of the form $\langle \theta, \phi, \eta \rangle$ where θ is a diagnose, ϕ is a symptom and $\eta \in [0, 1]$.

Most rules of type *diagnose-symptom* in *KR* are not used by the inference engine, only those of type **ao** are used by it.

The Inference Engine. CADIAG2 gets started with medical information about the patient. Such information is formally given by a set of basic medical entities present in the patient, each one together with a number in the interval $[0, 1]$ which, in principle, is intended to represent the degree to which such entity is present (i.e., its degree of presence). These values are, in most of the literature on CADIAG2, interpreted as membership degrees in the context of fuzzy set theory and respond to the possibly vague nature of medical entities in CADIAG2.

Values assigned to compound medical entities in the system (in principle only for those that are relevant for the inference) are generated according to the following rules, for θ, ϕ any medical entities:

- The assignment to $\theta \wedge \phi$ is obtained as the minimum between the corresponding assignments to θ and ϕ.
- The assignment to $\theta \vee \phi$ is obtained as the maximum between the corresponding assignments to θ and ϕ.
- The assignment to $\sim \theta$ is obtained as the difference between 1 and the assignment to θ.

After the initial medical information about the patient is obtained and entered into the system the rules in the knowledge base come into play. All the rules triggered by the initial information about the patient are used during the inference process. At each step in the inference process a rule of type **c**, **me** or **ao** is applied (that is done, in principle, in no particular order). Rules of these types are triggered as follows, for general entities θ, ϕ:

- A rule $\langle \theta, \phi, \eta \rangle$ of type **c** can be triggered at some step in the inference process if a strictly positive value has been previously assigned to θ. The use of the rule $\langle \theta, \phi, \eta \rangle$ will generate a new assignment for ϕ, calculated as the minimum between the value assigned to θ that triggers the rule and η.
- A rule $\langle \theta, \phi, 0 \rangle$ of type **me** can be triggered during the inference process if certainty about the presence of θ in the patient (i.e., the assignment 1) has been previously concluded. The application of $\langle \theta, \phi, 0 \rangle$ allows us to conclude certainty about the absence of ϕ in the patient (i.e., the assignment 0).
- A rule $\langle \theta, \phi, 1 \rangle$ of type **ao** can be triggered if certainty about the absence of ϕ has been previously concluded. The application of the rule $\langle \theta, \phi, 1 \rangle$ will allow us to conclude certainty about the absence of θ in the patient.

The inference process goes on until the system comes to the stage where neither new medical entities nor new assignments for those already generated can be inferred. CADIAG2 yields as outcome of the inference the set of diagnoses generated during the inference process along with the maximal value (with respect to the ordering $\preceq$ defined above) assigned to them during the inference.

It has to be mentioned that, according to part of the literature on CADIAG2 – for example [1]–, the original inference process in CADIAG2 works in a slightly different way. The update in the value of the distinct sentences involved in the inference is done as soon as two different values for the same sentence are produced by the system. The value chosen in the update for atomic sentences in L is the maximal one (with respect to the ordering $\preceq$). Notice though that this feature has a highly undesirable result (unless further restrictions on the rules or on the order in which the rules are used are imposed), which is that the outcome of a run of the inference mechanism can depend on the order in which the rules are applied. Such a drawback is easily avoided by assuming (as we do for this paper) that the chosen value, the maximal among all those produced along the inference with respect to the partial ordering $\preceq$, is only computed at the end of the process.

Notice that the system can generate what is called a *runtime inconsistency* given the ordering $\preceq$, produced when both values 0 and 1 are assigned to a medical entity along the inference process. In such case the system stops and produces an error message.

22.4 A Formalization of the Inference Process

In this section we provide a logical formalization of the inference process in CADIAG2 by means of a complete set of rules aimed at describing the possible steps along the inference.

Let L be a finite propositional language and SL the set of sentences obtained from L as its closure under conjunction ($\wedge$), disjunction ($\vee$) and negation ($\sim$). In the context of CADIAG2, the set $\{p_1, \ldots, p_l\}$ of basic medical entities will be a subset of L and the compound medical entities that can be obtained from L will be a subset of SL.

Let $\Gamma = \{\phi_1, ..., \phi_n\} \subset SL$, for some $n \in \mathbb{N}$. We will denote the sentence $\phi_1 \wedge ... \wedge \phi_n$ by $\bigwedge \Gamma$.

Definition 29. *A graded statement in L is a pair of the form* (ϕ, η), *with* $\phi \in SL$ *and* $\eta \in [0,1]$.

In the context of CADIAG2 a graded statement of the form (ϕ, η) represents the medical entity ϕ together with the value assigned to it, η, either at the outset (i.e., if ϕ is part of the initial information with which CADIAG2 gets started) or during the inference process.

22.4.1 The Calculus CadL

In this subsection we summarize results in [6] and present, in a slightly simplified version, the calculus **CadL** aimed at formalizing the inference process in CADIAG2.

First we define the notion of theory of **CadL**:

Definition 30. *A theory* $\mathcal{T}$ *of* **CadL** *is a pair of the form* (Φ, R) *characterized as follows:*

- Φ *is a finite set of graded statements in L.*
- $R = R^c \cup R^{me} \cup R^{ao}$, *with* R^c, R^{me} *and* R^{ao} *finite collections of rules of type* **c**, **me** *and* **ao** *respectively.*

In the context of CADIAG2 Φ would be given by the input of the system (i.e., the initial information about the patient) and R would be given by KR.

Let $\mathscr{T} = (\Phi, R)$ be a theory of **CadL**. We have the following rules:

- **Reflexivity rule**

$$(REF) \quad \frac{(\phi,\eta) \in \Phi}{\mathscr{T} \vdash (\phi,\eta)}$$

- **Evaluation rules**

$$(AND) \quad \frac{\mathscr{T} \vdash (\phi,\eta) \qquad \mathscr{T} \vdash (\theta,\zeta)}{\mathscr{T} \vdash (\phi \wedge \theta, \min(\eta,\zeta))}$$

$$(OR) \quad \frac{\mathscr{T} \vdash (\phi,\eta) \qquad \mathscr{T} \vdash (\theta,\zeta)}{\mathscr{T} \vdash (\phi \vee \theta, \max(\eta,\zeta))}$$

$$(NOT) \quad \frac{\mathscr{T} \vdash (\phi,\eta)}{\mathscr{T} \vdash (\sim \phi, 1-\eta)}$$

- **Manipulation rules**

$$(C) \quad \frac{\langle \theta,\phi,\eta \rangle \in R^c \qquad \mathscr{T} \vdash (\theta,\zeta)}{\mathscr{T} \vdash (\phi, \min(\eta,\zeta))} \quad \text{for } \zeta > 0$$

$$(ME) \quad \frac{\langle \theta,\phi,0 \rangle \in R^{me} \qquad \mathscr{T} \vdash (\theta,1)}{\mathscr{T} \vdash (\phi,0)}$$

$$(AO) \quad \frac{\langle \theta,\phi,1 \rangle \in R^{ao} \qquad \mathscr{T} \vdash (\phi,0)}{\mathscr{T} \vdash (\theta,0)}$$

REF simply aims at formalizing for general theories of the form (Φ, R) that a graded statement that belongs to Φ (i.e., to the input in CADIAG2) is itself inferred as a consequence (i.e., as part of the output in CADIAG2). The evaluation rules AND, OR and NOT aim at formalizing the assignments to compound medical entities along the inference process in a run of the inference mechanism of CADIAG2 and the rules C, ME and AO correspond to the use of rules of type **c**, **me** and **ao** respectively during the inference process, as explained in the previous section.

Given a theory $\mathscr{T}$ of **CadL** and a graded statement (ϕ,η), a *proof* of (ϕ,η) from $\mathscr{T}$ in **CadL** is defined as a finite sequence of *sequents* of the form

$$\mathscr{T} \vdash (\phi_1,\eta_1), \ldots, \mathscr{T} \vdash (\phi_n,\eta_n)$$

with $(\phi_n,\eta_n) = (\phi,\eta)$ and where, for $i \in \{1,\ldots,n\}$, each (ϕ_i,η_i) in $\mathscr{T} \vdash (\phi_i,\eta_i)$ follows from $\mathscr{T}$ by the application of one of the rules above, from graded statements in previous sequents.

We say that there exists a *maximal proof* of (ϕ,η) from $\mathscr{T}$ in **CadL** if there exists a proof of (ϕ,η) from $\mathscr{T}$ and there is no proof from $\mathscr{T}$ of (ϕ,ζ) with $\eta \prec \zeta$.

Let us now consider the theory $\mathscr{T} = (\Phi, R)$, with $R = KR$, ϕ a diagnose in L and $\eta \in [0,1]$. As should be clear from the description of the inference mechanism of CADIAG2 given in Section 22.3, the medical entity ϕ along with the value η would be given as an outcome in a run of the inference process of CADIAG2 on input Φ only if there exists a maximal proof of (ϕ,η) from $\mathcal{T}$ in **CadL** –for more details on this point see [6]–. In **CadL** a runtime inconsistency generated by the system would imply the existence of maximal proofs of $(\theta,0)$ and $(\theta,1)$ from $\mathcal{T}$, for some medical entity θ.

22.5 Towards a Semantics for CadL

In this section we look at the interpretation of the inference process in CADIAG2. We consider two possible alternatives in our attempt: probabilistic semantics and fuzzy semantics.

22.5.1 Probabilistic Semantics

The motivation for a probabilistic interpretation of the inference in CADIAG2 comes from the identification of the degrees of confirmation of rules in KR with frequencies or, more generally, probabilities and the rules in KR themselves with probabilistic conditional statements.

In this subsection we will assume that rules of the form $\langle\theta,\phi,\eta\rangle \in KR$ represent probabilistic conditional statements, where θ is the conditioning event or evidence, ϕ the uncertain event and η the probability of ϕ given that θ is true or that it occurs.

In order to set the inference process on probabilistic grounds and analyze its adequacy with probability theory we need also a suitable probabilistic interpretation of the graded propositions taken as input and generated along the process by the system. Recall that the value η in a statement of the form (ϕ,η) in the input of CADIAG2 is intended to represent the degree of presence of ϕ in the patient, normally identified with a membership degree in the context of fuzzy set theory (i.e., with a degree of truth). Here though we will adopt a probabilistic interpretation for these values.

We will focus our analysis on the binary fragment of KR (i.e., on the binary rules in KR), which we will denote by KR^{bin}. The vast majority of rules in KR are, as mentioned earlier, binary and they constitute the most characteristic fragment of CADIAG2 when seen as a representative example of a certain type of expert system. This restriction means leaving the evaluation rules in **CadL** aside. We will focus our analysis of the inference engine and thus of **CadL** on the manipulation rules.

Before going any further we need to introduce some preliminary notation and definitions.

Definition 31. *Let* $\omega : SL \longrightarrow [0,1]$*. We say that* ω *is a probability function on L if the following two conditions hold, for all* $\theta,\phi \in SL$*:*

- *If* $\models \theta$ *then* $\omega(\theta) = 1$*.*
- *If* $\models\sim(\theta\wedge\phi)$ *then* $\omega(\theta\vee\phi) = \omega(\theta)+\omega(\phi)$*.*[2]

[2] Here and throughout $\models$ represents classical entailment.

The first clause of the definition simply states that if θ is always true (or if it always occurs) then its probability must be 1 whereas the second one states that if ϕ and θ are never true at once (or that they never occur together) then the probability of $\theta \vee \phi$ is equal to the sum of the probabilities of θ and ϕ.

From Definition 31 the standard properties of probability functions on propositional languages follow. We give some without proof –for a proof and more details on probability functions see for example [17]–. For ω a probability function on L and $\theta, \phi \in SL$,

- $\omega(\theta \vee \phi) = \omega(\theta) + \omega(\phi) - \omega(\theta \wedge \phi)$,
- $\omega(\sim \theta) = 1 - \omega(\theta)$,
- if $\theta \models \phi$ then $\omega(\theta) \leq \omega(\phi)$.

For the next definition let us consider $\langle \theta, \phi, \eta \rangle$ to be a conditional probabilistic statement, for $\theta, \phi \in SL$ and $\eta \in [0,1]$.

Definition 32. *We say that a probability function ω on L satisfies $\langle \theta, \phi, \eta \rangle$ if*

$$\frac{\omega(\theta \wedge \phi)}{\omega(\theta)} = \eta.$$

If there exists such a probability function we then say that $\langle \theta, \phi, \eta \rangle$ is *satisfiable*.

As seen in the previous section, the inference mechanism in CADIAG2 gets started with a set of graded statements of the form (q, η), with $q \in L$ a basic medical entity present in the patient. Let us consider as an example the medical entity '*reduced glucose in serum*'. Let us assume that the value assigned at the outset in a run of the inference engine by the evaluation system in CADIAG2 to the statement '*Patient A has reduced glucose in serum*' out of the evidence given by the corresponding measurement of the amount of glucose in Patient A is η, for some $\eta \in [0,1]$. As an example, we could interpret such value as the *degree of belief* that a medical doctor has in the truth of the statement given the evidence. As such η could be interpreted as a probability. The probabilistic interpretation is certainly favoured by the discretization applied to medical concepts in CADIAG2 (for example, the concept '*glucose in serum*' generates five distinct medical entities in CADIAG2: '*highly reduced glucose in serum*', '*reduced glucose in serum*', '*normal glucose in serum*', '*elevated glucose in serum*' and '*highly elevated glucose in serum*'). Notice that such an interpretation places us within the subjective probabilistic frame and thus, for the sake of coherence, the knowledge base *KR* should also be interpreted subjectively. Other interpretations are also possible though. For example, one could regard such values as the ratio given by the number of doctors that agree on the truth of the statement out of all the doctors involved in the assessment. In order to accommodate such values into a coherent probabilistic frame along with the statements in *KR* one could justify them as being subjective probabilities assessed by a group of experts –see [9] or [16] for an analysis and justification of such concept–.

Formally, let $q \in L$ represent a basic medical entity present in the patient and assume that $\eta \in [0,1]$ is the initial value assigned to it by the evaluation system of

CADIAG2. We can identify the graded statement (q,η) with a probabilistic conditional statement of the form $\langle\kappa,q,\eta\rangle$, where $\kappa \in SL$ is the evidence that supports the presence of q in the patient.

Let us assume that the input of the system consists of

$$\langle\kappa_1,q_1,\eta_1\rangle,...,\langle\kappa_n,q_n,\eta_n\rangle,$$

for some $q_1,...,q_n$ basic medical entities and $\eta_1,...,\eta_n \in [0,1]$. Under this view, the set $\Omega = \{\kappa_1,...,\kappa_n\} \subset SL$ constitutes the initial *evidence* about the patient, which is then propagated along the inference process by the application of the rules in KR^{bin}.

Within our probabilistic interpretation the reflexivity and manipulation rules in **CadL** adopt the following form, for input Φ in $\mathscr{T}$ now formally given by the above conditional statements:

$$(REF^*) \quad \frac{\langle\kappa,\phi,\eta\rangle \in \Phi}{\mathscr{T} \vdash \langle\kappa,\phi,\eta\rangle}$$

$$(C^*) \quad \frac{\langle\theta,\phi,\eta\rangle \in R^c \qquad \mathscr{T} \vdash \langle\kappa,\theta,\zeta\rangle}{\mathscr{T} \vdash \langle\kappa,\phi,\min(\eta,\zeta)\rangle} \quad \text{for } \zeta > 0$$

$$(ME^*) \quad \frac{\langle\theta,\phi,0\rangle \in R^{me} \qquad \mathscr{T} \vdash \langle\kappa,\theta,1\rangle}{\mathscr{T} \vdash \langle\kappa,\phi,0\rangle}$$

$$(AO^*) \quad \frac{\langle\theta,\phi,1\rangle \in R^{ao} \qquad \mathscr{T} \vdash \langle\kappa,\phi,0\rangle}{\mathscr{T} \vdash \langle\kappa,\theta,0\rangle}$$

Within this frame, final outputs of the form (ϕ,η) produced by the inference engine shall be interpreted as conditionals of the form $\langle\bigwedge\Omega,\phi,\eta\rangle$ (i.e., as the probability of ϕ given all the medical evidence available about the patient). In order to make such interpretation operative and formalize it we need to extend **CadL** by introducing two new inference rules (the extended system will be denoted by **CadL***). The first of these rules formalizes the maximization process done by the system in order to yield as output the set of medical entities (diagnoses) along with the maximal value generated by it, with respect to the ordering $\preceq$:

$$(MAX) \quad \frac{\mathscr{T} \vdash \langle\bigwedge\Delta_1,\phi,\eta\rangle \qquad \mathscr{T} \vdash \langle\bigwedge\Delta_2,\phi,\zeta\rangle}{\mathscr{T} \vdash \langle\bigwedge(\Delta_1 \cup \Delta_2),\phi,\max^*(\eta,\zeta)\rangle}$$

for $\Delta_1,\Delta_2 \subseteq \Omega$.

An additional rule is necessary to produce the desired outcome:

$$(EX) \quad \frac{\mathscr{T} \vdash \langle\bigwedge\Delta,\phi,\eta\rangle \qquad \mathscr{T} \nvdash \langle\kappa,\phi,\zeta\rangle \text{ for all } \zeta \in [0,1]}{\mathscr{T} \vdash \langle\kappa \wedge \bigwedge\Delta,\phi,\eta\rangle}$$

for $\Delta \subset \Omega$ and $\kappa \in \Omega$.

This last rule, which we call *EX* as abbreviation of '*exhaustive*', simply states that, if κ is a piece of evidence that says nothing about the presence of ϕ in the patient (i.e., that κ and ϕ are *independent*) then the probability of ϕ given Δ should stay the same if in addition we consider the piece of evidence κ (i.e., $\Delta \cup \{\kappa\}$).

Consider now the theory $\mathscr{T} = (\Phi, R)$, with $R = KR^{bin}$ and Φ the input of the system which, as mentioned earlier, under our probabilistic interpretation takes the form of a collection of conditional probabilistic statements

$$\langle \kappa_1, q_1, \eta_1 \rangle, ..., \langle \kappa_n, q_n, \eta_n \rangle,$$

for some $q_1, ..., q_n$ basic medical entities, $\eta_1, ..., \eta_n \in [0,1]$ and $\Omega = \{\kappa_1, ..., \kappa_n\} \subset SL$ the initial evidence about the patient. The diagnose ϕ along with the value η would be given as an output in a run of the inference process of CADIAG2 on input Φ only if there exists a maximal proof (defined for **CadL*** essentially as for **CadL**) of $\langle \bigwedge \Omega, \phi, \eta \rangle$ from $\mathscr{T}$ in **CadL***. In our probabilistic interpretation, a run-time inconsistency in CADIAG2 can be manifested by the existence of maximal proofs of $\langle \bigwedge \Omega, \phi, 0 \rangle$ and $\langle \bigwedge \Omega, \phi, 1 \rangle$ from $\mathscr{T}$, for some medical entity ϕ, or by the non-existence of a proof of $\langle \bigwedge \Omega, \phi, \eta \rangle$ together with the existence of a proof of a statement of the form $\langle \kappa, \phi, \zeta \rangle$ from $\mathscr{T}$ (due to the fact that max^* is not defined for $(0,1)$) –for more details on all these issues see [19]–.

CadL* and Probabilistic Soundness

Among the manipulation rules in **CadL***, probabilistic soundness of ME^* is clear (i.e., that any probability function on L that satisfies $\langle \kappa, \theta, 1 \rangle$ and $\langle \theta, \phi, 0 \rangle$ also satisfies $\langle \kappa, \phi, 0 \rangle$). So is soundness of AO^*. However, C^* is certainly not sound with respect to probabilistic semantics. Among the two new additional rules in **CadL*** introduced to provide a probabilistic interpretation of the inference, *MAX* is clearly not sound and *EX* assumes some probabilistic independence among entities that may not actually be independent. Overall, **CadL*** does not score well within probability theory. This is no surprise. The computation of conditional probabilistic statements in a compositional way, as done by CADIAG2 primarily by means of the *min* and *max** operators, is clearly bound to be probabilistically unsound. One may wonder though what could be done in order to improve the inference on probabilistic grounds from a knowledge base like KR^{bin}. The answer seems to be 'not much'. Certainly a KR^{bin}-like knowledge base (i.e., a knowledge base given by some binary probabilistic conditional statements) is not the most convenient for inferential purposes in probability theory for medical applications like CADIAG2. As is well known, there are other knowledge-base structures better suited for that purpose, Bayesian networks being the most celebrated among them –see for example [5] or [18]–.

It is worth noting that **CadL*** satisfies what we can call *weak consistency* –called *weak soundness* in [11]–, defined as follows: if there is a maximal proof in **CadL*** of a statement of the form $\langle \bigwedge \Delta, \phi, 1 \rangle$ (or $\langle \bigwedge \Delta, \phi, 0 \rangle$) from some theory $\mathscr{T}$, with $\phi \in SL$ and $\Delta \subset SL$ then, if there is a maximal proof in **CadL*** of a statement of the form $\langle \bigwedge \Delta^*, \phi, \eta \rangle$, with $\Delta \subset \Delta^*$, then $\eta = 1$ (or $\eta = 0$ respectively). That is to say, if **CadL*** concludes certainty about the occurrence of some event or about the truth or falsity of some sentence then adding new evidence does not alter this certainty. Weak consistency is provided in **CadL*** and so in the inference mechanism of CADIAG2 by the operator max* defined over the ordering $\preceq$.

22.5.2 *Fuzzy (t-norm-Based) Semantics*

The motivation for an interpretation of the inference in CADIAG2 on the grounds of a *t-norm*-based semantics is motivated by the (fuzzy) methodology on which it is based and by the interpretation of the degree of presence η in a graded statement of the form (ϕ,η) in the input of CADIAG2 in the natural, most intuitive way: as a membership degree (i.e., truth degree) in the context of fuzzy set theory. However, in our attempt to provide a fuzzy interpretation of the inference in CADIAG2, we also need an interpretation of the rules in the system in those same terms. Although, as mentioned in previous sections, degrees of confirmation are intended to represent degrees of certainty about the presence of the corresponding diagnoses in the patient and are better characterized by means of uncertainty measures such as probability functions, in this section we will consider a characterization of the rules of the system and the corresponding degrees of confirmation in terms of truth degrees, arguably more suitable from the point of view of the intended fuzzy semantics (although the use of some fuzzy semantics to model uncertainty is not rare in the literature).

Graded statements in our settings become in this context what have been called *graded formulas* in [12]. Truth degrees in them will now be regarded as lower-bound thresholds (i.e., η in a graded statement of the form (ϕ,η) on L will now be regarded as a lower-bound threshold for the degree of truth of ϕ). Such an interpretation is not only motivated by the fact that it constitutes the common one to fuzzy logics but also by the inference in CADIAG2 itself when interpreted on fuzzy grounds: the choice of the maximal value with respect to the ordering $\preceq$ generated in relation to a certain diagnose as the output value for it goes well (i.e., is consistent) with the characterization of any values generated at each step in the inference as lower-bound thresholds.[3]

For our fuzzy semantics, the interpretation for conjunction ($\wedge$), disjunction ($\vee$) and negation ($\sim$) suggests itself by the values (degrees of truth in this context) that the system assigns to compound medical entities in *SL* along the inference process. Therefore, for $v : L \longrightarrow [0,1]$ a fuzzy valuation on L, we will have the following constraints, for $\phi,\theta \in SL$:

- $v(\phi\wedge\theta) = \min(v(\phi),v(\theta))$.
- $v(\phi\vee\theta) = \max(v(\phi),v(\theta))$.
- $v(\sim\phi) = 1 - v(\phi)$.

It is common in the field of fuzzy logic to interpret the conjunction by a *t-norm* (based on some natural, desirable properties that such interpretation should satisfy)

[3] This is not so in our probabilistic interpretation of the rules and graded statements involved in the inference process, as seen in the previous subsection. Recall that, in our probabilistic characterization, distinct values generated along the inference for the same diagnose (or, in general, medical entity) were intended to represent distinct degrees of certainty about the presence of such diagnose in the patient due mostly to differing amounts of evidence (i.e, subsets of what we denoted by Ω, explicitly formalized in our probabilistic characterization).

and the interpretation of the implication ($\rightarrow$) to its *residuum* –for more details on these notions see [12]–. Such identification places a further constraint on v:

$$v(\theta \rightarrow \phi) = \sup\{v(p) \,|\, v(\theta \wedge p) \leq v(\phi)\},$$

for $\theta, \phi \in SL$.

The identification of the interpretation of the conjunction ($\wedge$) with the Gödel *t-norm* (i.e., with the *minimum* operator) leads to the following interpretation of the implication ($\rightarrow$), for $\phi, \theta \in SL$:

$$v(\theta \rightarrow \phi) = \begin{cases} 1 & \text{if } v(\theta) \leq v(\phi) \\ v(\phi) & \text{otherwise} \end{cases}$$

In this framework we can identify an inference rule of the form $\langle \theta, \phi, \eta \rangle$ in the knowledge base of CADIAG2 –for $\theta, \phi \in SL$ and $\eta \in [0,1]$– with the graded statement $(\theta \rightarrow \phi, \eta)$.

Satisfiability of rules in *KR* and, in general, of any graded statements is defined in our framework as expected.

Definition 33. *The fuzzy valuation v on L is said to satisfy* (ϕ, η), *for some* $\phi \in SL$ *and* $\eta \in [0,1]$, *if* $v(\phi) \geq \eta$.

If such a valuation exists we say that (ϕ, η) is *satisfiable*.

CadL and Fuzzy Soundness

Among the manipulation rules in **CadL**, soundness of the rule *C* under the intended interpretation is clear (i.e., any fuzzy valuation v that satisfies (θ, ζ) and $(\theta \rightarrow \phi, \eta)$ also satisfies $(\phi, \min(\eta, \zeta))$) and so is soundness of *ME* and *AO*. The rule *C* responds to what is basically called *fuzzy modus ponens*, see for example [10]. As for the evaluation rules in **CadL**, *AND* and *OR* are sound with respect to the intended semantics but *NOT* is not sound (due to the characterization of the truth values in graded statements as lower-bound thresholds). As shown in [6], soundness of **CadL** can be basically provided by restricting the use of the rule *NOT* along the inference and by reinterpreting the intended role of the truth degrees in some graded statements: truth degrees in the graded statements that constitute the input in a run of the inference engine can be regarded as point values and also those in graded statements that are obtained from them by the application of any rules in **CadL** other than *C*. The rule *NOT* would only be applied to these statements (i.e., to graded statements where the truth degree is known to represent a point value). Thus, graded statements obtained as a result of the application of the rule *C* would not be used by the rule *NOT* –for more details on this point and, in general, on the content of this section see [6]–.

22.6 Conclusion

Two semantics have been taken as reference in our attempt to provide an interpretation of the inference process and output of the medical expert system CADIAG2:

probabilistic semantics and fuzzy (*t-norm*-based) semantics. The choice of probabilistic semantics was mostly motivated by the natural identification of the degrees of confirmation in the rules of the system with probabilities whereas the choice of a fuzzy semantics was mostly motivated by the natural identification of the input values of the input symptoms in a run of the inference engine with membership degrees in fuzzy set theory and by the inference methodology itself. In order to set the inference process on probabilistic grounds a probabilistic interpretation of the input values was needed and thus its natural interpretation, (arguably) more in keeping with a fuzzy semantics, had to be overlooked. On the other hand, in order to set the inference process fully on the grounds of a fuzzy semantics the degrees of confirmation in the rules of the system needed to be interpreted accordingly, despite the fact that such degrees are better represented by uncertainty measures such as probabilities. This granted, we showed that both semantics could account well for several steps along the inference process, in particular the attempted *t-norm*-based fuzzy semantics –based on the decision to use the *minimum* operator as the *t-norm*– yet, overall, none of them proved fully suitable as the intended interpretation of the system.

Acknowledgement. This work was partially supported by the Vienna Science and Technology Fund (WWTF). Grant MA07-016.

References

1. Adlassnig, K.-P., Kolarz, G., Scheithauer, W., Grabner, H.: Approach to a Hospital Based Application of a Medical Expert System. Medical Informatics 11(3), 205–223 (1986)
2. Adlassnig, K.-P., Kolarz, G.: Effenberger, Harald and Helmut Grabner: CADIAG: Approaches to Computer-assisted Medical Diagnosis. Computers in Biology and Medicine 15, 315–335 (1985)
3. Adlassnig, K.-P.: Fuzzy Set Theory in Medical Diagnosis. IEEE Transactions on Systems, Man and Cybernetics 16(2), 260–265 (1987)
4. Buchanan, B.G., Shortliffe, E.H. (eds.): Rule-Based Expert Systems: The MYCIN Experiments of the Stanford Heuristic Programming Project. Addison-Wesley, Reading (1984)
5. Castillo, E., Gutiérrez, J.M., Hadi, A.S.: Expert Systems and Probabilistic Network Models. Springer, New York (1997)
6. Ciabattoni, A., Vetterlein, T.: On the Fuzzy (Logical) Content of CADIAG2. Fuzzy Sets and Systems 161(14), 1941–1958 (2009)
7. Ciabattoni, A., Rusnok, P.: On the Classical Content of Monadic $G^{\sim}$ and its Application to a Fuzzy Medical Expert System. In: Proceedings of the 12th International Conference on the Principles of Knowledge Representation and Reasoning, KR 2010 (2010)
8. Daniel, M., Hájek, P., Nguyen, P.H.: CADIAG2 and MYCIN-like systems. Artificial Intelligence in Medicine 9, 241–259 (1997)
9. Genest, C., Zidek, J.V.: Combining Probability Distributions: A Critique and an Annotated Bibliography. Statistical Science 1(1), 114–135 (1986)
10. Gerla, G.: Fuzzy Logic. Kluwer Academic Press, Dordrecht (2000)

11. Hájek, P.: Towards a Probabilistic Analysis of Mycin-like Expert Systems. In: COMP-STAT 1988 Proceedings, Physica-Verlag, Heidelberg (1988)
12. Hájek, P.: Metamathematics of Fuzzy Logic. Kluwer Academic Press, Dordrecht (1998)
13. Hájek, P., Valdes, J.J.: An analysis of MYCIN-like expert systems. Mathware and Soft Computing 1, 45–68 (1994)
14. Heckerman, D.: Probabilistic interpretations for MYCIN's certainty factors. In: Uncertainty in Artificial Intelligence, pp. 167–196. North-Holland, Amsterdam (1986)
15. Klir, G.J., Folger, T.: Fuzzy Sets, Uncertainty and Information. Prentice-Hall International, Hemel Hempstead (1988)
16. Osherson, D., Vardi, M.Y.: Aggregating Disparate Estimates of Chance. Games and Economic Behavior 56, 148–173 (2006)
17. Paris, J.B.: The Uncertain Reasoner's Companion – A Mathematical Perspective. Cambridge Tracts in Theoretical Computer Science, vol. 39. Cambridge University Press (1994)
18. Pearl, J.: Probabilistic Reasoning in Intelligent Systems. Morgan Kaufman, San Mateo (1988)
19. Picado Muiño, D.: A Probabilistic Interpretation of the Medical Expert System CADIAG2. Soft Computing 15(10), 2013–2020 (2011)
20. Seising, R.: The Fuzzification of Systems. The Genesis of Fuzzy Set Theory and Its Initial Applications – Developments up to the 1970s. STUDFUZZ, vol. 216. Springer, Heidelberg (2007)
21. Shortliffe, E.H.: Computer-Based Medical Consultations: MYCIN. Elsevier, New York (1976)
22. Valdes, J.: An Integrated Environment for Uncertainty Processing using Graphical Models. IPMU 92 proceedings (1992)
23. Zadeh, L.A.: Fuzzy sets. Information and Control 8, 338–353 (1965)
24. Zadeh, L.A.: Fuzzy Logic and Approximate Reasoning. Synthese 30, 407–428 (1975)
25. Zimmermann, H.-J.: Fuzzy Set Theory and its Applications. Kluwer Academic Press, Amsterdam (1991)

23

Electronic Health Records Interoperability by Archetype Based Contexts

Belén Prados-Suárez, Carlos Molina,
Miguel Prados de Reyes, and Carmen Peña-Yañez

23.1 Introduction

The use of Electronic Health Records (EHR) has become a reality in the everyday practice of most of the hospitals, so it is possible to find in the literature a great variety of proposals to implement the EHR in different specialities like pediatrics, nursery, family care, emergencies, radiology, elder care or outpatient consultation (as can be seen in [14, 20, 22, 25, 36, 46] and [54], respectively); and also, under different regulations depending on the country, like in the Korean or the Czech medical systems (in [13] and [39], respectively).

In the last decades the necessity to improve the access to these systems and the communication between them have arose as important issues to be solved. The last one has been called *Interoperability* and a lot of efforts is applied to solve it. We claim that both problems have to be solve together.

However in most of these proposals, as well as in other studies regarding the satisfaction of the users about the implantation of the EHR like [38, 48, 51, 54] and [52]; or even about the comparison of different EHR systems as [4] and [21], there is a remarked problem: the great amount of information that is accumulating in the EHRs is making arise problems of access. Since all the information is always available, it is becoming really difficult to access a concrete information item required, even in relatively simple situations. It becomes really serious for situations like the urgencies, where the decisions must be taken within seconds and the relevant information for the concrete case should be immediately available to support them. Even more, the problem will get worse due to the increasing use of new medical machines and devices like PACs, that automatically generate documents to be included in the EHRs [43, 44].

To solve this situation the storage and access can't be restricted only to information with high clinical value, since depending on the assistance act the information needed may change. This problem is so relatively recent, that up to this moment it

R. Seising and M.E. Tabacchi (Eds.): *Fuzziness and Medicine*, STUDFUZZ 302, pp. 339–361.
DOI: 10.1007/978-3-642-36527-0_23

is quite difficult to find proposals that really face its whole extent. Most of them just focus on the definition of data structures and documents to organize the information provided by the EHR, offering navigation systems on it, like [30] and [38]. However they don't constitute a solution, since they allow logical and structured access to the information, but they don't avoid the uncomfortable selections steps and the successive screen-shots to reach the desired information [53].

In the medical research community it is clear that "having a good access to the information needed benefits the quality of the attention received by the patients" [1]. In addition, it is being pointed the importance of taking into account the situation or *context* from which the access is being performed [55], as a means to improve the access to the EHRs.

As an example, [16] propose to use an *infobutton* engine to manage the clinician and patient context in order to provide concise answers to frequent questions posed by clinicians. "Infobuttons are information retrieval tools that help clinicians to fulfill their information needs by providing links to on-line health information resources from within an electronic medical record (EMR) system" [18]. These models are usually based on classification models to predict clinician's decisions. However, these models are restricted to very concrete topics like the "medication infobutton data, used to predict medication-related content topics (e.g., dose, adverse effects, drug interactions, patient education) that a clinician is most likely to choose while entering medication orders in a particular clinical context" [18].

Other proposals related to the definition of contexts don't face explicitly nor directly the problem posed. They are mainly focused on the knowledge mobilization [47] and the the ubiquitous computation [32, 34]; or on the standardization of Hospital Information Systems and the exchange on information between them [10, 26, 40]. Proposals in the first cases, can rarely be applied to the Hospital Information Systems, since they are mainly based in the use of sensors to identify the context [34] or to provide information according to the device used so other applications can perform pervasive computing [32]. In addition, none of these proposals are designed nor useful for the immense databases of EHR. Proposals in the second case, instead of focusing on identifying the information that is really needed to be exchanged, are centered on adapting the system, its structures, contents and interfaces to different regulations and standards like HL7 [17], DICOM [27], [42], SNOMED-CT [41], or the most recent proposal of the European Committee for Standardization: the ISO 13606 regulation. It leads them to forget and even obviate the needs of the health professionals, who are the real users of the system, and whose work improvements have more repercussion and impact in the quality of the medical assistance provided to the patients.

Nevertheless, the problem of the access to concrete information items of interest in huge databases, do is addressed explicitly in other environments, like business, legacy and e-government (in [11, 37] and [6], respectively). A German office of digital services to the citizens has detected the problem through deep studies [6], but still hasn't proposed a solution to it. In the business framework this situation has also arose, as indicated by [11] and [8], and the proposals to solve it are based on the improvement of the information retrieval by the definition of different contexts and business models (as in [33]), changing the actual access mode and adapting it to the real information needs of the acceding user. However, these proposals are too young and are still in their first development phases, so it is soon to extend and adapt them to other type of systems.

This is why we propose to analyze the daily practice of the medical staff, and follow the same philosophy as these solutions, to improve their access to the information in the EHR based on the information they usually request in each assistance act. Following the work of a doctor we can find a great variety of situations with different purposes: from a deep study of a complex diagnosis process in his office, to a simple revision of the last consultation inform in a control of evolution process, passing through the requirement of very concrete data in the response to an emergency. As can be seen, we face a wide variety of activity contexts, with quite different requirements of information. In other words, we have different sets of relevant documents or information items of the EHR, depending on the *context* we are involved in.

Our proposal is based on the study of the access patterns so the information showed to the user can be *context-sensitive*. This way the system would only show to the doctor the information that is relevant to his/her present context. However it must be taken into account that the information needs are not static, and they may change along the time, so it is possible that a piece of information that today is important will be useless in the future. Moreover, the age of the data has influence too: there are cases like some analysis that must be repeated if the last result of the same type of analysis is older than a few months, since the results may change. Hence, all of these aspects must be considered when defining the *pertinence* of the information items to the *contexts*.

According to all of it three problems must be faced. First, it is necessary to identify the contexts of access. Second, the information relevant for each of them must be identified. And last, the information must be accessible to remote systems. To solve the first problem can be found some proposals focused on the context modeling like [5, 11, 19, 23] and [15]; but most of them are just theoretical models too complicated to be integrated in an existing system, and also require such complex algorithms that make them not suitable for an hospital information system. Even more if the system has to be updated continually to adapt to new needs. Proposals to face the second problem are mainly oriented to identify the relevant information inside documents as [9, 29, 31] and [35] propose; but due to the great amount of data involved in the Hospital Information Systems (hundreds of millions of records) it is not possible to use them. We need a very efficient way to contextualize the access and decide which information is relevant on each situation. The third one, the interoperability, has been faced separated from the other with solution that allow the system to understand each others.

In this chapter we present a proposal to faced the three problems inside an unify solution that is compatible with the new interoperability regulations. Next section present the background of the proposal presenting the system used for the development and the normal structure of the EHR systems. The next one present the interoperability regulation in Europe. Next, a proposal for contextualized access to EHR and the adaptation to interoperability is presented. The last section is dedicated to conclusions.

23.2 Background

First of all we must indicate that the proposal presented here has been developed in collaboration with the University Hospital San Cecilio from Granada, and that we have based their Electronic Health Record System, and used it as reference.

This system stores around 800.000 EHR, containing more than 50 millions documents. In the future it is expected to have a fast increase in the size, due to the inclusion of new types of documents from two sources: old documents that still have not been digitalized (scanned images, MRI, etc.) and new documents generated from the recently and future acquired devices and equipments like PAC's.

In this section we briefly show the characteristics of this EHR system, as well as the structure of the Electronic Health Records stored on it.

23.2.1 Electronic Health Records Structure

The information stored in the EHR is structured according to the *Reference Model* given by the [28]. According to this standard, the elements of the hospital information systems are organized according to an Ontology with a class *structure* that gives rise to the following classes:

- *Folder*: This class represents the divisions at the highest level inside the clinical history. In our case these divisions are the *assistance acts* and the *pathologies*, so all the documents in the EHR are grouped into assistance acts or pathologies, and both classifications coexist.
- *Section*: This class of the standard represents logical groupings of information, each one representing a set of data with an uniform informative clinical guidance (Figure 23.1), and corresponds to each *document* stored in the EHR. Examples of documents are from a blood analysis to a preanaesthetic study, or from an admission document to a X-ray test.
- *Entry*: According to the standard each entry represents a clinical observation or a set of them. It corresponds to what we call *data groups* (i. e. the hematology information in a blood analysis).
- *Cluster* and *Element*: These classes correspond to what we call *data items*. The difference between these classes is that the first one is used to represent an unique observation or action (a data item) that requires a complex structure like a list, a table or a temporal series (i.e. an electrocardiogram); whereas the second class represents a unique and simple value, instance of some of the types defined by it (i.e. the percentage of hematocrit in a blood analysis).

As indicated in [43] and [45], each document is characterized by a set of properties like:

- the type (exploration, anamnesis, epicrisis, checkup, nursing control, intervention, external,...).
- the specialty (medical specialty as surgery, cardiology and so on, nursing, administrative, etc.).
- the pathological or clinical process (documents about pregnancy, cataract, diabetes,...).
- ...

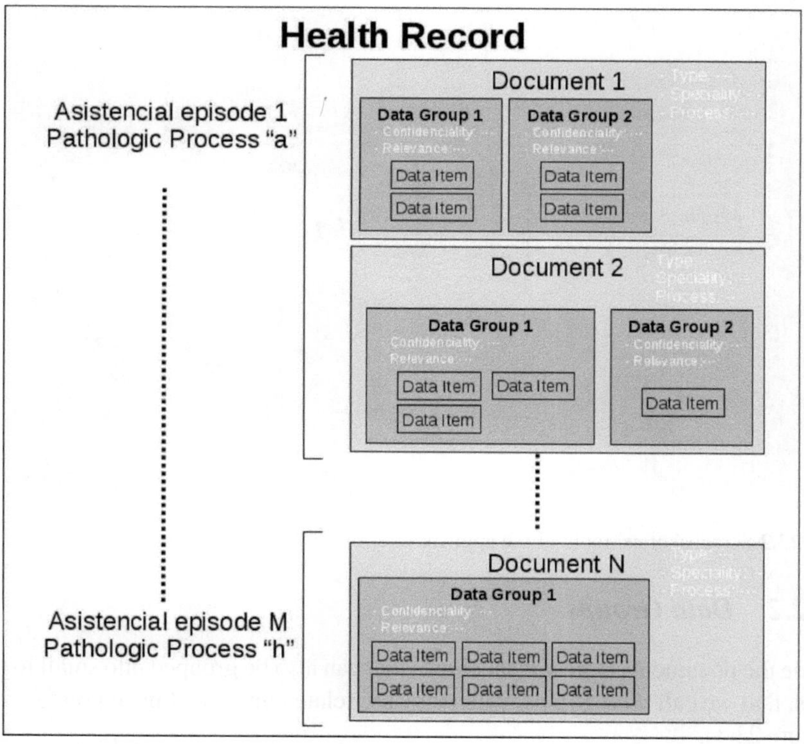

Fig. 23.1 Logical Organization of the EHRs

In our system, documents are organized according to *assistance episodes* (admissions, outpatient consultation, emergency assistance, day hospital,...) in a chronological or medical ordering, depending on the assistance processes. The documents are classified according to the types, considering 1500 different documents classes in the system: intervention sheet, progress sheet, nursing sheet, pregnancy process, diabetes protocol, radiological report, and so on. An example of it can be seen on Figure 23.2, where the interface that the medical personnel use to access the EHR is shown.

When a doctor is looking for a concrete data item, from an specific test made to the patient, he/she must select (on the square marked with a number 1 inside a circle in Figure 23.2) the type of assistance act that is performing. Then a search in the square marked with 2 in Figure 23.2 must be done, according to the date of the test or the medical specialty in which it was done. Once the assistance act in which the test was made is found, the doctor has to find among the documents generated in that act, the one with the results of the test, in the interface part marked with 3 in Figure 23.2. With it the document is recovered and finally it must be scanned to find the item of interest, by clicking on the tab marked with a number 4 in Figure 23.2. Though it is possible to use different ordering criteria (marked with number 5 in Figure 23.2).

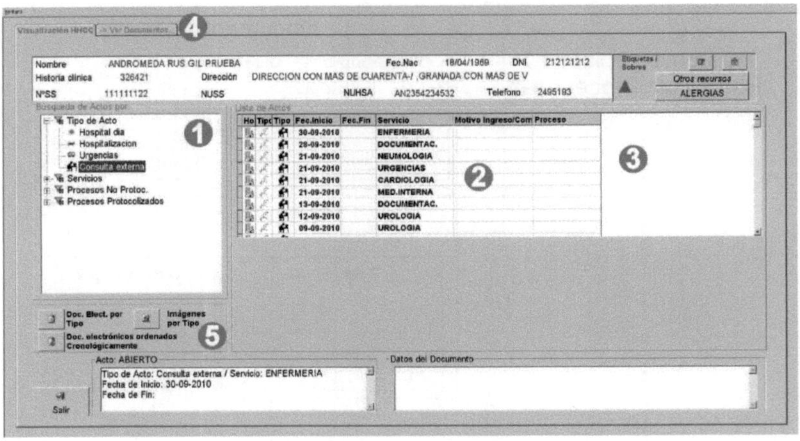

Fig. 23.2 Screenshot example of the applications

23.2.2 *Data Groups*

Inside the documents there are data items that can also be grouped into small logical units, that we call *data groups*, when they are related under a clinical point of view (Figure 23.1).

Each data group inherits the general properties of the document where it is contained. In addition, as shown in Figure 23.1, each data group has its own specific properties, like the relevance level (for the concrete patient and episode), the confidentiality level, etc.

Examples of data items for a blood analysis or a preanaesthetic study are: erythrocyte, hemoglobin, corpuscular volume, amylase, GGT, HDL-cholesterol, LDL-cholesterol or VLDL-cholesterol, in the first case; and Hypertension, cardiopathy, electrocardiogram, radiologic study or echography, in the second case. These data items can be grouped into the data groups general biochemistry and lipid information, for the first type of document; and risk factors or additional tests, for the second type. Here we would like to remark that the information of EHR and patient's identification is a "special" data group, common to all the documents. Due to it, it is discarded from the processes explained later.

This logical organization of documents and their content, allows the processing and analysis of the information, as much at *document* level as at individual *data items* level or *data group* level. Here we consider the data groups as the minimum unit of information, since a single data item can be managed as a data group with just one element.

23.2.3 EHR Information System

The structure of the system is shown in Figure 23.3. The users access the system using medical workstations. These are normal PCs, light PCs (or net PCs), medical devices like the X-Ray systems or the ultrasound scans, or the most recently incorporated terminals as the Tablet PCs and PDAs. The user then log on the system and access to a Citrix[1] farm of servers where the applications are executed. All the data are stored in a data base cluster using Oracle DBMS[2]. The screen-shot of the Doctor's interface once logged is shown in Figure 23.2.

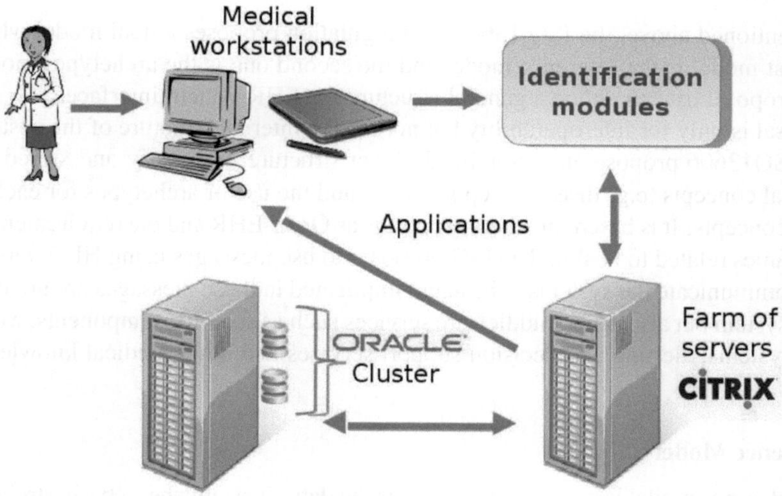

Fig. 23.3 Structure of the system

This system, as legally demanded, stores each access to the EHR, indicating the data acceded and, in case of modification, the modified data; the staff member acceding; and the assistance situation (called *"controlled assistance situation"*) in which the access occurs. From now on, we will call this access data base as

[1] `http://www.citrix.com`
[2] `http://www.oracle.com`

Retrospective Access Data Base (RADB). The number of records stored in the RADB is in the order of hundreds of millions.

We support the work proposed here on the registers of this data base since, as we will see next, their analysis allows to know which information has been acceded and the related context.

23.3 Interoperability

In the last decades, the EHR has been developed in most of the hospitals but without any coordination. Now the problem of communicating the systems has arisen and there are some proposals to solve it. All of them are based on the communications of the systems (machine-to-machine) so the EHR systems have to be adapted to understand an unified language. These solution are based on the use of archetypes as the information unit to be transmitted and languages to represent them.

In Europe, a regulation has been proposal for this problem. In next sections we briefly present the proposal.

23.3.1 CEN/ISO ISO 13606

As mentioned above, the ISO 13606 [28] regulation proposes a dual model where the first model is the reference model and the second one is the archetypes model. The proposal tries to define a general structure for EHR system interfaces. So, the proposal is only for interoperability but not for the internal structure of the system. The ISO13606 propose an hierarchical object structure to classify and stored the medical concepts (e.g. diseases, reports, etc.) and the use of archetypes for each of these concepts. It is based on others proposals as Open-EHR and the requirement by companies related to health. The ISO proposes to use messages using HL 7 version 3 to communicate the systems. The agent implicated in these messages are not only EHR system but also other middleware services such as security components, workflow systems, alerting and decision support services and other medical knowledge agents.

Reference Model

The reference model is proposed to structure the data. It establishes a basic structure using an object-oriented paradigm. It defines the main classes with the characteristics to store for each one. The classes are structured in a hierarchical manner considering from a set of documents (folder) to each value on an single analysis. It is based on a class called "structure" that gives rise to the following hierarchy of members:

- Folder: It represents the divisions at the highest level inside the extracts of the clinical history.
- Composition: It is the set of annotations related to a unique given clinical session or document.

- Sections: They are groupings in a clinical session.
- Entry: Each one represents a clinical observation or a set of them.
- Cluster: It is used when the representation of a unique observation or action requires a complex data structure, like a list, a table or a temporal series.
- Element: It contains a unique value that must be instance of some of the types defined by it.

Archetypes

The second model sets the Archetypes [2, 3, 7, 12, 50] as a way to define the clinical concepts managed by the systems. The archetypes are definitions of sets of clinical information items, that have a concrete clinical meaning; and they are created using the components defined in the ISO 13606.

Examples of these archetype may be:

- Pathological processes: Cataract.
- Protocols: Pregnancy.
- Documents: Blood analysis, Radiography and Prescription.
- Archetype can also be a group of items (biochemistry or lipid information) or a single item (HDL-cholesterol, LDL-cholesterol or VLDL-cholesterol) in a document.

So an Archetype is any information item or group of items related under a clinical point of view.

However this regulation just sets the basis and general description on which everything is opened and must be concreted, which is what we do in this paper.

23.3.2 Analysis

As the reader can see, the proposal is developed for machine-to-machine understanding, so the goal is to integrate the information on another system inside the institution EHR system. The proposal means a great efforts of developing and implementation because the complete system has to be change to support the archetype language so all the information can be exchange. In real situation, medical staff does not need to access the complete EHR of the patient but a portion of it related to the act involved. The CEN/ISO 13606 does not achieve this problem and only propose a translation of data and structure between systems.

The real user of the systems (the medical staff) is omitted from the solution (the local system will adapt the information sent to the local user). Medical staff does not need to access the complete EHR but a portion of it, so a complicated structure is not really needed in most of the external accesses. In that cases, a method to retrieve the important information needed would be better. In next section we present a proposal to retrieve this important information and adapt it to the interoperability problem.

23.4 Context-Based Access

In this section we present the contest-based access that is the start point for our proposal. In next sections, we present the definition of context, and the mechanisms to work with them in the EHR system. Later we will present how to use them in the interoperability problem.

23.4.1 Contexts

We call *Context* to a situation in the Doctor-Patient relationship inside an assistance act, requiring an access to the information previously stored in the EHR.

To contextualize the access to the EHR we first need to establish the set of possible situations or *contexts* where that access may occurs. Then, to exploit the contextualized access system, it is necessary to count on a mechanism to identify the context in which the medical staff is involved.

Context Definition

The contexts can be defined under three criteria or a combination of them:

- Pathological process: In this case the contexts are defined based on a diagnosed pathology that requires monitoring and it is included in the EHR as such process. Some of these processes are defined by the Regional Health Administration and others by the hospital services themselves. It must be taken into account that several medical specialities can be involved in the same process. Some examples are the pregnancy process, the cataract process, the diabetes process,...
- Medical specialty: Here the contexts are defined according to the specificity of each medical specialty (pediatrics, gynecology, nursery, cardiology,...).
- Kind of assistance: The context definition here is based on the environment where the assistance process takes places. The following cases can be distinguished:
  - Diagnostic study.
  - Surgical intervention.
  - Post-surgical revision.
  - Evolutive revision.
  - Room visit.
  - Treatment revision of outpatient consultation.
  - Analytical control.
  - Urgent assistance situation.

According to these three criteria, we ask to different medical doctors to identify the contexts on each speciality. The set of contexts obtained has been reviewed by different groups of medical doctors to validate the results for their corresponding specialty.

Context Identification

Once we have the contexts, it is necessary to have an automatic method to identify when a medical doctor accesses an EHR in a given context. By means of different interviews with the medical staff we have identified some characteristics of the accesses they perform, that are important in this process:

- Specialty of the medical staff like cardiology, ophthalmology, internal medicine, emergency, administration, nursing, and so on.
- Position of the medical staff. There are different positions for each type of medical personnel like. Some examples are: resident (from first to fifth year), facultative, section manager or head of service for the medical doctors; the categories of management technician, administrative technician, section manager or head of service for the administrative personnel; or the nursing position or nursing supervisor in that department.
- Type of the medical workstation. The data about the type of terminal used to perform the access, gives a lot of information about the type of assistance act in which the medical staff is involved. This attribute has several parts:
  - The type of the terminal. This value gives information about the hardware used (PC, PDA, patient's room terminal, computer associated to a concrete equipment like the X-ray machines or ultrasound scan, etc).
  - The medical unit associated. Each terminal is associated to an unit (gynecology, pediatrics, etc.) for management reasons; but this information helps to identify the context. As an example if a cardiologist is acceding an EHR from a computer associated to the emergency unit, the context could be a cardiology emergency.
  - Physical Location. It helps to concrete even more the type of context in which the medical staff is involved. In the previous example, if the terminal acceded is located in the observation room in emergencies, the context is different from the case when the access is performed from the surgery room.
- The kind of the present patient's appointment. For each appointment with a doctor, the information about its type is stored. There are around 50 usual types of appointments like first visit, checkup, scheduled visit, urgent visit, extern emergency, admission, several types for the different complementary tests and explorations, inter-consultation, movement between services, and so on. There are also some other types less usual or even rare but also considered in the system, like radiologic surgery.
- Last visit of the patient. This information in some cases helps to predict the cause of the next appointment. As an example, always after a surgical intervention there is a post-surgical checkup.

23.4.2 Pertinence

Once the set of considered contexts is defined it is necessary to identify the relevant information for each one. The relevance of a concrete data group for a given context is what we call *pertinence*: the more needed or interesting the data group is for the context, the higher is its pertinence to the context.

There is a great variety of factors to consider to compute this pertinence like:

- The regulations about each clinical process. Usually the information relevant for each act of some pathologies (not of all), is fixed by protocols set by governmental institutions, by the hospitals or by the medical services.
- The opinion of the concrete doctor. In addition to the regulations, each doctor can consider that, from his/her point of view, there are other items that must also be taken into account.
- The own history of a concrete patient. Some data groups without significance for the majority of the patients, may have a great and especial importance for a given patient.
- The aging of the information. With the time there are tests that loose their validity, because they are too old or because there are new tests of the same type.
- The access patterns. It is possible that the medical staff starts to access frequently a concrete data group for a given situation, and that they are not informed or "conscious" of it, so they don't include it through any of the previous ways. Taking into account this aspect of the pertinence, new patterns of access can be discovered and also the system can also automatically adapt to them.

The system must be capable of representing and bringing together all these aspects of the pertinence. The way we propose to do it is shown in next sections, where we present a method to capture and calculate each of these aspects of the pertinence.

Static Pertinence: Regulations, Doctors and Patients

As static pertinence we understand those set by medical criteria or given by the medical staff. Therefore, we consider three types of static pertinence, corresponding to three of the its aspects mentioned above:

On one hand, the medical criteria and regulations that determine which information must be always taken into account for a given process or pathology.

On the other hand, there personal opinions or even research studies of the doctors, that lead them to find a specific information item especially relevant for all the patients they see in a concrete *context*.

In addition, must be considered the concrete data group is particularly important for a given patient but not for the rest.

Hence, we include in the system three degrees of pertinence defined by doctors or medical criteria: one associated to the regulations ($P^R_{Dc} \in [0,1]$), another one related to the personal opinion of the doctor ($P^C_{Dc} \in [0,1]$) and the other one associated to the specific patient ($P^P_{Dc} \in [0,1]$).

Time Pertinence

The pertinence of a group of data (and the implicit document) will depend too on the date of creation. It is logic that the results of an analysis will be more important if it was completed a few days before than if it was performed a year ago.

However the influence of the age will not be the same for all document types: some type of analysis may be valid for several months meanwhile others are valid for years.

Hence we propose to modify the pertinence of the document depending on a established age threshold in months. If the document is younger than the threshold we want the time pertinence to be high (value grater than 0.7). If it is older, we want the time pertinence to decrease and give a low value.

To fulfill this restriction we propose the next definition.

Definition 34. *Been* D *a document and* A *the age of the it (express in months), we calculate the* Time pertinence of document D *as*

$$P_T(D) = e^{-\frac{log_B(A)}{e}} \tag{23.1}$$

where $B \in]1, +\infty]$ *is a parameter defining the decreasing strength.*

Figure 23.4 shows the behavior of the function according to the value B. Let note that the value of B is the point where the function has the first value under 0.7 (high pertinence).

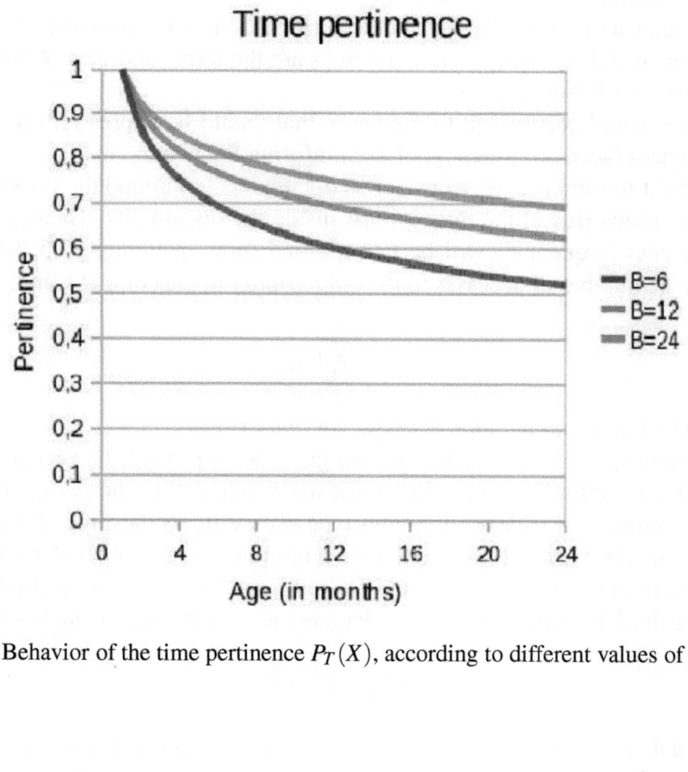

Fig. 23.4 Behavior of the time pertinence $P_T(X)$, according to different values of B

Dynamic Pertinence

In most of the situations the doctors will not give a static pertinence for a document neither a patient. So we need to learn the pertinences. Hence we propose to do it according to the accesses stored in the RADB database.

Due to the great number of records in the RADB database we need a very efficient process. If we consider that we want the system to be dynamic and to update on-line the pertinences according to the new accesses, the efficiency requirement is even more important.

As we have mentioned, different methods to calculated the relevance of preferences can be found in literature but the great complexity that they have, makes them not valid for our system. It has lead us to propose the new method explained next.

To calculate to pertinence we propose to use an adaptation of the Vector Space Model [49]. This technique comes from the Documentary Computing, concretely from the automatic indexation methods and retrieval systems [24]. It is used to determine which descriptors are more specific or discriminate better between documents.

The discrimination value classifies terms in the text according to their capability to distinguish some documents from others in a given collection; i.e., the discrimination value of a term depends on how the average distance between the documents changes when a content identification is set for the term. Therefore, the best words are those resulting in a higher distance.

The basic idea of this model lays in the construction of a matrix or table of information items and documents, where the rows are the terms and the columns correspond to the documents acceded.

The rows would correspond to the terms that would be expressed according to the occurrences (access frequency) of each information item.

Applying it to our case, we consider as documents (columns) the possible *Contexts* and as terms (rows) the *data groups* inside the documents. Hence, the table with the access frequencies will be like the one show in Figure 23.5, where tf_{ij} represents the number of accesses to the *data group i* in the *context j*, and

$$tf_j = \sum_{i=1}^{N} tf_{ij} \tag{23.2}$$

gives information about the total accesses for *context j*.

However in our situation it is not enough, since we need the recent accesses have to a higher influence than older ones when calculating the pertinence. This is why we propose to measure the relevance according to the time as the weight function shown in Figure 23.6. Let D_R be a reference date to consider relevant or not the information for the system and D_A represent the access date. In that case, we propose the following function to calculate the weight for a given date (D_A):

$$W(D_A) = 2^{\frac{D_A - D_R}{365}} \tag{23.3}$$

where the date difference is calculated in days. This way an access made today will have more influence that the accesses of the last year but, as the time goes by, less

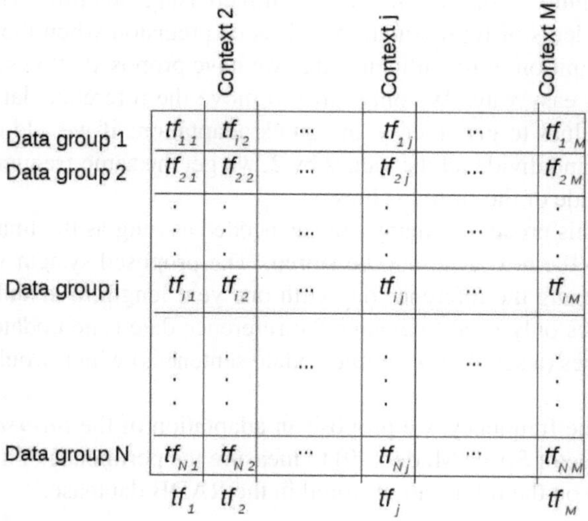

Fig. 23.5 Frequency table for *data groups* and *Contexts*

influence than future accesses. The equation establishes that given two accesses with a year of difference, the newer one will have double influence than the older one.

This definition introduces in the system two important and useful capabilities:

- The pertinences will be updated according to the aging of the access and the decreasing relevance.
- The system will be adapted automatically to future accesses patterns and needs, that can even allow us to define new contexts.

Then the system will update the pertinence of the data groups having more influence the newer accesses and enable the system to adapt to future needs.

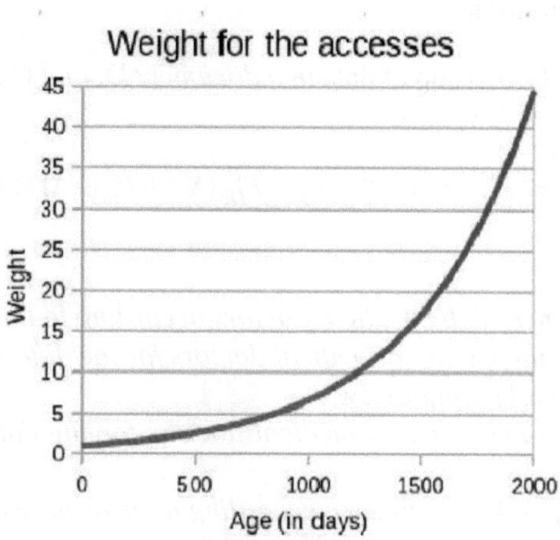

Fig. 23.6 Evolution of the influence according to the distance in days to the reference date

As shown in Figure 23.6, the influence is an increasing function. This may introduce some problems of representation or loss of precision when the values are very high. The definition of the influence that we have proposed allows us to avoid this problem in an easy way. We only have to move the reference date (D_R) and adapt the stored values to get an easy and quick adaptation: if we add one year to the reference date and divide all the values by 2, we get the same frequency and we reduce the magnitude of the stored values.

We can repeat this process as many time as needed as long as the final reference date is previous to the next access to be stored. The proposed system will do this each new year keeping the reference day with one year length to actual date. The update of the values only need to change the reference date (one update sentence) and the stored values (a set of very simple update sentences) which would need just a short time.

Now we have the frequency, we propose an adaptation of the *inverse document frequency* of the Vector Space Model [49] to measure the pertinence of a data group to a context, based on the information stored in the RADB database.

Definition 35. *Let C be a context and X a data groups, the* restrospective pertinence *is*

$$P_R^C(X) = [\frac{tfxc}{tfc}]^{1/4} \tag{23.4}$$

The idea behind this pertinence is to consider relevant a *data group* if the number of accesses to it is high in comparison to the total number of accesses.

Global Pertinence

Once we have the different considered aspects about the pertinence and defined a way to compute them them, we need to aggregate the information given by them into a single value. To do it, we obtain a global pertinence of a data group to a given context as in next definition.

Definition 36. *Let* X *be a* group of data *in a document* D, *and* C *a* context, *we define the* global pertinence of X to C *as*

$$P_G^C(X) = (P_{Dc}^R(X) \oplus P_{Dc}^C(X) \oplus P_{Dc}^P(X) \oplus P_R^C(X)) \otimes P_T(D) \tag{23.5}$$

where

- P_{Dc}^R *is the pertinence set by medical doctors according to the regulations,*
- $P_{Dc}^C(X)$ *is the pertinence set by medical doctors for the data group to the context under their personal point of view,*
- $P_{Dc}^P(X)$ *is the pertinence set by medical doctors for the data group to a given patient,*
- $P_R^C(X)$ *the retrospective pertinence according to prior accesses,*
- $P_T(X)$ *the pertinence considering the age of the document,*
- $\oplus$ *and* $\otimes$ *a t-conorm and a t-norm respectively.*

For the system we have chosen the *maximum* and the *minimum* as t-conorm and t-norm because of their simplicity, and therefore, efficient and fast calculation as well as they are quite extended.

Hence, we include in the system three degrees of pertinence defined by doctors or medical criteria: one associated to the regulations ($P^R_{Dc} \in [0,1]$), another one related to the personal opinion of the doctor ($P^C_{Dc} \in [0,1]$) and the other one associated to the specific patient ($P^P_{Dc} \in [0,1]$).

23.4.3 Contextualized Access System

With all the elements to implement the contextualized access to the EHR, we show next how we propose to provide this access by presenting the use of the proposed method, as well as the update process that allows the system to automatically adapt to new needs.

Access to the System

An scheme of the access process in shown in Figure 23.7.

- The doctor starts the process by logging in the system.
- Using the information about the terminal and the schedule of the doctor, the system gets the *context* for this access using the simple rule system.
- The doctor identifies the patient in the system to access his/her EHR.
- The system gets the EHR and queries the static and dynamic pertinences for all the data groups that appear in his/her EHR. The result of aggregating these pertinences and the time pertinence as shown in equation 23.5 is used to order the data.
- Finally, the system selects the first data groups and returns them to the doctor ordered y priority, as well as a way to access the other data groups if the doctor needs them.

Update Process

The system is updated on each access so the pertinences are adapted continually to reflect doctors' needs. In this process no manual intervention is needed and a few records are changed so it needs a short time to be executed. The update process is as follow:

- When the doctor logs in the system, the context of the access is calculated as mentioned above.
- The doctor asks for a data group of a specific patient.
- The system then gets the required data and returns them to the doctor. At the same time the system logs the access in the RADB table and updates the frequency table used to obtain the *retrospective pertinence* with this new access. Only two records are changed: the accesses to the data group in this particular context (tf_{ij}) and the total number of accesses to the context (tf_j).

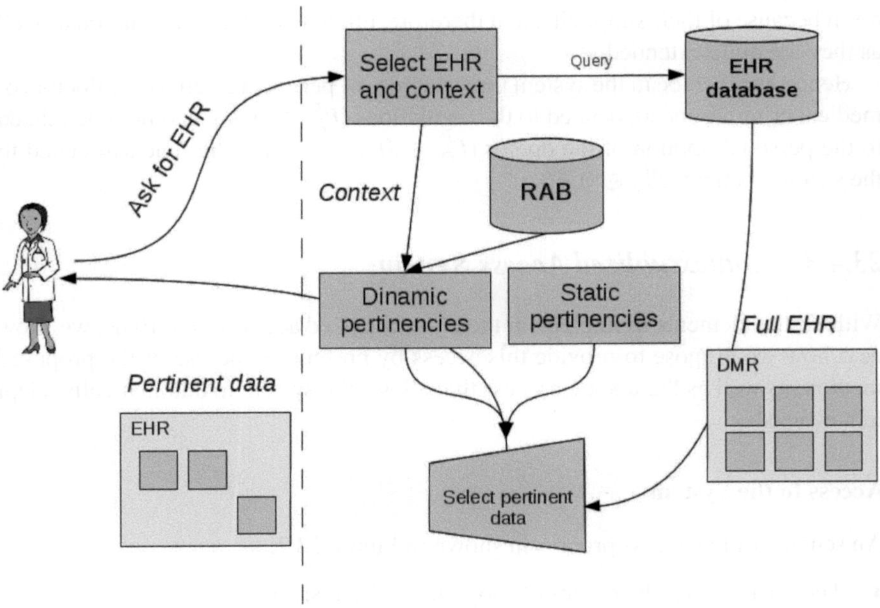

Fig. 23.7 Scheme of the contextualized query process

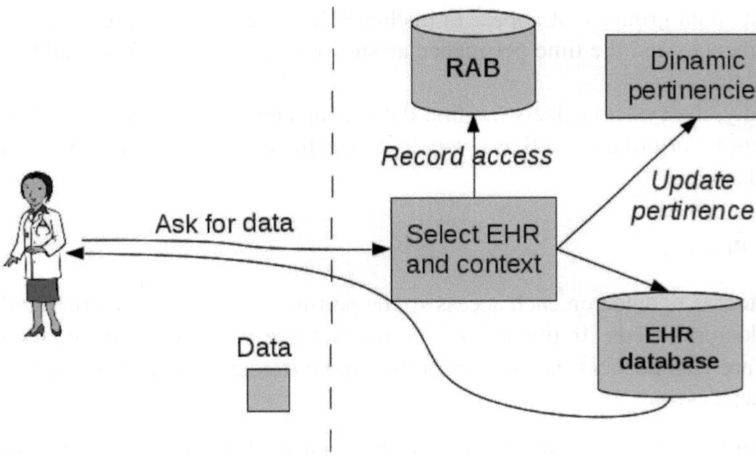

Fig. 23.8 Scheme for pertinences update process

A scheme summarizing of the process is shown in Figure 23.8.

After every access to the system, the dynamic pertinence is automatically updated so the next time a context is acceded the pertinence of the data groups to the context is computed considering the most updated information. As can be seen it is done with a very low computation cost. In addition this updating process allows, not only to give the most updated information, but also to discover new patterns of accesses, which give us the chance to define new contexts.

23.5 Interoperability by Archetype-Based Contexts

Once we have presented the context-based access we will present the proposal for interoperability. The proposals in this field are based on the interoperability between systems but forgetting the real users of the system. We want to change the approach to give more importance to the users than the systems but allowing these to communicate.

The main idea is to apply the context-bases access to the communication between systems. In this case, we have to adapt the proposal to the especial situation where the user and the information are in different hospitals or institutions. The contexts on both hospitals are almost the same due to the medical praxis is very similar in most of the institutions. We need to adapt the way to identify the context and the representation for the information transmitted.

In the first case, in most of the country some information about the medical staff that accesses the information has to be stored due to law obligation. Using this information we can try to identify the context of the access. In this point we have to differentiate three situations:

- If this access is the first time that both systems interact, then it is complicated to identify the context due to the normal differences between institutions. In this case (Non-trained system) the system will give as answer a list of context related to the medical staff specialty.
- If there are some interactions in the past, the system can infer the context but an error may occur so the system will answer the most probable context and a short list of less probable context according to the past history (System under test).
- If both systems have interacted previously in the past, enough to be be almost sure about the context, the system will answer just the most probable context (Trained system).

To implement this solution we only need three aspects: stored the previous accesses (normally obligated by law), an API between the system (very simple) and a way to send the archetypes. This is the last problem to solve: how to send the information. As in the previous case, the solution depends on the systems that interact: if both systems support an archetype language, then the information can be sent using this language. In other case, a standard format for medical documents can be used (DICOM [27] for images and PDF or XML for textual information).

With this points, all the aspects to adapt the solution are presented.

23.6 Conclusions

In this chapter we have presented a proposal for the problem of interoperability between EHR system. It is based on the use of an contextualized access system developed for local access adapted to the interoperability issues. The proposal can be used in systems with any degree of implementation of any interoperability solution due to it is a layer over the system that connects directly the medical staff with the remote system. If both systems use the same language for archetype, the proposal can use it to send the information needed. In other case, standard formats are used. In both cases, the access of remote EHR is improved reducing the navigation needed to access the remote information.

Acknowledgement. The research reported in this paper was partially supported by the Andalusian Government (Junta de Andalucía) under project P07-TIC03175 "Representación y Manipulación de Objetos Imperfectos en Problemas de Integración de Datos: Una Aplicación a los Almacenes de Objetos de Aprendizaje", by the Spanish Government (Science and Innovation Department) under project TIN2009-08296, and also by project UJA11/12/56. We would also like to thank their collaboration to the medical personnel that is participating in the development of the system.

References

1. Adams, A., Adams, R., Thorogood, M., Buckingham, C.: Barriers to the Use of e-Health Technology in Nurse Practitioner-patient Consultations. Informatics in Primary Care 15(2), 103–109 (2007)
2. Beale, T.: Archetypes: Constraint-based Domain Models for Future-proof Information Systems. In: OOPSLA 2002 Workshop on Behavioural Semantics. Citeseer (2002)
3. Bicer, V., Kilic, O., Dogac, A., Laleci, G.B.: Archetype-based Semantic Interoperability of Web Service Messages in the Health Care Domain. International Journal on Semantic Web and Information Systems 1(4), 1 (2005)
4. Bisbal, J., Berry, D.: An Analysis Framework for Electronic Health Record Systems. Methods of Information in Medicine 48(1) (2009)
5. Bobillo, F., Delgado, M., Gómez-Romero, J.: Representation of Context-dependant Knowledge in Ontologies: A Model and an Application. Expert Systems with Applications 35, 1899–1908 (2008)
6. Bohm, K., Wolf, E., Krcmar, H.: Context Oriented Structuring of Egovernment Services – An Empirical Analysis of the Information Demand of Expatriates in Germany. In: 43rd Hawaii International Conference on System Sciences (HICSS), pp. 1–10 (2010)
7. Brass, A., Moner, D., Hildebrand, C., Robles, M.: Standardized and Flexible Health Data Management With an Archetype Driven EHR System (ehrflex). Studies in Health Technology and Informatics 155, 212 (2010)
8. Buchholz, T., Hochstatter, I., Linnhoff-Popien, C.: Distribution Strategies for the Contextualized Mobile Internet. Electronic Commerce Research and Applications 6(1), 40–52 (2007)

9. Cao, Y., Xu, J., Liu, T.-Y., Li, H., Huang, Y., Hon, H.-W.: Adapting Ranking svm to Document Retrieval. In: SIGIR 2006: Proceedings of the 29th Annual International ACM SIGIR Conference on Research and Development in Information Retrieval, pp. 186–193. ACM, New York (2006)
10. Cayir, S., Basoglu, A.N.: Information Technology Interoperability Awareness: A Taxonomy Model Based on Information Requirements and Business Needs. In: International Conference on Management of Engineering Technology, PICMET 2008, Portland, pp. 846–855 (2008)
11. Chaker, H., Chevalier, M., Soule-Dupuy, C., Tricot, A.: Improving Information Retieval by Modelling Business Context. In: Third International Conference on Advances in Human-Oriented and Personalized Mechanisms, Technologies and Services (CENTRIC), pp. 117–122 (2010)
12. Chen, R., Klein, G.O., Sundvall, E., Karlsson, D., Åhlfeldt, H.: Archetype-based Conversion of EHR Content Models: Pilot Experience With a Regional EHR System. BMC Medical Informatics and Decision Making 9(1), 33 (2009)
13. Cho, I., Kim, J.A., Kim, J.H., Kim, H.Y., Kim, Y.: Design and Implementation of a Standards-based Interoperable Clinical Decision Support Architecture in the Context of the Korean EHR. International Journal of Medical Informatics 79(9), 611–622 (2010)
14. Cho, I., Staggers, N., Park, I.: Nurses' Responses to Differing Amounts and Information Content in a Diagnostic Computer-based Decision Support Application. Computers, Informatics, Nursing: CIN 28(2), 95–102 (2010)
15. Chu, W.W., Johnson, D., Kangarloo, H.: Hooshang Kangarloo: A Medical Digital Library to Support Scenario and User-tailored Information Retrieval. IEEE Transactions on Information Technology in Biomedicine 4(2), 97–107 (2000)
16. Collins, B., Speedie, S.: Attaching Context Sensitive Infobuttons to an EHR Options and Issues. In: AMIA, Annual Symposium Proceedings / AMIA Symposium AMIA Symposium, p. 914 (2008)
17. HL7 Data Exchange Standard (2011), `http://www.hl7.org`
18. Del Fiol, G., Haug, P.J.: Classification Models for the Prediction of Clinicians' Information Needs. Journal of Biomedical Informatics 42(1), 82–89 (2009)
19. Ehsan, M.A., Amini, M., Jalili, R.: Handling Context in a Semantic-based Access Control Framework. In: International Conference on Advanced Information Networking and Applications Workshops, WAINA 2009, pp. 103–108 (2009)
20. Erdal, S., Catalyurek, U.V., Payne, P.R., Saltz, J.H., Kamal, J., Gurcan, M.N.: A Knowledge-anchored Integrative Image Search and Retrieval System. Journal of Digital Imaging: The Official Journal of the Society for Computer Applications in Radiology 22(2), 166–182 (2009)
21. Zuniga, F., Enrique, A., Win, K.T., Susilo, W.: Functionalities of Free and Open Electronic Health Record Systems. International Journal of Technology Assessment in Health Care 26(4), 382–389 (2010)
22. Gagnon, M.-P., Desmartis, M., Labrecque, M., Légaré, F., Lamothe, L., Fortin, J.-P., Rancourt, J.-F., Duplantie, J.: Implementation of an Electronic Medical Record in Family Practice: A Case Study. Informatics in Primary Care 18(1), 31–40 (2010)
23. Garcia-Morchon, O., Wehrle, K.: Efficient and Context-aware Access Control for Pervasive Medical Sensor Networks. In: 2010 8th IEEE International Conference on Pervasive Computing and Communications Workshops (PERCOM Workshops), pp. 322–327 (2010)

24. Gil-Leyva, I., Rodríguez-Muñoz, J.V.: Tendencias en los sistemas de indización automática, Estudio Evolutivo. Revista Española de Documentación Científica 19(3), 273–291 (1966)
25. Ginsburg, M.: Pediatric Electronic Health Record Interface Design: The Pedone System. In: 40th Annual Hawaii International Conference on System Sciences, HICSS 2007, p. 139 (2007)
26. Leppanen, J., Lahteenmaki, J., Kaijanranta, H.: Interoperability of Personal Health Records. In: Proceedings of the International Conference of the IEEE Engineering in Medicine and Biology Society, pp. 1726–1729 (2009)
27. DICOM Image Storage Standard (2011), `http://www.medical.nema.org`
28. ISO-13606. Iso 13606: Electronic Health Record Communication (2008)
29. Järvelin, K., Kekäläinen, J.: IR Evaluation Methods for Retrieving Highly Relevant Documents. In: SIGIR 2000: Proceedings of the 23rd Annual International ACM SIGIR Conference on Research and Development in Information Retrieval, New York, NY, USA, pp. 41–48 (2000)
30. Jerding, D.F., Stasko, J.T.: The Information Mural: A Technique for Displaying and Navigating Large Information Spaces. IEEE Transactions on Visualization and Computer Graphics 4(3), 257–271 (1998)
31. Jones, K.S.: A Statistical Interpretation of Term Specificity and its Application in Retrieval. Journal of Documentation 60, 493–502 (2004)
32. Judd, G., Steenkiste, P.: Providing Contextual Information to Pervasive Computing Applications. In: Proceedings of the First IEEE International Conference on Pervasive Computing and Communications (PerCom 2003), pp. 133–142 (2003), doi:10.1109/PERCOM.2003.1192735
33. Jung, J.J.: Contextualized Query Sampling to Discover Semantic Resource Descriptions on the Web. Information Processing & Management 45(2), 280–287 (2009)
34. Kang, D.-O., Lee, H.-J., Ko, E.-J., Kang, K., Lee, J.: A Wearable Context Aware System for Ubiquitous Healthcare. In: Conference Proceedings: 28th Annual International Conference of the IEEE Engineering in Medicine and Biology Society, vol. 1, pp. 5192–5195 (2006)
35. Kanoulas, E., Pavlu, V., Dai, K., Aslam, J.: Modeling the Score Distributions of Relevant and Non-relevant Documents. In: Advances in Information Retrieval Theory, pp. 152–163 (2010)
36. Karahoca, A., Bayraktar, E., Tatoglu, E., Karahoca, D.: Information System Design for a Hospital Emergency Department: A Usability Analysis of Software Prototypes. Journal of Biomedical Informatics 43(2), 224–232 (2010)
37. Moa, J.-Y., Benbasat, I.: The Effects of Contextualized Access to Knowledge on Judgement. International Journal of Human-Computer Studies 55(5), 787–814 (2001)
38. McAlearney, A.S., Robbins, J., Hirsch, A., Jorina, M., Phil Harrop, J.: Perceived Efficiency Impacts Following Electronic Health Record Implementation: An Exploratory Study of an Urban Community Health Center Network. International Journal of Medical Informatics 79(12), 807–816 (2010)
39. Nagy, M., Hanzlćcek, P., Precková, P., Ríha, A., Dioszegi, M., Seidl, L., Zvárová, J.: Semantic Interoperability in Czech Healthcare Environment Supported by HL7 version 3. Methods of Information in Medicine 49(2), 186–195 (2010)
40. Nagy, M., Preckova, P., Seidl, L., Zvarova, J.: Challenges of Interoperability Using HL7 v3 in Czech Healthcare. Studies in Health Technology and Informatics 155, 122–128 (2010)

41. Snomed-CT nomenclature medical standard (2011), http://www.nlm.nih.gov/research/snomad/snomed_main.html
42. Open-EHR Open Electronical Health Rercords (2011), http://www.openehr.org
43. Prados, M.A., Yáñez, M.C.P.: Sistemas de Información hospitalarios. Organización y gestión de Proyectos. In: EASP (2003)
44. Prados, M.A., Yáñez, P., Carmen, M., Prados-Suárez, B., Martinez, B., Ortigosa, J.C., Delgado, A.C.: Electronical Health Record (EHR) Representation Through Ontology, Mobility, Accesibility and Interoperability Usefulness. In: 2010 EFMI Special Topic ConferenceSeamless Care — Safe Care: The Challenges of Interoperability and Patient Safety in Health Care, Reykjavik, Iceland, June 2-4 (2010)
45. Prados-Suárez, B., González Revuelta, E., Carmona Martínez, G., Yáñez, P., Carmen, M., Fernández, C.M.: Ontology Based Semantic Representation of the Reports and Results in a Hospital Information System. In: Prooeedings of the ICEIS 2008, pp. 300–306 (2008)
46. Pung, H.K., Gu, T., Xue, W., Palmes, P.P., Zhu, J., Ng, W.L., Tang, C.W., Chung, N.H.: Context-aware Middleware for Pervasive Elderly Homecare. IEEE Journal of Selected Areas in Communications 27, 510–524 (2009)
47. Ray, P., Wimalasiri, J.: The Need for Technical Solutions for Maintaining the Privacy of Ehr. In: Conference Proceedings: 28th Annual International Conference of the IEEE Engineering in Medicine and Biology Society, vol. 1, pp. 4686–4689 (2006)
48. Ross, S.E.: Results of a Survey of an Online Physician Community Regarding Use of Electronic Medical Records in Office Practices. The Journal of Medical Practice Management: MPM 24(4), 254–256 (2009)
49. Salton, G., Wong, A., Yang, C.-S.: A Vector Space Model for Automatic Indexing. Communications of the ACM 18(11), 613–620 (1975)
50. Serrano, P., Moner, D., Sebastián, T., Maldonado, J.A., Navalón, R., Robles, M., Gómez, Á.: Utilidad de los arquetipos iso 13606 para representar modelos clínicos detallados. RevistaeSalud.com 5(18) (2009)
51. Svanaes, D., Das, A., Alsos, O.A.: The Contextual Nature of Usability and its Relevance to Medical Informatics. Studies in Health Technology and Informatics 136, 541–546 (2008)
52. Vest, J.R., Jasperson, J.: What Should we Measure? Conceptualizing Usage in Health Information Exchange. Journal of the American Medical Informatics Association, JAMIA 17(3), 302–307 (2010)
53. Vila Miranda, M.A., Prados de Reyes, M., Yáñez, P., Carmen, M., Belen Prados Suárez, M.: Generation and Use of one Ontology for Intelligent Information Retrieval from Electronic Record Histories (2006)
54. Vishwanath, A., Singh, S.R., Winkelstein, P.: The Impact of Electronic Medical Record Systems on Outpatient Workflows: A Longitudinal Evaluation of its Workflow Effects. International Journal of Medical Informatics 79(11), 778–791 (2010)
55. Weinstock, M.: For Hospitals and Meaningful Use, Context is Everything. Hospitals & Health Networks / AHA 84(8), 20–21 (2010)

Part VI

Data Analysis and Decision Making

24
Fuzzy Pain Assessment in Musculoskeletal Disorder

Ernesto Araujo and Leandro Lazzareschi

24.1 Introduction

There are reports all over the world describing the struggle of human beings against the pain from ancient times [15]. In modern society, the presence of pain can mostly be explained by new lifestyle, increased longevity, severe medical conditions, traumatic surgical interventions, reduced tolerance of suffering by man etc.

According to the International Association for the Study of Pain (IASP), pain is defined as an "unpleasant emotional and sensory experience associated with actual or potential tissue damage or described in terms of such damage" [8]. Present in the majority of the diseases, pain is mostly related to individual experiences, be it physical or psychological, embracing cultural, sensory, cognitive, behavioral, and social aspects. Due to that, pain can be defined within a multifactorial event [6]. Further, many people accumulate more than one pain experience and perception regarding the same or different body regions. The great challenge is to find out a conclusive pain assessment necessary to prescribe the best treatment to reduce pain and suffering of patients.

Pain assessment is of special interest when dealing with chronic musculoskeletal pain. Skeletal muscles represent 40% of body weight being the most common functional organs of the human body. It is estimated that 40% of patients manifest chronic musculoskeletal pain at some point in life [6]. The disorders of the locomotor body system are the most common causes of pain [12]. Since the musculoskeletal system is the element that provides movement to the body as well as are the source of stability, support, and even form, it is an important source of research for measurement and treatment. This paper addresses the use of fuzzy set theory and fuzzy logic for musculoskeletal pain assessment. Such a formal and mathematical approach is a feasible manner to represent the inherent uncertainty, imprecision, and vagueness present in emotional, complex perceptual, subjective, and personal pain experiences as well as the difficulty to communicate it due to linguistic expression, frames of reference, and so on.

Mechanisms employed to quantify pain have been proposed during the last two decades. They enable patients and healthcare professionals to achieve a better

R. Seising and M.E. Tabacchi (Eds.): *Fuzziness and Medicine*, STUDFUZZ 302, pp. 365–377.
DOI: 10.1007/978-3-642-36527-0_24

communication and report regarding the (*i*) incidence, (*ii*) duration, and (*iii*) intensity of pain as well as the (*iv*) relief due to therapies [17]. There are diverse internationally accepted scales to measure pain [2, 10]. Unidimensional and multidimensional pain assessment mechanisms differ for the first being mostly related to pain intensity measurement meanwhile the second being simultaneously related to intensity, incidence and duration both of physical and psychological experiences. Nevertheless, pain assessment involves several levels of imprecision and uncertainty concerning both the subjectivity of pain perception and accuracy in mechanical or electrical devices. Despite being better known and applied, classic (Aristotelian) unidimensional pain scales still generate many controversies when interested in representing the subjectivity of their classification for the predictive indication of more effective treatment [13]. Classic (Aristotelian) multidimensional pain scales are also not able to assess the degree of the pain in terms of subjectivity and vagueness inherently present in reports and measurements. The objective herein is to develop a pain assessment mechanism based on previous fuzzy unidimensional pain scales [3] and fuzzy multidimensional professional-social-sexual scale [4] for being employed with any class of musculoskeletal pain assessment. The proposed approach advantages of being simultaneously, or not, employed with visual analog scale (VAS), numerical rating scale (NRS), face pain scale (FPS) and its fuzzy counterpart, i.e., fuzzy visual analog scale (FVAS), fuzzy numerical rating scale (FNRS), fuzzy face pain scale (FFPS) as measured input. The fuzzy qualitative pain scale (FQPS) is employed to compose a n–dimensional fuzzy input–output mapping for being employed in musculoskeletal clinical analysis and assessment, classification, and treatment.

24.2 Fuzzy Pain Assessment

To measure and classify pain constitutes a challenge to researchers worldwide mainly when taking into account the subjectivity, complexity and multidimensionality characteristics concerning such an unpleasant experience.

The more accurate is the pain assessment the more real is the description of its severity and also the appropriateness of a therapy for relief. Unidimensional pain scale has the advantage of easy applicability and low cost. Examples of classic (Aristotelian) unidimensional pain scales are visual analogue scale (VAS), numerical pain scale (numerical rating scale) (NPS), qualitative pain scale (verbal pain scale) (QPS); and face pain scale (FPS). Multidimensional pain scale, on the other hand, advantages of achieving greater scope for evaluating different levels of pain, embracing as sensory as affective qualities, as well as location and intensity [2]. Classic (Aristotelian) multidimensional scale is exemplified as McGill Pain Questionnaire. Nevertheless, such classic scales still generate much discussion and disagreement concerning the subjectivity of their classification in the evaluation of predictive degree of pain to achieve the most effective clinical analysis and assessment, classification, and treatment [3, 4, 13].

Fuzzy set theory and fuzzy logic are feasible alternatives to represent the inaccurate, unclear, uncertain, imprecise, vague information, as well as partial truths – i.e., imperfect information [19] – inherently associated to clinical aspects of pain and the subjectivity present in human nature. Different from classical sets, where an element, x, defined in an universe of discourse, X, belongs to a set, $M = \{x \in X\}$, or not, such that $\mu_M(x) \rightarrow \{0,1\}$, fuzzy sets employ membership functions to determine degrees varying from zero to one which an element belongs to a set [18]. A fuzzy set is, then, defined in a universe of discourse, X, representing the possibility, similarity, or conformity an element, x, belongs to a set, $M = \{x \in X\}$, according to a degree, $\mu_M(x)$, in the interval, $\mu_M(x) \rightarrow [0,1]$. An element mapping to the null value, $\mu_M(x) = 0$, means that it is not included in the fuzzy set, while mapping to the unitary value, $\mu_M(x) = 1$, describes a fully included member, and mapping into this interval, $0 < \mu_M(x) < 1$, represents a partial degree of membership. A fuzzy set is characterized by a support, $s(M(x))$, and a core, $c(M(x))$, of a membership function, $M(x)$, respectively, $s(M(x)) = \{x \in X | \mu_M(x) > 0\}$ and $c(M(x)) = \{x \in X | \mu_A(x) = 1\}$. While, the first is the set of all elements in X that belongs to the set $M(x)$ has positive membership function (are not null), the latter is the set of all elements whose degree of membership is unitary to the set $M(x)$.

24.2.1 Unidimensional Fuzzy Pain Intensity Scale

The internationally validated and accepted main classic pain intensity measurements are inherently crisp set representations. To best represent the inherent imprecision, uncertainty and vagueness related to the fifth vital sign/symptom of medical condition, the visual analog scale (VAS), numerical rating scale (NRS), qualitative rating scale (QRS), face pain scale (FPS) are extended to fuzzy set theory obtaining the fuzzy visual analog scale (FVAS), fuzzy numerical rating scale (FNRS), fuzzy qualitative pain scale (FQPS), fuzzy face pain scale (FFPS) in [3]. The fuzzy pain intensity scales use possibility distribution functions to represent the inherent imprecision, uncertainty and vagueness presented in the pain report and assessment.

Fuzzy Visual Analog Scale (FVAS)

The fuzzy visual analog scale consists of a 10 cm single line assigned in one border labeled *no pain* in opposition to the *maximum pain* in the other extremity (Fig. 24.1a). The patient marks this line with a cross, trace or any sign concerning pain intensity. The distance from beginning of the line (zero point) to the mark, x, is directly measured in centimeters by employing a ruler or by a computer program [5]. The mark in the line corresponds to the core of the membership function and, thus, to the maximum value of pain intensity, $\mu_M(x) = 1$. Since there is subjective, vague representation of the pain in the scale as well as there is no accuracy in utilizing a ruler in centimeters or the reading does not represents accurately the actual value, then a fuzzy set best represents the mark of the patient Fig. 24.1c. Approximately 2, and about 5 are, respectively, described by Gaussian and triangular fuzzy sets.

Fuzzy Numerical Rating Scale (FNRS)

The fuzzy numerical rating scale consists of a graded line scale identified by eleven numbers from 0 to 10 (Fig. 24.1b). The equivalence to pain intensity is obtained with *no pain* corresponding to 0 while *maximum pain* is related to 10. The patient marks this scale, x, with the pain intensity that better represents the assumed physical discomfort. Likewise FVAS, when there is a mark in the line it is related to the core of a membership function that assumes a full degree, $\mu_{A(x)} = 1$. Due to the subjective, vague representation of pain in the scale and no accuracy in reading the actual value, then the uncertainty and imprecision of marked value is best represented by a fuzzy set Fig. 24.1c. Similarly, approximately 2, and about 5 are, respectively, described by Gaussian and triangular fuzzy sets.

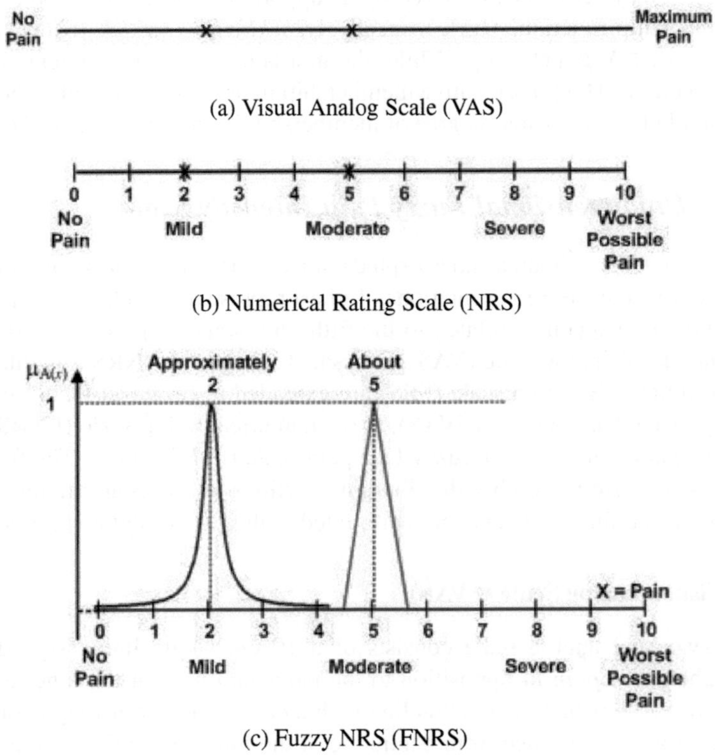

Fig. 24.1 Unidimensional Fuzzy Scales (FVAS) [3]

In a glimpse, observe that the Fuzzy Visual Analog Scale and the Fuzzy Numerical Rating Scale are twosome since VAS also maps the marked value in a numeric scale with the support of the ruler of computer program.

Fuzzy Qualitative Pain Scale (FQPS)

The Fuzzy Qualitative Pain Scale consists of a verbal rating scale in which categories are labeled with words. The patient is asked to classify the pain intensity according to linguistic expressions (adjectives) such as (1) *no pain*, (2) *light pain*, (3) *moderate pain*, (4) *intense pain*, (5) *maximum pain* that are registered for evaluation. The linguistic expressions for representing pain intensity may be directly represented by fuzzy sets as depicted in Fig. 24.2b, contrary to classical qualitative pain scale that uses crisp boundaries Fig. 24.2a. The absence of crisp boundaries in the membership function and the general theory of approximate reasoning address the interface between numbers and symbols by using the fuzzy set approach.

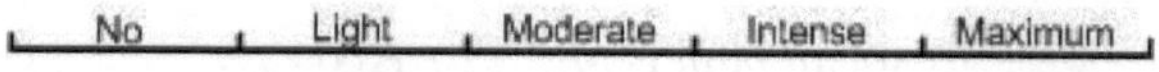

(a) Qualitative Pain Scale (QPS)

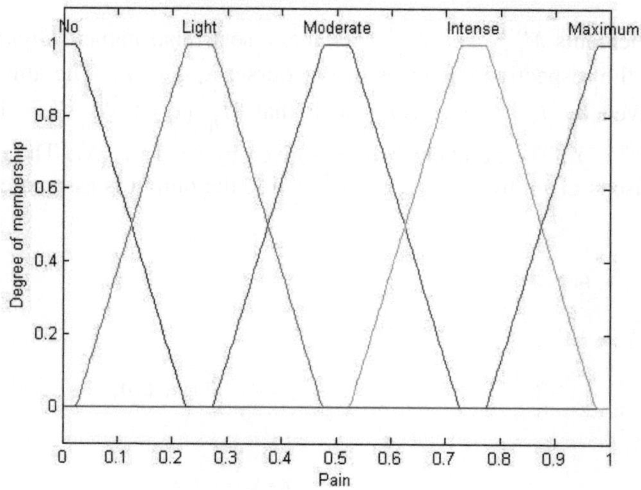

(b) Fuzzy QPS (FQPS)

Fig. 24.2 Unidimensional Fuzzy Qualitative Pain Scale (FQPS) [3]

24.2.2 *N–Dimensional Fuzzy Pain Scale*

A multi–criteria fuzzy pain assessment is further proposed in [4] by intertwining unidimensional fuzzy pain scales and the Mamdani fuzzy inference system. Base for a *n*–dimensional fuzzy pain assessment, it is able to represent the inherent physiological, behavioral, and psychological characteristics by taking into account the emotional, complex perceptual, subjective, and personal phenomenon involving all domains of an individual meanwhile can deal with cultural mechanisms within individual life experience.

Such an approach embodies sensorial information simultaneously that contextualize it within cultural aspects that permeate the human life, when behavior and disability aspects are taken into account. The main focus is to represent the professional, social, and sexual aspects concerned to the fifth vital sign/symptom of medical condition. Professional–social–sexual pain-related disabilities are simultaneously represented in a tridimensional premise space, as depicted in Fig. 24.3, and mapped into an output associated to pain assessment. The 3D Fuzzy PSS pain assessment is represented as IF-THEN *fuzzy rules*, in the general form:

$$\begin{aligned} \mathrm{R}_i : \mathrm{IF} & \left\langle \textit{professional pain} \text{ is } M_{ij_{professional}}^{professional} \right\rangle \text{ AND } \ldots \\ & \left\langle \textit{social pain} \text{ is } M_{ij_{social}}^{social} \right\rangle \text{ AND } \ldots \\ & \left\langle \textit{sexual pain} \text{ is } M_{ij_{sexual}}^{sexual} \right\rangle \\ & \text{THEN } \left\langle \textit{disability pain} \text{ is } N_{ij_{disability-pain}}^{disability-pain} \right\rangle , \end{aligned} \tag{24.1}$$

where the elements $M_{ij(\cdot)}^{(\cdot)}$ and $N_{ij(\cdot)}^{(\cdot)}$ are fuzzy sets (also named *linguistic terms*) partitioning the respective universes of discourse, X_k and Y. The amount of partitions is given by $j(\cdot) = 1,\ldots,m_{(\cdot)}$ such that $M_{j_{(\cdot)}}^{(\cdot)}(x_k) \subset X_k \; \forall k = 1,\ldots,n$ and $N^{disability-pain} \subset Y$. The number of rules is given by $i = 1,\ldots,N_r$. The input vector of the premise is given by $x = [x_1, x_2, x_3]^T$, while the output is associated to y. The

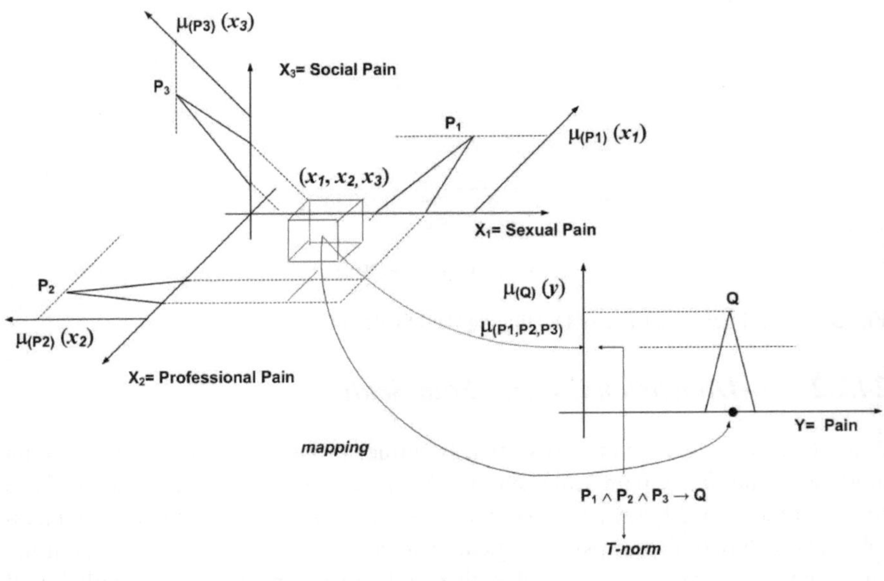

Fig. 24.3 Tridimensional Fuzzy Pain Measurement [4]

input variables are *professional pain* $\in X_1$, *social pain* $\in X_2$, *sexual pain* $\in X_3$ while the output variable is *disability pain* $\in Y$. Resulting system and detailed information is obtained in [4].

24.3 Multi–criteria Fuzzy Pain Assessment for Patients with Musculoskeletal Disorder

The musculoskeletal system is mainly composed of bones (skeleton), muscles, cartilage, tendons, ligaments, and joints. Such a locomotor system is able to perform movements that range from more intense and complex to simple and refined. Human movements are controlled and monitored by the nervous system that, at first, identify the muscles used for a particular motion for, in sequence, generating stimulus that will develop the strength to their activation. The majority of the joint movements act as a lever system, such that each joint presents a range of motion which characterizes an adequate operation and determines their mobility and thus of the human being.

The analysis of movements depends on a correct description of the joint movements. The skeletal muscle has in common with the smooth muscle the composition of the musculoskeletal system but being the only one able to move the body. Characterized as being elastic, the skeletal muscle can be lengthened or shortened by performing different functions that directly depend on the bone structure and a joint component. Together, they are extremely important for achieving an efficient performance of the human body movement [7]. The relation between the body movement and musculoskeletal pain is directly associated to the manner that individuals use their muscles and joints. Their overuse or improper use brings harmful effects to the body, affecting the range of motion and leading individuals to the world of pain.

Another important aspect of musculoskeletal pain concerns the reduction of range of motion, which can generate some temporary loss of function, affecting the social life. As a result of musculoskeletal pain, the range of motion decreases, and may cause a temporary or permanent disability [14]. The musculoskeletal pain is more evident in adults and is the leading cause of chronic pain throughout society, creating an impact on quality of life, interfering with daily activities in 66.6% of patients and thus a public health problem worldwide [11].

The range of motion of the human body occurs due to a complex system of articulated segments in static or dynamic balance. The movement is caused by internal forces acting outside the joint axis causing angular displacement of the segments, and by forces outside the body. This measurement is usually based on records or in verbal descriptors commonly used by patients to describe the pain they are experiencing at the moment.

Mechanical or digital goniometer as well as by digital image processing are alternatives to measure the range of motion. The angle of measurement corresponds to the range of motion. In spite of the mechanism employed for obtaining the range of motion, the perception of pain is approximate and subjective, respectively, due to the imprecision and uncertainty introduced by the mechanism of measurement and the dependence on personal experience and skill of the evaluator, be it the proper patient, be it a healthcare professional. Further, it must be emphasized that when using such classical measurement approaches, the flexion and the extension are information that are most of time analyzed isolatedely instead of intertwined during the clinical assessment.

Subject to various characteristics, musculoskeletal pain implies in subjective and multifactorial measurements that should be took into account for evaluation and treatment [11].

24.3.1 Fuzzy Musculoskeletal Pain Assessment for Patients with Reduction of Motion on the Shoulder Sagittal Plane

The musculoskeletal system encompasses diverse joint movements. The fuzzy musculoskeletal pain assessment is applied for shoulder joint pain measurement, as a practical example, when interested in dealing with reduction of range of motion in the sagittal plane. Such a mathematical and formal proposed approach innovates, first, in aggregating the input variables of range of motion for shoulder extension and shoulder flexion by employing logical connectives and, second, by mapping them into fuzzy pain output classes resulting in a novel mechanism for musculoskeletal pain assessment.

The shoulder joint is a spheroid type, having movements in (*i*) sagittal, (*ii*) frontal, and (*iii*) transverse planes, being one of the most important in human for accomplishing surviving tasks. The shoulder joint is composed of three bones (humerus, scapula, and clavicle), four joints (sternoclavicular, acromioclavicular, glenohumeral, and scapular-thoracic), ligaments that provide stability, and sixteen muscles involved with the shoulder complex system [1].

The movements in the sagittal plane correspond to flexion and extension, while the frontal plane movements concerns abduction and adduction, and in the transverse plane, movements occur perpendicular to the soil. This paper will focus on sagittal plane for flexion–extension (FE) motion, as depicted in Fig. 24.4. Flexion is the bending motion of a bone on the other causing a decrease in joint angle, $\theta_{flexion}$. The normal tour of motion occurs from 0 to 180 degrees. The extension is the movement that occurs inversely to bending. It is the straightening of a bone on the other, causing an increased angle of articulation, $\theta_{extension}$. Its normal movement is from 0 to 45 degrees.

The input variables for the fuzzy sagittal shoulder joint pain assessment are the range of motion for shoulder flexion, X_1, and the range of motion for shoulder extension, X_2, resulting a Cartesian product, $X_1 \times X_2$, related to the input space. The linguistic terms $M^{flexion}_{j_{flexion}}$, and $M^{extension}_{j_{extension}}$, respectively, with $j_{flexion} = j_{extension} = 1,\ldots,5$, yield a set of 25 fuzzy regions in the bidimensional input space. In general, this input space is mapped into an output universe of discourse by using a fuzzy IF-THEN inference mechanism (mapping). The output variable is the quantification of pain (severity of disorder), Y, according to the area of interest, with linguistic terms, $M^{pain/severity}_{j_{pain/severity}}$, such that $j_{pain/severity} = 1,\ldots,5$. All the universes of discourse are equivalent in structure to Fuzzy Qualitative Pain Scale. Each of the input and output universes of discourse can, thus, adopt the same number of partitions. The set of linguistic terms and their associated membership functions are distributed in the universe of discourse for the range of motion for shoulder flexion as $X_1 = [0,220]$, while the universe of discourse for the range of motion for shoulder extension is $X_2 = [0,55]$, and the quantification of pain (severity of disorder) is $Y = [0,10]$.

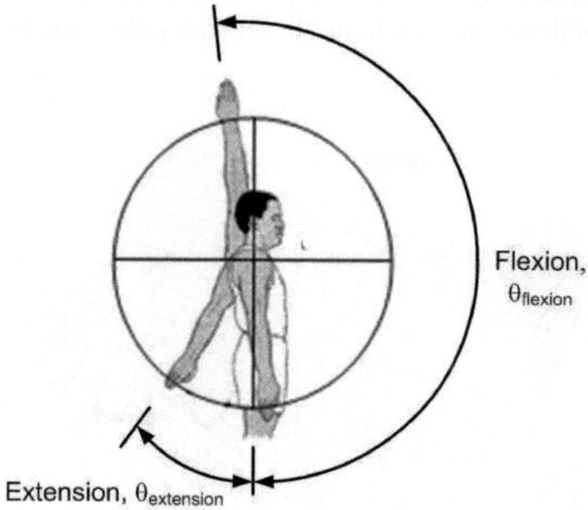

Fig. 24.4 Range of Motion for shoulder flexion and shoulder extension (adapted from [9])

Mamdani inference method is employed to represent the heuristic knowledge to build the fuzzy IF–THEN rule base:

$$
\begin{aligned}
R_1 :\ & \text{IF } \langle \textit{Flexion} \text{ is } \textit{No} \rangle \text{ AND } \langle \textit{Extension} \text{ is } \textit{No} \rangle \\
& \qquad \text{THEN } \langle \textit{Pain / Disorder} \text{ is } \textit{Maximum} \rangle \\
R_2 :\ & \text{IF } \langle \textit{Flexion} \text{ is } \textit{No} \rangle \text{ AND } \langle \textit{Extension} \text{ is } \textit{Light} \rangle \\
& \qquad \text{THEN } \langle \textit{Pain / Disorder} \text{ is } \textit{Maximum} \rangle \\
& \ldots \\
R_{24} :\ & \text{IF } \langle \textit{Flexion} \text{ is } \textit{Maximum} \rangle \text{ AND } \langle \textit{Extension} \text{ is } \textit{Intense} \rangle \\
& \qquad \text{THEN } \langle \textit{Pain / Disorder} \text{ is } \textit{Intense} \rangle \\
R_{25} :\ & \text{IF } \langle \textit{Flexion} \text{ is } \textit{Maximum} \rangle \text{ AND } \langle \textit{Extension} \text{ is } \textit{Light} \rangle \\
& \qquad \text{THEN } \langle \textit{Pain / Disorder} \text{ is } \textit{Normal} \rangle \ .
\end{aligned}
\tag{24.2}
$$

The linguistic terms part the input universes of discourse, *angle of flexion*, $X_1 = \theta_{flexion}$, and *angle of extension*, $X_2 = \theta_{extension}$, respectively, such that for $M_j^{flexion}$

they are $No = \langle 0,0,4.5,40.5\rangle$, $Light = \langle 4.5,40.5,49.5,85.5\rangle$, $Moderate = \langle 49.5,85.5,94.5,130.5\rangle$, $Intense = \langle 94.5,130.5,139.5,175.5\rangle$, and $Maximum = \langle 139.5,175.5,184.5,220\rangle$, while for $M_j^{Extension}$ they are $No = \langle 0,0,1.1, 10.1\rangle$, $Light = \langle 1.1,10.1,12.4,21.4\rangle$, $Moderate = \langle 12.4,21.4,23.6,32.6\rangle$, $Intense = \langle 23.6,32.6,34.9,43.9\rangle$, $Maximum = \langle 34.9,43.9,46.1,55\rangle$. The linguistic terms that part the output universe of discourse, *intensity of pain* (*severity of disorder*), Y, for $M_j^{pain/disorder}$ are $Normal = \langle 0,0,0.3,2.4\rangle$, $Light = \langle 0.3,2.4,2.9,5.1\rangle$, $Moderate = \langle 2.9,5.1,5.7, 7.8\rangle$, $Intense = \langle 5.7,7.8,8.4,10.5\rangle$, and $Maximum = \langle 8.4,9.5,12,12\rangle$. The overlapping of those linguistic terms, in general, yields a graduated and smooth classification.

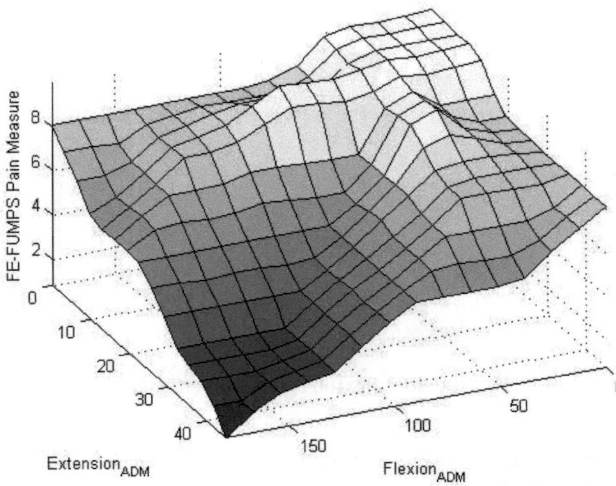

Fig. 24.5 Fuzzy Musculoskeletal Pain Scale (FUMPS) dealing with Flexion–Extension (FE) Shoulder Range of Motion Analysis (FE–FUMPS)

The surface of the fuzzy model corresponding to (24.2) determines the correlation of the range of motion in shoulder flexion and extension when mapped into the severity of pain or disorder as depicted in Fig. 24.5. The surface generated from the fuzzy model corresponds to the decision to stratify the level of pain as well as the disorder severity. The proposed fuzzy model reveals the direct relation between the significance of the pain level and the range of motion achieved by the patient. The last third of each range of motion for shoulder flexion and shoulder extension reach maximum levels of pain, corresponding to the patient functional limitation, affecting the muscle and joint component, as available in [1, 16].

24.3.2 Experimental Results

Experimental data are collected in a random population of patients diagnosed with pain on the shoulder region regardless the kind of medication in use, clinical intervention and phase of pain. This study is approved by the Research Ethics Committees of the University of Taubaté, Brazil (no. 139/11). Patients with no exclusion criteria are included in the present study. They are submitted to evaluation of amplitude of movement concerning shoulder flexion and shoulder extension rating the intensity of the pain according to a classic numeric (rating) pain scale (NRS). The range of motion is obtained by using a mechanical goniometer.

The comparison between the Numerical Rating Scale (NRS) and the proposed Fuzzy Musculoskeletal Pain Scale (FUMPS) dealing with Flexion–Extension (FE) Shoulder Range of Motion Analysis (FE–FUMPS) is available in Table 24.1. Observe that the proposed FE–FUMPS achieves levels of pain close to those reported by the patients when using the NRS. The FE–FUMPS advantages of not being influenced by the subjectivity of the patient's pain perception. In so doing, the proposed approach becomes a more accurate mechanism for pain measurement than those reported by patients because it directly relates pain to its ability to perform free motion.

Table 24.1 Results comparison between the Numerical Rating Scale (NRS) and the proposed Fuzzy Musculoskeletal Pain Scale (FUMPS) dealing with Flexion–Extension (FE) Shoulder Range of Motion Analysis (FE–FUMPS)

Patient	Range of Motion		Pain / disorder	
	Flexion [^{o}]	Extension [^{o}]	NRS	FUMPS
1	160	45	2	2.16
2	160	35	2	2.69
3	150	40	2	2.5
4	145	30	3	3.56
5	140	40	3	2.69
6	100	35	4	4.89
7	100	25	5	4.89
8	90	20	6	5.91
9	65	20	7	7.12
10	55	20	8	8.39

According to results, the fuzzy musculoskeletal pain scale becomes an affordable, simple, fast and comprehensive approach that may be an effective alternative in respect to the subjectivity of the evaluation of musculoskeletal pain.

24.4 Conclusions

The proposed fuzzy decision support system for musculoskeletal pain assessment is characterized by being comprehensive and consistent to clinical practice. Able to assist in decision making and automatically incorporating inaccurate, unclear, vague and partial truths inherently associated with the clinical aspects of pain and the subjectivity present in human nature, such a system presents to be a natural alternative to represent the inherent complexity of pain assessment.

The fuzzy system reveals how it is possible to analyze the subjectivity related to inaccurate and subjective pain perception, and provides an important tool in its measurement, contributing to a better clinical approach. Further, the proposed Fuzzy System Musculoskeletal Pain Assessment advantages by its ability to explain the direct relationships of musculoskeletal pain that are not linguistically well understood and the freedom of movement leading to an effective pain assessment tool.

References

1. Abad, C.C.C., Ito, L.T., Barroso, R., Ugrinowitsch, C., Tricoli, V.: Effect of classic massage in the subjective perception of pain, swelling, range of motion and maximum force after delayed onset muscle soreness induced by exercise. Revista Brasileira de Medicina no Esporte 16(1), 36–40 (2010) (in Portuguese)
2. Abou-Setta, A.M., Beaupre, L.A., Jones, C.A., Rashiq, S., Hamm, M.P., Sadowski, C.A., Menon, M.R.G., Majumdar, S.R., Wilson, D.M., Karkhaneh, M., Wong, K., Mousavi, S.S., Tjosvold, L., Dryden, D.M.: Pain Management Interventions for Hip Fracture: Comparative Effectiveness Review, No. 30. Agency for Healthcare Research and Quality. AHRQ Publication No. 11-EHC022-EF
3. Araujo, E., Miyahira, S.A.: Unidimensional fuzzy pain scale. In: International Conference on Fuzzy Systems, pp. 185–190. FUZZ-IEEE (2009)
4. Araujo, E., Miyahira, S.A.: Tridimensional fuzzy pain assessment. In: IEEE International Conference on Fuzzy Systems, pages pre–print (2011)
5. Bocato, E.S., Araujo, E., Miyahira, S.: Fuzzy system for pain assessment by using api swing and java computational tools. In: Brazilian Congress of Health Informatics, SBIS (2010) (in Portuguese)
6. Convington, E.: Chronic pain management in spine disordersE. Neurologic Clinics 25(2), 539–566 (2007)
7. Enoka, R.M.: Neuro-mechanical bases of Kinesiology. Manole, São Paulo (2000) (in Portuguese)
8. International Association for the Study of Pain. Pain terms: A list with definitions and notes on usage. Pain, 6, 249–252 (1979); recommended by an IASP subcommittee on Taxonomy
9. Hamill, J., Knutzen, K.M.: Biomechanical Basis of Human Movement. Williams & Wilkins, Baltimore (2009)
10. ICSI Health Care Guideline. Assessment and Management of Chronic Pain (2009)
11. Merskey, H., Teasell, R.W.: Problems with Insurance–based Research on Chronic Pain. The Medical Clinics of North-America 91(1), 31–43 (2007)

12. Mullaney, M.J., McHughand, M.P., Johnson, C.P., Tyler, T.F.: Reliability of Shoulder Range of Motion Comparing a Goniometer to a Digital Level. Physiotherapy Theory and Practice 26(5), 327–333 (2010)
13. de Mattos-Pimenta, C.A., de Almeida Lopes Monteiro da Cruz, D.: Tools for Pain Assessment: What's New in Our Midst. Arquivos Brasileiros de Neurocirurgia 17(1), 15–24 (1998)
14. Siqueira, J.T.T., Teixeira, M.J.: Dor orofacial: Diagnóstico, Terapêutica e Qualidade de Vida. Maio, Curitiba (2001)
15. Skevington, S.M.: Investigating the Relationship Between Pain and Discomfort and Quality of Life using the WHOQOL. Pain 76, 395–406 (1998)
16. Stochkendahl, M.J., Christensen, H.W.: Chest Pain in Focal Musculoskeletal Disorders. The Medical Clinics of North-America 94, 259–273 (2010)
17. Teixeira, M.J., Figueiró, J.A.B.: Pain: Epidemiology, Pathophysiology, Assessment, Pain Syndromes and Treatment. Moreira Jńior, São Paulo (2001) (in Portuguese)
18. Zadeh, L.A.: Fuzzy Sets. Information and Control 8, 338–353 (1965)
19. Zadeh, L.A.: A Theory of Approximate Reasoning. In: Hayes, J.E., Michie, D., Mikulich, L.I. (eds.) Machine Intelligence, pp. 149–194. Ellis Horwood Limited, Chinchester (1979)

25

Fuzzy Logic in Diagnostics of Rare Diseases

Tatiana Kiseliova, Maka Korinteli, and Karaman Pagava

25.1 Introduction

Rare disease is any disease that affects a small percentage of the population. There is no single, widely accepted definition for rare diseases (RDs).

In the United States, a rare disease is strictly defined according to prevalence, specifically "any disease or condition that affects less than 200,000 persons in the United States," or about 1 in 1,500 people.

In Japan, the legal definition of a rare disease is one that affects fewer than 50,000 patients in Japan, or about 1 in 2,500 people.

The European Commission on Public Health defines rare diseases as "life-threatening or chronically debilitating diseases which are of such low prevalence that special combined efforts are needed to address them." The term low prevalence is later defined as generally meaning fewer than 1 in 2,000 people. The definitions used in the medical literature and by national health plans are ranging from 1/1,000 to 1/200,000 [9].

About 80 % of rare diseases are of genetic nature. The great majority of the RDs are manifesting in childhood. The specific share of the RD within the children and adolescent morbidity structure is increasing all over the world, particularly, in the developed countries. The precise data are hardly available.

The general practitioners, perhaps, to more extent in developing countries and countries with transitional economy, usually are not well-acquainted with the RDs, and this predetermines the omission of the necessary investigations and vice-versa - the prescription of a multitude of unnecessary and potentially hazardous invasive diagnostic interventions. Because of the rarity of this group of diseases and insufficient implementation of the evidence based medicine principles as well as the absence of special algorithms, the correct diagnose is usually belated; quite frequently it is not made at all. It is noteworthy, that according to the available data, there is no software worldwide (at least within the field of pediatrics), which could be applied for a purposeful diagnostics of clusters of various RDs.

The treatment and, generally, the management of these diseases cannot be considered as adequate and efficient. This fact is particularly jeopardizing the children's

R. Seising and M.E. Tabacchi (Eds.): *Fuzziness and Medicine*, STUDFUZZ 302, pp. 379–399.
DOI: 10.1007/978-3-642-36527-0_25

and adolescents' health. It is also noteworthy that due to the rareness of the RDs, it is not financially reasonable for pharmaceutical companies to produce medicines to treat them; therefore, the relevant research and production are quite limited. Because of the limited number of cases it is quite difficult to establish the efficiency of the therapeutic interventions by employing the classical methods. This fact in its turn indicates the advisability of elaborating new methods and means of treatment and assessing their efficacy [15]. The current situation indicates the gravity of the problem and the necessity to find the ways to solve it, not only in a particular country, but globally as well.

25.2 Description of the Approach

The main goal of our investigation is to elaborate a methodological approach that can be used in computer-assisted diagnosing to help a physician to suspect the RD. This can be a part of an algorithm, to be used as a basis for a computer-assisted medical decision support system. For our purposes we choose the fuzzy logic framework (the reason will be explained later in this section).

We do not consider rare disease's cases when the outstanding symptoms directly exhibit a disease, rather we deal with cases when the RD is masked by a common disease.

We assume, that a process to suspect the RD in a given patient is as follows.

In daily practice, it is very seldom, that a patient will be given an exact diagnosis about the presence of some RD during his/her first visit to a practitioner: "a rare disease has such a low prevalence in a population that a physician in a busy general practice would not expect to see more than one case a year" [27]. Moreover, quite frequently the description of the RD is related to very expensive and invasive lab tests, investigations, etc., and it is not realistic to expect all the patient to undergo such non-standard procedures.

In our approach we assume, that a patient was given a preliminary diagnosis (that could be wrong), but some hesitation about "normality" of the proposed diagnosis was evident. Then a physician would ask a computer system, if there are any deviations from the "normal" (typical) case. If deviations were confirmed by the system, it could be considered as a sign of possible RD.

Thus, a physician (who uses the computer decision-support system) should be alarmed by a computer program about a possible rare disease. Our task is to describe an appropriate algorithm for such computer program, i.e, the program should warn the user about the possible abnormal cases, which are "outside" of the scope of the possible diagnoses of the system. It can be considered as a first step, and the next step might be monitoring incl. performing of additional investigations, using the special search machines in order to decide finally whether we have only atypical case of the common disease or some other diseases, including a rare one.

A search of the RD can be continued in the specific databases. For instance, one can found a description of RDs in the database like ORPHANET [23], some other web portals [5], [22]. A search for an appropriate case can be continued there.

In our approach we use a methodology of fuzzy logic, as the elements of the diagnostic process (symptoms, diagnoses, connections between both) and a diagnostic process itself are mostly described imprecisely and approximately. Moreover, a "normal" disease (with typical clinical picture/course) is not a unique (crisp) concept. A "normal" disease can be also categorized as, for example, confirmed, possible, etc. Thus, we should define deviations from non-uniquely defined "normal" diseases that can be interpreted as a marker of the RD.

In our work we restrict ourselves to a limited number of child/adolescent diseases, particularly, pneumonia, bronchitis, atopic dermatitis, some others.

We obtain a description of these diseases from the experts (manuals): preliminary information about "normal" diseases is summarized in linguistic and numerical form (the details will be given below). This description is done based on the following criteria:

a) *general* properties that include, for example, the following parameters: gender, age, etc.
b) *interior* properties, that include how a patient himself describes his/her state. The problem is that in pediatrics it is difficult to obtain such description from children younger than $5-7$ years old.
c) *exterior* properties are obtained from
   a) persons who observed a child (parents, relatives, etc.)
   b) physician's observation.
   c) lab and instrumental tests.
d) observation of a disease duration and reaction on a treatment.

Subjectivity is present in most of these criteria.

25.3 Preliminaries

25.3.1 Notions and Denotations

As was already discussed [12–14], four components - symptom-disease relation, patient information, patient-disease relation and an inference mechanism with corresponding denotation $\langle R_{SD}, S_p, D_p, \circ \rangle$ - should be defined to describe a medical decision-support system within the fuzzy logic framework.

Let the knowledge base of the proposed decision support system consists of fuzzy $IF-THEN$ rules that describe the relationships between symptoms/signs, test results and findings - for all these medical entities we use a term "symptom/sign" or its abbreviation "S"; and diseases, diagnoses - with denotation "D". Thus, our rules look like "IF S THEN D". Fuzzy relations between symptoms/signs and diseases can be defined as

$$R_{SD} : \Sigma \times \Delta \to [0,1] \tag{25.1}$$

To build these fuzzy relations the crisp sets of patients $\Pi = \{p_1, \ldots, p_r\}$, symptoms/signs $\Sigma = \{s_1, \ldots, s_m\}$ and diseases $\Delta = \{d_1, \ldots, d_n\}$ under consideration are used. For example, Δ can denote more typical child/adolescence diseases in Georgia, Σ are symptoms/signs of these diseases, and Π are investigated patients for the diseases.

It is a formalized representation of the fuzzy IF-THEN rules mentioned above. For example, two types of symptom/sign-disease relations -*confirmation* R^c_{SD} and *occurrence* R^o_{SD} relations - can be used in the knowledge base of a system [4, 8]. These fuzzy relations estimate each symptom/sign-diagnose connection from two perspectives: strength of confirmation (the degree to which a symptom/sign S confirms the presence of disease D) and frequency of occurrence of symptom/sign S with disease D.

These relations can be defined as follows.

$R^o_{SD}(s_i,d_j)$ and $R^c_{SD}(s_i,d_j)$ are derived from relative frequencies, i.e., numerically [8]:

$$R^o_{SD}(s_i,d_j) = f(s_i|d_j) \quad (25.2)$$

and

$$R^c_{SD}(s_i,d_j) = f(d_j|s_i) \quad (25.3)$$

where $f(s_i|d_j) = \frac{f(d_j \cap s_i)}{f(d_j)}$, $f(d_j|s_i) = \frac{f(d_j \cap s_i)}{f(s_i)}$; $f(s_i|d_j)$ is a conditional frequency of s_i given d_j, $f(d_j|s_i)$ is a conditional frequency of d_j given s_i, $f(d_j \cap s_i)$ is the absolute frequency of joint occurrence of d_j and s_i, $f(d_j)$ and $f(s_i)$ are absolute frequencies of d_j and s_i, correspondingly. We call this numerical interpretation.

A linguistic way opens a possibility to estimate relations *occurrence* and *confirmation* R^o_{SD} and R^c_{SD} (linguistic variables) using fuzzy sets (values of linguistic variables), e.g., presented in the Table 25.1.

Table 25.1 Linguistic values

never	very seldom	seldom
sometimes	unspecified	occasionally
often	very often	always

The fuzzy sets (Table 25.1) are defined as mappings from $[0,1]$ to $[0,1]$. An example of a linguistic description of symptom/sign - disease connection is presented in the Table 25.2. Additionally we assume that a negation of a fuzzy set is defined as usual, e.g., $not\ often(x) = 1 - often(x), x \in [0,1]$.

Table 25.2 Linguistic representation of symptom/sign - disease connections

	d_1	d_2	...	d_n
s_1	often	always	...	never
s_2	never	often	...	always
$\vdots$	$\vdots$	$\vdots$		$\vdots$
s_m	often	seldom	...	always

Assume, that linguistic values from Table 25.1 are predefined. In general, fuzzy relations R^o_{SD} and R^c_{SD} can be defined as follows:

$$R^{\{o,c\}}_{SD} : \Sigma \times \Delta \rightarrow \mathscr{F}([0,1]) \qquad (25.4)$$

where $\mathscr{F}([0,1])$ is a power set of $[0,1]$; denotes the set of all ordinary fuzzy sets that can be defined within the universal set $[0,1]$ [16, 17].

Each linguistic value can be defined by an expert [24]. For example, an expert can define a fuzzy set *often* and supports his/her interpretation with the following sentence: symptom/sign and disease meet each other often, if it happens in, approximately, 60%. Here we deal with fuzzy relations of type II [16]. An example of linguistic values from the Table 25.1 as trapezoidal fuzzy sets [16] is shown in the Table 25.5.

Another possibility to define linguistic values is to assign to them an ordered set of numbers from $[0,1]$ as shown, e.g,, in the Table 25.3.

Table 25.3 Representation of linguistic terms as numbers

never	*very seldom*	*seldom*	*sometimes*	*unspecified*	*occasionally*	*often*	*very often*	*always*
0	0.2	0.25	0.4	0.5	0.6	0.75	0.8	1.0

Table 25.4 Representation of linguistic terms as intervals

never	*very seldom*	*seldom*	*sometimes*	*unspecified*	*occasionally*	*often*	*very often*	*always*
[0,.2)	(.2,.25]	(.25,.4]	(.4,.5)	[.5,.5]	(.5,.6]	(.6,.75]	(.75,.8]	(.8,1]

Table 25.5 Representation of linguistic terms as trapezoidal fuzzy sets

never	*very seldom*	*seldom*	*sometimes*	*unspecified*
(0,0,0,0.2)	(0,0.0,0.2,0.25)	(0.0,0.2,0.25,0.4)	(0.2,0.25,0.4,0.5)	(.25,.4,.5,.6)
occasionally	*often*	*very often*	*always*	
(0.4,0.5,0.6,0.75)	(0.5,0.6,0.75,0.8)	(0.6,0.75,0.8,1.0)	(0.75,0.8,1.0,1.0)	

The possibility to define the fuzzy relations as intervals (e.g., presented in the Table 25.4) was discussed in [18]. It is based on the assumption, that different patient settings influence all-purpose consultant systems.

Besides above described fuzzy relations R^o_{SD} and R^c_{SD} there can be another type of a symptom/sign-disease relation due to the expert estimations, e.g., an *exclusion* relation $R^e_{SD} : \Sigma \times \Delta \rightarrow [0,1]$. The value $R^e_{SD}(s_i, d_j)$ indicates the degree in which the present symptom/sign (combination) excludes (or disconfirms) the disease d_j (it is so called negative knowledge [8]). A proposal, that symptoms/signs cannot at the same time confirm and exclude the diagnosis, may lead to the following assumption: $R^e_{SD}(s_i, d_j) = 0$ or (but not "and"!) $R^c_{SD}(s_i, d_j) = 0$ at a given time. Notice, that it is only one of the possible pre-definitions. For example, there might not be enough information about R_{SD} and in that case we may even have $R^c_{SD} = R^e_{SD}$ = some low value (including 0 if there is no information at all about a given disease).

Notice, that the exclusion relation R^e_{SD} was introduced in [8] to define Conorm-Cadiag to be able to establish a correspondence between CADIAG and MYCIN-like systems. CADIAG-like and MYCIN-like are computer assisted medical diagnosis systems for different applications. CADIAG-like systems are based on fuzzy rules and an inference procedure – a composition of fuzzy relations – is applied. MYCIN-like systems use combining functions to calculate the global weights (degrees) of suggested diagnoses [8, 12].

We intend here to show different types of $S-D$ relations, given by an expert as initial information, and we do not discuss a possibility to substitude R^e_{SD} by, for example, $1-R^c_{SD}$.

We may introduce another type of relation $R^t_{SD}(s_i,d_j)$ - *temporal* or *time of manifestation*. This relation shows to which degree it is true that exhibition of a symptom s leads to immediate manifestation of a disease d (or a disease d is manifested after some period of time). Notice, that this relation may be also estimated by linguistic values from Table 25.1.

Thus, it can be seen that relations between symptoms/signs and diseases can be of different type (occurrence, confirmation, exclusion, temporal, etc.). And in general, it depends what information is available, what estimations are given by expert-physicians.

25.3.2 The Patient Information

To use an approximate reasoning mechanism to infer a diagnosis, information about a patient to whom a diagnosis will be established has to be available. Although medical knowledge concerning $S-D$ relationship constitutes one source of imprecision and uncertainty in the diagnostic process, the knowledge concerning the state of the patient constitutes another [16].

Information about patients' symptoms/signs is presented in the form of a fuzzy set $S_p : \Sigma \to [0,1]$, where each element of the fuzzy set S_p shows to which degree it is true, that a patient p has symptom/sign s_i, or a degree of possibility of the presence of the symptom, or its severity; symbol D_p is used for the final diagnosis for a patient p, $D_p : \Delta \to [0,1]$, where each element of the fuzzy set D_p shows to which degree it is true, that a patient p has a given disease d_j, or a degree of possibility with which we can attach each relevant diagnostic label to the patient [16].

In the Section 2 we have described criteria that are used for diseases description. Due to our denotations, these criteria are used for construction of a knowledge-base of type, e.g., R^o_{SD}, R^c_{SD}, R^e_{SD}, R^t_{SD} and also these criteria represent symptoms/signs of a patient to be estimated. Notice, that in our approach we use linguistic scale (Table 25.1) and its simple numerical representation (Table 25.3) for $S-D$ relations and, correspondingly, the same estimations (linguistic and numerical) are assumed for a degree of truth, that a patient p has symptom s_i'. Additionally note, that, although we assume that a state of an investigated patient is described with the same linguistic values (Table 25.1) as $S-D$ relationships, practically often only three of them are used: *always (yes), never (no)* and *unspecified.*

25.3.3 The Inference Mechanism

A max − min composition of fuzzy relations [26, 32] or its generalised version t-conorm-t-norm composition can be used for medical diagnosing. Thus,

$$D_P =_{\text{def}} S_P \circ R_{SD} \tag{25.5}$$

is a composition of a fuzzy set and a fuzzy relation and $\forall d_j \in \Delta$

$$D_P(d_j) =_{\text{def}} \bigvee_{s_i \in \Sigma} \wedge \{S_P(s_i); R_{SD}(s_i, d_j)\} \tag{25.6}$$

where $D_P : \Delta \to [0,1]$ are inferred possible diagnoses for the patient and $\vee$ is a t-conorm, $\wedge$ is a t-norm.

In general, the aggregation operators can be used in this inference mechanism [16].

25.3.4 Interpretation of Inference Results

As can be seen from Section 25.3.3, we have obtained a fuzzy set D_P and with each d_j its membership degree is associated. An appropriate defuzzyfication method allows us to choose the reliable diagnosis. It is one way.

Another possibility ("because of features of physicians' thinking" [4, 8]) is to differentiate in advance several types of inference rules/compositions for a final diagnosis, e.g.,:

- confirmation (by present symptoms/signs): $D_P^1 =_{\text{def}} S_P \circ R_{SD}^c$,
- exclusion (by present symptoms/signs): $D_P^2 =_{\text{def}} S_P \circ (1 - R_{SD}^c)$,
- exclusion (by absent symptoms/signs): $D_P^3 =_{\text{def}} (1 - S_P) \circ R_{SD}^o$,
- possible (by present symptoms/signs): $D_P^4 =_{\text{def}} S_P \circ R_{SD}^o$,
- possible (by present symptoms/signs): $D_P^5 =_{\text{def}} S_P \circ R_{SD}^t$,
- exclusion (by present symptoms/signs): $D_P^6 =_{\text{def}} S_P \circ R_{SD}^e$

The results for different types of a symptom/sign-disease relation have to be interpreted for obtaining the patient(s) diagnosis. For example, a diagnosis d_i is confirmed (by D_P^1) iff there exists a fully present symptom/sign s_j ($S_P(s_j) = 1$) which has full/maximal contribution to the diagnosis, i.e., $R_{SD}^c(s_j, d_i) = 1$. A diagnosis d_i is excluded by a present symptom/sign (by D_P^2) iff there exists a fully present symptom/sign s_j ($S_P(s_j) = 1$) which has 0 (i.e. negative) contribution to the diagnosis, i.e., $R_{SD}^c(s_j, d_i) = 0$. A diagnosis d_i is excluded by an absent symptom/sign (by D_P^3) iff there exists a fully absent symptom/sign s_j ($S_P(s_j) = 0$) which has full/maximal occurrence for the diagnosis, i.e., $R_{SD}^o(s_j, d_i) = 1$.

Note, that an estimation of each diagnosis (under the presence of R^c_{SD}, R^o_{SD}) from three perspectives (confirmed, excluded, possible) just defined in this section, depends on the choice of a designer. In general, it can be also accepted degrees of exclusion or confirmation, i.e., the reals between 0 and 1.

If an exclusion relation R^e_{SD} is defined then an excluded diagnosis: $D^e_p =_{\text{def}} S_p \circ R^e_{SD}$.

The final diagnosis (a *total* degree) under the presence of the exclusion relation can be calculated as follows:

$$D^{tot}_p(d_j) =_{\text{def}} D^1_p(d_j) \oplus -D^6_p(d_j) \tag{25.7}$$

where $\oplus$ is a group operation with particular properties [8, 12]. Thus, for every diagnosis its confirmation is decreased according to its exclusion, represented as negative confirmation. Notice, that the group operator $\oplus$ is defined on $[-1,1]$ and it should be used in accordance with definition of fuzzy relations on $[0,1]$.

Another possibility, we may include in our set of possible diagnostic hypotheses for patient p any diseases d_j $j = 1,\ldots,n$ such that inequality

$$0.5 < \max\{D^4_p(d_j), D^1_p(d_j)\} \tag{25.8}$$

is satisfied.

Let us summarize. Several possibilities to infer a diagnosis have been described above: first, a diagnosis can be chosen by a defuzzyfication method from (25.6); second, all $d_j \in \Delta$ can be classified in the following classes - confirmed, excluded, and possible - and, third, a total degree can be found due to (25.7), where each element of the fuzzy set D_p shows to which degree it is true, that a patient p has disease d_j.

25.4 How to Suspect a Rare Disease

Working with a decision-support system, a physician expects from a computer program a tip, a help, what diagnosis it can be for a patient at hand. In this way, the system should alarm if some things are outside of its normal functioning, i.e., if the case is neither confirmed nor possible, for example; or, the total degree from (25.7) has "strange" values, or (25.8) is not satisfied. Thus, such behaviour of a system could be considered as a sign of a possible RD.

Our approach is based on the assumption, that to be able to suspect the RD, the computer program should fix deviations from the "normal"(typical) case. For example, one patient was diagnosed "Gastroesophageal reflux", and another patient was assigned with the diagnosis "Acute poststreptococcal Glomerulonephritis". But a physician hesitated about the diagnoses. Then a physician asked a computer system to estimate deviations from the "normal case", presented in the knowledge base (Table 25.6, Table 25.7) relatively to the exhibition of patient's symptoms/signs. If the estimation (as a result of applying the inference procedure described in the previous sections) showed, that a case in hand was excluded, or, neither confirmed nor possible, for example, a sign of non-normality existed. If it showed, that the case was at least possible or even confirmed, physician's opinion was supported.

Another possible criteria to estimate deviations are discussed in Section 25.4.1.

Our approach naturally mimics the behaviour of a physician making diagnoses - s/he first checks the common (normal) diagnoses and if they are not confirmed - continues to surf among the RDs. Note, that this approach is considered when there are no outstanding symptoms/signs for the RD, but rather the RD being masked as a common disease. In this case none of physicians starts to look for the RD right from the beginning. RDs are encountered very rarely, thus it is rational to begin diagnostic with considering of common diseases. First, the normal cases are taken into consideration, some kind of preliminary separation should be done. Afterwards, the monitoring of the proposed disease is undergone and then the final diagnosis is established. We follow this line to model our approach.

Table 25.6 Possible degrees for "normal" disease GER

	Gastroesophageal reflux (GER) in infants and young children
crying and/or irritability	very often
Apnea	seldom
bradycardia	seldom
Poor appetite	sometimes
Vomiting	often
Wheezing	some times
Stridor	often
Weight loss or poor growth	seldom
Recurrent pneumonitis	seldom
Sore throat	sometimes
Chronic cough	seldom
Bilious or forceful vomiting	seldom
Hematemesis or hematochezia	seldom
concomitant diarrhea	very seldom
Abdominal tenderness or distension	as a rule no

It is known [8], that the results of rule-based systems, considered in this paper, are based on the compositionality where effects (contributions) of the rules are composed and a numerical result is attached to the diagnosis. We relay on this compositionality (although it has been undergone a criticism by several authors [8]), because such systems are well performed systems [25]. Recently, there are attempts to introduce a firm mathematical (logical) formalization in such systems to be able to manage the propositions reasonably [30].

Let us show on examples, how to alarm the RD. It is obvious that conclusions about the patient's diagnosis with a help of a computer program is made based on the information available, in particular, what initial information is contained in

Table 25.7 Possible degrees for a "normal" disease Acute poststreptococcal Glomerulonephritis (APG)

	Acute poststreptococcal Glomerulonephritis (APG)
Significant hypertension	not very often
Significant edema	not very often
Significant abdominal pain	some times
Abdominal complaints	seldom
Recurrence of clinical signs	very seldom
Massive proteinuria in the beginning	seldom
Leukocytosis	some times
Hyaline and/or granular casts in urine	almost always

the knowledge base and what information about a patient at hand we have. In the following section we consider how to suspect the RD under the presence of different initial information, in our denotation R^o_{SD}, R^c_{SD}, R^e_{SD} or R^t_{SD}.

25.4.1 Under the Presence of R^o_{SD}, R^c_{SD}, R^e_{SD}, R^t_{SD}

We illustrate the following description by examples. Assume, that a knowledge base contains R^o_{SD} as, for example, in the Table 25.8 and corresponding numerical form (due to the scale Table 25.3) is in the Table 25.9. In this case $\Delta = \{d_1, d_2\}$, $\Sigma = \{s_1, s_2, \ldots, s_6\}$. We assume that the RD is not in the knowledge base, it means, that it is not in Δ. Notice, that technically we can synthesize the initial tables (Table 25.6, Table 25.7, Table 25.8) within one table similar to Table 25.2. Actually, we assume, that a physician has already established a diagnosis (one from the Δ, without a help of computer system), but has some hesitations. In this case s/he checks him/herself on a particular diagnosis, maybe on two, as, for example, considered in the Table 25.8.

First assume, that the process of inference is presented in the usual way (see (25.6)). As was discussed above (see Section 25.3.4), the results of a diagnostic process can be classified in confirmed, excluded and possible diagnoses.

As we speak about the RD, excluded and possible diagnoses are a subject of interest for us: we consider how "far" is this case from the common representation.

For example, if after an inference process all of the considered diagnoses from Δ are classified as excluded (due to our classification, done preliminary), it can be considered as a sign for the RD for the case at hand: a patient possibly has the RD.

As we have seen from Section 25.3.4 excluded diagnoses are defined if a symptom is fully present/absent with a corresponding full occurrence/absent of occurrence. Simply speaking, at least one element of the Table 25.9 should be 1 or 0 and at least one membership degree of fuzzy set S_P should be 1 or 0 as well. It means,

Table 25.8 Linguistic descriptions for "normal" diseases *Bronchitis/Pneumonia*

	Bronchitis	*Pneumonia*
wheezing	sometimes	occasionally
breathlessness	very seldom	often
anosmia	seldom	seldom
fever	sometimes	often
sinusitis	sometimes	sometimes
chronic otitis	seldom	seldom

Table 25.9 Corresponding numerical descriptions for "normal" diseases Bronchitis and Pneumonia (Table 25.8)

	d_1	d_2
s_1	0.4	0.6
s_2	0.2	0.75
s_3	0.25	0.25
s_4	0.4	0.75
s_5	0.4	0.4
s_6	0.25	0.25

that, to define such case, we need a crisp information. It is a clear situation, but is not always a case.

The difficulty to suspect the RD is because of its symptomatic similarity to the "normal cases". Therefore, another alarm can be represented by possible diagnoses. If a physician has enough experience with a computer program, s/he usually has been working, and s/he mentions that the values for possible diagnoses are much below or much above the usual representation, it can be also the sign of alarm "a rare disease" for a physician.

We need to define appropriate operations and thresholds (that allow to detect a deviation from the "normal" case). If we take max-min composition of fuzzy relations (25.6), it restricts the maximum membership degree of possible diseases for a patient by values in Table 25.9. For example, if a patient at hand has

$$S_p^1 = \{(s_1, 0.4), (s_2, 0.2), (s_3, 0.25), (s_4, 0.4), (s_5, 0.4), (s_6, 0.25)\} \tag{25.9}$$

the possible diagnosis d_1 has the membership degree 0.4 (see (25.11)). If a patient at hand has

$$S_p^2 = \{(s_1, 1.0), (s_2, 1.0), (s_3, 0.2), (s_4, 0.25), (s_5, 0.2), (s_6, 0.2)\} \tag{25.10}$$

the possible diagnosis d_1 has the membership degree 0.4 as well.

Table 25.10 Linguistic and numerical descriptions of a rare disease *Primary Ciliary Diskinesia*

	Primary Ciliary Diskinesia	d_3
wheezing	often	0.75
breathlessness	often	0.75
anosmia	often	0.75
fever	often	0.75
sinusitis	very often	0.8
chronic otitis	often	0.75

$$D_p(d_1) = \max \left\{ \begin{array}{l} \min\{0.4, 0.4\} \\ \min\{0.2, 0.2\} \\ \min\{0.25, 0.25\} \\ \min\{0.4, 0.4\} \\ \min\{0.4, 0.4\} \\ \min\{0.25, 0.25\} \end{array} \right\} = 0.4 \tag{25.11}$$

This standard $\max - \min$ composition in our case guarantees that the degree of occurrence can be less than 0.4, but not more. If we take the *absolute difference* (for two numbers a and b their *absolute difference* is defined as $|a-b|$) instead of min-operation (max-operation remains unchanged) we obtain more flexibility to detect deviations. For example, for S_p^1 the membership degree of d_1 in this case is 0 and for S_p^2 we obtain 0.8. If instead of the *max* operator we take another aggregation operator, such as the *arithmetic mean* of deviations (the *arithmetic mean* of $a_1, a_2, \dots, a_n$ is $\frac{a_1+a_2+\dots+a_n}{n}$), for d_1 in the case of S_p^1 we obtain 0 as well and 0.3 in the case of S_p^2. We interpret 0 as a sign of most believable diagnosis, and every deviation from 0 points less believable diagnosis. The question is, as always in applications, how to detect a threshold, under (or above) which a suspicious of the RD arises. If we take *max-absolute difference* composition of S_p and R_{SD} and a result is different from 0, the final value shows that at least one symptom/sign differs from the normal case, but does not say anything about the rest of symptoms. When the RD can be pointed by a representative symptom (i.e., such symptom which presence/absence is a sure sign of the non-normality of a diagnosis, as was mentioned above, outstanding symptoms/signs) max- *absolute difference* is suitable.

The *mean-absolute difference* composition of S_p and R_{SD} shows the mean value of all deviations. As it is often with RDs, they are described with the same symptoms/signs as "normal" diseases and only a certain deviation can point the RD, the application of *mean-absolute difference* composition of S_p and R_{SD} seems to be reasonable. Notice, that in general, $p - mean$ and/or other distance metrics can be considered. We can also instead of *absolute difference* operation consider *prod* operation.

To continue to discuss a question about a threshold, let extend our example and assume, that a description of a rare disease Primary Ciliary Diskinesia is available and differs from the normal Bronchitis, Pneumonia (see Table 25.8) linguistically and numerically as presented in the Table 25.10. We choose this example only for illustration, to show deviations of a "normal" case from a rare case, recalling, that our approach is to suspect the RD.

Due to the *mean-absolute difference* composition a possible degree for d_3 under the presence of S_p^1 is 0.44 and under the presence of S_p^2 is 0.45.

Let us see values for d_1, d_2 if a patient has the complete picture of a rare disease *Primary Ciliary Diskinesia*, i.e.,

$$S_p^3 = \{(s_1, 0.75), (s_2, 0.75), (s_3, 0.75, (s_4, 0.75), (s_5, 0.8), (s_6, 0.75)\}$$

The possible degrees for d_1, d_2 under S_p^3 are 0.44 and 0.28 correspondingly.

The possible degrees for d_1, d_2 and d_3 under S_p^1, S_p^2, S_p^3 are presented in the Table 25.11 and Table 25.12.

Table 25.11 Possible degrees for "normal" diseases

	d_1	d_2
S_p^1	0.0	0.18
S_p^2	0.31	0.24
S_p^3	0.44	0.28

Table 25.12 Possible degrees for the RD

	d_3
S_p^1	0.47
S_p^2	0.45
S_p^3	0.0

For this particular example 0.25 can be chosen as a threshold to point a suspicion of the RD, i.e., if all numbers in one string in the Table 25.11 are above 0.25 a physician should think about "non-normality" of a possible diagnosis for a patient at hand. It means, that we found an approach to suspect the RD if the diagnoses from the initially defined list seems to be possible. The choice of a threshold remains on experts. There are many ways to formalize this procedure [7, 11, 20], and what approach to use is a subject of a separate investigation.

It can be argued that one number, as a threshold, does not reflect a flexibility in diagnostics: interval- and fuzzy sets estimations of linguistic expressions show more flexibility for the RD diagnostic problem.

Several additional ways to warn non-normality of a diseases can be added. In some systems a possibility of diagnostic contradictions and not generated diagnoses are predefined: in the first case a diagnosis is confirmed and excluded at the same time, whereas in the second case the membership value of each disease in the set of confirmed diagnosis is below the predefined threshold: $0 < D_p(d_j) < \varepsilon$. If all investigated diseases d_j from Δ are classified as diagnostic contradictions and/or not generated diagnoses, then a suspicion of the RD exists.

In these situations a physician that is working with such computer-assisted system should start to do monitoring of the supposed disease and look for a particular diagnosis (As was already told above, this search can be done in the specific databases [5, 22, 23]).

If the available initial information contains R^e_{SD} and R^c_{SD} and the total degree of a diagnosis is calculated as was defined in (25.7), then the following observation can be done. If the total degree is not much different from meanings of R^e_{SD}, that can be considered as an alarm of the RD.

25.4.2 A Comparison with Mamdani and TSK Methods of Fuzzy Inference Process

Let us make several remarks concerning the proposed *mean-absolute difference* inference mechanism and well-known fuzzy inference methods such as Mamdani [19] and Takagi-Sugeno-Kang (TSK)[29]. The main difference between the Mamdani and TSK methods lies in the consequent of fuzzy rules. Mamdani fuzzy systems use fuzzy sets as rule consequent whereas TSK fuzzy systems employ linear functions of input variables as rule consequent. All the existing results on fuzzy systems as universal approximators deal with Mamdani fuzzy systems only and no result is available for TSK fuzzy systems with linear rule [28]. Let us consider the Mamadani inference process in a simplified form as it shown below, using denotations introduced in this paper.

$$\begin{aligned}
&\mathfrak{R}_1 : IF\ S_1 THEN\ D_1\\
&also\\
&\mathfrak{R}_2 : IF\ S_2 THEN\ D_2\\
&\text{fact: } s_0\\
&-----------\\
&\text{consequence: } D
\end{aligned}$$

In Mamdani inference fuzzy implication is considered as min operator, *also* is interpreted as max operator.

Moreover, the following operations are predefined:

- The firing levels of the rules

$$\alpha_1 = S_1(s_0),\ \alpha_2 = S_2(s_0)$$

- the individual rule outputs are obtained by

$$D_1'(d) = (\alpha_1 \wedge D_1(d)),\ D_2'(d) = (\alpha_2 \wedge D_2(d))$$

- The overall system output:

$$D(d) = D_1'(d) \vee D_2'(d) = (\alpha_1 \wedge D_1(d)) \vee (\alpha_2 \wedge D_2(d)))$$

- Any defuzzification method to obtain a deterministic control action.

In our case we have already formal representation of rule-base as R^o_{SD}, R^c_{SD}, R^e_{SD}, or R^t_{SD}, so we do not construct these relations, they are given by experts. If D_2 coinsides with D_1, in particular case, and S_1, S_2 and $s_0 = S_p$ are estimated by linguistic terms (Table 25.1) and their numerical equavalent (Table 25.3), the firing levels of the rules and individual rule outputs are substituted by the following expressions: $D_1' = (S_p \wedge R_{S_1D_1})$, $D_1'' = (S_p \wedge R_{S_2D_1})$ and $D = D_1' \vee D_1''$. If S_1 and S_2 are fuzzy sets (see Table 25.5) and S_p is a singleton, a fuzzification is a necessary step of Mamdani case. If S_p is a triangle or trapezoidal fuzzy set, max and min operations are used to find the individual rule outputs. Thus, a step with firing levels of the rules is, in general, calculated using max and min operators and this as usually (see, for example, fuzzy Matlab Toolbox) predefined in fuzzy control systems, mostly using Mamdani and TSK inference process.

25.5 Simulation with Fuzzy Markup Language

We have done a simulation of proposed approach with the help of Fuzzy Markup Language (FML) [1, 2, 31]. Fuzzy Markup Language is a XML-based domain-specific language proposed by Acampora and Loia [2] whose main aim is to model fuzzy systems by directly dealing with fuzzy concepts, fuzzy rules and fuzzy inference engines [8]. In the last years, FML (Fuzzy Markup Language) is emerging as one of the most efficient and useful language to define a fuzzy control thanks to its capability of modeling Fuzzy Logic Controllers in a human-readable and hardware independent way, i.e., the so-called Transparent Fuzzy Controllers (TFCs) [3]. In particular, it is used to model two well-known kind of fuzzy controllers: Mamdani and Takagi-Sugeno-Kang (TSK).

We show how FML mechanism can be adjusted to suspect the RD [1]. Due to the discusion from Section 25.4.2 some adjustments of FML to the given problem are needed.

Using results discussed in the Section 25.4.1, remarks from the Section 25.4.2 the rule-base of six input variables (wheezing, breathlessness, anosmia, fever, sinusitis, chronic otitis) and two output variables (Bronchitis and Pneumonia) is presented as it is shown in the Figure 25.1.

Results of execution of FML under S_p^1 (see (25.9)) for d_1 (Bronchitis) is presented in the Figure 25.2.

In the Listing 25.1 a portion of the FML-based fuzzy controller to suspect the RD is presented.

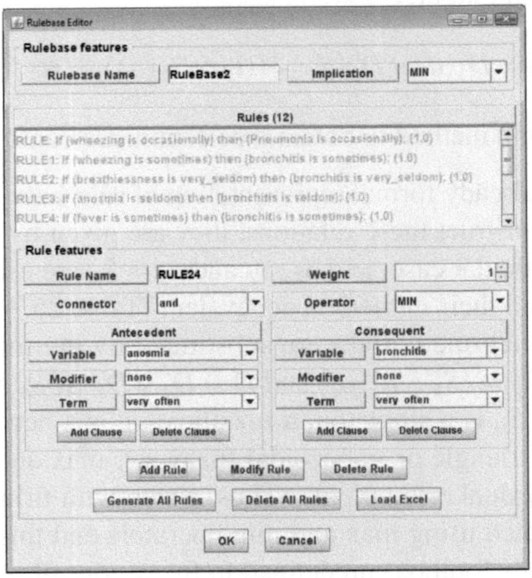

Fig. 25.1 12 rules describing relation of six symptoms and two diseases in FML

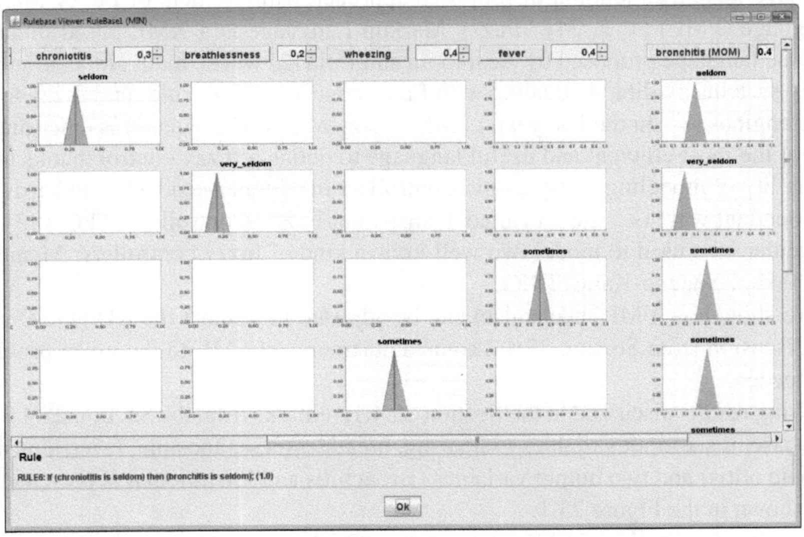

Fig. 25.2 Results of execution of FML under S_p^1 for d_1

```xml
<?xml version="1.0" encoding="UTF-8"?>
<FuzzyController name="Mamdani_controller" ip="127.0.0.1">
    <KnowledgeBase>
        <FuzzyVariable name="wheezing" domainleft="0.0" domainright="1.0" scale=""
                                        type="input">
            <FuzzyTerm name="always" complement="false">
                <TriangularShape Param1="0.8" Param2="0.9" Param3="1.0"/>
            </FuzzyTerm>
            <FuzzyTerm name="never" complement="false">
                <TriangularShape Param1="0.0" Param2="0.1" Param3="0.2"/>
            </FuzzyTerm>
            <FuzzyTerm name="occasionally" complement="false">
                <TriangularShape Param1="0.5" Param2="0.6" Param3="0.7"/>
            </FuzzyTerm>
            <FuzzyTerm name="often" complement="false">
                <TriangularShape Param1="0.6" Param2="0.7" Param3="0.8"/>
            </FuzzyTerm>
            <FuzzyTerm name="seldom" complement="false">
                <TriangularShape Param1="0.2" Param2="0.3" Param3="0.4"/>
            </FuzzyTerm>
            <FuzzyTerm name="sometimes" complement="false">
                <TriangularShape Param1="0.3" Param2="0.4" Param3="0.5"/>
            </FuzzyTerm>
            <FuzzyTerm name="unspecified" complement="false">
                <TriangularShape Param1="0.4" Param2="0.5" Param3="0.6"/>
            </FuzzyTerm>
            <FuzzyTerm name="very_often" complement="false">
                <TriangularShape Param1="0.7" Param2="0.8" Param3="0.9"/>
            </FuzzyTerm>
            <FuzzyTerm name="very_seldom" complement="false">
                <TriangularShape Param1="0.1" Param2="0.2" Param3="0.3"/>
            </FuzzyTerm>
        </FuzzyVariable>
        ......
        <FuzzyVariable name="bronchitis" domainleft="0.0" domainright="1.0"
                                        scale="" defaultValue="0.0" accumulation="MEAN"
                                        defuzzifier="MOM" type="output">
            <FuzzyTerm name="always" complement="false">
                <TriangularShape Param1="0.8" Param2="0.9" Param3="1.0"/>
            </FuzzyTerm>
            <FuzzyTerm name="never" complement="false">
                <TriangularShape Param1="0.0" Param2="0.1" Param3="0.2"/>
            </FuzzyTerm>
            <FuzzyTerm name="occasionally" complement="false">
                <TriangularShape Param1="0.5" Param2="0.6" Param3="0.7"/>
            </FuzzyTerm>
            <FuzzyTerm name="often" complement="false">
                <TriangularShape Param1="0.6" Param2="0.7" Param3="0.8"/>
            </FuzzyTerm>
            <FuzzyTerm name="seldom" complement="false">
                <TriangularShape Param1="0.2" Param2="0.3" Param3="0.4"/>
            </FuzzyTerm>
            <FuzzyTerm name="sometimes" complement="false">
                <TriangularShape Param1="0.3" Param2="0.4" Param3="0.5"/>
            </FuzzyTerm>
            <FuzzyTerm name="unspecified" complement="false">
                <TriangularShape Param1="0.4" Param2="0.5" Param3="0.6"/>
            </FuzzyTerm>
            <FuzzyTerm name="very_often" complement="false">
                <TriangularShape Param1="0.7" Param2="0.8" Param3="0.9"/>
            </FuzzyTerm>
            <FuzzyTerm name="very_seldom" complement="false">
                <TriangularShape Param1="0.1" Param2="0.2" Param3="0.3"/>
            </FuzzyTerm>
        </FuzzyVariable>
        ......
    </KnowledgeBase>
    <RuleBase name="RuleBase1" andMethod="MIN" orMethod="MAX"
                    activationMethod="MIN" type="mamdani">
        <Rule name="RULE1" connector="and" operator="MIN" weight="1.0">
            <Antecedent>
                <Clause>
                    <Variable>wheezing</Variable>
                    <Term>sometimes</Term>
                </Clause>
            </Antecedent>
            <Consequent>
                <Clause>
                    <Variable>bronchitis</Variable>
                    <Term>sometimes</Term>
                </Clause>
            </Consequent>
        </Rule>
        ........
    </RuleBase>
</FuzzyController>
```

Listing 25.1 FML code to model a portion of the FML-based fuzzy controller to suspect a rare disease

25.6 Concluding Discussion and Future Development

Whenever possible, standard methodological approaches should be applied in the design and analysis of a clinical trial that warrant adequate informative value. However, there are circumstances when the number of experimental subjects is unavoidably small. In such circumstances it is justified to consider abandoning standard statistical methodology in place of alternative approaches [6].

The problem to suspect the RD (in particular, in pediatrics) with a help of computer - assisted system is an important problem and till now it was not investigated well enough. This problem is connected with the absence, insufficiency, uncertainty and imprecision of the information and, therefore, belongs to the category of problems, that can be solved by fuzzy logic approaches.

Our main idea to suspect the RD is based on the assumption, that the deviation from a "normal" disease is a sign to warn the RD. Thus, adequate acquaintance with normal diseases leads to a recognition of the RD. We suppose, that a physician has already established a preliminary diagnosis for a patient, but s/he hesitates about its correcteness. Then a physician, based on the patient's data, checks the deviations from the "normal" cases, and if these deviations reach certain level, a suspicion of the RD arises, i.e., our approach is not for final diagnostic, the main aim of proposed algorithm is to raise suspicion on an abnormality of the common diseases, consequently on a possibility of RD.

We assume that RDs are not in the knowledge base of a decision support computer system, that we have developed. If a suspicious of the RD arises, a user can search for in an appropriate database [5, 22, 23], where several thousand of RDs are described. Notice that because of immense number of RDs in WWW data banks, it seems to be reasonable to choose an appropriate subsets for certain regions/countries (e.g., for Georgia).

"Normal" diseases is not a crisp concept. And recognition of "normal" diseases is a subject of investigation of many researches dealing with a problem of decision making in medicine. A "normal" disease can be classified into different categories such as possible, excluded, confirm and some others. These classification depends, in general, on the initial information available. In the paper we have investigated, under which conditions these classifications are not a case. We use an aggregation operators based approximate reasoning mechanism, in particular, *mean-absolute difference* composition. Such composition reflects our intent to deal with deviations from normal cases. For example, if all elements from Δ are considered as excluded, or the value of membership of a diagnoses in the class of possible diagnoses is less than the a priory defined threshold, then it is at the border of possible and non-possible diagnoses. Thus, once again, if we know what do the "normal" diseases imply and how they are exhibited, we have investigated in existing systems the cases of the "abnormal" exhibition.

We illustrate our approach with examples from daily practice - more or less sufficient. It would be better to have the full list of deviations and their evaluation. But it will be rather difficult and time-consuming job because of insufficient information about RDs. Two directions of future investigations for RDs recognition can be outlined here: rare event simulation [21] and class imbalance problems [10].

The obtained results would facilitate the optimisation of RDs management in children and adolescents, particularly in terms of a substantial improve in the diagnostics and treatment. Application of fuzzy logic approaches provide a significant input in clinical medicine and particularly in pediatrics. In our opinion, it would be quite useful for further perfection of the children and adolescent health care system improvement.

The following categories of population should be considered as the beneficiaries of this research: up to 5-6% of children population, who might have some RD, their family members and care-givers. From the scientific point of view, the creation of the management algorithms based on new approaches as well as the receipt of new evidence in the area of the public health care, in particular, for resolving the RDs related problems, would be a great novelty. The obtained materials could be used as a database for health care management, for conducting a pre-marketing research and clinical trials by pharmaceutical companies in order to establish the efficiency of some medicines.

Acknowledgement. This work was supported by Science and Technology Center in Ukraine and Sh. Rustaveli National Foundation, Grant STCU-GNSF #5015; Sh. Rustaveli National Foundation and Ministry of Education and Science of Georgia, Grant GNSF/ST08/6-460,

References

1. Acampora, G., Kiseliova, T., Pagava, K., Vitiello, A.: Towards Application of FML in Suspicion of Non-Common Diseases. In: 2011 IEEE International Conference on Fuzzy Systems, Taipei, Taiwan, pp. 2073–2079 (2011)
2. Acampora, G., Loia, V.: Fuzzy Control Interoperability and Scalability for Adaptive Domotic Framework. IEEE Transactions on Industrial Informatics 1(2), 97–111 (2005)
3. Acampora, G., Loia, V., Vitiello, A.: Enhancing Transparent Fuzzy Controllers through Temporal Concepts: An Application to Computer Games. In: 2010 International Conference on Technologies and Applications of Artificial Intelligence, pp. 405–412 (2010)
4. Adlassnig, K.-P., Kolarz, G.: CADIAG-II: Computer-assisted Medical Diagnosis using Fuzzy Subsets. In: Gupta, M.M., Sanchez, E. (eds.) Approximate Reasoning in Decision Analysis, pp. 495–505. North Holland Publishing Company (1982)
5. Children's r.a.r.e disease network, `http://www.crdnetwork.org/`
6. de la Paz, M.P., Groft, S.C. (eds.): Rare Diseases Epidemiology. Springer (2010)
7. Grzymala-Busse, J.W.: Managing Uncertainty in Expert Systems. The Kluwer International Series in Engineering and Computer Science. Kluwer Academic Publishers, Boston (1991)
8. Daniel, M., Hájek, P., Nguyen, H.P.: CADIAG-2 and MYCIN-like systems. Artificial Intelligence in Medicine 9, 241–259 (1997)

9. Internet Portals: http://www.siope.eu/SIOPE-EU/English/SIOPE-EU/Advocacy-Activities/Rare-Diseases/page.aspx/148, Rare Disease Act of 2002, Rare diseases: what are we talking about?, "Useful Information on Rare Diseases from an EU Perspective". European Commission (retrieved May 19, 2009). "Rare Diseases: Understanding This Public Health Priority". European Organisation for Rare Diseases (EURORDIS) (November 2005) (retrieved May 16, 2009)
10. Japkowicz, N.: Learning from Imbalance Data Sets: A comparison of Various Solutions. In: Japkowicz, N. (ed.) AAAI 2000 Workshop on Learning from Imbalanced Data Sets, AAAI Press (2000)
11. Kandel, A.: Fuzzy Expert Systems. CRC Press, Boca Raton (1991)
12. Kiseliova, T.: A theoretical comparison of Disco and CADIAG-II-like systems for medical diagnoses. Kybernetika 42(6), 723–748 (2006)
13. Kiseliova, T., Pagava, K.: New approach to estimate different drugs and/or other medical interventions effectiveness based on fuzzy logic principles. Georgia Medical News 3(156), 65–68 (2008)
14. Kiseliova, T., Pagava, K.: Modelling uncertainty in the connection of socio-economic factors and health-related behavior of adolescents in Georgia. In: Proceedings of the 28th North American Fuzzy Information Processing Society Annual Conference (NAFIPS 2009), Cincinnati, OH, USA, pp. 41–46 (2009)
15. Kiseliova, T., Pagava, K., Korinteli, I., Maka, K., Shonvadze, D.: Purposefulness of using fuzzy logic approaches in the rare disease clinical trials. Georgian Medical News 193(4), 22–24 (2011)
16. Klir, G.J., Yuan, B.: Fuzzy Sets and Fuzzy Logic. Theory and Applications. Prentice Hall PTR (1995)
17. Lee, K.H.: First Course on Fuzzy Theory and Applications. Springer (2005)
18. Leitich, H., Adlassnig, K.-P., Kolarz, G.: Evaluation of two different models of semi-automatic knowledge acquisition for the medical consultant system CADIAG-II/RHEUMA. Artificial Intelligence in Medicine 25, 215–225 (2002)
19. Ebrahim, M., Assilian, S.: An experiment in linguistic synthesis with a fuzzy logic controller. Int. J. Man Mach. Stud. 7(1), 1–13 (1975)
20. Naylon, C.: How to build an inferencing engine. In: Forsyth, R. (ed.) Expert Systems, Principles and Case Studies, pp. 85–105. Champman and Hall (1989)
21. Newman, R.L., Foyle, D.C.: Test Scenarios for Rare Events. In: Twelfth International Symposium on Aviation Psychology, pp. 873–882. Wright State University, Dayton (2003)
22. NORD-National Organisation for Rare Disorder, http://www.rarediseases.org/search/rdblist.html
23. The Portal for Rare Diseases and Orphan Drugs, http://www.orpha.net/consor/cgi-bin/index.php?lng=EN
24. Phagava, H.: Numerical estimates of probability expressions to be used in medical expert programs. Georgian Medical News 2, 130–134 (2002)
25. Sakaguchi, S., Takifuji, K., Arita, S., Yamaue, H.: Development of an early Diagnostic System using Fuzzy Theory for Postoperative Infection in Patients with Gastric Cancer. Digestive Surgery 21, 210–214 (2004)
26. Sanchez, E.: Medical diagnosis and composite fuzzy relations. In: Gupta, M.M., Ragade, R.K., Yager, R.R. (eds.) Advances in Fuzzy Set Theory and Applications, pp. 437–444. North-Holland, New York (1979)
27. Sleep-EVAL Research, http://www.sleepeval.com/fuzzy_logic.htm

28. Sivanandam, S.N., Sumathi, S., Deepa, S.N.: Introduction to Fuzzy Logic using MATLAB. Springer, Heidelberg (2007)
29. Michio, S.: Industrial Applications of Fuzzy Control. Elsevier, Amsterdam (1985)
30. Vetterlein, T., Agata, C.: On the (Fuzzy) Logical Content of CADIAG-2. Fuzzy Sets and Systems 161, 1941–1958 (2010)
31. Wang, M.H., Lee, C.S., Hsieh, K.L., Hsu, C.Y., Acampora, G., Chang, C.: Ontology-based Multi-agents for Intelligent Healthcare Applications. Journal of Ambient Intelligence and Humanized Computing 1(2) (2010), doi:10.1007/s12652-010-0011-5
32. Zadeh, L.A.: The Concept of a Linguistic Variable and its Application to Approximate Reasoning, Part I, Part II, Part III. Information Sciences 8, 9, 199–249, 301–357, 43–80 (1975)

26

Category Theoretic Ontology for Representation of Assessment Scales and Consensus Guidelines in Elderly Care

Patrik Eklund

26.1 Introduction

Kazem Sadegh-Zadeh's approach [19] to *medical language* is a first true and complete attempt to provide concrete and detail insight into clinical practice and medical decision-making based on practiced morality and normative ethics. His 'language of medicine' is combined with 'medical praxiology' in a very subtle way not seen before in these contexts. Our discussion on ontology in this paper can be seen, in the small, to relate to epistemological aspects in Sadegh-Zadeh's presentation on epistemology, and his book at large will be a continuous inspiration for our further efforts in this area. Our discussion is not broadly in medicine, and, in fact, not within medicine only. Ageing and elderly care is a typical <area where 'medical' and 'social' needs to join forces, and we will point out hopefully some interesting aspects in this borderline.

The reason for this paper is at least two-fold. On the one hand, we build upon the extension of general logic, into the so called generalized general logic [10], and commit ourselves to be extremely aware of the roles as represented by metalanguage for logic and object language actually describing all building blocks of logic. On the other hand, we show how such a pure category theoretic approach to ontology provided by this generalized general logic can be used for uncertainty based information and knowledge representation and, accordingly, how it is used in decision-making in health and social care. Our examples are drawn from management of assessment scales and consensus guidelines in care of older people. In doing this, we then also point out the informal logic character of international standards of medical ontology, and explain e.g. why logical modelling of uncertainty becomes too ambiguous in such informal frameworks.

Computerized decision-making in social and health care is traditionally viewed with ontology not as part of underlying logics for decision-making, but rather as standards and terminologies including skeletons and frameworks of informal

R. Seising and M.E. Tabacchi (Eds.): *Fuzziness and Medicine*, STUDFUZZ 302, pp. 401–413.
DOI: 10.1007/978-3-642-36527-0_26

relational information structures. We bring these views to the point where data and information are seen residing in the underlying signatures of logic, thus providing a strict basis for producing terms and sentences, in turn appearing in reasoning empowered by a selected proof calculus.

Perhaps the most important point here is that there is not a single logic to model all information and knowledge, and respective professional and ontology user cannot be expected to adapt to one such universally chosen logic. This is not a question about a professional not being able to adapt to such a chosen logic, but rather supports the view that context of decision-making is not related to semantics of data, but to appropriate and necessary selections of underlying logics of reasoning. The realm of general logic also and in particular in its generalized form makes explicit use of mappings from one logic to another, so that the status of mutual understanding between professional, possibly using different logics, resides in those morphisms between respective logics.

The paper outline is as follows. We first recall some history of logic and developments of formal logic, and how we arrive at using our framework for generalized general logic. In doing so, we then also provide the overall scope of that formal logic framework. We then provide some related views on existing medical ontology in order to show how these ontologies are logically very restricted and informal. This is followed by a section on ageing, where we provide necessary background to health and social care of older people, and also provide some detailed information e.g. on assessment scales used in these *observe-assess-decide* processes in a care of older people. The following section then goes into the strictly formal aspects of generalized general logic, and we will see how assessment scale based information, knowledge representation and reasoning can be managed in this purely categorical framework. This also reveals where and how modelling of uncertainty can be formally incorporated into this machinery.

26.2 Logic Defines Ontology

Programming in logic is manipulation of terms, and substitution with terms. Classical terms won't suffice. An ontology building upon classical terms, trying to enhance missing parts in the underlying structures by being clever about inference, becomes logically sterile and basically useless in formal frameworks. We also need to make a distinction between imprecise or vague information, and being formal and accurate in reasoning with vague values. Furthermore, a value may be vague as produced by a crisp operation, or a value is vague since the underlying operation is vague.

From formal point of view this is all about underlying categories and monads, and in this paper we will continue investigations [7] showing how the signatures reside in term monads over chosen categories. Our approach is thus monadic, and we consider monads over suitable categories.

Ontology can be informal of formal, and our approach is that ontology must be nothing but formal and mathematically unambiguous. To be more precise concerning *logic*, let us describe *what* logic is and *how* logic is defined.

Firstly, there is not a single logic for everything. Secondly, we need to distinguish logic as the basis for mathematical reasoning from logic as dedicated to theory development and programming of rule bases. In all this, it is important to understand what is the object language for logic, and what is the metalanguage supporting that object language.

The logic for mathematical reasoning goes back to Aristotle and even before those times to pre-Socratic times when e.g. reductio ad absurdum was used by Zeno. Mathematicians, like Szabó [22], say Aristotle didn't say all that much that influenced modern developments of logic, whereas philosophers, like Hintikka, read lots between the lines and provide far going interpretation about what Aristotle said e.g. about deictics (syntactic, roughly speaking) and apodeictics (semantics, roughly speaking). Our take on logic must be the mathematical one, since the philosophical approach doesn't primarily support formalism and ontology based strict representations. Logic becomes formal logic during late nineteen century when Frege [12] defines what we now call *first-order logic*. This logic was originally intended as logic only for mathematical reasoning, i.e. logic for mathematics. At the change of the century, Hilbert pointed out the difficulties concerning natural numbers and logic, and the question was "Which comes first?". The metalanguage for this first-order logic is not existing *per se*, but we rather have a situation where the non-meta based object language for logic is constructed, and leading to formal difficulties and even paradoxes, which are then rendered, and the formal basis for the object language is reiterated to avoid these difficulties. This process of finding difficulties followed by rendering these difficulties continued for decades, and when Hilbert some fifty years later (with Bernays) was finishing work on set theory and foundations of mathematics [13, 14], the question remained still unanswered. Between Frege's *Begriffsschrift* and Hilbert-Bernays' *Grundlagen*, lots of things happen in the discussion on logic. Peano [17] did his axioms for natural numbers, Russell entered the debate through paradoxes and many others contributed to these discussions. Some computationally interesting things happen also late at those times, e.g. by Schönfinkel [20], a frequent visitor to Hilbert in Göttingen, and his work on combinatory logic, later transformed by Curry in his thesis [5] (supervised by Hilbert and Bernays) providing groundwork for λ-calculus, using only a subset of Schönfinkel's combinators, and thereby type theory was born. Curry together with Howard later showed how propositions can be interpreted as types, an observation that has seduced computer scientist almost a century now.

Logic as dedicated to theory development builds upon a very precise meaning of what logic really is. Formally (and computationally) speaking, logic consists of

- its signature with sorts (types) and operators,
- algebras providing the meaning of the signature,
- all terms constructed (syntactically) using operators in the signature, and the resulting algebraic interpretations (semantics) of these terms,

- all sentences having terms as building blocks, and again equipped with the corresponding meaning (algebras) of these sentences,
- all theoremata being conglomerates of sentences as used in reasoning,
- entailment as the relation between theoremata representing what we already know, and sentences representing knowledge we are trying to arrive at,
- satisfaction as the semantic counterpart to entailment providing the notion of valid conclusions,
- axioms saying what we take for granted at start,
- inference rules saying how we can jump to conclusions in a chain of entailments, and these rules being selected so as to ensure equality (i.e. the so called soundness and completeness of the logic) between the entailment and satisfaction relations (equality cannot always be achieved as the completeness part of logic is sometimes difficult to reach).

In a subsequent section we will make all these notions precise using category theory as metalanguage.

At this point, note how the signature and terms are ingredients for information (as "data") in databases and database theory, where further inclusions of sentence and theoremata are ingredients for knowledge ("representation"). Entailment and inference rules are then finally need in order to "compute" of "infer" with knowledge. This means that we must be careful when we speak about "guidelines" since we must reveal whether we speak only about the knowledge representations involved or also about how to deduce new knowledge using these known representations. Unfortunately, most guidelines are only knowledge representative.

For this notions to enable unambiguous formalism, category theory plays a fundamental role as the metalanguage (in turn with the Zermelo-Fraenkel set theory as the metalanguage for category theory, and so on, hierarchically) for logic formalism, as the formal (and computable) notions of *term*, *sentence* and *theoremata* are given by functors extendable to *monads*, and in the case of theoremata even to *partially ordered monads* [9].

An important part of this approach to ontology is also its capacity and capability to embrace modelling of uncertainty and non-determinism.

At this point we should again underline that we do not have a single logic, as dedicated to theory development, covering reasoning within all applications. The situation is very much the opposite, namely, in that site response and site management must be allowed to use different logics, and crisis response and management logic again differs rather significantly from site response and management logics. The important property in these respects is that there are mappings between these logics so that knowledge, represented in a particular logic, can be carried over to be represented in another logic, understood by other users and stakeholders. The categorical and monadic approach to logic is critical in particular for these homomorphic transformations as represented enabled by functors and represented mostly by natural transformations between them.

We thus define ontology as information and knowledge encoded using a particular logic.

To summarize our main claim in this section, we see logic for mathematics being the first-order approach developing hand in hand with axiomatic set theory, providing ZFC, Zermelo-Fraenkel's set theory including the Axiom of Choice, as the metalanguage (including appropriate intuitions for *conglomerates* and *universe*) for the object language *category theory*. In turn, when we move over to defining *formal logic*, category theory becomes the metalanguage for the object language *generalized general logic*.

In this strictly hierarchical approach we forbid moving back and forth, as Gödel frequently did, and indeed remain strict when representation terms, sentences and proofs in logic. Gödel's numbering indeed comes to a proof calculus, using proof trees and provides numberings for sentences appearing in proof trees, then producing predicates involving these numberings, and goes back to the set of sentences and throws this new sentences into the bag of old sentences. This was allowed one hundred years ago, and some still allow it. We don't, and indeed for our families of logic enabled by the framework of generalized general logic. Whatever happened before ZFC became ZFC, is here not of our concern. We trust ZFC and we trust ZFC as the metalanguage, not *a* metalanguage, for category theory. And generalized general logic must use categorical notions only, and as such based on ZFC. No by-passing of this principle is allowed.

26.3 Ontology in the Medical Domain

Obviously, ontology as traditionally known e.g. in the medical domain as built upon standards like HL7, SNOMED CT and openEHR, or OWL and RDF for web ontology, are not fully logical. They are only partially logical in that even the underlying signature for encoding their vocabularies is treated informally with concepts being more like atoms, and sentence constructions as typically represented by relations, like `IS_A` in SNOMED CT, e.g. in statements like `open fracture of foot IS_A fracture of foot IS_A injury of foot IS_A disorder of foot`. The term `open fracture of foot` is then more typically used in first response for decision-making related to pre-hospital interventions for open fractures, whereas `disorder of foot` more levels involving expertise for orthopedics.

OWL and SNOMED CT have adopted variants of description logics for their partial ontologies. The variant EL++ is favored in OWL, and has recently (because of that use within OWL) also been adopted for SNOMED CT. However, OWL is more tightly bound to EL++, whereas SNOMED CT is still only intentionally bound to EL++.

It should also be noted that description logic is not a formal logic as described above. Description logic doesn't even have a formal involvement of signature as they use *concept* as a primitive notion. Concepts are used as terms and sentences are relational only, which means description logics appear (intentionally) as kind of an informal subset of first-order logic. Description logic further does not really recognize the distinction between logic as the basis for mathematical reasoning from logic as dedicated to theory development and programming of rule bases. It is surely intended for the latter, but it is constructed in the manner like the former. Even worse, description logic has severe difficulties to include reasoning mechanisms, which means that this logic as a partial ontology remains on the logic levels including signatures, terms and sentences only, and even being rather informal about them.

Partial ontology is taken to mean information (databases) and knowledge (guidelines) encoded in logic where parts of the logic structure are missing. The traditional meaning of ontology, such as in web ontology, indeed either completely neglects or is intentionally informal in particular about the sentential and inferential parts of logic. Partial ontology, in particular as seen in the case of SNOMED CT, is more like a mereology since the meronomic type hierarchies in SNOMED CT still seek to find a proper inclusion of deductive elements, and therefore in some sense disqualifies to be called ontology. Another way of speaking is to say that nomenclature is not sufficient, since we need a *calculus of nomenclature*[1].

26.4 Ageing

The overall objectives of the Observe-Assess-Decide (OAD) process in elderly care is to provide a complete system for observation, assessment and decision-making focused on home care and prolongation of independent living, by providing a necessary and sufficient ontology and assessment scale based information, thereby enabling well-founded predictions and continuous monitoring of decline and progrediation on both individual as well as group level. OAD aims to facilitate both dynamical settings of individual care level for care provision at point-of-need as well as demographic change based accurate socio-economic modelling supporting strategic regional management of ageing.

The lack of regional strategies together with scattered and unstructured guidelines for prevention, detection and intervention related to older persons' decline in cognitive and functional capabilities, are the most serious obstacles in the way of a sustainable development of supportive environments for the elderly. Further, the lack of well-structured guidelines and well-organized utility of assessment and, in particular, rigorous assessment based decision-making and care provisioning, leads to overlaps and inefficiency, and even worse, to subjective decision-making and care processes that cannot be measured nor evaluated.

There are assessment scales that are more suitable for home care, where other scales might be seen more suitable for nursing homes, and so on and so forth. For example, on non-cognitive aspects of dementia, some of the first parts of NPI might be more effectively used in home care, whereas Behave-AD and CMAI (focusing on agitation) are more useful in residential care and hospital wards.

[1] Stanislaw Lesniewski (1886-1939), a Polish logician contemporary with Alfred Tarski and Jan Lukasiewicz, used ontology in the sense of a *calculus of names* in his Grundzüge [15].

Optimal use of OAD's gerontechnological platform[2] relies on the specific competences as represented by respective professionals and professional groups. Elderly care includes personnel of various fields, skills and expertise e.g. social workers, nurses, gerontologists, therapists, psychologists and physicians, general practitioners, neurologists and geriatricians. It should be noted that the home care staff in its vast majority consists of a selected mix of social workers and nurses, and thus social care becomes comparably important together with health care. Also in residential and nursing homes, social and health care should be in balance, while in hospital wards the provision of health/medical care is usually seen more important.

In comparison with the working population, older people are more likely to suffer from a wider range of diseases. Public diseases, including problems caused by, and related to metabolic syndromes, diabetes, obesity, malnutrition and sleep deprivation, usually appear accompanied with cardiovascular diseases (cardiac failure, atherosclerosis, vascular disease and hypertension). Ageing then comes more and more with cerebrovascular disease, COPD (Chronic Obstructive Pulmonary Disease), and various frailty syndromes including osteoporosis and sarcopenia, with the risk of a potential fall to be on the increase, having severe effects on the care levels. For instance after a fall, the need for physical exercise and rehabilitation increases. Furthermore, various forms of cancer appear more frequently, and palliative treatment in the last stages of cancer is one of the main reasons why a transfer to domestic environment is often preferred by the patient.

While monitoring of health condition and follow-up of interventions can be supported by devices and ubiquity (e.g. glucose meters for diabetes and monitoring sleep disorders by using sensors implanted in beds), the detecting and monitoring of cognitive decline and psycho-geriatric diseases require assessment scales.

Cognitive decline in MCI (Mild Cognitive Impairment) stages and as appearing in different severity degrees in Alzheimer's disease and other dementia types are typical for old age, and are further accompanied by psycho-geriatric problems such as depression, delirium, and various non-cognitive[3] symptoms.

Figure 26.1 illustrates the minimal set of assessment scales, which usually comprises of some ADL (Activities of Daily Living) scales combined with suitable cognitive scales like MMSE [11]. Combination scales, like the CDR [16]

---

[2] `http://www.fourcomp.com/oad/`

[3] We prefer the neutral and widely accepted term "non-cognitive symptoms of dementia", even if the concept of Behavioral and Psychological Symptoms in Dementia (BPSD) has been defined e.g. by the International Psychogeriatric Association (IPA). BPSD was intended to cover a heterogeneous range of psychological reactions, psychiatric symptoms, and behavior occurring in people with dementia of any aetiology. However, BPSD has became controversial as it invites to treating a syndrome or disorder, thus neglecting distinctions between individual symptoms. Aetiological homogeneity in these respects is now seen to be rather unlikely. Research and trials on BPSD might even lack external validity since pharmacological trials showing the effectiveness of psychotropic drugs in treating these symptoms have been based on summations representing the variety of BPSD symptoms rather than using particular scales. Notably, BPSD is not included as a term in medical databases.

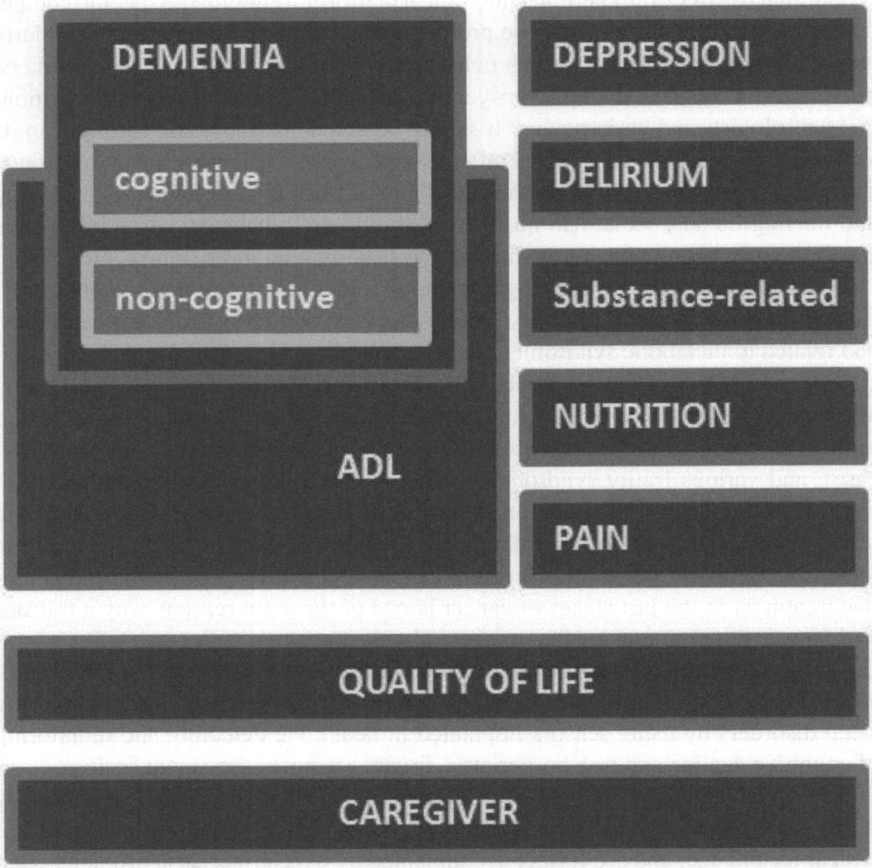

Fig. 26.1 Framework for assessment scales

(Clinical Dementia Rating) for ADL/DEMENTIA, are also widely used. Non-cognitive signs are captured e.g. by NPI [4] (Neuropsychiatric Inventory), CMAI [3] (Cohen-Mansfield Agitation Inventory) and BEHAVE-AD [18]. NPI is particularly useful in home care [21]. Depression is usually captured in its own right as a non-cognitive aspect of dementia, where e.g. GDS [23] (Geriatric Depression Scale) is widely used in home care. Depression is known to accelerate cognitive decline. Nutrition scales are important, as are the scales for social conditions, and so on and so forth.

The selection of assessment scales to be used is of utmost importance and must be optimized with respect to professional resources available in the particular service field where the OAD gerontechnological platform is to be installed and used.

Accurate monitoring of assessment scale based data supports also dementia differential diagnosis [6] according to guidelines as provided e.g. by DSM-IV [1] and NINCDS-ARDRA. Early detection of dementia is important e.g. to achieve favorable effects of pharmacologic treatment by cholinesterase inhibitors (for Alzheimer's disease and Lewy body dementia).

26.5 Generalized General Logic

A signature $\Sigma = (S, \Omega)$ consists of sorts (types) in S and operators in Ω. Here S is a *set* in the sense of ZFC. On the other hand, Ω is not just a set, but in fact an object in an underlying category. If this category is Set, the ordinary category of sets and functions, in the sense of ZFC, then Ω is a set just like S also is just a set.

Now let answer $\in S$ be a sort, and let no, yes $:\to$ answer be two constant (0-ary operators) of sort answer. In GDS, the first question is "*Are you basically satisfied with your life?*". The observation about the target older person may be *Yes*. This gives no room for representing uncertainty about the observation.

For each sort $\mathtt{s} \in S$, the algebra $\mathfrak{A}$ provides the sort with a domain $\mathfrak{A}(\mathtt{s})$, which typically is seen as a set, i.e. an object in Set. Operators $\omega : \mathtt{s}_1 \times \cdots \times \mathtt{s}_n \to \mathtt{s}$ are then provided with a meaning $\mathfrak{A}(\omega) : \mathfrak{A}(\mathtt{s}_1) \times \cdots \times \mathfrak{A}(\mathtt{s}_n) \to \mathfrak{A}(\mathtt{s})$, i.e. a morphism in Set. Again, there is no a priori reason why Set must be fixed as the underlying category for algebras of signatures.

In order to see the difference in using other underlying categories than Set, let us first look at the term functor $\mathsf{T}_\Sigma : \mathtt{Set} \to \mathtt{Set}$. The term functor can be constructed in a strict categorical fashion [9], so that $\mathsf{T}_\Sigma X$ becomes the set of all terms over the set X of variables, i.e. X being an object of Set.

To continue the example above, the term yes is recorded as the observation. Let now the underlying category be changed to $\mathtt{Set}(L)$, the Goguen category, where L is a suitable lattice. Objects in $\mathtt{Set}(L)$ are pairs (A, α) where $\alpha : A \to L$ is a mapping. Morphisms $f : (A_1, \alpha_1) \to (A_2, \alpha_2)$ are mappings $f : A_1 \to A_2$ such that $\alpha_2(f(a)) \geq \alpha_1(a)$ for all $a \in A_1$. Note that Set is not isomorphic to $\mathtt{Set}(\{0,1\})$. Assume for instance that $L = \{\mathtt{absent}, \mathtt{possible}, \mathtt{probable}, \mathtt{present}\}$, with the names for the elements in L really being just names or symbols for points in L. The set S of sorts remains a set, but the 'set' of operators becomes an object of $\mathtt{Set}(L)$, so we now have (Ω, ϑ), for some $\vartheta : \Omega \to L$, as the operator object in $\mathtt{Set}(L)$. The constant no $:\to$ answer is now recorded as $\vartheta(\mathtt{no}) \in L$. Even more so, ϑ should now be seen as *specific for an observer*. There may indeed be (at least) two observers, Flo and Rence, so that $\vartheta_{\mathtt{Flo}}$ and $\vartheta_{\mathtt{Rence}}$ bind uncertainty values of yes to the specific observer. Thus, we may have $\vartheta_{\mathtt{Flo}} = \mathtt{present}$ and $\vartheta_{\mathtt{Rence}} = \mathtt{absent}$. Flo, an experienced home carer may have recorded the observation after having cared for the patient over the past five years, whereas Rence a primary care physician may have seen the patient for the first time in relation to updating a prescription for hypertension.

The term functor is now $\mathsf{T}_\Sigma : \mathtt{Set}(L) \to \mathtt{Set}(L)$, and in fact, these functors can be extended to monads, and we speak of the term monad over $\mathtt{Set}(L)$.

At this point we are able to see alternatives for incorporating models of uncertainty. An operator $\omega : \mathtt{s}_1 \times \cdots \times \mathtt{s}_n \to \mathtt{s}$ residing in (Ω, ϑ) is *fully*[4] fuzzy, and $\vartheta(\omega)$ represents the uncertainty of that particular operator. We can then speak about *fuzzy operators*. If our underlying signature is the signature for natural numbers, i.e. $S = \{\mathtt{nat}\}$ and $\Omega = \{\mathtt{0} :\to \mathtt{nat}, \mathtt{succ} : \mathtt{nat} \to \mathtt{nat}\}$, then $\vartheta(\mathtt{0})$ and $\vartheta(\mathtt{succ})$ are equipped with uncertainties, and the uncertainty of a term like $\mathtt{succ}(\mathtt{succ}(\mathtt{succ}(\mathtt{0})))$ can be computed from the basic uncertainties of the operators. Note here also that a 'set' Y of variables is an object of $\mathtt{Set}(L)$, so $Y = (X, \beta)$ with $\beta : X \to L$. This means not only that a variable is uncertain but variable substitutions, and computing as based on variable substitutions become uncertain. This view of a basis for *fuzzy arithmetic* is entirely different from traditional set-theoretic notions of uncertainty.

An alternative way to incorporate modelling of uncertainty as compared with *uncertain computation* is to enable *computing with uncertainties*. This is essentially done with composing suitable monads with the term monad over Set. Indeed let $\mathsf{T}_\Sigma : \mathtt{Set} \to \mathtt{Set}$ be the term monad over $\mathtt{Set}$, as used above, and let $\phi : \mathtt{Set} \to \mathtt{Set}$ be another monad over $\mathtt{Set}$ that is *composable*[5] with the term monad in the sense of the composed functor $\varphi \circ \mathsf{T}_\Sigma : \mathtt{Set} \to \mathtt{Set}$ being extendable to a monad. In case of *fuzzy*, φ is typically selected to be the fuzzy powerset functor L. Now a variable set X is an object of $\mathtt{Set}$, as just an ordinary set, but substitution is e.g. a morphism $\sigma : X \to \mathsf{L}\mathsf{T}_\Sigma X$ that maps $x \in X$ into $\sigma(x) = \{0/0.7, \mathtt{succ}(0)/0.5, \mathtt{succ}(\mathtt{succ}(0))/0.2\}$, using Zadeh's original notation for fuzzy sets and assuming $L = [0,1]$, the unit interval. In this substitution we have x is bound to '0' with uncertainty value 0.7, x is bound to '1' with uncertainty value 0.5 and to '2' with uncertainty value 0.2. Note how this then eventually leads to *arithmetic with fuzzy*, entirely distinct conceptually from fuzzy arithmetic. In the case of fuzzy arithmetic it is further far from clear that we can do with the nat sort only, or if we need some additional fuznat sort, or even some form of type constructor $\mathtt{fuz} : \mathtt{type} \to \mathtt{type}$ on a second level of signatures, where nat would be integrated as a constant operator $\mathtt{nat} :\to \mathtt{type}$, and we obtain a new type $\mathtt{fuz}(\mathtt{nat})$ for which the algebra then is something like $\mathfrak{A}(\mathtt{fuz}(\mathtt{nat})) = \mathfrak{A}(\mathtt{fuz})(\mathfrak{A}(\mathtt{nat}))$. If $\mathfrak{A}(\mathtt{fuz}) = L$ and $\mathfrak{A}(\mathtt{nat}) = N$, then clearly $\mathfrak{A}(\mathtt{fuz}(\mathtt{nat})) = \mathsf{L}N$, which shows that the meaning of algebra also becomes extended when going in these generalizing directions. This can in fact be formalized, as is done in forthcoming papers. The distinction between *computing with uncertainty* and *uncertain computation* is indeed a first step towards identifying various paradigms for substitutions [8] that are underlying for the whole machinery of generalized general logic.

For assessment scales, like e.g. the GDS scale for depression with a total of 30 questions, or one of its subsets GDS-15, GDS-10, or even GDS-4 with just 4 questions. At least two 'positive' answers out of 4 "raises a flag". This is not saying depression is there, and clearly this is not a step in mood diagnostics of depression e.g. according to the DSM-IV guidelines. It is saying "pay attention" since we

4 According to Lawrence Neff Stout's vocabulary.

5 Composability of monads is subject to certain conditions, so called *distributive laws*, first studied by Jon Beck [2].

have something here that falls under the umbrella of depression, and we know that depression accelerates memory loss.

We will not formally define sentences, but here only draw the attention to sentences being defined by a sentence functor Sen with domain being the category of monads over a fixed underlying category. The typical example is $\mathsf{Sen}(\mathsf{T}_\Sigma) = \mathsf{id}^2 \circ \mathsf{T}_\Sigma$ in the case of producing sentence for equational logic. First-order logic and various extensions can be defined in the context of generalized general logic, and this first-order logic must not be confused with the first-order logic appearing together with ZFC. Note also that natural numbers can be made to "reappear" e.g. in equational logic as defined above, and this Peano arithmetics is then not to be confused with Peano's arithmetic as appearing in the realm of ZFC, for which Gödel's self-referential numbering approaches are accepted.

At this point we can proceed to be extremely formal, but this requires writing space far beyond what is available for this paper. We may for the purpose of this paper, a bit informally, picture sentences like GDS-4(number_of_'positive'_answers) ≥ 2, and then we intuitively see how the 'truth' of this sentence is related to our observations.

Suppose we are faced with a dementia case, and we want to differentiate between Alzheimer's Disease (AD) and a Vascular Dementia (VaD). Inhibiting drugs may be used for AD, but they are not suitable for VaD. Also the progrediation of AD differs from that of VaD, so a long-term treatment plan for AD may differ from a corresponding plan for VaD, since e.g. behavioral syndromes related to a VaD patient may be more clear than for a AD patient. We may then have sentences formulated based on observations of depression (e.g. by a GDS scale), hypertension, information about a previous stroke, and memory loss (e.g. by the MMSE scale). Depending on how many of these sentences tend to show 'truth', we will make a basic judgment about VaD and AD, which may be very useful e.g. for home care decision-making before possible neurological statements are at hand.

Concerning entailment, and even more informally speaking, we then have conclusions like

$$\{\mathtt{depression}, \mathtt{stroke}, \mathtt{hypertension}\} \vdash \mathtt{VaD}$$

Now the premises, called *theoremata*, fit into a logic shared by a particular professional. Back to `Flo` and `Rence`, we can then imagine the respective conclusions

$$\{\mathtt{depression}_{\mathtt{Flo}}, \mathtt{stroke}_{\mathtt{Flo}}, \mathtt{hypertension}_{\mathtt{Flo}}\} \vdash_{\mathtt{Flo}} \mathtt{VaD}_{\mathtt{Flo}}$$

$$\{\mathtt{depression}_{\mathtt{Rence}}, \mathtt{stroke}_{\mathtt{Rence}}, \mathtt{hypertension}_{\mathtt{Rence}}\} \vdash_{\mathtt{Rence}} \mathtt{VaD}_{\mathtt{Rence}}$$

where $\mathtt{depression}_{\mathtt{Flo}}$ and $\mathtt{depression}_{\mathtt{Rence}}$ embrace observations $\varsigma_{\mathtt{Flo}}(\mathtt{no}) = \mathtt{present}$ and $\varsigma_{\mathtt{Rence}}(\mathtt{no}) = \mathtt{absent}$ for the first question in GDS-4. Important here is that the entailment $\vdash_{\mathtt{Flo}}$ resides in the logic adopted by `Flo`, and $\vdash_{\mathtt{Rence}}$ resides in the logic adopted by `Rence`. The question of which conclusion is 'correct' is rather irrelevant. The interesting aspect is whether or not there is a mapping $\vdash_{\mathtt{Flo}} \rightarrow \vdash_{\mathtt{Rence}}$, or in general a morphism between the logics adopted, respectively, by `Flo` and `Rence`.

The theoremata $\Gamma = \{'\texttt{depression}', '\texttt{stroke}', '\texttt{hypertension}'\}$ has a very special form as it is a subset of $\mathsf{Sen}(\mathsf{T}_\Sigma)X$, where X is a variable 'set', usually many-sorted. For P denoting the powerset functor, which is extendable to a monad, we have $\Gamma \in \mathsf{PSen}(\mathsf{T}_\Sigma)X$. There is no reason why theoremata couldn't be given by significantly more complicated monads Φ than just P.

Generalized general logic is $\texttt{LOGIC} = (\texttt{Sign}, \mathsf{Sen}, \mathsf{Mod}, \Phi, L, \vdash, \models, \texttt{ProofCalc})$, where Sign is the category of signature, Sen is the sentence functor, Mod is the functor capturing the generalized notion of corresponding algebras, Φ is the theoremata monad, L is a lattice of external truth values, not to be confused with a possible lattice K appearing in the Goguen category $\texttt{Set}(K)$. We may have $K = L$, but it is not necessary. The entailment relation is $\vdash$ and the satisfaction relation is $\models$. ProofCalc represents functors and natural transformations adding up to a generalized proof calculus. Details are and must be omitted in this paper, but part of this framework was published by Eklund and Helgesson in 2010 [10], and further detail are under preparation.

We may construct the category of generalized general logics with corresponding morphisms, so that e.g. $\Xi : \texttt{LOGIC}_{\texttt{Flo}} \to \texttt{LOGIC}_{\texttt{Rence}}$ captures some kind of *understanding* between Flo and Rence. The interesting thing here is that $\texttt{LOGIC}_{\texttt{Flo}}$ is obviously 'owned' by Flo and $\texttt{LOGIC}_{\texttt{Rence}}$ by Rence, but who owns the morphism Ξ? It may perhaps be seen as a convergent dialectics between Flo and Rence.

References

1. American Psychiatric Association: Diagnostic and Statistical Manual of Mental Disorders, 4th edn. (DSM-IV-TR®), Text Revisions, American Psychiatric Association (2000)
2. Beck, J.: Distributive laws. In: Seminars on Triples and Categorical Homology Theory, 1966/1967. Lecture Notes in Mathematics, vol. 80, pp. 119–140. Springer (1969)
3. Cohen-Mansfield, J., Marx, M.S., Rosenthal, A.S.: A Description of Agitation in a Nursing Home. Journal of Gerontology 44, M77–M84 (1989)
4. Cummings, J.L., Mega, M., Gray. K. Rosenberg-Thompson, S., Carusi, D.A., Gornbein, J.: The Neuropsychiatric Inventory: Comprehensive Assessment of Psychopathology in Dementia. Neurology 44, 2308–2314 (1994)
5. Curry, H.B.: Grundlagen der kombinatorischen Logik. American Journal of Mathematics 52, 509–536, 789–834 (1930)
6. Eklund, P.: Assessment Scales and Consensus Guidelines Encoded in Formal Logic. In: 19th IAGG World Congress of Gerontology and Geriatrics, Paris (2009); Journal of Nutrition, Health & Aging 13(suppl. 1), S558–S559
7. Eklund, P.: Signatures for Assessment, Diagnosis and Decision-Making in Ageing. In: Hüllermeier, E., Kruse, R., Hoffmann, F. (eds.) IPMU 2010, Part II. CCIS, vol. 81, pp. 271–279. Springer, Heidelberg (2010)
8. Eklund, P., Galán, M.Á., Helgesson, R.: Paradigms for Many-sorted Non-classical Substitutions. In: 41st IEEE International Symposium on Multiple-Valued Logic (ISMVL 2011), pp. 318–321 (2011)

9. Eklund, P., Gähler, W.: Fuzzy Filter Functors and Convergence. In: Rodabaugh, S.E., Klement, E.P., Höhle, U. (eds.) Applications of Category Theory to Fuzzy Subsets. Theory and Decision Library B: Mathematical and Statistical Methods, vol. 14, pp. 109–136. Kluwer, Dordrecht (1992)
10. Eklund, P., Helgesson, R.: Monadic Extensions of Institutions. Fuzzy Sets and Systems 161, 2354–2368 (2010)
11. Folstein, M.F., Folstein, S.E., McHugh, P.R.: "Mini Mental State", A Practical Method for Grading the Cognitive State on Patients for the Clinician. Journal of Psychiatry Research 12, 189–198 (1975)
12. Frege, G.: Begriffsschrift: Eine der arithmetischen nachgebildete Formelsprache des reinen Denkens. Verlag von Louis Nebert, Halle (1879)
13. Hilbert, D., Bernays, P.: Grundlagen der Mathematik. I. Die Grundlehren der mathematischen Wissenschaften, vol. 40. Springer, Berlin (1934)
14. Hilbert, D., Bernays, P.: Grundlagen der Mathematik. II. Die Grundlehren der mathematischen Wissenschaften, vol. 50. Springer, Berlin (1934)
15. Lesniewski, S.: Grundzüge eines Neuen Systems der Grundlagen der Mathematik. Fundamenta Mathematicae XIV, 1–81 (1929)
16. Morris, J.C.: The Clinical Dementia Rating (CDR): Current Version and Scoring Rules. Neurology 43, 2412–2414 (1993)
17. Peano, G.: Arithmetices Principia, Nova Methodo Exposita. Fratres Bocca (1889)
18. Reisberg, B., Borenstein, J., Salob, S.P., Ferris, S.H., Franssen, E., Georgotas, A.: Behavioral Symptoms in Alzheimer's Disease: Phenomenology and Treatment. International Journal of Geriatric Psychiatry 48(suppl.), 9–15 (1987)
19. Sadegh-Zadeh, K.: Handbook of Analytic Philosophy of Medicine. Philosophy and Medicine, vol. 113. Springer, Heidelberg (2012)
20. Schönfinkel, M.: Über die Bausteine der mathematischen Logik. Mathematische Annalen 92, 305–316 (1924)
21. Selbaek, G., Kirkevold, Ø., Engedal, K.A.: The Prevalence of Psychiatric Symptoms and Behavioural Disturbances and the Use of Psychotropic Drugs in Norwegian Nursing Homes. International Journal of Geriatric Psychiatry 22(9), 843–849 (2007)
22. Szabó, Á.: The Beginnings of Greek Mathematics. Reidel, Dordrecht (1978)
23. Yesavage, J.: Development and Validation of Geriatric Depression Screening Scale: A preliminary report. Journal of Psychiatry 17, 37–49 (1983)

27

Fuzzy Cognitive Map Decision Support System for Successful Triage to Reduce Unnecessary Emergency Room Admissions for the Elderly

Voula C. Georgopoulos and Chrysostomos D. Stylios

Abstract. This work presents a Fuzzy Cognitive Map Medical Decision Support System (FCM-MDSS) for the hospital admission procedure of elderly patients. The FCM-MDSS is applied to the Emergency Department (ED), where elderly patients arrive requesting medical assistance. Here a new hybrid methodology is introduced to develop FCM-MDSS exploiting human experience and accompanied by available bibliographic information. It is based on the widely applied Triage complex decision-making process and the generally accepted procedures while trying to minimize unnecessary admissions as well as over/under-triaging. The FCM-MDSS is evaluated for known cases of real patients arriving at the ED from the literature.

27.1 Introduction

Triaging involves an initial sorting of patients who arrive at the emergency room, usually called emergency department (ED), by rapidly identifying patients requiring immediate care due to urgent, life-threatening conditions as well as assessing the severity of the problem so as to ensure that care is appropriate and timely [11].

Triage is a complex decision-making process, and as a result several triage scales have been designed corresponding to decision support systems [5] to guide the triage nurse to a correct decision.

Unfortunately, in the emergency room elderly patients, as a general rule, undergo more diagnostic testing and have longer length of stays than younger ones, [4, 42] because of their multiple health problems and as a result, they usually use more resources. The Emergency Department (ED) all over the world is faced with a continuous increase in visits [22], partly due to its excessive use for non-urgent problems. The elderly frequently visit the ED because of their increased prevalence to chronic-degenerative diseases, susceptible to frequent exacerbations. Since the aging population is destined to increase further, providing quality

R. Seising and M.E. Tabacchi (Eds.): *Fuzziness and Medicine*, STUDFUZZ 302, pp. 415–436.
DOI: 10.1007/978-3-642-36527-0_27

cost-effective care of these patients with multiple, complex conditions is a very crucial problem [36, 40].

Elderly patients are admitted to the hospital, most of the times, unnecessarily due to the complexity of decision-making about their health conditions (since the clinical problems and needs of older patients are often substantially different from those of younger patients) and they may be accompanied by cognitive or functional deterioration. In addition to this, many older patients have multiple co-morbidities, polypharmacy and further complex health and social care needs. Thus, they have higher readmission rates. Many physicians and junior doctors are not specially trained in geriatric medicine so they may have difficulty in assessing the patient's condition as being of an intermediate risk or requiring just monitoring and observation [8, 9, 26].

Besides the various clinical tests and laboratory exams run in the ED and the medical history taking, various questionnaires are used to assess patient status. For example, risk factors known to have often-adverse health outcomes are used by the questionnaire Identification of Seniors at Risk tool to detect impaired functional status and depression at the evaluation [37].

It is significant to mention that in a sample of 50 randomly selected cases of ED admissions patients 65 years or older, discrepancies were found between the medical staff and expert nurses in 20 cases: where staff nurses had undertriaged 13 patients and overtriaged 7 patients [23].

Nowadays, the new technological advances, the utilization of ICT in the hospital and all the new technology based diagnostic tests produce a huge amount of data being available to make decisions. But under the tight time constraints, as is the case of Emergency Department, only part of this data is utilized. On the other hand, the limited number of medical professionals requires the efficient exploitation of human resources to make the right decisions and leads to the need to develop automatic decision making systems, such as in the process of triage in the emergency departments.

Generally speaking, Medical Decision Support Systems have a crucial role in today's complex health systems, since it is required to combine the human clinical experience acquired through hospital practice with widely accepted systematic analytic approaches. Such hybrid methods that combine both of them are in favor of medical professionals. One such approach is the soft-computing modeling methodology of Fuzzy Cognitive Maps, which is discussed in the next section.

The aims of this research is to present a Fuzzy Cognitive Map Medical Decision Support System (FCM-MDSS) for supporting in the triaging of elderly patients arriving in the emergency room for medical assistance while trying to minimize unnecessary admission and/or over/undertriaging. A Fuzzy Cognitive Map MDSS architecture is developed and described here based on existing medical protocols on patient triaging, along with the consultation and support of emergency care nurses and physicians.

27.2 Fuzzy Cognitive Maps

Fuzzy Cognitive Maps (FCMs) belong to Soft Computing approaches that are introduced to create advanced modeling systems aiming to resemble human-like reasoning. FCMs have successfully been applied to a wide range of problems in many engineering application domains, mainly to model complex systems and develop advanced diagnosis and/or decision support systems. Human knowledge and experience is reflected in the creation procedure and the infrastructure of FCMs, making them suitable for modeling the decision-making and reasoning approach in a human-like manner. Especially in the medical field, the decision-making procedure is often crucial and must be achieved in a timely manner.

Fuzzy Cognitive Maps with their modifications integrate aspects of fuzzy logic, neural networks, semantic networks, expert systems and they are usually supplemented with other soft and hard computing methodologies. An FCM is illustrated as a causal graphical representation consisting of interrelated concepts [19]. FCMs are fuzzy signed directed graphs permitting feedback, where the weighted edge w_{ij} from causal concept C_i to affected concept C_j describes the degree with which the first concept influences the latter, as is illustrated in Fig. 27.1. FCMs are characterized as fuzzy feedback models of causality, where the weighted interconnections among concepts of the FCMs present causality among concepts and creating an interconnected network of interrelated entities, like an abstract mental model. Feedback interconnections are permitted along with if-then inferencing; that permits FCMs to model complex nonlinear dynamic systems. FCMs have the ability to include hidden nonlinear dynamics.

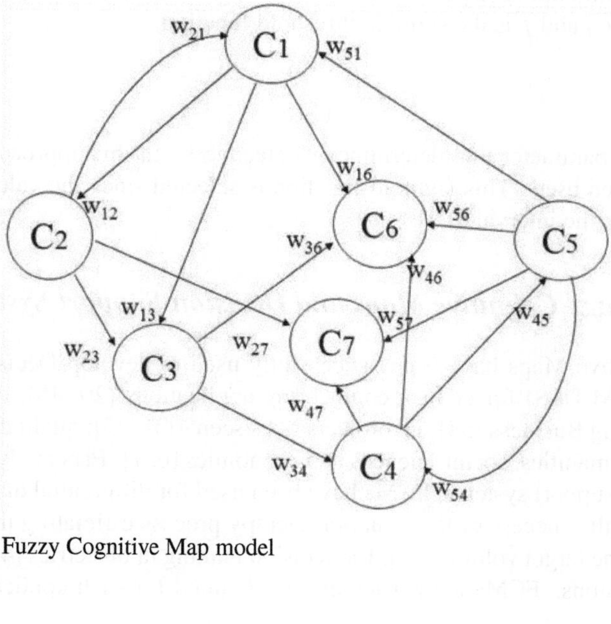

Fig. 27.1 The Fuzzy Cognitive Map model

The concepts of the Fuzzy Cognitive Model stand for the main characteristics comprising an abstract model of any system; each concept of the FCM represents a granular entity such as state, variable, input, output, event, action, goal, trend of the system that is modeled as an FCM. The value of every concept C_i is A_i and it results from the transformation of the real fuzzy value of the system's variable, for which this concept stands for, in the interval $[0,1]$. Thus, when the initial concept value is produced, then this value is updated as it is computed through the interaction of the interconnected concepts with the corresponding weights. Generally, between two concepts there are three possible types of causal relationships that express the type of influence from one concept to the other. The weight of the arc between concept C_i and concept C_j could be positive ($W_{ij} > 0$) which means that an increase in the value of concept C_i leads to the increase of the value of concept C_j, and a decrease in the value of concept C_i leads to the decrease of the value of concept C_j. Or there is negative causality ($W_{ij} < 0$) which means that an increase in the value of concept C_i leads to the decrease of the value of concept C_j and vice versa. The value A_i of concept C_i expresses the degree of its corresponding physical value. Fuzzy Cognitive Map is used to model the behavior of a system; during the simulation step, the value A_i of a concept C_i is calculated by computing the influence of the interconnected concepts C_j's on the specific concept C_i following the calculation rule:

$$A_i^{(k+1)} = f(A_i^{(k)}) + \sum_{j=1, j\neq i}^{N} A_j^{(k)} \cdot w_{ji} \tag{27.1}$$

where $A_i^{(k+1)}$ is the value of concept C_i at simulation step $k+1$, $A_i^{(k)}$ is the value of concept C_i at simulation step k, w_{ij} is the weight of the interconnection from concept C_i to concept C_j and f is the sigmoid threshold function:

$$f = \frac{1}{1+e^{-\lambda x}} \tag{27.2}$$

where λ is a parameter that determines its steepness. In this approach, the value $\lambda = 1$ has been used. This sigmoid function is selected since the values A_i of the concepts lie in the interval $[0,1]$.

27.2.1 Fuzzy Cognitive Maps and Decision Support Systems

Fuzzy Cognitive Maps have been successfully used to develop Decision Support Systems (FCM-DSS) for control engineering applications [20, 45]; urban design [55] in banking Business [54]; IT projects risks scenarios [35]; qualitative dynamic systems in humanities, social sciences and economics [6, 7]. Especially in the medical decision support systems, FCMs have been used for differential diagnosis [13], to determine the success of the radiation therapy process estimating the final dose delivered to the target volume [30]; for decision making in obstetrics [43] and many other applications. FCMs are particularly well suited for such applications, since medical systems are complex systems involving inexact, uncertain, imprecise and ambiguous information [15].

Fuzzy Cognitive Maps have been successfully used to develop Medical Decision Support System (MDSS). A specific type for Medical Diagnosis is the Competitive Fuzzy Cognitive Map (CFCM) [14, 15] which consists of two main types of concepts: diagnosis-concepts and factor-concepts. Fig. 27.2 illustrates an example CFCM model that is used to perform medical diagnosis. Here the concepts of the FCM and the causal relations among them that influence concepts and determine the value of diagnosis concepts indicating final diagnosis are illustrated.

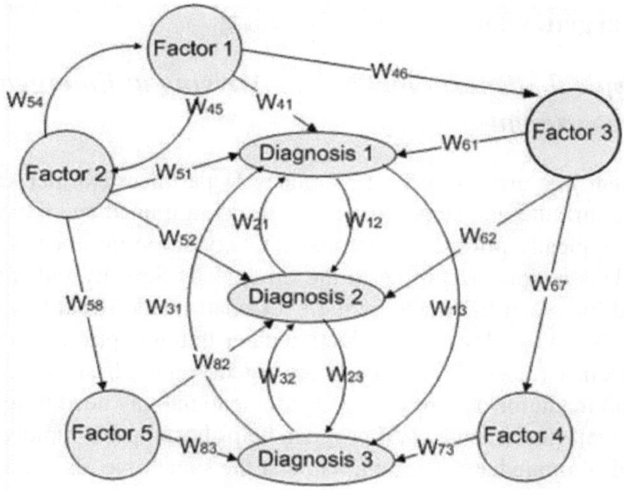

Fig. 27.2 A CFCM model for Medical Diagnosis

In the CFCM model each diagnosis concept represents a single diagnosis, which means that these concepts must be mutually exclusive because the main intention is to infer always only one diagnosis. This is the case of most medical applications, where, according to symptoms, medical professionals conclude to only one diagnosis and then they decide accordingly the most appropriate the treatment. Actually, this comes from the medical axiom: "every patient has only one disease" but may represent many symptoms related to different diseases but all are results of the primitive disease. The general diagnosis procedure is a complex process that has to take under investigation a variety of interrelated factors, symptoms and functions. Usually, in any real world diagnosis and decision problem, many different factors have to be taken into consideration to conclude the most appropriate diagnosis. In accomplishing any diagnosis process, some of these factors are complementary, others are similar and even others are conflicting.

In the Competitive Fuzzy Cognitive Map model, the factor-concepts represent inputs into the MDSS, their values correspond topatient data, observed symptoms, patient records, experimental and laboratory tests etc. These can be dynamically updated based on the system interaction, whereas the decision-concepts are considered as outputs where their estimated values outline the possible diagnosis for the patient. It should be mentioned that the real strength of FCMs is their ability to model and describe complex systems and handle successfully with situations where there are feedback relationships and interrelationships between the factor concepts. Thus, interrelations between factor-concepts can be included in the proposed medical decision-support model. Such interconnections are shown in Fig. 27.2 where the "competitive" interconnections between diagnosis concepts are also illustrated.

27.3 Emergency Department Triaging

27.3.1 Typical Scenario for Patient Arriving at Emergency Department

When a patient first arrives in the Emergency Department (former known as the emergency room), the first stop is triage. In triage, a trained and experienced registered nurse typically prioritizes each patient's condition into one of five general categories. This is done according to the Emergency Severity Index (ESI) which was designed for use in ED triage by the US Department of Health & Human Services. The ESI is a five-level categorization algorithm that prioritizes patients into five groups from 1 (most urgent) to 5 (least urgent) on the basis of acuity (i.e. seriousness) and the number of resources that the patient may need to receive proper care [53]. A well-implemented ESI program helps hospital ED rapidly identify patients in need of immediate attention, while at the same time also identify patients who could safely and more efficiently be transferred to other departments rather than the Emergency Department. Triage staff use specific criteria to determine each patient's acuity. For example they rapidly interview the patient, take patient's vital signs (blood pressure, pulse, oxygen saturation level and respiratory rate). If the patient is complaining about pain they are asked to self-assess on a scale of 1-10 and to identify the location of the pain. Additionally, nurses ask them what the major complaint was that brought them into the ED. From the above and other information collected, the triage nurse produces an Emergency Severity Index (ESI) score [16], assessing the patient's condition. Based on the ESI score, the clinical staff schedules to check back with the patient on a timely basis based on the patient's condition [52].

27.3.2 Emergency Department Triaging Details

To ensure patient safety and provide quality services, hospitals must be certain that each patient entered to the emergency department (ED) receives the appropriate care at the right time. Triage is a means by which this is ensured. An experienced triage nurse evaluates the patient's condition, as well as any changes, and determines their priority for admission to the ED and their need for treatment [3]. This is necessary to make patient assessments in order to properly anticipate the resources needed for each patient and recognize abnormal vital signs; thus, tools such as the ESI are "only as good as the person using them" [39]. For example, a study conducted among 305 triage ratings comparing triage nurses' ratings to retrospective ratings assigned by an expert panel of emergency department triage nurses revealed an agreement in approximately half of the cases [47].

Of course the primary goal of triage is to decrease morbidity and mortality for all ED patients. However, a gap in the knowledge exists regarding the real time reasoning process of clinical decision making that occurs during ED triage [5, 17].

The ESI uses the following scale based on decision points to determine its categories [3, 16]:

- *ESI category 1-Emergent:* patient intubated, without pulse or respiration, or unresponsive. i.e the patient requires immediate life-saving intervention so as to prevent loss of life, limb, or eyesight,
- *ESI category 2-Urgent:* patient is in a high-risk situation, or confused, lethargic or disoriented, or in severe pain, or danger zone vital signs.
- *ESI category 3-Acute:* patient is in need of many resources to be taken care of. These may include, for example, Laboratory Tests, ECG, X-rays, CT-MRI-ultrasound-angiography, IV fluids, specialty consultation, complex procedures etc.
- *ESI category 4-Routine:* patient is in need of one resource.
- *ESI category 5-Non urgent:* patient is in need of no resources.

It is interesting to note that specific guidelines do not exist within the triage procedure and a great deal is relied on the experience of the triaging nurse. For example the Joint Commission on Accreditation of Healthcare Organizations does not specifically state a standard for vital signs. The organization does assert that physiologic parameters should be assessed as determined by patient condition but JCAHO does not require vital signs to be done during triage. Vital signs are usually recorded if the triage nurse determines they may be useful [16].

27.3.3 *Triaging Elderly Patients*

In a study of 929 Emergency Department visits of patients older than 65, it was found that in general the ESI algorithm demonstrates validity. However, patients, particularly elderly ones (but not only), frequently present to emergency departments (EDs) with non-specific complaints (NSCs) such as "not feeling well," "feeling weak," "being tired," feeling "dizzy,"or simply being unable to cope with usual daily activities [49]. Studies have shown that up to 20% of older individuals presenting to the ED have no specific complaints [50] while 50% of older individuals without specific complaints suffered from an acute medical problem [33] and were at a particularly high-risk group for adverse outcomes (e.g. functional decline, dependence, and death) [24]. The difficulty arising from the uncertainty in the diagnostic process for these patients may lead to ineffective or suboptimal triage of these patients [27].

Weakness is a common presenting symptom in patients in the emergency department (ED), and is an obvious challenge to ED physicians [28]. A number of all non-trauma patients (19.7%) admitted to the ED complained of some form of weakness easily recognized by ED nurses and ED physicians. Localized weakness is well described and may be called a "stroke-like symptom" [34]. Generalized weakness is most often caused by serious disease requiring immediate attention [28].

Frail elderly patients admitted without specific complaints are at risk of inappropriate or delayed evaluation due to undertriage at the door of the ED. A more specific geriatric assessment should be integrated early in the triage process of these patients. Emergency department admission decisions for elderly adults rely on various medical and social factors, along with the availability of timely follow-up [31]. These may include:

- *Patient data and test results* (e.g., Age, ESI level, Heart rate, Diastolic blood pressure, lab results)
- *Patient Chief complaints* (e.g. General weakness, Fainting (syncope), Chest pain, Neurologic weakness, Shortness of breath, Labored or difficult breathing, Vomiting, Abdominal pain, Decreased appetite, Blood in stool, Blood in urine, Painful urination, Patient History (e.g.Nonischemic heart disease, Cerebrovascular disease (stroke), Pneumonia, Anemia, Diabetes)
- *Cognitive/Psychiatric state*
- *Injury* (e.g. Leg / hip fracture / dislocation, Head / neck / facial injury)
- *Index scores* (e.g. Charlson Comorbidity Index Score)
- *Other factors such as:* patient lives alone, suspected elderly abuse/neglect, recently discharged, polypharmacy, adverse drug affects, alcohol abuse.

These general components contribute with varying degrees to the decision an emergency care physician makes to admit or discharge the elderly patient after a visit to the ED.

27.3.4 Decision Support Systems for ED Triage

The significance of the ED triage assessment has lead researchers to investigate and developed Decision Support Systems for ED Triage. A Web-based triage decision support tool (eTRIAGE) based on the Canadian Triage and Acuity Scale (CTAS) has been developed in Canada and is now used in a number of ED regional hospitals. Decision support, such as an electronic triage tool, can assist the medical staff performing triage by displaying the key elements for each complaint, so that to help define the criteria for each triage level. It is expected that experienced triage staff are better able to estimate a triage level based on their initial clinical assessment than those with less experience, giving them greater confidence to override the tool if required [56].

Wilkes and colleagues [52] proposed a system of cognitive agents and a supervisor, dubbed the TriageBot System that would gather both logistical and medical information, as well as take diagnostic measurements, from an incoming patient for later use by the triage team. TriageBot would also give tentative, possible diagnoses to the triage nurse, along with recommendations for non-physician care.

San Pedro and colleagues [38] proposed a Mobile Decision Support for Triage in Emergency Departments based on decision support strategies that include the use of heuristic and fuzzy reasoning that allow the system to support nurse's ability to use his/her expert judgment and justify his/her decision using natural language.

Finally, Aronsky et al. [1] described an integrated, computerized triage application which exchanges information with other information systems, including the ED patient tracking board, the longitudinal electronic medical record, the computerized provider order entry, and the medication reconciliation application. The application includes decision support capabilities such as assessing the patients' acuity level, age-dependent alerts for vital signs, and clinical reminders.

Research using empirical results from a clinical trial of an emergency DSS with a decision model based on expert knowledge has shown [18] that there are differences in how clinician groups of the same specialty, but different level of expertise, elicit necessary emergency DSS input variables and use these variables in their clinical decisions.

The following sections will introduce a novel development approach for a Decision Support System based on Fuzzy Cognitive Maps and will describe, in detail, how to include actual factors taken into consideration, as well as to present the outcomes for case studies presented to the emergency room.

27.4 Fuzzy Cognitive Maps Designing and Development Procedure

Since the ESI instrument categorizes ED patients into 5 mutually exclusive categories, the type of Fuzzy Cognitive Map that will be used here is the Competitive Fuzzy Cognitive Map (CFCM) where the possible decision outcomes are mutually exclusive and compete with each other [14, 15].

Many different approaches have been proposed to develop and construct FCMs either based only to human experts who are invited to design conceptual structures that correspond the operation and model of a system or based on available quantitative historical data or both of them [25, 41, 44, 45]. The construction methodology and the possible implementation of learning algorithm has great importance to sufficiently model any system. Here a new hybrid method for it is proposed developing Fuzzy Cognitive Map Decision Support Systems (FCM-MDSS) mainly based on a group of experts who are used to transform their reasoning approach on inferring decision into an aggregated decision making model. The proposed methodology extracts the knowledge from the experts and exploits their experience on decision-making and evaluating diagnosis [44] and it is further complemented with generally expected bibliographic input.

The proposed approach here is not only based on the human experts, but, also, it introduces the use of existent widely accepted procedures and bibliographic data, constituting a hybrid methodology. It is proposed to use the experience and human reasoning procedure, in order to determine the importance of every factor and so its degree of influence on the corresponding assignment. Usually every individual, in order to conclude to a decision, doesn't take into consideration all the possible factors but focuses on the most important factors, a procedure that is dependent on the specific conditions; that means the same expert, in another case, may select another set of essential factors.

In order to generalize the procedure and produce a generic decision making procedure, the following approach is introduced. First, the possible factors that may influence a decision are determined based on bibliographic and general accepted methodologies, then specific cases are presented to a group of experts, asking them to select the most important factors for each case and coming to a decision based on these factors. Thus, for every case, each expert usually selects 3-5 factors, based on his or her experience, from which decision/ diagnosis is concluded. So for every factor / concept, we introduce its *importance weight*, which will be used then to determine its influence to the final decision:

$$iw = \frac{\text{\# of experts considering this factor}}{\text{total number of cases}}. \tag{27.3}$$

Moreover, we introduce a complementary second weight, the "influence to specific decision" *specific weight – sw*, which represents how much the specific factor leads towards a specific decision / diagnosis. The procedure to calculate the is the following, every expert who considers one factor as important and he takes it into consideration, he is asked to present the degree with which the specific factor leads the expert to select one decision. Every expert describes the degree of influence of one factor towards one decision using a linguistic variable, such as "strong influence", "medium influence", "weak influence", etc.

More specifically, the causal interrelationships from one factor/ concept towards a decision/ diagnosis concept are declared using the variable *Influence* which is interpreted as a linguistic variable taking values in the universe $U = [-1, 1]$. Its term set *T(influence)* is suggested to comprise nine variables so that to permit to experts to explicitly describe the degree of influence, actually using nine linguistic variables, an expert can describe in detail the influence of factor concept towards decision concept and can discern between different degrees of influence. The nine variables used here are: *T(influence)* = negatively very strong, negatively strong, negatively medium, negatively weak, zero, positively weak, positively medium, positively strong and positively very strong. The corresponding membership functions for these terms are shown in Figure 27.3 and they are μ_{nvs}, μ_{ns}, μ_{nm},μ_{z},μ_{pw},μ_{pm},μ_{ps}, and μ_{pvs}.

Thus, every expert describes the *specific weight sw* of each interconnection with a fuzzy linguistic variable from the above mentioned set, which stands for the relationship between the two concepts and determines the grade of causality between the two concepts. Then, all the proposed linguistic weights for one interconnection suggested by experts are aggregated using the SUM method and an overall linguistic weight is produced. The overall linguistic weight with the defuzzification method of Center Of Gravity (COG) [21], is transformed to a numerical weight *sw*, belonging to the interval $[-1,1]$. A similar approach was initially presented for the description of the development of FCM model in [45].

Then the overall weight describing the influence from one factor concept towards a decision concept is calculated using the form:

$$w_{ji} = sgn(sw)\,(l_1 * iw + l_2 * |sw|) \qquad (27.4)$$

where the two parameters l_1, l_2 are introduced to represent the participation of the *importance weight iw* and the *specific weight sw*, on the overall weight describing the influence of every factor concept towards the decision/diagnosis concept. It is mentioned that the value of w_{ii} has to be normalized in the interval $[-1,1]$, where the weight takes values.

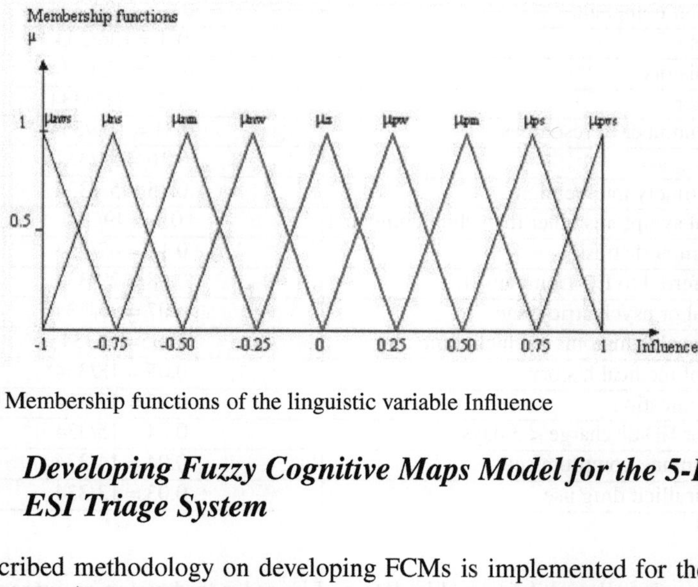

Fig. 27.3 Membership functions of the linguistic variable Influence

27.4.1 *Developing Fuzzy Cognitive Maps Model for the 5-Level ESI Triage System*

The described methodology on developing FCMs is implemented for the case of constructing a medical decision making system for the 5-level Emergency Severity Index (ESI) triage system [10, 16, 46, 53]. The ESI describes the main factors and based on them provides a standardized algorithm for the triage process using a systematic approach and utilizes both intuitive and analytical approaches to clinical decision making.

Based on the literature as presented in sections 27.3.2 and 27.3.3, as well as a study of 18 triage nurses [12], a series of factor concepts were concluded to be part of the Competitive Fuzzy Cognitive Map Medical Decision Support System for ESI (CFCM-ESI) for triage. Twenty-two (22) factors are selected that represent the potential concepts of the Fuzzy Cognitive Map decision model, but they do not all have the same importance in order to infer an assignment on the severity of the patient based on the 5-level triage system.

In the research of Garbez et al. [12], only ESI level 2 or level 3 were studied, where triage nurses were asked to select 3 to 4 factors that they rated as important in their clinical decision making process as they assigned an acuity level for each individual patient. Examples of these cases are shown in Table 27.1 as well as the calculation of the corresponding *iw* values (# of experts of considering this fac-tor)/(total number of patient cases, i.e. 334), which will be included as factor concepts of the CFCM-ESI, according to equation 27.3.

Table 27.1 The *importance weight iw* for Factor Concepts

Physical meaning	$iw = \frac{\text{\# of experts considering this factor}}{\text{total number of cases}}.$
Patient chief complaint	0.67 = 224/334
Vital signs	0.4 = 136/334
Medical history	0.35 = 120/334
Other factor	0.32 = 110/334
Expected number of resources	0.31 = 106/334
Patient age	0.16 = 54/334
Required timely intervention	0.15 = 53/334
Additional symptoms other than chief complaint	0.14=49/334
Severe pain or distress	0.12 = 42/334
Patient referred to ED from outside	0.08 = 29/334
Behavioral or psychiatric issue	0.07 = 25/334
No additional symptoms to chief complaint	0.05=18/334
Absence of medical history	0.05 = 18/334
Patient medications	0.05 = 17/334
Hospital or ED discharge < 3 days	0.04 = 15/334
Patient immune-compromised	0.04 = 14/334
Alcohol or illicit drug use	0.03 = 13/334

However, based on bibliographic data and in order to develop an integrated advanced FCM-ESI, some additional Factor Concepts mostly related to the other 3 ESI levels but not exclusively are included:

- Life or organ-threatening condition, $iw = .45$. It is concluded based on prevalence statistics of emergency room triaging of elderly [32] in conjunction with the fact that this is a very significant determining factor for ESI level 1.
- Limb threatening state $iw = 0.40$, based on prevalence statistics of limb loss in the general population [29] and elderly visits to the ED in conjunction with the fact that this is a very significant determining factor for ESI level 1.
- Weakness, $iw = 0.20$ [28]
- No recent change mental state, $iw = 0.75$ [51]
- Patient can walk or sit for prolonged periods $iw = 0.12$, based on non-urgent presentations [2]

The *importance weight*, *iw*, values for these factors were calculated on incidence % of arrivals in an ED and refers to patients over 65 years of age.

It is concluded that the CFCM-ESI will consist of these total 22 Factor Concepts and thus, based on them, a possible triage Decision will be assigned. More accurately each patient is assigned one of the 5 ESI levels, therefore the CFCM-MDSS will include 5 Decision Concepts (DC), each one for every ESI level:

Table 27.2 Decision Concepts

Decision concept (DC)	Physical meaning
DC1	ESI Level 1 (ESI1)
DC2	ESI Level 2 (ESI2)
DC3	ESI Level 3 (ESI3)
DC4	ESI Level 4 (ESI4)
DC5	ESI Level 5 (ESI5)

After determining the concepts of the Fuzzy Cognitive Map, the most important issue is the assignment of the influence among concepts, which is the second step of FCM development [45]. The FCM development procedure is very important since this model is then used for decision making and diagnosis. Here, we further apply the designing methodology presented in section 27.4 in order to assign weight values between the Factor Concepts (FC) and the Decision Concepts (DC).

This designing methodology utilizes the data used and provided in the study of Garbez et al., [12], where 334 cases of patients were examined and 18 experts assigned them to ESI levels. According to this designing methodology, the first stage is the assignment of the *importance weight*, at every concept using equation 27.3, which is depicted in Table 27.1. Then the *specific weight*, *sw*, representing the influence from a Factor Concept FC to a Decision Concept DC must be determined. Subsequently equation 27.4 is applied in order to calculate the weight from Factor Concept to Decision Concepts. Here, for this case, in order to calculate the overall weight from FCs to DCs, a simplified version of equation 27.4 is used along with the normalization to 1, where $l_1 = 1$ and $l_1 = 0.5$. Thus:

$$w_{ji} = sgn(sw)\,(iw + 0.5 * |sw|) \tag{27.5}$$

The overall weight after the normalization to 1, is then fuzzified according to the membership functions of Fig 27.3. The weights from FCs to DCs are depicted in Table 27.3 which are used to produce the CFCM-ESI illustrated in Figure 27.4.

At this stage of the research we only assign weights from Factor Concepts to Decision Concepts, but the FCM capabilities permit us to introduce weights among the Factor Concept themselves, that create a more accurate but too complex model, which is part of ongoing research.

The weights of Table 27.3 are based on membership functions of Figure 27.3:

- VVS positive very very strong (high end of the *pvs* membership function)
- VS positive very strong (*pvs* membership function)
- S positive strong (*ps* membership function)
- MS positive medium strong (high end of the *pm* membership function)
- M positive medium (*pm* membership function)
- - M negative medium (*nm* membership function)
- MW positive medium weak (low end of the *pm* membership function)
- W positive weak (*pw* membership function)
- -W negative weak (*nw* membership function)
- VW positive very weak (*pvw* membership function)
- VVW positive very weak (low end of the *pvw* membership function)

Table 27.3 Specific weights sw from FCs to DCs of the CFCM-ESI

FC#	Name of concept	ESI1	ESI2	ESI3	ESI4	ESI5
FC1	Life threatening	VVS	0	0	0	0
FC2	Limb threatening	VVS	0	0	0	0
FC3	Patient chief complaint	0	MS	MS	0	0
FC4	Vital signs	0	M	MW	0	0
FC5	Medical history	0	MW	MW	0	0
FC6	Other factor	0	MW	MW	0	0
FC7	Expected number of resources	0	W	MW	-W	-M
FC8	Patient age	0	W	VW	0	0
FC9	Required timely intervention	0	W	VW	-W	-M
FC10	Weakness	0	VS	S	VVW	0
FC11	Additional symptoms other than chief complaint	0	W	VW	0	0
FC12	Severe pain or distress	0	VW	VW	0	0
FC13	Patient referred to ED from outside	0	VVW	VW	0	0
FC14	Behavioral or psychi-atric issue	0	VVW	VVW	0	0
FC15	No additional symptoms to chief complaint	0	VVW	VVW	M	MS
FC16	Absence of medical history	0	VVW	VVW	0	0
FC17	Patient medications	0	VVW	VVW	0	0
FC18	Hospital or ED discharge 3days	M	VVW	VVW	0	0
FC19	Patient immunocompromised	M	VVW	VVW	0	0
FC20	Alcohol or illicit drug use	0	VVW	VVW	0	0
FC21	No recent change mental state	0	0	0	M	M
FC22	Patient can walk or sit	0	0	W	VS	VVS

In the following subsection the CFCM-ESI is applied to real patient cases, arriving at the Emergency Department.

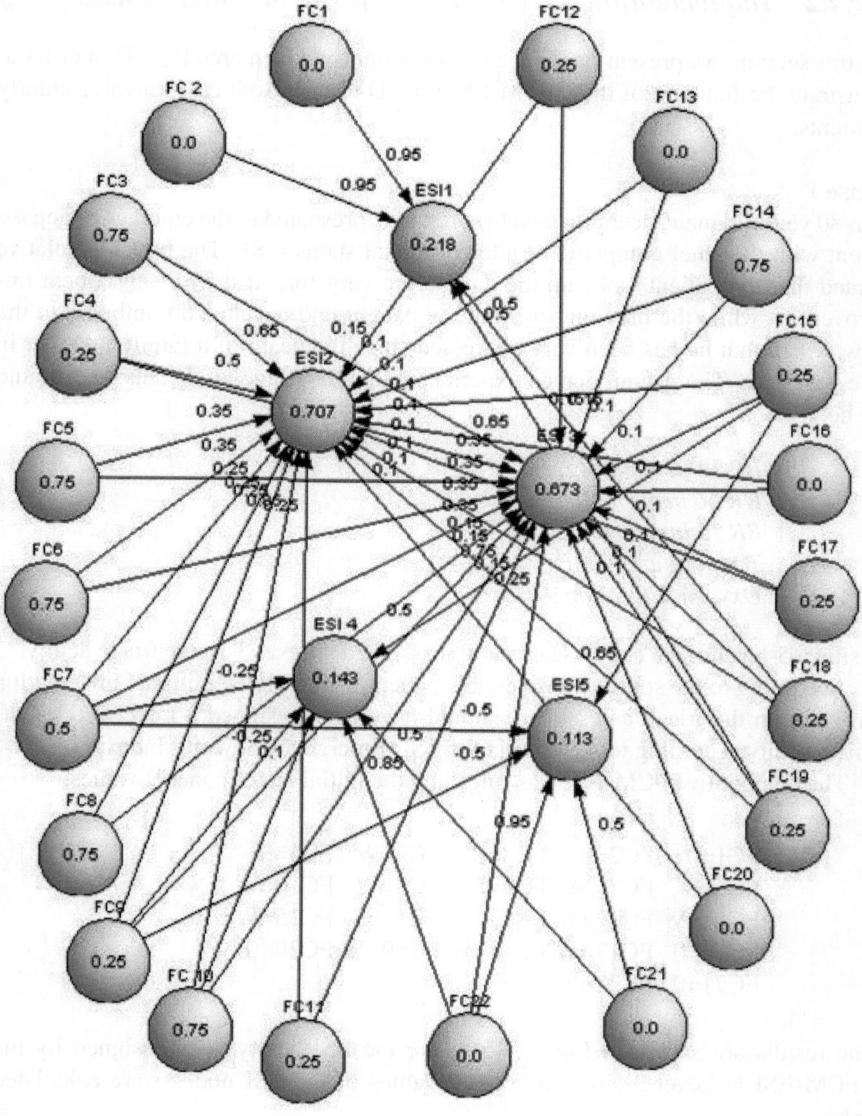

Fig. 27.4 The CFCM-ESI for the first case

27.4.2 Implementing the CFCM-ESI for Real Patient Cases

In this section, we present two real cases of patients who entered the ED in order to illustrate the function of the CFCM-ESI for ED triage. Both cases involve elderly patients.

Case 1
An 80 year-old male, accompanied by a relative, presented to the emergency department with the chief complaint of altered mental status [48]. The patient's relative stated that the patient woke up the day before very forgetful with subsequent improvement while the previous evening the patient had developed numbness to the jaw. Also, that he has been very depressed since the death of a family member in the past year. The patient denied experiencing pain. Triage vital signs were found to be:

BP 138/78 mm Hg,
HR 66 beats/min,
RR 16 breaths/min,
Temperature 97.8F (36.5C),
Oxygen saturation 97%.

Using a 5-level triage acuity scale he was assigned a Level 3-Acute triage acuity.

According to the source however, this patient, based on the minimal information provided in the triage assessment, should have been assigned a Level 2 (Urgent) triage acuity according to the criteria for ESI (Emergency Severity Index).

The competitive FCM-ESI was run using the initial factor concept values:

FC1=0 FC2=0 FC3=S FC4=W FC5=S
FC6=S FC7=M FC8=S FC9=W FC10=S
FC11=W FC12=W FC13=0 FC14=S FC15=W
FC16=0 FC17=W FC18=W FC19=W FC20=0
FC21=0 FC22=0

The results are shown in Fig. 27.5 where the ESI acuity level assigned by the CFCM-ESI is Level 2 since the output values of the ESI nodes were calculated to be:

ESI 1 = 0.2181
ESI 2 = 0.7072
ESI 3 = 0.6726
ESI 4 = 0.1432
ESI 5 = 0.1131

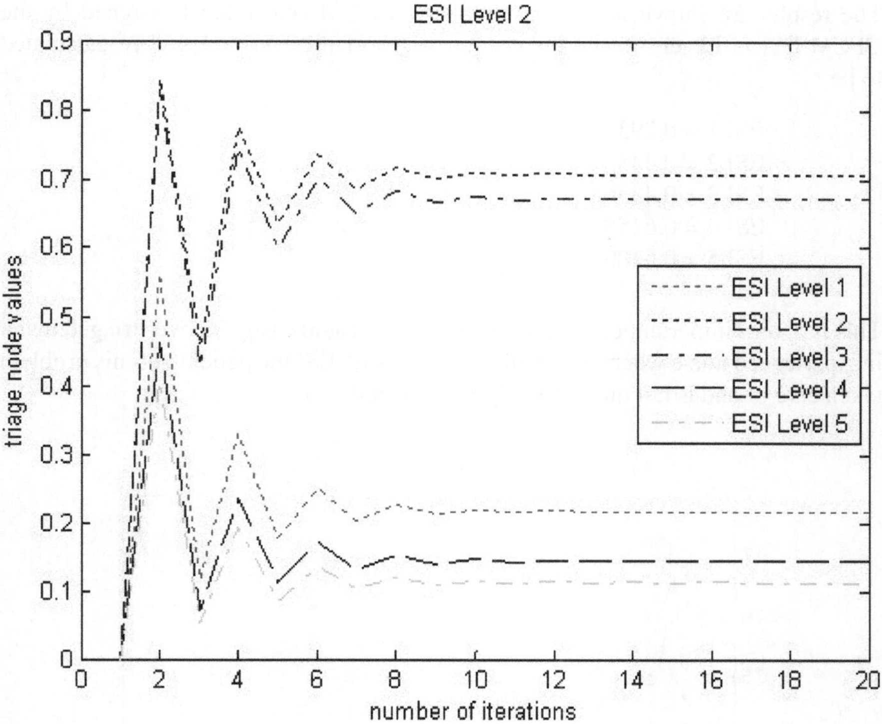

Fig. 27.5 CFCM-ESI output for case 1, patient is correctly triaged at ESI2

Case 2

A 63-year-old cachectic male was brought to the ED from the nursing home because his feeding tube fell out again. The patient is usually unresponsive and has been in the nursing home since he suffered a massive stroke about 4 years ago [16].

The patient was triaged at ESI level-4-Routine, which means that the patient was sent back to the nursing home after the feeding tube was reinserted. There was no acute change in his medical condition, even though he was unresponsive, since that is the patient's baseline mental status and so he was not triaged at ESI level 1.

The Competitive FCM-ESI was run using the initial fuzzy factor concept values based on the case information:

FC1=0	FC2=0	FC3=0	FC4=W	FC5=W
FC6=W	FC7=W	FC8=S	FC9=W	FC10=0
FC11=W	FC12=0	FC13=0	FC14=S	FC15=W
FC16=0	FC17=W	FC18=0	FC19=W	FC20=0
FC21=VVS	FC22=0			

The results are shown in Fig. 27.6 where the ESI acuity level assigned by the CFCM-ESI is Level 4 since the output values of the ESI nodes were calculated to be:

ESI 1 = 0.2931
ESI 2 = 0.4483
ESI 3 = 0.4356
ESI 4 = 0.6158
ESI 5 = 0.5109

This is a very important case because the patient could easily be over-triaged by an inexperienced nurse whereas consulting the CFCM-ESI the patient gets his problem taken care of and is not unnecessarily hospitalized.

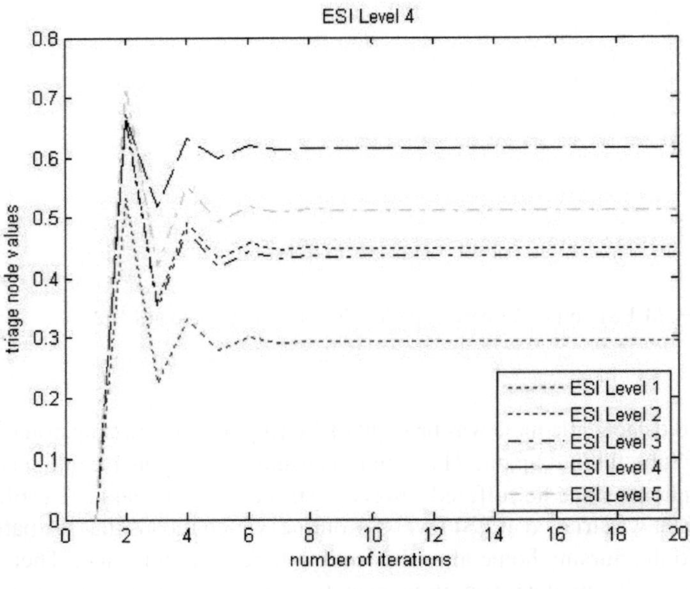

Fig. 27.6 FCM DSS output for case 2, patient is correctly triaged at ESI4

27.5 Conclusions

Here, the Soft Computing methodology of Fuzzy Cognitive Maps (FCMs) is applied for the first time to develop a Medical Decision Support Systems for the ESI Triage, a significant procedure during patient admission at the Emergency Department (ED) of hospitals. The main focus of this application is the older patients, who are admitted quite frequently at the ED suffering from chronic problems, presenting many complementary and/or controversial symptoms and not presenting a high level communication ability that increases the complexity of any assessment and decision about their health condition, the emergency and the required treatment.

FCMs have been successfully used to develop Medical Decision Support Systems and here the general framework of Competitive FCM is used. In addition to this, here a novel hybrid design methodology for FCM is applied that combines the knowledge and experience of human experts along with information and bibliographic data, in order to create a more efficient CFCM-MDSS.

The clinical decision support system based on CFCM for the 5-level ESI triage scale was developed and presented in detail: it considers 22 factors and concludes to one of the 5 ESI triage levels. The CFCM for ESI triage was tested using real patient cases from the literature and the assessment results showed that it reached the correct triage decision. It is considered that the CFCM is an efficient modeling method for the complex decision-making process of triage, and it is developed and evaluated into an advanced CFCM-ESI system for the ED. This advanced CFCM-ESI, following the designing methodology presented here, will take into consideration more factors and will also interaction between factors, so that to create a generic integrated CFCM-MDSS. This CFCM-ESI was tested and its accuracy was compared with the rating of experienced triage nurse. Further, comparison of CFCM-ESI to the rates of undertriage and overtriage will be analyzed, in future work.

Acknowledgement. This work is partially supported by the programme "Greece-Czech Joint Research and Technology projects 2011-2013" of the General Secretariat of Research & Development, Greek Ministry of Education, Lifelong Learning and Religious Affairs co-financed by the Greece and the European Union.

References

1. Aronsky, D., Jones, I., Raines, B., Hemphill, R., Mayberry, S.R., Luther, M.A., Slusser, T.: An Integrated Computerized Triage System in the Emergency Department. In: AMIA Symposium Proceedings, pp. 16–20 (2008)
2. Australian Institute of Health and Welfare, Australian Hospital Statistics 2009-10: EmergencyDepartment Care and Elective Surgery Waiting Times (2010), `http://www.aihw.gov.au/publications/index.cfm/title/12271` (accessed on September 30, 2010)
3. Barbee, G.A., Berry-Cabán, C.S., Daymude, M.L., Oliver, J., Gay, S.: The Effect of Provider Level Triage in a Military Treatment Facility Emergency Department. Journal of Emergency Primary Health Care (JEPHC) 8, Article 990386 (2010)
4. Baum, S.A., Rubenstein, L.Z.: Old people in the Emergency Room: Age-related Differences in Emergency Department Use and Care. Journal of the American Geriatrics Society 35, 398–404 (1987)
5. Benner, P., Tanner, C.: Clinical Judgment: How Expert Nurses Use Intuition. American Journal of Nursing 87, 23–31 (1987); Bullard, M.J., Unger, B., Spence, J., Grafstein, E.: Revisions to the Canadian Emergency Department Triage and Acuity Scale (CTAS) Adult Guidelines. Canadian Journal of Emergency Medicine (CJEM) 10, pp. 136–151 (2008)
6. Carvalho, J.P.: On the Semantics and the Use of Fuzzy Cognitive Maps and Dynamic Cognitive Maps in Social Sciences. Fuzzy Sets and Systems (2012), `http://dx.doi.org/10.1016/j.fss.2011.12.009`

7. Carvalho, J.P.: Rule Based Fuzzy Cognitive Maps in Humanities, Social Sciences and Economics. In: Seising, R., Sanz González, V. (eds.) Soft Computing in Humanities and Social Sciences. STUDFUZZ, vol. 273, pp. 297–308. Springer, Heidelberg (2012)
8. Conroy, S., Cooper, N.: Acute Medical Care of Elderly People. British Geriatrics Society, London (2004)
9. Dempsey, J.: The Appropriateness of Admissions and the Influences on a Decision to Admit. Journal of Quality in Clinical Practice 20, 95–99 (2000)
10. Eitel, D., Travers, D.A., Rosenau, A.M., Gilboy, N., Wuertz, R.: The Emergency Severity Index Algorithm Version 2 is Reliable and Valid. Academic Emergency Medicine 10, 1070–1080 (2003)
11. Emergency Nurses Association (ENA): Making the Right Decision: A triage Curriculum (2nd ed.), Des Plaines, IL (2001)
12. Garbez, R., Carrieri-Kohlman, V., Stotts, N., Chan, G., Neighbor, M.: Factors Influencing Patient Assignment to Level 2 and Level 3 Within the 5-Level ESI Triage System. Journal of Emergency Nursing 37(6), 526–532 (2012)
13. Georgopoulos, V.C., Malandraki, G.A., Stylios, C.D.: A Fuzzy Cognitive Map Approach to Differential Diagnosis of Specific Language Impairment. Artificial Intelligence in Medicine 29, 261–278 (2003)
14. Georgopoulos, V.C., Stylios, C.D.: Augmented Fuzzy Cognitive Maps Supplemented with Case Based Reasoning for Advanced Medical Decision Support. In: Nikravesh, M., Zadeh, L.A., Kacprzyk, J. (eds.) Soft Computing for Information Processing, pp. 388–389. Springer, Heidelberg (2005)
15. Georgopoulos, V.C., Stylios, C.D.: Complementary Case-based Reasoning, Competitive Fuzzy Cognitive Maps for Advanced Medical Decisions. Soft Computing 12, 191–199 (2008)
16. Gilboy, N., Tanabe, P., Travers, D.A., Rosenau, A.M., Eitel, D.: Emergency Severity Index, Version 4: Implementation Handbook. Agency for Healthcare Research and Quality, Publication No. 05-0046-2, Rockville, MD (2005), `http://www.ahrq.gov/research/esi/`
17. Goransson, K.E., Ehrenberg, A., Markland, B., Ehnfors, M.: Emergency Department Triage: Is there a Link Between Nurses' Personal Characteristics and Accuracy in Triage Decisions? Accident and Emergency Nursing 14, 83–88 (2006)
18. Hine, M.J., Farion, K.J., Michalowski, W., Wilk, S.: Decision Making by Emergency Room Physicians and Residents: Implications for the Design of Clinical Decision Support Systems. International Journal of Healthcare Information Systems and Informatics 4, 17–36 (2009)
19. Kosko, B.: Fuzzy Cognitive Maps. International Journal of Man-Machine Studies 24, 65–75 (1986)
20. Kottas, T.L., Boutalis, Y.S., Christodoulou, M.A.: Fuzzy Cognitive Network: A Generalized Framework. Intelligent Decision Technologies 1, 1–14 (2007)
21. Lin, C.-T., George Lee, C.S.: Neural Fuzzy Systems: A Neuro-Fuzzy Synergism to Intelligent Systems. Prentice-Hall, Upper Saddle River (1996)
22. McCaig, L.F., Nawar, E.W.: National Hospital Ambulatory Medical Care Survey: 2004 Emergency Department Summary. Advance Data 372, 1–32 (2006)
23. McCall, B., Travers, D., Platts-Mills, T., Biese, K.: Mistriage of Elderly in the Emergency Department. Connecting the Dots: Geriatric Nursing, Education, and Clinical Simulation. Chapel Hill, NC (2009)

24. McCusker, J., Verdon, J., Tousignant, P., de Courval, L.P., Dendukuri, N., Belzile, E.: Rapid Emergency Department Intervention for Older People Reduces Risk of Functional Decline: Results of a Multicenter Randomized Trial. Journal of the American Geriatric Society 49, 1272–1281 (2001)
25. Miao, Y., Miao, C., Tao, X., Shen, Z., Liu, Z.-Q.: Transformation of Cognitive Maps. IEEE Transactions on Fuzzy Systems 18, 114–124 (2010)
26. Mozes, B., Schiff, E., Modan, B.: Factors Affecting Inappropriate Hospital Stay. Quality Assurance in Health Care 3, 211–217 (1991)
27. Nemec, M., Koller, M.T., Nickel, C.H., Maile, S., Winterhalder, C., Karrer, C., Laifer, G., Bingisser, R.: Patients Presenting to the Emergency Department with Non-specific Complaints: The Basel Non-specific Complaints (BANC) Study, vol. 17, pp. 284–292. Academic Emergency Medicine (2010)
28. Nickel, C.H., Nemec, M., Bingisser, R.: Weakness as Presenting Symptom in the Emergency Department. Swiss Medical Weekly 139, 271–272 (2009)
29. NLLIC Staff: National Limb Loss Information Center fact Sheet: Amputation Statistics by Cause, Limb Loss in the United States, National Limb Loss Information Center (2008), http://www.amputee-colaition.org/fact_sheet/amp_stats_cause.html
30. Papageorgiou, E., Stylios, C., Groumpos, P.P.: An Integrated Two-level Hierarchical System for Decision Making in Radiation Therapy Using Fuzzy Cognitive Maps. IEEE Transactions on Biomedical Engineering 50, 1326–1339 (2003)
31. Pines, J.M., Mongelluzzo, J., Hilton, J.A., Hollander, J.E., Shofer, F.S., Souder, J., Synnestvedt, M., Weiner, M.G., Datner, E.M.: Postdischarge Adverse Events for 1-Day Hospital Admissions in Older Adults Admitted From the Emergency Department. Annals of Emergency Medicine 56, 253–257 (2010)
32. Platts-Mills, T.F., Travers, D., Biese, K., McCall, B., Kizer, S., LaMantia, M., Busby-Whitehead, J., Cairns, C.B.: Accuracy of the Emergency Severity Index Triage Instrument for Identifying Elder Emergency Department Patients Receiving an Immediate Life-saving Intervention. Academic Emergency Medicine 17, 238–243 (2010)
33. Rutschmann, O.T., Chevalley, T., Zumwald, C., Luthy, C., Vermeulen, B., Sarasin, F.P.: Pitfalls in the Emergency Department Triage of Frail Elderly Patients Without Specific Complaints. Swiss Medicine Weekly 135, 145–150 (2005)
34. Safwenberg, U., Terént, A., Lind, L.: Differences in Long-term Mortality for Different Emergency Department Presenting Complaints. Academic Emergency Medicine 15, 9–16 (2008)
35. Salmeron, J.L.: Augmented Fuzzy Cognitive Maps for modelling LMS Critical Success Factors. Knowledge Based Systems 22, 275–278 (2009)
36. Salvi, F., Morichi, V., Grilli, A., Giorgi, R., De Tommaso, G., Dessì-Fulgheri, P.: The Elderly in the Emergency Department: A Critical Review of Problems and Solutions. Internal and Emergency Medicine 2, 292–301 (2007)
37. Samaras, N., Chevalley, T., Samaras, D., Gold, G.: Older Patients in the Emergency Department: A Review. Annals of Emergency Medicine 56, 261–269 (2010)
38. San Pedro, J., Burstein, F., Cao, P., Churilov, L., Zaslavsky, A.B., Wassertheil, J.: Mobile Decision Support for Triage in Emergency Departments. In: Decision Support in an Uncertain and Complex World: The IFIP TC8/WG8.3 International Conference, pp. 714–723 (2004)
39. Shelton, R.: The Emergency Severity Index 5-level Triage System. Dimensions of Critical Care Nursing 28, 9–12 (2009)

40. Soar, J., Yuginovich, T., Whittaker, F.: Reducing Avoidable Hospital Admissions of the Frail Elderly Using Intelligent Referrals. eJHI - electronic Journal of Health Informatics 2, e3 (2007)
41. Stach, W., Kurgan, L.A., Pedrycz, W.: Numerical and Linguistic Prediction of Time Series With the Use of Fuzzy Cognitive Maps. IEEE Transactions on Fuzzy Systems 16, 61–72 (2008)
42. Strange, G.R., Chen, E.H., Sanders, A.B.: Use of Emergency Departments by Elderly Patients: Projections from a Multicenter Data Base. Annals of Emergency Medicine 21, 819–824 (1992)
43. Stylios, C.D., Georgopoulos, V.C., Malandraki, G.A., Chouliara, S.: Spyridoula Chouliara: Fuzzy Cognitive Map Architectures for Medical Decision Support Systems. Applied Soft Computing 8, 1243–1251 (2008)
44. Stylios, C.D., Groumpos, P.P.: Fuzzy Cognitive Maps in Modeling Supervisory Control Systems. Journal of Intelligent & Fuzzy Systems 8, 83–98 (2000)
45. Stylios, C.D., Groumpos, P.P.: Modeling Complex Systems Using Fuzzy Cognitive Maps. IEEE Transactions on Systems, Man and Cybernetics: Part A Systems and Humans 34, 155–162 (2004)
46. Tanabe, P., Gimbel, R., Yarnold, P.R., Adams, J.G.: The Emergency Severity Index (version 3) 5-level Triage System Scores Predict ED resource consumption. Journal of Emergency Nursing 30, 22–29 (2004)
47. Travers, D., Waller, A.E., Bowling, J.M., Flowers, D., Tintinalli, J.: Fivelevel Triage System more Effective than Three-level in Tertiary Emergency Department. Journal of Emergency Nursing 28, 395–400 (2002)
48. Triage first (2008), http://www.triagefirst.com/newsletter/2008Q3/casepresentation.html
49. van Bokhoven, M.A., Koch, H., van der Weijden, T., Dinant, G.-J.: Special Methodological Challenges when Studying the Diagnosis of Unexplained Complaints in Primary Care. Journal of Clinical Epidemiology 61, 318–322 (2008)
50. Vanpee, D., Swine, C., Vandenbossche, P., Gillet, J.B.: Epidemiological Profile of Geriatric Patients Admitted to the Emergency Department of a University Hospital Localized in a Rural Area. European Journal of Emergency Medicine 8, 301–304 (2001)
51. Wilber, S.T.: Altered Mental Status in Older Emergency Department Patients. Emergency Medicine Clinics of North America 24, 299–316 (2006)
52. Wilkes, D.M., Franklin, S., Erdemir, E., Gordon, S.M., Strain, S., Miller, K., Kawamura, K.: Heterogeneous Artificial Agents for Triage Nurse Assistance. In: IEEE-RAS International Conference on Humanoids Robots, pp. 130–137 (2010)
53. Wuerz, R.: Emergency Severity Index Triage Category is Associated With Six-month Survival, ESI triage study group. Academic Emergency Medicine 8, 61–64 (2001)
54. Xirogiannis, G., Glykas, M., Staikouras, C.: Fuzzy Cognitive Maps in Banking Business Process Performance Measurement. In: Glykas, M. (ed.) Fuzzy Cognitive Maps. STUDFUZZ, vol. 247, pp. 161–200. Springer, Heidelberg (2010)
55. Xirogiannis, G., Stefanou, J., Glykas, M.: A Fuzzy Cognitive Map Approach to Support Urban Design. Journal of Expert Systems with Applications 26, 257–268 (2004)
56. Zimmermann, P.G.: The Case for a Universal, Valid, Reliable 5-tier Triage Acuity Scale for US Emergency Departments. Journal of Emergency Nursing 27, 246–254 (2001)

Authors

Alberto Alvarez-Alvarez received the B.S. degree from the Universidad de Oviedo, Spain, in 2006 and the M.S. degree from the Universidad Autónoma de Madrid, Spain, in 2008, both in physics. In July 2010, he received the M.S. degree in soft computing and intelligent data analysis organized from the European Centre for Soft Computing and the University of Oviedo. He is currently working toward the Ph.D. degree in computer science with the same university. Since September 2008, he has been a Research Assistant with the "Cognitive Computing: Computing with Perceptions" research unit at the European Centre for Soft Computing. He has published twelve papers in international journals and peer-reviewed conferences and registered one patent. His main research interests include the use of sensors to obtain and manage data from the physical context, analyze them using computational intelligence techniques, and produce accurate models close to natural language. Mr. Alvarez-Alvarez's three contributions have received the Best Special Session Student Paper Award in the 11th International Conference on Intelligent Systems Design and Applications (Córdoba, Spain, 2011), the IEEE Computational Intelligence Society 2011 Outstanding Paper Award at the 5th IEEE International Workshop on Genetic and Evolutionary Fuzzy Systems (Paris, France, 2011), and the Best Presentation Award at the International Open Workshop Fuzziness and Medicine (Mieres, Spain, 2011).

Ernesto Araujo: Ph.D. in Computer Science from Brazilian National Space Research Institute (INPE), MSc. Degree in Electronic Engineering and Computer from Technical Institute for Aeronautics (ITA), and undergraduate degree in Electrical Engineering from Pontifical Catholic University (PUC). Currently, work as Professor at the Universidade Federal de Sao Paulo (UNIFESP), in the Health Informatics Dpt. (DIS) since 2007, being also Professor at the Faculdade de Ciências Médicas de Minas Gerais (FCMMG), in the Post-Graduation and Research Institute (IPG), as well as is with the Unimed Cooperativa de Trabalhos Médicos (UNIMEDBH) as Research and Development Expert. At the Hospital Municipal Dr. José de Carvalho Florence (HMJCF) worked as Researcher and Project Coordinator from 2008 to 2012, where was also as Technical Director of its Center of

Research/Studies Fábio Schmidt Goffi (CEFSG). At the National Space Research Institute (INPE) was Professor in the Space Mechanics and Control Dpt. (DMC) from 2005 to 2010 and worked at the Integration and Testing Lab. (LIT) from 1995 to 2010. Yet, was Training Director at the Instrumentation, System and Automation Society (ISA) from 2006-2008. Also works as referee of international and national journals related to IEEE, Elsevier, SBA, Pesquisa Naval, RBM only to mention few. Presents experience in Computational Intelligence and Artificial Intelligence, in the fields of Engineering, Computer Science, and Medicine, taking into account cognitive aspects of human nature, working in control design, modeling, automation, and decision support systems. Themes of interest encompass fuzzy logic, artificial neural network, particle swarm optimization (PSO), genetic algorithm (GA), intelligent agents, cybernetics, dynamic systems, and chaos theory. Areas of interest and work are medicine and health care, engineering, humanities (social sciences, economics, politic).

Luis Argüelles Ménendez holds an MSc degree in Astronomy (High Distinction) from the Swinburne University of Technology, Melbourne, Australia. In March, 2010, he received a Master of Business Administration degree from the ITEAP Institute, Malaga, Spain. He has worked as the R+D department's director in a private coal mining company in Spain along 20 years, directing and/or coordinating more than 30 research projects, covering regional, national and European frames of research. Inside these projects he has developed discrete event simulation based models, virtual reality systems and soft computing based models for geology and mining engineering. Luis is a pioneer in developing intelligent models for double stars in observational astronomy, having explored also the utility of fuzzy-sets theory in galactic morphology. His fields of interest cover the use and application of fuzzy-logic based techniques in astronomy, industrial processes and organizational management, specially in the field of total quality management (TQM). Since 2011 he is an Affiliated Researcher at the European Centre for Soft Computing.

Txetxu Ausín is Tenured Scientist and Chair of the Unit of Applied Ethics at Spanish National Research Council (CSIC), Madrid. He received his Ph.D. in Philosophy and First Prize for the year from the University of the Basque Country in 2000. His research focuses are deontic logic, bioethics, ethics of communication, and human rights. He is Editor of the web and journal about Applied Ethics DILEMATA: www.dilemata.net and Main Researcher of KONTUZ! Project about precautionary principle (FFI2011-24414): www.kontuz.weebly.com

Najib T. Ayas graduated from the University of Alberta in 1992. He completed an Internal Medicine Residency at the Mayo Clinic in 1996, and post-graduate training in Respiratory, Sleep, and Critical Care Medicine at Brigham and Women's Hospital/Harvard Medical School in 2000. He was on staff at Brigham and Women's Hospital for two years and also completed his Masters Degree in Public Health from the Harvard School of Public Health in 2002. In September 2002 Dr. Ayas joined the Respiratory Division at Vancouver General Hospital and was appointed on staff at the Sleep Disorders Program. Shortly thereafter, Dr. Ayas joined the Division of Critical Care Medicine. In 2007, Dr. Ayas was promoted to Associate Professor in the Department of Medicine at UBC and was appointed as Head, Divisions of Critical Care Medicine for UBC, VGH and PHC in 2009. Dr. Ayas' research interests include the investigation of the public health and safety consequences of sleep disorders, including both respiratory sleep disorders (such as sleep apnea) and sleep deprivation. He has received research funding from a number of national and provincial agencies, and has published in numerous, highly respected medical journals.

Clara Barroso Jerez has a Ph.D. in Philosophy and Education Science from the University of La Laguna, Spain where is Associated Professor at the Dpt. of Logic and Moral Philosophy at the same university. She has made research stays at the Institute of Philosophy of CSIC, the Centre d'Estudis Avançats of Blanes, the Institut de Investigació en Intelligencia Artificial of CSIC and University of Edinburgh Her areas of interest are in general related to the field of Science, Technology and Society and, in particular, to the application of information technologies to teaching and learning processes and knowledge representation.

Silvia Bortot has a Ph. D. in Mathematics for Economic Decisions from the University of Trento, Italy. She is currently an Assistant professor in the Department of Computer and Management Sciences at University of Trento, Italy. Her research interests are in Decision Theory, particularly in the multiagent and multicriteria decision frameworks.

Humberto Bustince, (M'08) is a Full Professor at the Department of Automatics and Computation, Public University of Navarra, Spain. He holds a Ph.D. degree in Mathematics from Public University of Navarra from 1994. He is a board member of the European Society for Fuzzy Logic and Technology (EUSFLAT). His research interests are fuzzy logic theory, extensions of Fuzzy sets (Type-2 fuzzy sets, Interval-valued fuzzy sets, Atanassov's intuitionistic fuzzy sets), Fuzzy measures, Aggregation functions and fuzzy techniques for Image processing. He is author of over 95 published original articles and involved in teaching Artificial Intelligence for students of Computer Sciences. Moreover, he is Editor-in-Chief of the *Mathware & Soft Computing Magazine*.

Agata Ciabattoni is Professor for Nonclassical Logics in Computer Science at the Vienna University of Technology. She is currently the head of the research projects "Fuzzy Logic: from Mathematics to Medical Applications" (2008-2012) and "Nonclassical Proofs: Theory, Applications and Tools" (2011-2017). The latter was funded as a START prize from the Austrian Science Fund (FWF).

Patrik Eklund, is a professor at Umeå University, Department of Computing Science, Umeå, Sweden. He received his PhD in mathematics, wrote over 100 scientific publications, is involved in research both on the theoretical as well the applied side. Software developments include crisis management, distributed systems, group decision support, plant project management, and medical decision support. The overall scope and motivation is to enhance methodological issues to support effective and efficient development of guidelines and workflows. Software engineering methodologies are developed to support handling of platform independencies, web services and provide effective techniques for handling client-server and human-computer interactive applications. Patrik Eklund has experience, since 1992, from participation in several European FP (DIDOS, CHIN, HANSA), COST (COST15, COST274) and Interreg (BRB, eAW, Bel-HMI) projects.

Mario Fedrizzi has been working since 1986 as Full Professor of Mathematical Methods for Economics at the Department of Computer and Management Sciences, University of Trento, Italy. His fields of interest are utility and risk theory, group decision making, fuzzy decision analysis, and soft computing. He has authored more than 150 papers, appeared in peer reviewed international journals, edited volumes and proceedings of international conferences. He is member of the editorial boards of *International Journal of Uncertainty Fuzziness and Knowledge-Based Systems*, *International Journal of General Systems*, *Group Decisions and Negotiation*, *Control and Cybernetics*, *Applied Computational Intelligence* and *Soft Computing*.

Itziar García-Honrado (Gijón, Spain, 1985) obtained a M.Sc. degree in Mathematics with specialization in Statistics at the University of Oviedo in 2007. That year she joined the Unit of Fundamentals of Soft Computing at the European Centre for Soft Computing, where she carried out the research for her Ph.D. Dissertation entitled "Contribution to the Ordinary Reasoning and Computing with Words", presented in 2011 at the University of León. Currently she is a member of the department of "Statistics, Operations Research and Mathematics Education" at the University of Oviedo, and teaches in the section of Mathematics Education. She has published around 25 papers in international journals, international and national conferences, and in several book chapters. These publications mainly deal with models of Conjectures, Hypotheses and Consequences (CHC models), mathematical representations of linguistic imprecise terms, and on the analysis of schemes of classical reasoning in the context of Fuzzy Logic. Since 2012 she is an Affiliated Researcher of the European Centre for Soft Computing

Voula C. Georgopoulos holds a Diploma in Electrical Engineering from the University of Thrace, Greece (1984), an SM in Electrical Engineering and Computer Science (1987) and an Engineer's Professional Degree from the Massachusetts Institute of Technology (1988), and a Ph.D. in Electrical Engineering from Tufts University (1992). In May 1988 she joined the MITRE Corporation, Bedford, MA, as a Member of Technical Staff. Between April 1994 and December 1995 she worked as a research scientist in the Electrical Engineering Department of the University of Patras, Greece. In January 1996 she joined the faculty of the School of Electrical Engineering and Computer Science of Ohio University, as an Assistant Professor. As of September 1998 she is Professor of Informatics in the Dept. of Speech and Language Therapy at the Technological Educational Institute of Patras in Greece. Her current research interests include differential diagnosis and medical decision support systems and speech signal processing using advanced techniques.

She has authored/co-authored more than 80 publications in peer reviewed journals and conference proceedings.

Juan Carlos Hernández Clemente is a Associate Professor of Medical Humanities in the Department of Psychiatry. Faculty of Medicine of the Universidad Autónoma de Madrid.

Karin Hutflötz is teaching philosophy at the Academy of Fine Arts and at the Hochschule für Philosophie S.J. in Munich. After studying chemistry, mathematics and philosophy she received her M.S. degree and Ph.D. in philosophy at the university in Munich. Her main research topics are philosophical anthropology, dealing with questions of metaphysics and phenomenology of the human person, philosophy of nature and science, and aesthetics.

Julia Inthorn is a medical ethicist with a background in philosophy. She holds a diploma in mathematics and statistics from the University of Munich and postgraduate degrees in adult's education and philosophy. She gained her Ph.D. in philosophy with a study on research methods in social sciences from the Munich School of Philosophy. She is currently a research assistant at the Department for medical ethics and history of medicine at the University Medical Centre Göttingen. Her main research interests are Intercultural Bioethics and Empirical Ethics, especially in the field of End-of-Life Decisions, Ethics of Genetic Testing as well as Perspectives on Health and Justice.

Aranzazu Jurio received the M.Sc. degree in Computer Sciences from the Public University of Navarra, Pamplona, Spain, in 2008. She currently holds a research position at the Department of Automatics and Computation where she is working towards the Ph.D. degree. Her research interests are image processing, focusing on magnification and segmentation, and applications of fuzzy sets and their extensions.

Lukas Kaelin is currently Research Fellow at the Institute for Ethics and Law in Medicine, University of Vienna, Austria. His research in bioethics and the philosophy of medicine focuses on the intercultural dimensions of medical practice.

Krzysztof Kielan received his Medical Diploma from Medical University of Silesia, Poland, in 1988. He completed his clinical training in psychiatry and he received the PhD degree in medicine in 1995. He is currently a Consultant Psychiatrist at the Department of Psychiatry, Harrison House, Peaks Lane, Grimsby, UK, and an honorary senior lecturer at Hull & York Medical School. His clinical practice and research interests include: brain mapping, QEEG assessment, new ways of working within acute setting, rehabilitation of cognitive functions, ADD/ADHD and Asperger spectrum, dynamic psychotherapy, and computer-based medical decision support systems.

Tatiana Kiseliova is an Assistant Professor at the Department of Exact and Natural Sciences, Iv. Javakhishvili Tbilisi State University, Georgia, where she currently teaches "Mathematical Logic and Discrete Mathematics", "Fuzzy Logic with

Applications". She has received her PhD and DSc in Computer Sciences and Applied Mathematics from the same University in 1995 and 2006, respectively. Her research mainly focuses on applications of fuzzy (in particular) and soft computing (in general) methodologies for medical diagnoses, time series analysis as well as theoretical and practical aspects of many-valued logics, temporal logics, fuzzy logics.

Maka Korinteli, MD. Graduated from the Tbilisi State Medical University in 2005. Worked as a physician in different clinics and as a medical advisor with pharmaceutical companies. Since 2011 PhD student at the Tbilisi State Medical University.

Mila Kwiatkowska received the MA degree in Interdisciplinary Studies of Polish Philology and Informatics from the University of Wroclaw in Poland, the MSc degree in Computing Science from the University of Alberta in Canada, and the PhD degree in Computing Science from Simon Fraser University in Canada. She is currently an Associate Professor in the Computing Science Department at Thompson Rivers University (TRU) in Kamloops, Canada. Her research interests include medical data mining, medical decision systems, clinical prediction rules, knowledge representation, fuzzy logic, semiotics, and case-based reasoning. She is author or co-author of over 30 peer-reviewed publications. She teaches courses in database systems, data mining, web-based systems, and biomedical informatics.

José Lázaro (born in La Coruña, Spain), Doctor of Medicine, teaches Medical Humanities as a full time Professor, Universidad Autónoma de Madrid. He has pursued in the past two lines of research: the history of psychoanalytic concepts and the history of Spanish psychiatry. He is currently studying the relation (both past and present) between the scientific search for objectivity (Evidence Based Medicine) and clinical recognition of subjectivity (personal, social, and cultural values), as well as the physiopathology of violence. E-mail: jose.lazaro@uam.es

Leandro Lazzareschi is at the Department of Physiotherapy, University of Cruzeiro do Sul and University of Mogi das Cruzes, Brazil.

von Krzysztof Michalik is a Professor in the Department of Knowledge Engineering, University of Economics, Katowice, Poland. His research interests include fuzzy logic, knowledge management, and medical expert systems. He is a founder of an AI software company, AITECH. His hybrid expert system, SPHYNX, has been utilized in many medical and financial applications.

Carlos Molina received his M.S. degree in Computer Science in 2002 and his Ph.D. in Computer Science in 2005, both from the University of Granada. He is an assistant professor in the Department of Computer Science of the University of Jaen since 2004. His current main research interests are in the fields of Multidimensional Model, Data Mining and Soft Computing.

Takehiko (Take) Nakama received two Ph.D.s from The Johns Hopkins University in Baltimore, Maryland, USA. He completed his first Ph.D. program in 2003 by conducting quantitative neurophysiological research at The Johns Hopkins Krieger Mind/Brain Institute. In 2009, he completed his second Ph.D. program in the Department of Applied Mathematics and Statistics by conducting research on stochastic processes that mathematically characterize stochastic search and optimization algorithms. In 2010, he completed the master's program at the European Center for Soft Computing and joined Enrique Ruspini's research unit as a postdoctoral researcher. His research interests include measure-theoretic probability, stochastic processes (Markov chains in particular), statistics for Hilbert-space-valued data (including fuzzy data), stochastic optimization, analysis of algorithms, system identification, mathematical foundations of fuzzy logic, and reasoning under uncertainty.

Vesa Niskanen is Dr. Docent at the University of Helsinki, Department of Economics & Management, Helsinki, Finland. He has studied fuzzy systems since the 1970's. He has focused on the methodology of the human sciences. He acted as the Secretary of IFSA two periods in 1999-2003. He is conducting two BISC Special Interest Groups at the UC Berkeley.

Karaman Pagava, MD, PhD, DSc. Graduated from the Tbilisi State Medical Institute. Received PhD from the same institution in 1975, DSc - from the Moscow Institute of Pediatrics of the Academy of Medical Sciences of the USSR in 1990. Since 1996 Professor at the Department of Pediatrics of the Tbilisi State Medical University. Author of about 300 scientific publications, incl. monographs and manuals. Supervised 24 doctoral theses. Areas of scientific interests: anatomical and physiological peculiarities of growing organism, clinical trials, adolescent medicine, usage of mathematical methods, incl. fuzzy logic approaches, in clinical medicine.

Miguel Pagola received the M.Sc. degree in industrial engineering and the Ph.D. degree, both from the Public University of Navarra (UPNa), Pamplona, Spain, in 2000 and 2008, respectively. He is currently an Associate Lecturer with the Department of Automatics and Computation, UPNa. He is the author of more than 20 published original articles in WoS and is involved in teaching artificial intelligence for students of computer sciences. His research interests include fuzzy techniques for image processing, fuzzy set theory, medical image segmentation, and medical data mining. Dr. Pagola is member of the European Society for Fuzzy Logic and Technology.

Daniel Paternain received the M.Sc. degree in Computer Sciences from the Public University of Navarra, Pamplona, Spain, in 2008. He is currently working towards the Ph.D. degree with the Department of Automatics and Computation, Public University of Navarra. He is currently a Teaching Assistant with the Department of Automatics and Computation, Public University of Navarra. His research interests include image processing, focusing on image reduction, and applications of aggregation functions, fuzzy sets, and extensions of fuzzy sets.

Carmen Peña-Yañez, M.S. degree in Physics from University of Granada, is actually the Technical Director of the Department of Computer Science in San Cecilio Hospital in Granada. She is the author of several research papers in the fields of Healthcare Information Systems and Artificial Intelligence applied to health activities.

David Picado Muiño gained several degrees (*management and accounting* in 1997, *economics* and *philosophy* in 2002 and *mathematics* in 2005). He wrote his Phd thesis at the University of Manchester on uncertain reasoning and probability logic. From 2009 to 2011 he worked as a postdoctoral researcher at the *Technische Universität Vienna*, Austria in a project related to the analysis and improvement of a medical knowledge-based system (CADIAG 2). Since April 2011 he is a postdoctoral researcher in the *Intelligent Data Analysis and Graphical Models* group at the European Centre for Soft Computing.

Miguel Prados de Reyes, Ph.D. in Mathematics from the University of Granada, is currently Head of the Department of Informatics in San Cecilio Hospital in Granada and associate professor in the Department of Computer Science and A.I. at the University of Granada. He is also Professional Association of Health Informatics in Andalucia, member of various committees and scientific societies and author of several research papers in the field of Healthcare Information Systems and Artificial Intelligence applied to health activities.

Belén Prados-Suárez was born in Granada. She received her M.S. degree in Computer Science in 2001 and her Ph.D. in Computer Science in 2006, both from the University of Granada. She was an assistant professor in the Department of Computer Science of the University of Jaen from 2004 to 2006, and since then in the Department of Software Engineering in the University in Granada. Her current main research interests are in the fields of Context Information Retrieval, Healthcare Information Systems, Image Processing and Soft Computing.

Cristina Puente Águeda, born in 1978 in Madrid (Spain), received her M.S. degree in Computer Engineering in 2001 (ICAI-Pontificia Comillas University, Madrid, Spain). She is Phd. student (ICAI-Pontificia Comillas University, Madrid, Spain). Principal Employment and Affiliations: From 2005: Associate Professor of the Department of Telecommunications, SEK (IE) University, Segovia, Spain. From 2006: Professor of the Department of Computer Science, ICAI -Pontificia Comillas University, Madrid, Spain. From 2007: Professor of the Department of Mathematics, ICAI -Pontificia Comillas University, Madrid, Spain.

Kazem Sadegh-Zadeh, born in 1942, is an analytic philosopher of medicine. He studied medicine and philosophy at the German universities of Münster, Berlin, and Göttingen with Internship and residency 1967-1971, assistant professor and lecturer 1972-1982, full professor of philosophy of medicine at the University of Münster 1982-2004. Sadegh-Zadeh was born in Tabriz, Iran, and is a German citizen. He is the founder of the analytic philosophy of medicine. He has been working in this area since 1970. He is the founding editor of the international journals *Metamed*, founded in 1977 (current title: *Theoretical Medicine and Bioethics*, published by Springer Verlag) and *Artificial Intelligence in Medicine*, founded in 1989 (published by Elsevier). His work includes: *Handbook of Analytic Philosophy of Medicine* (2011), "The Prototype Resemblance Theory of Disease" (2008), theory of fuzzy biopolymers (2000), and theory of the Machina Sapiens (2000). From: $http://en.wikipedia.org/wiki/Kazem_sadegh-Zadeh$

Rudolf Seising, born 1961 in Duisburg, Germany, received an MS degree in mathematics from the Ruhr University of Bochum in 1986, a Ph.D. degree in philosophy of science from the Ludwig Maximilians University (LMU) of Munich in 1995, and a postdoctoral lecture qualification (PD) in history of science from the LMU of Munich in 2004 for his book on the history of the theory of fuzzy sets (*The Fuzzification of Systems*, Springer-Verlag, 2007). He has been scientific assistant for computer sciences at the University of the Armed Forces in Munich (1988-1995) and for history of sciences at the same university (1995-2002). He was scientific assistant in the Core unit for medical statistics and informatics at the University Vienna Medical School (2002-2008), which in 2004 became the Medical University of Vienna. Since 2005 he is also college lecturer in the faculty of History and Arts at the LMU of Munich. He was acting as a professor (substitute) for the history of science at the Friedrich-Schiller-University Jena (2008) and at the LMU of Munich (2008/2009). He was several times visiting scholar at the University of California at Berkeley, CA (2000-2003) and at the University of Turku, Finland (2008). In 2009 and 2010 he was Visiting Researcher at the European Centre for Soft Computing in Mieres, Spain where he is Adjoint Researcher since 2011.

Alejandro Sobrino Cerdeiriña is Ph. D. in Philosophy from the University of Santiago de Compostela, Spain. Currently is Associated Professor at the Dpt. of Logic and Moral Philosophy at the same university, where he teaches 'Formal Grammars' and 'Logic Programming'. His areas of interest are: vagueness, fuzzy logic and (vague) natural language processing.

Chrysostomos D. Stylios is an Assistant Professor at the Department of Informatics and Telecommunications Technology, Technological Educational Institute of Epirus; he is a senior researcher at Telematics Center Department of Computer Technology Institute & Press. He was a visitor assistant professor at the Computer Science Department of the University of Ioannina. He received his Ph.D from the Department of Electrical & Computer Engineering University of Patras in 1999. He received the diploma in Electrical & Computer Engineering from the Aristotle University of Thessaloniki in 1992. He has published over 100 journal and conference papers, book chapter and technical reports. His main scientific interests include: Fuzzy Cognitive Maps, Soft Computing techniques, Computational Intelligence Techniques, Evolutionary methods, Neural Networks, Support Vector Machines, Knowledge Hierarchical Systems and intelligent data fusion and Decision Support Systems for Medical application. His major contribution is investigating new models of Fuzzy Cognitive Maps and exploring their utilization for developing intelligent systems and Decision Support Systems.

Marco Elio Tabacchi is currently the Scientific Director of Istituto Nazionale di Ricerche Demopolis, as well as a Research Assistant at the Soft Computing Research group of the Dipartimento di Matematica ed Informatica – Università degli Studi di Palermo, Italy. He holds a joint PhD in Mathematics and Information Science and Science and Technologies of Information, Telecommunication and Systems awarded from Università degli Studi di Palermo and Université de Paris Sud XI. His main scientific interest are in the field of complexity evaluation and comparison in artificial vision using the soft computing framework, and the general problem of dealing with complexity when gathering subjective information, as well as the recursive aspect of reality. His work has been recently focused on the problem of replicating, with the use of algorithms, the human reaction in terms of cognitive load to variation in visual complexity, evaluated through the use of indirect indicators such as the perception of passing time.

Settimo Termini is Professor of Theoretical Computer Science at the University of Palermo and has directed from 2002 to 2009 the Istituto di Cibernetica "Eduardo Caianiello" of the CNR (National Research Council). Among his scientific interests, we mention: the introduction and formal development of the theory of (entropy) measures of fuzziness; an analysis in innovative terms of the notion of vague predicate as it appears and is used in Information Sciences, Cybernetics and AI. He has been interested also in the problem of the connections between scientific research and economic development of a country. Recently he has extended his interest on the conceptual foundations of Fuzzy Sets and Soft Computing in the analysis of the role that Fuzzy Set Theory can play in the "interface" between, Hard Sciences and Humanities. He is Fellow of the *International Fuzzy System Association* and of the *Accademia Nazionale di Scienze, Lettere ed Arti* of Palermo. Main books: *Aspects of Vagueness*, Reidel (1984), edited with E. Trillas and H. J. Skala; *Imagination and Rigor*, Springer (2006); *Contro il declino, Codice edizioni* (2007), coauthored with Pietro Greco; *Memoria e progetto*, Edizioni GEM (2010), edited with Pietro Greco.

Enric Trillas (Barcelona, 1940) is Emeritus Researcher at the European Centre for Soft Computing (Mieres, Asturias, Spain). He got a Ph.D. on Sciences from the University of Barcelona and he became Professor at the Technical University of Catalonia in 1974. In 1988 moved to the Technical University of Madrid, where he was Professor at the Department of Artificial Intelligence until September 2006. Formerly, and among other positions, he was Vice-Rector of the Technical University of Catalonia, President of the High Council for Scientific Research (CSIC), Director General of the National Institute for Aerospace Technology (INTA), Secretary General of the National Plan for Scientific and Technological Research, and Chairman of the company Aerospace Engineering and Services (INSA). Other than several distinctions and medals, he is Fellow of the International Fuzzy Systems Association (IFSA), got the Fuzzy Pioneers Award of the European Society for Fuzzy Logic and Technologies, the Fuzzy Systems Pioneer Award of the IEEE

Computational Intelligence Society, the Spanish National Prize on Computer Sciences in 2007, the Kampé de Fériet Award in 2008 and the IFSA Outstanding Achie vement Award 2011. He has published over two hundred fifty papers in Journals, Conference's Proceedings, and editor's books,as well as several books. He serves in the Editorial Board of many International Journals. His current research interests are, Fundamentals of Fuzzy Set Theories, and Fuzzy Logic, Methods of reasoning: conjectures, hypotheses and consequences.

Gracian Triviño, 1982 M.S., 2000 Ph.D. Electrical Engineering, Polytechnic University of Madrid (Spain). From 1982 to 1999 he occupied several positions managing R&D projects in the industry. Areas covered during this professional activity include: Industrial Control, Nuclear Power Plants Control, Telecommunications, Avionics, and Software Engineering. From 1999 to 2006 he occupied the position of Associated Professor at the Computer Science School of the Polytechnic University of Madrid. Topics covered were: Intelligent building control, Control of physical processes, Electronic instrumentation, Photonic devices, Development of computational systems, and Architectures for robotics. Since January 2007 he occupies the position of principal researcher in Computing with Perceptions at the European Centre for Soft Computing.

Thomas Vetterlein studied mathematics in Heidelberg and wrote his PhD thesis at the Slovak Academy of Sciences in the field of quantum structures. Since several years his work has focused on fuzzy logic. From 2007 to 2010 he was employed at the Medical University of Vienna, Austria; at present, he works in the Department of Knowledge-Based Mathematical Systems at the Johannes Kepler University in Linz, Austria.

MIX
Papier aus verantwortungsvollen Quellen
Paper from responsible sources
FSC® C105338
FSC
www.fsc.org

If you have any concerns about our products,
you can contact us on
ProductSafety@springernature.com

In case Publisher is established outside the EU,
the EU authorized representative is:
Springer Nature Customer Service Center GmbH
Europaplatz 3, 69115 Heidelberg, Germany

Printed by Libri Plureos GmbH
in Hamburg, Germany